D1093787

Guide to
Natural Healing

Guide to
Natural Healing

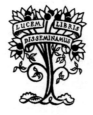

Contents

1

Therapies for Body and Soul

The therapies in this section are primarily concerned with treatment of the body through massage and manipulation, sometimes through its energy channels or meridians. The mystical influence in many of the treatments has its origins in eastern medicine and philosophy. The therapies are therefore not merely treatments for one physical ailment or one part of the body, but are holistic ones, treating the patient as a physical and spiritual whole.

Acupuncture

Origins

Acupuncture is an ancient Chinese therapy that involves inserting needles into the skin at specific points of the body. The word 'acupuncture' originated from a Dutch physician, William Ten Rhyne, who had been living in Japan during the latter part of the 17th century and it was he who introduced it to Europe. The term means literally 'prick with a needle'. The earliest textbook on acupuncture, dating from approximately 400 BC, was called *Nei Ching Su Wen*, which means 'Yellow Emperor's Classic of Internal Medicine'. Also recorded at about the same time was the successful saving of a patient's life by acupuncture, the person having been expected to die whilst in a coma. Legend has it that acupuncture was developed when it was realized that soldiers who recovered from arrow wounds were sometimes also healed of other diseases from which they were suffering. Acupuncture was very popular with British doctors in the early 1800s for pain relief and to treat fever. There was also a specific article on the successful treatment of rheumatism that appeared in *The Lancet*. Until the end of the Ching dynasty in China in 1911, acupuncture was slowly developed and improved, but then medicine from the west increased in popularity. However, more recently there has been a revival of interest and it is again widely practised throughout China. Also, nowadays the use of laser beams and electrical currents is found to give an increased stimulative effect when using acupuncture needles.

The specific points of the body into which acupuncture needles are inserted are located along 'meridians'. These are the pathways or energy channels and are believed to be related to the internal organs of the body. This energy is known as *qi* and the needles are used to decrease or increase the flow of energy, or to unblock it if it is impeded. Traditional Chinese medicine sees the body as being comprised of two natural forces known as the *yin* and *yang*. These two forces are complementary to each other but also opposing, the yin being the female force and calm and passive and also representing the dark, cold, swelling and moisture. The yang force is the male and is stimulating and aggressive, representing the heat and light, contraction and dryness. It is believed that the cause of ailments and diseases is due to an imbalance of these forces in the body, e.g. if a person is suffering from a headache or hypertension then this is because of an excess of yang. If, however, there is an excess of yin, this might result in tiredness, feeling cold and fluid retention.

The aim of acupuncture is to establish whether there is an imbalance of yin and yang and to rectify it by using the needles at certain points on the body. Traditionally there were 365 points but more have been found in the intervening period and nowadays there can be as many as 2,000. There are 14 meridians (12 of which are illustrated on page 12), called after the organs they represent, e.g. the lung, kidney, heart and stomach as well as two organs unknown in orthodox medicine—the triple heater or warmer, which relates to the activity of the

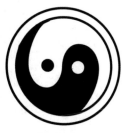

yin and yang

11

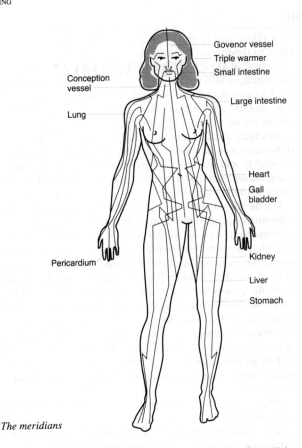

Govenor vessel
Triple warmer
Small intestine
Conception vessel
Large intestine
Lung
Heart
Gall bladder
Pericardium
Kidney
Liver
Stomach

The meridians

endocrine glands and the control of temperature. In addition, the pericardium is concerned with seasonal activity and also regulates the circulation of the blood. Of the 14 meridians, there are two, known as the *du,* or governor, and the *ren,* or conception, which both run straight up the body's midline, although the du is much shorter, extending from the head down to the mouth, while the ren starts at the chin and extends to the base of the trunk.

There are several factors that can change the flow of qi (also known as shi or ch'i), and they can be of an emotional, physical or environmental nature. The flow may be changed to become too slow or fast, or it can be diverted or blocked so that the incorrect organ is involved and the acupuncturist has to ensure that the flow returns to normal. There are many painful afflictions for which acupuncture can be used. In the west, it has been used primarily for rheumatism, back pain and arthritis, but it has also been used to alleviate other disorders such as stress, allergy, colitis, digestive troubles, insomnia, asthma, etc. It has been claimed that withdrawal symptoms (experienced by people stopping smoking and ceasing other forms of addiction) have been helped as well.

Qualified acupuncturists complete a training course of three years duration and also need qualifications in the related disciplines of anatomy, pathology, physiology and diagnosis before they can belong to a professional association. It is very important that a fully qualified acupuncturist, who is a member of the relevant professional body, is consulted because at the present time, any unqualified person can use the title 'acupuncturist'.

The treatment

At a consultation, the traditional acupuncturist uses a set method of ancient rules to determine the acupuncture points. The texture and colouring of the skin, type of skin, posture and movement and the tongue will all be examined and noted, as will the patient's voice. These different factors are all needed for the Chinese diagnosis. A number of questions will be asked concerning the diet, amount of exercise taken, lifestyle, fears and phobias, sleeping patterns and reactions to stress. Each wrist has six pulses, and each of these stand for a main organ and its function. The pulses are felt (known as palpating), and by this means acupuncturists are able to diagnose any problems relating to the flow of qi and if there is any disease present in the internal organs. The first consultation may last an hour, especially if detailed questioning is necessary along with the palpation.

The needles used in acupuncture are disposable and made of a fine stainless steel and come already sealed in a sterile pack. They can be sterilized by the acupuncturist in a machine known as an autoclave but using boiling water is not adequate for this purpose. (Diseases such as HIV and hepatitis can be passed on by using unsterilized needles.) Once the needle is inserted into the skin it is twisted between the acupuncturist's thumb and forefinger to spread or draw the energy from a point. The depth to which the needle is inserted can vary from just below the skin to up to 12 mm (half an inch) and different sensations may be felt, such as a tingling around the area of insertion or a loss of sensation at that point. Up to 15 needles can be used but around five is generally sufficient. The length of time that they are left in varies from a few minutes to half an hour and this is dependent on a number of factors such as how the patient has reacted to previous treatment and the ailment from which he or she is suffering.

Patients can generally expect to feel an improvement after four to six sessions of therapy, the beneficial effects occurring gradually, particularly if the ailment has obvious and long-standing symptoms. Other diseases such as asthma will probably take longer before any definite improvement is felt. It is possible that some patients may not feel any improvement at all, or even feel worse after the first session and this is probably due to the energies in the body being over-stimulated. To correct this, the acupuncturist will gradually use fewer needles and for a shorter period of time. If no improvement is felt after about six to eight treatments, then it is doubtful whether acupuncture will be of any help. For general body maintenance and health, most traditional acupuncturists suggest that sessions be arranged at the time of seasonal changes.

How does it work?

There has been a great deal of research, particularly by the Chinese, who have produced many books detailing a high success rate for acupuncture in treating a variety of disorders. These results are, however, viewed cautiously in the west as methods of conducting clinical trials vary from east to west. Nevertheless trials have been carried out in the west and it has been discovered that a pain message can be stopped from reaching the brain using acupuncture. The signal would normally travel along a nerve but it is possible to 'close a gate' on the nerve, thereby preventing the message from reaching the brain, hence preventing the perception of pain. Acupuncture is believed to work by blocking the pain signal. However, doctors stress that pain can be a warning that something is wrong or of the occurrence of a particular disease, such as cancer, that requires an orthodox remedy or method of treatment.

It has also been discovered that there are substances produced by the body that are connected with pain relief. These substances are called endorphins and encephalins, and they are natural opiates. Studies from all over the world show that acupuncture stimulates the release of these opiates into the central nervous system, thereby giving pain relief. The amount of opiates released has a direct bearing on the degree of pain relief. Acupuncture is a widely used form of anaesthesia in China where, for suitable patients, it is said to be extremely effective (90 per cent). It is used successfully during childbirth, dentistry and for operations. Orthodox doctors in the west now accept that heat treatment, massage and needles used on a sensitive part of the skin afford relief from pain caused by disease elsewhere. These areas are known as trigger points, and they are not always situated close to the organ that is affected by disease. It has been found that approximately three-quarters of these trigger points are the same as the points used in Chinese acupuncture. Recent research has also shown that it is possible to find the acupuncture points by the use of electronic instruments as they register less electrical resistance than other areas of skin. As yet, no evidence has been found to substantiate the existence of meridians.

Auricular therapy

Auricular therapy is a method of healing using stimulation of different acupuncture points on the surface of the ear. Auricular therapists claim that there are over 200 points on the ear that are connected to a particular organ, tissue or part of the body. If a disorder is present, its corresponding point on the ear may be sensitive or tender to touch and pressure, or there may even be some kind of physical sign such as a mark, spot or lump. Stimulation of the ear is carried out by means of acupuncture needles, or minute electric currents or a laser beam may be used.

It is claimed that auricular therapy is helpful in the treatment of various chronic conditions such as rheumatism and arthritis and also problems of addiction. During a first consultation, the auricular therapist obtains a detailed picture of the patient's state of health, lifestyle and family background. A physical examination of the ears is carried out and any distinguishing features are recorded. The therapist passes a probe over the surface of the ear to find any sensitive points that indicate the areas requiring treatment.

The practice of manipulating needles in the ear to cure diseases in other parts of the body is a very ancient one. It has been used for many hundreds of years in some eastern and Mediterranean countries and in China. Although the method of action is not understood, auricular therapy is becoming increasingly popular in several countries of the world including Great Britain.

The Alexander Technique

Breaking the habit of bad posture

The Alexander Technique is a practical and simple method of learning to focus attention on how we use ourselves during daily activities. Frederick Mathias Alexander (1869–1955), an Australian therapist, demonstrated that the difficulties many people experience in learning, in control of performance, and in physical functioning are caused by unconscious habits. These habits interfere with your natural poise and your capacity to learn. When you stop interfering with the innate coordination of the body, you can take on more complex activities with greater self-confidence and presence of mind. It is about learning to bring into our conscious awareness the choices we make, as we make them. Gentle hands-on and verbal instruction reveal the underlying principles of human coordination, allow the student to experience and observe their own habitual patterns, and give the means for release and change.

Armouring

Most of us are unconsciously armouring ourselves in relation to our environment. This is hard work and often leaves us feeling anxious, alienated, depressed and unlovable. Armouring is a deeply unconscious behaviour that has probably gone on since early childhood, maybe even since infancy. Yet it is a habit we can unlearn in the present through careful self-observation. We can unlearn our use of excess tension in our thoughts, movements, and relationships.

Correct posture

The Alexander technique is based on correct posture so that the body is able to function naturally and with the minimum amount of muscular effort. F. M. Alexander was also an actor and found that he was losing his voice when performing but after rest his condition temporarily improved. Although he received medical help, the condition was not cured and it occurred to him that whilst acting he might be doing something that caused the problem. To see what this might be he performed his act in front of a mirror and saw what happened when he was about to speak. He experienced difficulty in breathing and lowered his head, thus making himself shorter. He realized that the strain of remembering his lines and having to project his voice, so that people furthest away in the audience would be able to hear, was causing him a great deal of stress and the way he reacted was a quite natural reflex action. In fact, even thinking about having to project his voice made the symptoms recur and from this he concluded that there must be a close connection between body and mind. He was determined to try to improve the situation and gradually, by watching and altering his stance and posture and his mental attitude to his performance on stage, matters improved. He was able to act and speak on stage and use his body in a more relaxed and natural fashion.

In 1904 Alexander travelled to London where he had decided to let others know about his method of retraining the body. He soon became very popular with other actors who appreciated the benefits of using his technique. Other

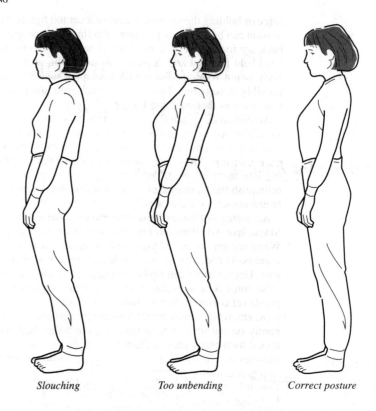

Slouching   *Too unbending*   *Correct posture*

public figures, such as the author Aldous Huxley, also benefited. Later he went to America, achieving considerable success and international recognition for his technique. At the age of 78 he suffered a stroke but by using his method he managed to regain the use of all his faculties — an achievement that amazed his doctors.

The treatment

The Alexander technique is said to be completely harmless, encouraging an agreeable state between mind and body and is also helpful for a number of disorders such as headaches and back pain. Today, Alexander training schools can be found all over the world. A simple test to determine if people can benefit is to observe their posture. People frequently do not even stand correctly and this can encourage aches and pains if the body is unbalanced. It is incorrect to stand with round shoulders or to slouch. This often looks uncomfortable and discomfort may be felt. Sometimes people will hold themselves too erect and unbending, which again can have a bad effect. The correct posture and balance for the body needs the least muscular effort but the body will be aligned correctly. When walking one should not slouch, hold the head down or have the shoulders stooped. The head should be balanced correctly above the spine with the shoulders relaxed. It is suggested that the weight of the body should be felt being transferred from one foot to the other whilst walking.

Once a teacher has been consulted, all movements and how the body is used will be observed. Many muscles are used in everyday activities, and over the years bad habits can develop unconsciously, with stress also affecting the use of muscles. This can be demonstrated in people gripping a pen with too much force or holding the steering wheel of a car too tightly whilst driving. Muscular tension can be a serious problem affecting some people and the head, neck and back are forced out of line, which in turn leads to rounded shoulders with the head held forward and the back curved. If this situation is not altered and the body is not re-aligned correctly, the spine will become curved with a hump possibly developing. This leads to back pain and puts a strain on internal organs such as the chest and lungs.

An Alexander teacher guides a person, as he or she moves, to use less tension. The instructor works by monitoring the student's posture and reminding him or her to implement tiny changes in movement to eradicate the habit of excess tension. Students learn to stop bracing themselves up, or to stop collapsing into themselves. As awareness grows, it becomes easier to recognize and relinquish the habit of armouring and dissolve the artificial barriers we put between ourselves and others.

An analogy of this process can be seen in the now familiar three-dimensional Magic Eye Art. With our ordinary way of looking we see only a mass of dots. When we shift to the 'Magic Eye' way of seeing, a three-dimensional object appears. Through the Alexander technique a similar type of experience is available. But the three-dimensional object we experience is ourselves.

No force is used by the teacher other than some gentle manipulation to start pupils off correctly. Some teachers use light pushing methods on the back and hips, etc, while others might first ensure that the pupil is relaxed and then pull gently on the neck, which stretches the body. Any bad postures will be corrected by the teacher and the pupil will be shown how best to alter this so that muscles will be used most effectively and with the least effort. Any manipulation that is used will be to ease the body into a more relaxed and natural position. It is helpful to be completely aware of using the technique not only on the body but also with the mind. With frequent use of the Alexander technique for posture and the release of tension, the muscles and the body should be used correctly with a consequent improvement in, for example, the manner of walking and sitting.

The length of time for each lesson can vary from about half an hour to three quarters of an hour and the number of lessons is usually between 10 and 30, by which time pupils should have gained sufficient knowledge to continue practising the technique by themselves. Once a person has learned how to improve posture, it will be found that he or she is taller and carrying the body in a more upright manner. The technique has been found to be of benefit to dancers, ath-

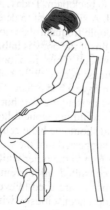

Slumped posture

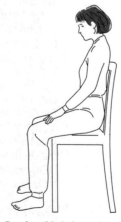

Comfortably balanced posture

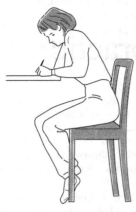

Bad posture

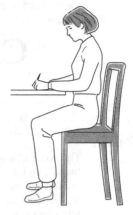

Good, balanced posture

letes and those having to speak in public. Other disorders claimed to have been treated successfully are depressive states, headaches caused by tension, anxiety, asthma, hypertension, respiratory problems, colitis, osteoarthritis and rheumatoid arthritis, sciatica and peptic ulcer.

The Alexander technique is recommended for all ages and types of people as their overall quality of life, both mental and physical, can be improved. People can learn how to resist stress and one eminent professor experienced a great improvement in a variety of ways: in quality of sleep; lessening of high blood pressure and improved mental awareness. He even found that his ability to play a musical instrument had improved.

The Alexander technique can be applied to two positions adopted every day, namely sitting in a chair and sitting at a desk. To be seated in the correct manner the head should be comfortably balanced, with no tension in the shoulders, and a small gap between the knees (if legs are crossed the spine and pelvis become out of line or twisted) and the soles of the feet should be flat on the floor. It is incorrect to sit with the head lowered and the shoulders slumped forward because the stomach becomes restricted and breathing may also be affected. On the other hand, it is also incorrect to hold the body in a stiff and erect position.

To sit correctly while working at a table, the body should be held upright but in a relaxed manner with any bending movement coming from the hips and with the seat flat on the chair. If writing, the pen should be held lightly and if using a computer one should ensure that the arms are relaxed and feel comfortable. The chair should be set at a comfortable height with regard to the level of the desk. It is incorrect to lean forward over a desk because this hampers breathing, or to hold the arms in a tense, tight manner.

There has been some scientific research carried out that concurs with the beliefs that Alexander formed, such as the relationship between mind and body (the thought of doing an action actually triggering a physical reaction or tension). Today, doctors do not have any opposition to the Alexander technique and may recommend it on occasions.

Although the Alexander technique does not treat specific symptoms, you can encourage a marked improvement in overall health, alertness, and performance by consciously eliminating harmful habits that cause physical and emotional stress, and by becoming more aware of how you engage in your activities.

Chiropractic

Origins

Daniel Palmer

The word chiropractic originates from two Greek words *kheir*, which means 'hand', and *praktikos*, which means 'practical'. A school of chiropractic was established in about 1895 by a healer called Daniel Palmer (1845–1913). He was able to cure a man's deafness that had occurred when he bent down and felt a bone click. Upon examination Palmer discovered that some bones of the man's spine had become displaced. After successful manipulation the man regained his hearing. Palmer formed the opinion that if there was any displacement in the skeleton this could affect the function of nerves, either increasing or decreasing their action and thereby resulting in a malfunction i.e. a disease.

Pain relief by manipulation

Chiropractic is used to relieve pain by manipulation and to correct any problems that are present in joints and muscles but especially the spine. Like osteopathy, no use is made of surgery or drugs. If there are any spinal disorders they can cause widespread problems elsewhere in the body such as the hip, leg or arm and can also initiate lumbago, sciatica, a slipped disc or other back problems. It is even possible that spinal problems can result in seemingly unrelated problems such as catarrh, migraine, asthma, constipation, stress, etc. However, the majority of a chiropractor's patients suffer mainly from neck and back pain. People suffering from whiplash injuries sustained in car accidents commonly seek the help of a chiropractor. The whiplash effect is caused when the head is violently wrenched either forwards or backwards at the time of impact.

Another common problem that chiropractors treat is headaches, and it is often the case that tension is the underlying cause as it makes the neck muscles contract. Athletes can also obtain relief from injuries such as tennis elbow, pulled muscles, injured ligaments and sprains, etc. As well as the normal methods of manipulating joints, the chiropractor may decide it is necessary to use applications of ice or heat to relieve the injury.

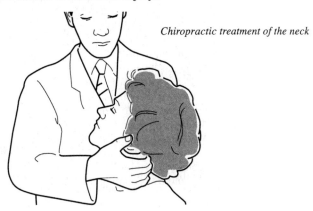

Chiropractic treatment of the neck

Children can also benefit from treatment by a chiropractor, as there may be some slight accident that occurs in their early years that can reappear in adult life in the form of back pain. It can easily happen, for example, when a child learns to walk and bumps into furniture, or when a baby falls out of a cot. This could result in some damage to the spine that will show only in adult life when a person experiences back pain. At birth, a baby's neck may be injured or the spine may be strained if the use of forceps is necessary, and this can result in headaches and neck problems as he or she grows to maturity. This early type of injury could also account for what is known as 'growing pains', when the real problem is actually damage that has been done to the bones or muscles. If a parent has any worries it is best to consult a doctor and it is possible that the child will be recommended to see a qualified chiropractor. To avoid any problems in adult life, chiropractors recommend that children have occasional examinations to detect any damage or displacement in bones and muscles.

As well as babies and children, adults of all ages can benefit from chiropractic. There are some people who regularly take painkillers for painful joints or back pain, but this does not deal with the root cause of the pain, only the symptoms that are produced. It is claimed that chiropractic could be of considerable help in giving treatment to these people. Many pregnant women experience backache at some stage during their pregnancy because of the extra weight that is placed on the spine, and they also may find it difficult keeping their balance. At the time of giving birth, changes take place in the pelvis and joints at the bottom of the spine and this can be a cause of back pain. Lifting and carrying babies, if not done correctly, can also damage the spine and thereby make the back painful.

It is essential that any chiropractor is fully qualified and registered with the relevant professional association. At the initial visit, a patient will be asked for details of his or her case history, including the present problem, and during the examination painful and tender areas will be noted and joints will be checked to see whether they are functioning correctly or not. X-rays are frequently used by chiropractors since they can show signs of bone disease, fractures or arthritis as well as the spine's condition. After the initial visit, any treatment will normally begin as soon as the patient has been informed of the chiropractor's diagnosis. If it has been decided that chiropractic therapy will not be of any benefit, the patient will be advised accordingly.

For treatment, underwear and/or a robe will be worn, and the patient will either lie, sit or stand on a specially designed couch. Chiropractors use their hands in a skilful way to effect the different manipulative techniques. If it is decided that manipulation is necessary to treat a painful lumbar joint, the patient will need to lie on his or her side. The upper and lower spine will then be rotated manually but in opposite ways. This manipulation will have the effect of partially locking the joint that is being treated, and the upper leg is usually flexed to aid the procedure. The vertebra that is immediately below or above the joint will then be felt by the chiropractor, and the combination of how the patient is lying, coupled with gentle pressure applied by the chiropractor's hand, will move the joint to its furthest extent of normal movement. There will then be a very quick push applied on the vertebra, which results in its movement being extended further than normal, ensuring that full use of the joint is regained. This is due to the muscles that surround the joint being suddenly stretched, which has the effect of relaxing the muscles of the spine that work upon the joint. This alteration should cause the joint to be able to be used more naturally and should not be a painful procedure.

There can be a variety of effects felt after treatment—some patients may feel sore or stiff, or may ache some time after the treatment, while others will experience the lifting of pain at once. In some cases there may be a need for multiple treatments, perhaps four or more, before improvement is felt. On the whole, problems that have been troubling a patient for a considerable time (chronic) will need more therapy than anything that occurs quickly and is very painful (acute).

Although there is only quite a small number of chiropractors in the UK—yet this numbers is increasing—there is a degree of contact and liaison between them and doctors. It is generally accepted that chiropractic is an effective remedy for bone and muscular problems, and the majority of doctors would be happy to accept a chiropractor's diagnosis and treatment, although the treatment of any general diseases, such as diabetes or asthma, would not be viewed in the same manner.

Hydrotherapy

The healing quality of water

Hydrotherapy is the use of water to heal and ease a variety of ailments, and the water may be used in a number of different ways. The healing properties of water have been recognized since ancient times, notably by the Greek, Roman and Turkish civilizations but also by people in Europe and China. Most people know the benefits of a hot bath in relaxing the body, relieving muscular aches and stiffness, and helping to bring about restful sleep. Hot water or steam causes blood vessels to dilate, opens skin pores and stimulates perspiration, and relaxes limbs and muscles. A cold bath or shower acts in the opposite way and is refreshing and invigorating. The cold causes blood vessels in the skin to constrict and blood is diverted to internal tissues and organs to maintain the core temperature of the body. Applications of cold water or ice reduce swelling and bruising and cause skin pores to close.

Physiotherapy

In orthodox medicine, hydrotherapy is used as a technique of physiotherapy for people recovering from serious injuries with problems of muscle wastage. Also, it is used for people with joint problems and those with severe physical disabilities. Many hospitals also offer the choice of a water birth to expectant mothers, and this has become an increasingly popular method of childbirth. Hydrotherapy may be offered as a form of treatment for other medical conditions in *naturopathy,* using the techniques listed above. It is wise to obtain medical advice before proceeding with hydrotherapy, and this is especially important for elderly persons, children and those with serious conditions or illnesses.

Treatment techniques in hydrotherapy
Hot baths

Hot baths are used to ease muscle and joint pains and inflammation. Also, warm or hot baths, with the addition of various substances such as seaweed extract to the water, may be used to help the healing of some skin conditions or minor wounds. After childbirth, frequent bathing in warm water to which a mild antiseptic has been added is recommended to heal skin tears.

Most people know the relaxing benefits of a hot bath. A bath with the temperature between 36.5°C and 40°C (98°F and 104°F) is very useful as a means of muscle relaxation. To begin with, five minutes immersion in a bath of this temperature is enough. This can be stepped up to ten minutes a day, as long as no feelings of weakness or dizziness arise. It is important to realize that a brief hot bath has quite a different effect from a long one.

There is nothing to be gained by prolonging a hot bath in the hope of increasing the benefit. Immersion in hot water acts not only on the surface nerves but also on the autonomic nervous system (which is normally outside our control), as well as the hormone-producing glands, particularly the adrenals, which become less active. A hot bath is sedative, but a hot bath that is prolonged into a long soak has quite the opposite effect.

Cold baths

Cold baths are used to improve blood flow to internal tissues and organs and to reduce swellings. The person may sit for a moment in shallow cold water with additional water being splashed onto exposed skin. An inflamed, painful part may be immersed in cold water to reduce swelling. The person is not allowed to become chilled, and this form of treatment is best suited for those able to dry themselves rapidly with a warm towel. It is not advisable for people with serious conditions or for the elderly or very young.

Neutral bath

There are many nerve endings on the skin surface and these deal with the reception of stimuli. More of these are cold receptors than heat receptors. If water of a different temperature to that of the skin is applied, it will either conduct heat to it or absorb heat from it. These stimuli have an influence on the sympathetic nervous system and can affect the hormonal system. The greater the difference between the temperature of the skin and the water applied, the greater will be the potential for physiological reaction. Conversely, water that is the same temperature as the body has a marked relaxing and sedative effect on the nervous system. This is of value in states of stress, and has led to the development of the so-called 'neutral bath'.

Before the development of tranquillizers, the most dependable and effective method of calming an agitated patient was the use of a neutral bath. The patient was placed in a tub of water, the temperature of which was maintained at between 33.5°C and 35.6°C (92°F to 96°F), often for over three hours, and sometimes for as long as twenty-four hours. Obviously, this is not a practical proposition for the average tense person.

As a self-help measure, the neutral bath does, however, offer a means of sedating the nervous system if used for relatively short periods. It is important to maintain the water temperature at the above level, and for this a bath thermometer should be used. The bathroom itself should be kept warm to prevent any chill in the air.

Half an hour of immersion in a bath like this will have a sedative, or even soporific, effect. It places no strain on the heart, circulation or nervous system, and achieves muscular relaxation as well as a relaxation and expansion of the blood vessels: all of these effects promote relaxation. This bath can be used in conjunction with other methods of relaxation, such as breathing techniques and meditation, to make it an even more efficient way of wiping out stress. It can be used daily if necessary.

Steam baths

Steam baths, along with saunas and Turkish baths, are used to encourage sweating and the opening of skin pores and have a cleansing and refreshing effect. The body may be able to eliminate harmful substances in this way and treatment finishes with a cool bath.

Sitz baths

Sitz baths are usually given as a treatment for painful conditions with broken skin, such as piles or anal fissure, and also for ailments affecting the urinary and genital organs. The person sits in a specially designed bath that has two compartments, one with warm water, the other with cold. First, the person sits in the warm water, which covers the lower abdomen and hips, with the feet in the cold water compartment. After three minutes, the patient changes round and sits in the cold water with the feet in the warm compartment.

Hot and cold sprays

Hot and cold sprays of water may be given for a number of different disorders but are not recommended for those with serious illnesses, elderly people or young children.

Wrapping

Wrapping is used for feverish conditions, backache and bronchitis. A cold wet sheet that has been squeezed out is wrapped around the person, followed by a dry sheet and warm blanket. These are left in place until the inner sheet has dried and the coverings are then removed. The body is sponged with tepid water (at blood heat) before being dried with a towel. Sometimes the wrap is applied to a smaller area of the body, such as the lower abdomen, to ease a particular problem, usually constipation.

Cold packs

Cold packs were described by the famous 19th-century Bavarian pastor, Sebastian Kniepp, in his famous treatise *My Water Cure*, in which he explained the advantages of hydrotherapy. A cold pack is really a warm pack—the name comes from the cold nature of the initial application.

For a cold pack you need:
A large piece of cotton material; a large piece of flannel or woollen (blanket) material; a rubber sheet to protect the bed; a hot water bottle; safety pins.

First, soak the cotton material in very cold water, wring it out well and place it on the flannel material that is spread out on the rubber sheet on the bed. Lay the person who is having the treatment on top of the damp material, fold it round his trunk and cover him up at once with the flannel material. Safety-pin it all firmly in place.

Now pull up the top bed covers and provide a hot water bottle. The initial cold application produces a reaction that draws fresh blood to the surface of the body; this warmth, being well insulated, is retained by the damp material. The cold pack turns into a warm pack, which gradually, over a period of six to eight hours, bakes itself dry. Usually lots of sweat will be produced, so it is necessary to wash the materials well before using again.

The pack can be slept in—in fact it should encourage deeper, more refreshing sleep. Larger, whole body packs can be used, which cover not only the trunk but extend from the armpits to the feet, encasing the recipient in a cocoon of warmth.

If a feeling of damp coldness is felt, the wet material may be inadequately wrung out, or the insulation materials too loose or too few.

Flotation

A form of sensory deprivation, flotation involves lying face up in an enclosed, dark tank of warm, heavily salted water. There is no sound, except perhaps some natural music to bring the client into a dream-like state. It is exceptionally refreshing and induces a deep, relaxing sleep.

Kinesiology

The function of kinesiology

Kinesiology is a method of maintaining health by ensuring that all muscles are functioning correctly. It is believed that each muscle is connected with a specific part of the body such as the digestive system, circulation of the blood and specific organs, and if a muscle is not functioning correctly this will cause a problem in its related part of the body. The word is derived from *kinesis*, which is Greek for 'motion'. Kinesiology originated in 1964 and was developed by an American chiropractor named George Goodheart who realized that while he was treating a patient for severe pain in the leg, by massaging a particular muscle in the upper leg, the pain experienced by the patient eased and the muscle was strengthened. Although he used the same method on different muscles, the results were not the same. Previous research done by an osteopath named Dr Chapman, in the 1900s, indicated that there were certain 'pressure points' in the body that were connected with particular muscles and, if these were massaged, lymph would be able to flow more freely through the body. Using these pressure points, Chapman found which point was connected to each particular muscle and realized why, when he had massaged a patient's upper leg muscle, the pain had lessened. The pressure point for that leg muscle was the only one that was situated above the actual muscle — all the other points were not close to the part of the body with which they were connected.

The use of pressure points

In the 1930s it was claimed that there were similar pressure points located on the skull and, by exerting a light pressure on these, the flow of blood to their related organs could be assisted. Goodheart tested this claim, which originated from an osteopath called Terence Bennett, and discovered that after only fingertip pressure for a matter of seconds, it improved the strength of a particular muscle. After some time he was able to locate sixteen points on the head, the back of the knee and by the breastbone that were all allied to groups of important muscles. Goodheart was surprised that so little force applied on the pressure point could have such an effect on the muscle, so to further his studies he then applied himself to acupuncture. This is a form of healing that also makes use of certain points located over the body but that run along specific paths known as meridians. After further study, Goodheart came to the conclusion that the meridians could be used for both muscles and organs. The invisible paths used in kinesiology are exactly the same as the ones for acupuncture.

Energy and lymph

A kinesiologist will examine a patient and try to discover whether there is any lack of energy, physical disorders or inadequate nutrition that is causing problems. Once any troublesome areas have been located, the practitioner will use only a light massage on the relevant pressure points (which, as mentioned, are generally not close to their associated muscle). For example, the edge of the rib cage is where the pressure points for the muscles of the upper leg are situated.

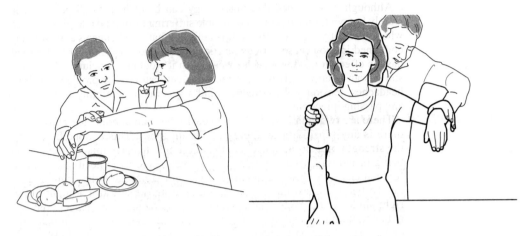

A— determining sensitivity or allergy to foods   *B—determining whether there is weakness in the shoulder muscle*

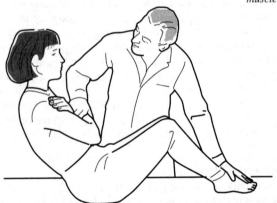

C—determining whether there are weak muscles in the stomach

In kinesiology it is maintained that the use of pressure points is effective because the flow of blood to muscles is stimulated and therefore a good supply of lymph is generated too. Lymph is a watery fluid that takes toxins from the tissues and if muscles receive a good supply of both lymph and blood they should function efficiently. As in acupuncture, it is maintained that there is an unseen flow of energy that runs through the body and if this is disrupted for any reason, such as a person being ill or suffering from stress, then the body will weaken due to insufficient energy being produced. The way in which a kinesiologist assesses the general health of a patient is by testing the strength of the muscles as this will provide information on the flow of energy. It is claimed that by finding any inbalance and correcting it, kinesiology can be used as a preventive therapy. If there is a lack of minerals and vitamins in the body or trouble with the digestive system, it is claimed that these are able to be diagnosed by the use of kinesiology. If a person is feeling 'below par' and constantly feels tired, it is believed that these conditions are aggravated by a sluggish flow of the internal body fluids such as the circulation of blood. Kinesiologists can treat the disorder by stimulating the flow of lymph and blood by massaging the pressure points.

Although it is claimed that kinesiology can be of help to all people, it is widely known for the treatment of people suffering from food allergies or those who are sensitive to some foods. It is believed that the chemicals and nutrients contained in food cause various reactions in the body, and if a particular food has the effect of making muscles weak, then it would be concluded that a person has an allergy to it. Allergic reactions can cause other problems such as headaches, tension, colds, tiredness and a general susceptibility to acquiring any passing infections.

There are two simple tests that can easily be tried at home to determine if there is any sensitivity or allergy to certain foods. This is done by testing the strength of a strong muscle in the chest, and to carry this out the person being tested will need the help of a partner. There is no need to exert real force at any time, just use the minimum amount needed to be firm but gentle. To test the chest muscle, sit erect, holding the left arm straight out at right angles to the body. The elbow should be facing outwards and the fingers and thumb drooping towards the table. The partner will then place his or her right hand on the person's nearest shoulder (the right) and the two fingers only on the area around the left wrist. A gentle downward pressure will then be exerted by the partner on the person's wrist who will try to maintain the level of the arm, whilst breathing in a normal fashion. This downward pressure should be exerted for approximately five seconds. If the person was able to resist the downwards pressure and the muscle felt quite firm, then the allergy test can be tried. However, if this was not the case and the person was unable to keep the arm level, the muscle would not be suitable for use in the subsequent test. It would therefore be advisable to use another muscle such as one in the arm. To do this, place an arm straight down at the side of the body with the palm of the hands facing outwards. The partner will then use the same amount of pressure to try to move the arm outwards, again for a similar amount of time. If the person is unable to keep the arm in the same position, then it would be advisable to get in touch with a trained kinesiologist.

To undertake the allergy test, hold the left arm in the same way as for testing the muscle (*see* page 26, figure A). If, for example, the food that is suspected of causing an allergy is chocolate, a small piece of this should be put just in the mouth, there is no need for it to be eaten. This time as well as applying the pressure on the wrist as before, the partner should put his or her first two digits of the left hand below the person's right ear. Once again, the person tries to resist the downwards force and if successful, it is claimed that there is no sensitivity or allergy connected with that food. However, if this does not happen and the arm is pushed downwards or even feels slightly weak, then kinesiology would suggest that this food, if eaten at all, should never be consumed in any great amount.

It is claimed that the use of kinesiology can be of benefit to people who suffer from irrational fears or phobias. An example of this is the recommendation that the bone below the eye, just level with the pupil, is softly tapped. Neck and back pain can be treated without any manipulation of joints and some of the methods can be learnt by patients for use at home. An example of this for the alleviation of back pain is for a patient to massage the muscle situated on the inside of the thigh.

A number of other practitioners, such as homoeopaths, herbalists and osteopaths make use of kinesiology, so if there is a problem connected with the ligaments, muscles or bones it may be advisable to contact a chiropractor or osteopath who is also qualified in kinesiology. If the problem is of a more emotional or mental nature, then it might be best to select a counsellor or psychotherapist who also practises kinesiology. It is important always to use a fully qualified practitioner and the relevant association should be contacted for information. At the first consultation, detailed questions will be asked concerning the medical history, followed by the therapist checking the muscles' ability to function effectively. For instance, a slight pressure will be exerted on a leg or arm while the patient holds it in a certain way. The patient's ability to maintain that position against the pressure is noted and if the patient is unable to do so, then the therapist will find the reason why by further examination. Once the areas in need of 'rebalancing' have been identified, he therapist will use the relevant pressure points to correct matters. It is believed that if some of the points are painful or sore to the touch, this is because there has been an accumulation of toxins in the tissues, and these toxins stop the impulses between muscles and the brain. If this is the case, the muscle is unable to relax properly and can cause problems in areas such as the neck and shoulders.

There are ways of identifying any possible problems. For example, if there is any weakness in the shoulder muscle it may be that there is some problem connected with the lungs. To test for this, the patient sits upright with one arm raised to slightly below shoulder level and the other arm lower and out to the front. The therapist grasps the patient's upper arm and presses gently downwards on the raised arm at the elbow (*see* page 26, figure B). If the mucle is functioning correctly then this downwards force should not be allowed to move the arm lower. If the patient is suffering from pain in the back, the probable cause lies with weak muscles in the stomach. To test for this, the patient sits on the floor with the knees raised, the arms crossed on the chest and then they lean backwards (*see* page 26 figure C). The therapist checks the stomach muscles' efficiency by pushing gently backwards on the patient's crossed arms. If all is well the patient should be able to maintain the position and not lean back any further.

After treatment by massage of the pressure points, there may well be some tenderness experienced for one or two days as the toxins in the tissues dissipate gradually. However, there should be an overall feeling of an improvement in health and in particular with the problem that was being treated.

Although there has been an increase in the use of kinesiology by doctors to help discover the cause of an ailment, there has been little scientific research carried out. Therefore, the majority of doctors using conventional medicine do not believe that the flow of electrical energy present in the body can be changed by the use of massage or similar methods.

Massage

Introduction

Origins

We massage ourselves nearly every day. The natural reaction to reach out and touch a painful part of the body—such as a sprain—forms the basis of massage. As long ago as 3000 BC massage was used as a therapy in the Far East, making it one of the oldest treatments used by humans. In 5 BC in ancient Greece, Hippocrates recommended that to maintain health, a massage using oils should be taken daily after a perfumed bath. Greek physicians were well used to treating people who suffered from pain and stiffness in the joints. The relaxation and healing powers of massage have been well documented over the past 5000 years.

The therapeutic value of applying oils and rubbing parts of the body to lessen pain and prevent illness was recognized among the ancient Mediterranean civilizations. In ancient times scented oils were almost always used when giving massages, creating an early form of aromatherapy massage.

Popularity

Massage increased in popularity when, in the 19th century, Per Henrik Ling, a Swedish fencing master and academic, created the basis for what is now known as Swedish massage. Swedish massage deals with the soft tissues of the body.

Swedish massage is a combination of relaxing effects and exercises that work on the joints and muscles, but it is still based on the form that was practised in ancient times. More recently, a work was published in the 1970s called *The Massage Book,* by George Downing, and this introduced a new concept in the overall technique of massage, that the whole person's state should be assessed by the therapist and not solely the physical side. The emotional and mental states should be part of the overall picture. Also combined in his form of massage were the methods used in reflexology (*see* page 55) and shiatsu (*see* page 90), and this was known as therapeutic massage. The aim of this is to use relaxation, stimulation and invigoration to promote good health.

Uses

Massage is commonly used to induce general relaxation, so that any tension or strain experienced in the rush of daily life can be eased and eliminated. It is found to be very effective, working on the mind as well as the body. It can be used to treat people with hypertension (high blood pressure), sinusitis, headaches, insomnia and hyperactivity, including people who suffer from heart ailments or circulatory disorders. At the physical level, massage is intended to help the body make use of food and to eliminate the waste materials, as well as stimulating the nervous and muscular system and the circulation of blood. Neck and back pain are conditions from which many people suffer, particularly if they have not been sitting correctly, such as in a slightly stooped position with their shoulders rounded. People whose day-to-day work involves a great deal of physical activity, such as dancers and athletes, can also derive a great deal of benefit from the use of massage. Stiffness can be a problem that they have after training or working, and this is relieved by encouraging the toxins that gather in the muscles to disperse. Massage promotes a feeling of calmness and serenity, and this is particularly beneficial to people who frequently suffer from bouts of depression or anxiety. Once the worry and depression have been dispelled, people are able to deal with their problems much more effectively and, being able to do so, will boost their self-confidence.

Medical use

An aid to recovery

In hospitals, massage has been used to ease pain and discomfort as well as being of benefit to people who are bedridden, since the flow of blood to the muscles is stimulated. It has also been used for those who have suffered a heart attack and has helped their recovery. A more recent development has been the use of massage for cancer patients who are suffering from the after-effects of treatment, such as chemotherapy, as well as the discomfort the disease itself causes. Indeed, there are few conditions when it is not recommended. However, it should not be used when people are suffering from inflammation of the veins (phlebitis), varicose veins, thrombosis (clots in the blood) or if they have a raised temperature such as occurs during a fever. It is then advisable to contact a doctor before using massage. Doctors may be able to recommend a qualified therapist, a health centre may be able to help or contact can be made with the relevant professional body.

Psychological benefits

Along with the diagnosis element of massage there are great psychological benefits—the enjoyment of touch and of being stroked and caressed by another person. During a massage the patient is coaxed from emotional and occupational stresses and brought into the intense arena of the here and now. The importance of this kind of one-on-one nonverbal communication can never be underestimated in our increasingly impersonal and detached society.

Massage has a wide range of uses for a variety of disorders. Its strengths lie in the easing of strain and tension and inducing relaxation and serenity, plus the physical contact of the therapist. Although doctors make use of this therapy in conjunction with orthodox medicine, it is not to be regarded as a cure for diseases in itself and serious problems could occur if this were the case.

Benefits

Massage affects the whole body through rhythmically applied pressure. Gentle pulling and stroking movements increase the circulation of the blood and cause the blood vessels to dilate. The stimulation of nerves and blood will also affect the internal organs. Lymph is a milky white liquid that carries waste substances and toxins away from the tissues via the lymphatic system. Inactivity can cause an unhealthy build-up of this substance, and as the circulation of the lymph is largely dependent on muscle contractions, so massage will help speed the lymph's progress through the system. Active people can also benefit from massage as strenuous activity burns up the muscle, producing an increase of waste products in the muscle tissue. Massage will help to balance the system in both cases and can increase oxygen capacity by 10–15 per cent.

By realigning our bodies, massage can go a long way to repairing our generally damaged postures. Inactive lifestyles and sedentary occupations have created a society of people with cramped, stooped and neglected postures. Not only does massage help to coax the spine and corresponding physiology back into position, it also makes us more aware of our bodies. Relieved of muscle tension, the body feels lighter and can therefore be borne more naturally and with more poise. Used in conjunction with postural therapies such as Pilates or the Alexander technique (*see* page 15), massage can help achieve a relaxed yet controlled posture.

Women in labour have found that the pain experienced during childbirth can be eased if massage is performed on the buttocks and back. The massage eases the build-up of tension in the muscles, encouraging relaxation and easing of labour pains. It is said to be more effective on women who had previously experienced the benefits and reassurance of massage.

Many of the benefits of massage come through the healer/patient contact. Our hands are one of the most sensitive parts of our body, and we experience much of our sense of touch through our hands. An experienced masseur is able to use his or her hands to communicate feelings of harmony and relaxation. A practised masseur will also be able to diagnose the patient through touch. He or she can 'listen' to tension and stress through the texture of the skin, knotted muscles and stiff joints. Old and current sprains, congestion and swelling should all be obvious to a good masseur. The actions of massage—the stroking, kneading and pulling—detoxify the body, improving circulation and lymphatic drainage. After tension and weaknesses in the body have been pinpointed and relieved, the patient is left feeling, relaxed and energized.

The massage session

Preparation

A session may be undertaken in the patient's home, or he or she can attend the masseur or masseuse at a clinic. At each session the client will undress, leaving only pants or briefs on, and will lie on a firm, comfortable surface, such as a table that is designed especially for massage. The massage that follows normally lasts from 20 minutes to one hour.

If performed by professionals, massage is not a technique for the unduly modest. It achieves best results if the person receiving the massage is either naked or else dressed in the scantiest of underwear. For anyone who is competent and wishes to provide some simple massage for a partner, there are some basic rules to follow. The room should be warm and peaceful. People will find it difficult to relax if they are cold, and the person performing the massage will be faced with a mass of goose pimples. The surface on which the person lies should be quite comfortable but firm. Use a mid-thigh level table or the floor. A futon (a quilted Japanese mattress) can be used, and to relieve the upper part of the body from any possible discomfort, a pillow should be placed underneath the torso. Any pressure that may be exerted on the feet can be dispelled by the use of a rolled-up towel or similar placed beneath the ankles. Both people should be relaxed, and to this end soft music can be played. All the movements of the hand should be of a continuous nature. It is suggested that the recipient always has one hand of the masseur or masseuse placed on him or her. If you wish you can buy a perfumed massage oil from a chemist or health shop, or mix your own using a blend of aromatherapy oils. Vegetable oil (about one teaspoonful) is suitable but should not be poured straight on to the person. It should be spread over the hands by rubbing, which will also warm it sufficiently for use. Should the masseur or masseuse get out of breath, he or she should stop for a rest, all the while retaining a hand on the person.

Basic techniques

Massage can be divided into four basic forms, and these are known as *percussion* (also known as drumming); *friction* (also called pressure); *effleurage* (also called stroking) and *petrissage* (also called kneading). These methods can be practised alone or in combination for maximum benefit to the patient.

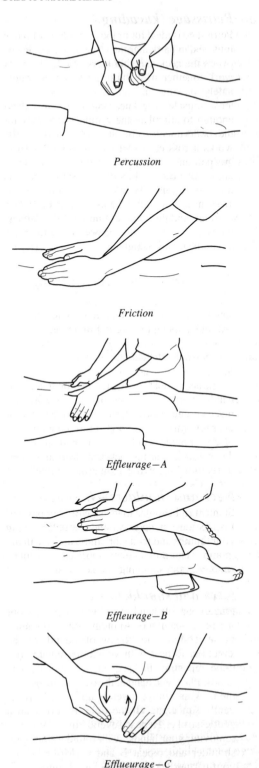

Percussion

Friction

Effleurage—A

Effleurage—B

Efflueurage—C

Percussion (drumming or tapotement)

Percussion is also called tapotement, which is derived from *tapoter*, a French word that means 'to drum', as of the fingers on a surface. As would be expected from its name, percussion is generally done with the edge of the hand with a quick, chopping movement, although the strokes are not hard. This type of movement would be used on places like the buttocks, thighs, waist or shoulders where there is a wide expanse of flesh.

Friction (pressure)

Friction strokes are used to penetrate into deep muscle tissue. Friction is often used on dancers and athletes who experience problems with damaged ligaments or tendons. This is because the flow of blood is stimulated and the movement of joints is improved. Friction can be performed with the base of the hand, some fingers or the upper part of the thumb. It is not advisable to use this method on parts of the body that have been injured in some way, for example where there is bruising.

Effleurage (stroking)

Effleurage is performed in a slow, rhythmical, controlled manner using both hands together with a small space between the thumbs (A). If the therapist wishes to use only light pressure he or she will use the palms of the hands or the tips of the fingers with light gliding strokes, working away from the heart. Light gliding strokes have a relaxing effect on the nervous system. For increased pressure the knuckles or thumbs will be used in an upwards stroking motion towards the heart. Stronger pressure has more of an effect on the blood circulation and the nervous system.

Effleurage can be used on the upper leg as far up as the hip on the outside of the leg. Once the person is lying face downwards (with support under the chest), continue to use effleurage movements on the back of the lower leg. Continue as before but work on the upper leg (B), avoiding the knee. The muscles in the buttocks can be worked upon with both hands to squeeze but making sure that the hands are moving in opposite ways (C).

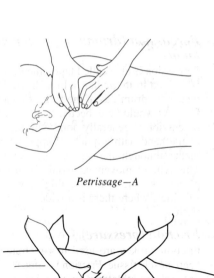

Petrissage—A

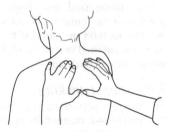

Petrissage—B

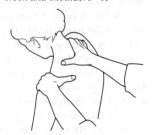

Neck and shoulders—A

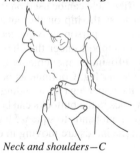

Neck and shoulders—B

Neck and shoulders—C

Petrissage (kneading)

Petrissage is ideal for unlocking aching or tense muscles, in particular the trapezium muscle between the neck and shoulders (A). Both hands work together in a rhythmic sequence, alternately picking up and gently squeezing the tense muscle. The kneading action gets deep enough to stimulate the lymph into removing the build-up of lactic acid. As the therapist works across each section, an area of flesh is grasped and squeezed, and this action stimulates the flow of blood and enables tensed muscles to relax. People such as athletes can have an accumulation of lactic acid in certain muscles, and this is why cramp occurs. Parts of the body on which this method is practised are along the stomach and around the waist (B).

Neck and shoulder massage

What follows can be used to relieve headaches, loosen the shoulder muscles and provide a general feeling of relaxation.

Neck and shoulders – A

Stand behind your seated partner. Begin with effleurage, applying firm pressure with both hands. Start at the bottom of the shoulder blades up each side of the spine to the base of the neck. Move your hands apart across the top of the shoulders and then bring them gently down to the starting position. Repeat several times, finishing with a light return stroke.

Neck and shoulders – B

Stand at right angles to the side of your partner. Locate tension spots in the shoulders using your thumbs and then work these areas with the thumbs. The pressure can approach your partner's pain threshold but not exceed it.

Neck and shoulders – C

Place your left hand in an 'L' shape on your partner's shoulder. Applying firm pressure, move it slowly up the whole length of the shoulder. Repeat with your other hand. Continue repeating the sequence using alternate hands. Place one hand at the base of the back of the neck and move it gently up to the hairline, gently squeezing all the time. Return with a gentle stroke. Repeat several times. Without removing your hands, walk round to the other shoulder and repeat B and C. Move behind your partner and repeat A several times.

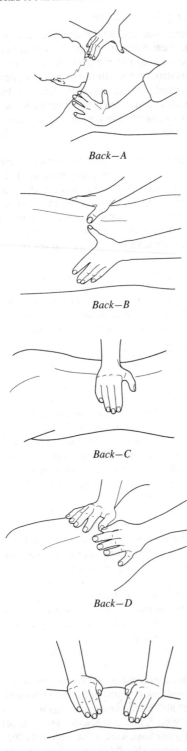

Back—A

Back—B

Back—C

Back—D

Limbs—A

Back massage

Back massage helps to relax the whole body. The strokes should be carried out smoothly, without lifting the hands from the back. Applying thumb pressure to the channels on either side of the spine on the upper back will help respiratory problems. The same stroke on the lower back can relieve constipation and menstrual discomfort.

Back – A

Place your hands, facing each other, on either side of the base of the spine. Move them up the back, using your body weight to apply pressure. Take your hands round the shoulders and return lightly down the sides of the body. Repeat several times before stopping to knead the shoulders. Work on one shoulder and then the other. Repeat the movement.

Back – B

Place your hands at waist level, with your thumbs in the hollows on either side of the spine and your fingers open and relaxed. Push your thumbs firmly up the channels for about 2 ins (6 cm), relax them, and then move them back about 1 in (2 cm). Continue in this way up to the neck. Then gently slide both hands back to the base of the spine. Repeat. Follow with the sequence in A.

Back – C

Place your hand flat across one side of your partner's back at the base of the spine. Apply firm palm pressure and work up to the shoulders. Follow closely with your other hand. Repeat using alternate hands. Work through the same sequence on the other side of the back, then repeat on both side several times. Finish by working through A.

Back – D

Place your hands, facing up the back, on either side of the spine. Applying firm palm pressure, work from the base of the spine to chest level. Turn your fingers outwards and move your hands apart to the sides of the body. Repeat this stroke at waist and hip levels. Repeat the first movement in A several times.

Limb massage

Limbs – A

Begin at the ankle and stroke vertically up the leg with one hand. Follow the same path with your other hand. Continue this sequence, using alternate hands.

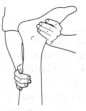

Limbs—B

Limbs – B

Raise your partner's foot and hold it with the knee at a right angle. Using the palm of your free hand, stroke firmly down the back of the leg from ankle to knee level. Use a light stroke to return to the ankle. Repeat the whole movement several times. If including the foot, work through D and E next before repeating the full sequence (A to B) on the other leg.

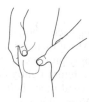

Limbs—C

Limbs – C

Help your partner to turn over, and begin by stroking with alternate hands up the whole leg, as in A. Then put your hands on either side of the knee and, using your thumbs to apply pressure, circle around the knee cap. If including the foot, bring your hands down to the ankle and use the sandwich stroke (D) on the front of the foot. Work through the full movement on the other leg.

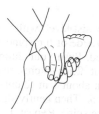

Limbs—D

Limbs – D

With your partner lying face down, take one foot between your hands, so that the palm of your upper hand is resting in the arch. Press firmly, and slowly draw your hands down to the tip of the foot. Use plenty of pressure for this 'sandwich' stoke.

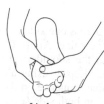

Limbs—E

Limbs – E

Hold the foot with your thumbs lying side by side behind the toes. Pull both thumbs back to the sides of the foot, then push them forward. Repeat this zig-zag movement as you work down to the heel. Then push firmly all the way back to the toes, keeping your thumbs side by side. Repeat the whole movement several times. Work through the whole sequence (D to E) on the other foot.

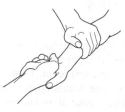

Limbs—F

Limbs – F

Take hold of your partner's hand as in a firm handshake, and lift the arm up slightly, as far as the elbow. Gently place the palm of your fee hand across the top of the wrist and close your fingers round the raised arm. Apply firm pressure and slide your hand up to the elbow, or as far as the shoulder. Move your palm underneath the arm and use a light stroke to return to the wrist. Repeat several times.

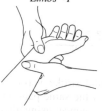

Limbs—G

Limbs – G

Place your thumbs across the inside of your partner's wrist. Applying pressure with both your thumbs, make wide circles around the wrist area. Repeat F. As you finish, relax your hold on the wrist and pull off firmly and slowly in a sandwich stroke, as in D. Repeat the full sequence (F to G) on the other arm, finishing with the hand variation of D.

Face and head massage

The following sequence encourages deep relaxation. Gentle stroking of the forehead (B) can help to relieve stress-related tension and headaches, while pressure applied to the sides of the nose and along the cheekbones (C) alleviates nasal congestion and sinus problems. Scalp massage (D) stimulates circulation.

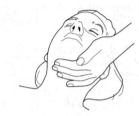

Face and head—A

Face and head – A

Use alternate hands to stroke up one side of the face, starting beneath the chin and working up towards the forehead. Work through the same movement on the other side of the face. Repeat several times. Finish by placing one palm across your partner's forehead, ready for the next stroke.

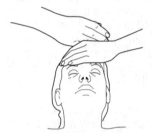

Face and head—B

Face and head – B

Begin by stroking up the forehead with alternate palms. Then place the pads of the middle three fingers of both hands in the centre of the forehead between the eyes. Draw them gently apart across the brow and round the outside corner of the eyes. Lift off the middle two fingers and use your fourth fingers only to return under the eyes towards the nose.

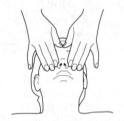

Face and head—C

Face and head – C

Position your thumbs on your partner's forehead. Using the three middle fingers of both hands, press firmly against the sides of the nose. Continue along the top of the cheekbone, until you reach the temple. Keeping your thumbs in position, return to the nose, pressing along the middle of the cheekbone.

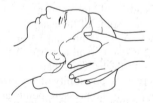

Face and head—D

Face and head – D

Spread out the fingers and thumbs of both hands and place them on your partner's scalp. Keep them in position and begin to move the scalp muscle over the bone by applying gentle pressure and circling slowly and firmly on the spot. Stop occasionally to move to a different area, then begin again, working gradually over the whole scalp.

Acupressure

This is an ancient form of healing combining massage and acupuncture, practised over 3,000 years ago in Japan and China. It was developed into its current form using a system of special massage points and is today still practised widely in the Japanese home environment.

Certain 'pressure points' are located in various parts of the body and these are used by the practitioner by massaging firmly with the thumb or fingertip. These points are the same as those utilized in acupuncture. There are various ways of working and the pressure can be applied by the practitioner's fingers, thumbs, knees, palms of the hand, etc. Relief from pain can be quite rapid at times, depending upon its cause, while other more persistent problems can take longer to improve.

Acupressure is said to enhance the body's own method of healing, thereby preventing illness and improving the energy level. The pressure exerted is believed to regulate the energy, qi, that flows along the meridians. As previously menntioned, the meridians are the invisible channels that run along the length of the body. These meridians are mainly named after the organs of the body such as the liver and stomach, but there are four exceptions, which are called the 'pericardium', 'triple heater', 'conception' and 'governor'. Specifically named meridian lines may also be used to treat ailments other than those relating to it.

Ailments claimed to have been treated successfully are back pain, asthma, digestive problems, insomnia, migraine and circulatory problems, amongst others. Changes in diet, regular exercise and certain self-checking methods may be recommended by your practitioner. It must be borne in mind that some painful symptoms are the onset of serious illness so you should always first consult your G.P.

Before any treatment commences, a patient will be asked details of lifestyle and diet, the pulse rate will be taken along with any relevant past history relating to the current problem. The person will be requested to lie on a mattress on the floor or on a firm table, and comfortable but loose-fitting clothing is best so that the practitioner can work most effectively on the energy channels. No oils are used on the body and there is no equipment. Each session lasts from approximately 30 minutes to 1 hour. Once the pressure is applied, and this can be done in a variety of ways particular to each practitioner, varying sensations may be felt. Some points may feel sore or tender and there may be some discomfort such as a deep pain or coolness. However, it is believed that this form of massage works quickly so that any tenderness soon passes.

The number of treatments will vary from patient to patient, according to how the person responds and what problem or ailment is being treated. Weekly visits may be needed if a specific disorder is being treated while other people may go whenever they feel in need. It is advisable for women who are pregnant to check with their practitioner first since some of the acupressure methods are not recommended during pregnancy. Acupressure can be practised safely at home although it is usually better for one person to perform the massage on another. Common problems such as headache, constipation and toothache can be treated quite simply although there is the possibility of any problem worsening first before an improvement occurs if the pressure points are over stimulated. You should, however, see your doctor if any ailment persists. To treat headache, facial soreness, toothache and menstrual pain, locate the fleshy piece of skin between the thumb and forefinger and squeeze firmly, pressing towards the forefinger. The pressure should be applied for about five minutes and either hand can be used. This point is known as 'large intestine 4'.

To aid digestive problems in both adults and babies, for example to settle infantile colic, the point known as 'stomach 36' is utilized, which is located on the outer side of the leg about 75 mm (3 ins) down from the knee. This point should be quite simple to find as it can often feel slightly tender. It should be pressed quite firmly and strongly for about five to ten minutes with the thumb.

When practising acupressure massage on someone else and before treatment begins, ensure that the person is warm, relaxed, comfortable and wearing loose-fitting clothing and that he or she is lying on a firm mattress or rug on the floor. To discover the areas that need to be worked on, press firmly over the body and see which areas are tender. These tender areas on the body correspond to an organ that is not working correctly. To commence massage using fingertips or thumbs, a pressure of about 4.5 kg (10 lbs) should be exerted. The massage movements should be performed very quickly, about 50 to 100 times every minute, and some discomfort is likely (which will soon pass) but there should be no pain. Particular care should be taken to avoid causing pain on the face, stomach or over any joints. If a baby or young child is being massaged then considerably less pressure should be used. If there is any doubt as to the correct amount, exert a downwards pressure on bathroom scales to ascertain the weight being used. There is no need to hurry from one point to another since approximately 5 to 15 minutes is needed at each point for adults, but only about 30 seconds for babies or young children.

Using the 'self-help' acupressure, massage can be repeated as often as is felt to be necessary with several sessions per hour usually being sufficient for painful conditions that have arisen suddenly. It is possible that as many as 20 sessions may be necessary for persistent conditions causing pain, with greater intervals of time between treatments as matters improve. It is not advisable to try anything that is at all complicated (or to treat an illness such as arthritis) and a trained practitioner will obviously be able to provide the best level of treatment and help. To contact a reputable practitioner who has completed the relevant training it is advisable to contact the appropriate professional body.

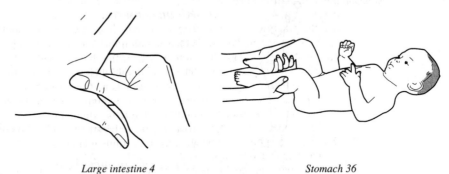

Large intestine 4   Stomach 36

Do-in

Do-in (pronounced doe-in) is another ancient type of massage that originated in China. It is a technique of self-massage and, as in other forms of alternative therapy, it is believed that there is a flow of energy throughout the body that travels along 'meridians' and that each of these is connected to a vital organ such as the lungs, liver and heart. Do-in has a connection with shiatsu (*see* page 90), and people of any age can participate, the only stipulation being that they are active and not out of condition. Clothing should not be tight or restrictive and adequate space is needed to perform the exercises.

If do-in is to be used as an invigorating form of massage, then the best time of day is as soon as possible after rising, but not after breakfast. After meals are the only times when do-in is to be avoided. It is generally recommended that people wishing to practise do-in should first go to classes so that when the exercises are done at home they are performed correctly. It is claimed that the use of do-in is preventive in nature since the vital organs are strengthened and therefore maintained in a healthy state.

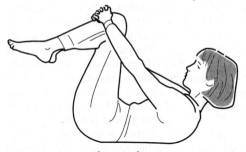

A—warming up

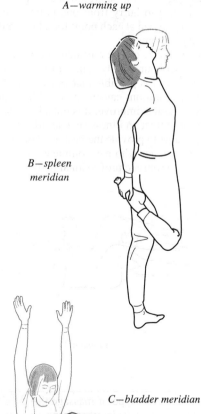

B—spleen
meridian

C—bladder meridian

Warming up

Before starting, it is best to do some warming-up exercises so that the body is not stiff. Begin by sitting on the ground with the knees up, grasp the knees and begin a rocking motion forwards and backwards. Then sit up, again on the floor, position the legs as if to sit cross-legged but put the soles of the feet touching each other. Hold the toes for a short time. These two exercises should help to make the body more supple (A).

Spleen meridian

For the *spleen meridian* exercise, which is connected with the stomach, stand as near as possible in front of a wall. Place one hand palm-downwards high up the wall so that there is a good stretching action and with the other hand grasp the foot that is opposite to the raised arm. The neck and head should be stretched backwards, away from the wall. Maintain this stretched position, inhale and exhale deeply twice and then relax. Repeat the procedure using the other arm and leg (B).

Bladder meridian

For the *bladder meridian* exercise, and thereby the kidneys, sit on the floor with the legs straight out in front and ensure that the toes are tensed upright. The arms should then be stretched above the head and a breath taken. After breathing out, bend forwards from the shoulders with the arms in front and hold the toes. Maintain this for the length of time it takes to breathe in and out three times. Repeat the procedure again (C).

Pericardium meridian

To do the exercise for the *pericardium meridian*, which affects the circulation, sit on the floor with feet touching, but one behind the other, ensuring that the hands are crossed and touching opposite knees. Grasp the knees and incline the body forwards with the aim of pushing the knees downwards on to the floor. Do this exercise again but with the hands on opposite knees and the other foot on the outside.

Large intestine meridian

Using the exercise that strengthens the *large intestine meridian* and in turn the lungs, stand upright

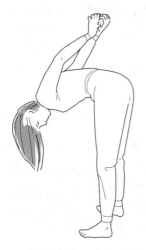

D—large intestine meridian

with the feet apart. Link the thumbs behind the back and then inhale. Exhale and at the same time place the arms outwards and upwards behind the back. To complete the exercise, lean forwards from the hips and then stand upright (D).

Gall bladder meridian

To strengthen the liver by stimulating the *gall bladder meridian*, sit upright on the floor with the legs the maximum distance apart. Then inhale, passing the arms along the length of the right leg so that the base of the foot can be held. There should be no movement of the buttocks off the floor. Maintain this stretched position while breathing deeply twice. Repeat the exercise using the other leg.

After all exercises have been accomplished, lie flat out on the floor with the legs apart and the arms stretched at the sides, palms uppermost. Then lift the head so that the feet can be seen and then put the head back on the floor again. The head and body should then be shaken so that the legs, arms and neck are loosened. To complete the relaxation, the eyes should be closed and the person should lie quietly for a few minutes.

Osteopathy

Introduction

An alternative medical treatment

Osteopathy is a technique that uses manipulation and massage to help distressed muscles and joints and make them work smoothly.

The profession began in 1892 when Dr Andrew Taylor Still (1828–1917), an American farmer, inventor and doctor, opened the USA's first school of osteopathic medicine. He sought alternatives to the medical treatments of his day which he believed were ineffective as well as often harmful.

Still's new philosophy of medicine, based upon the teachings of Hippocrates, advocated that 'Finding health should be the purpose of a doctor. Anyone can find disease.' Like Hippocrates, Still recognized that the human body is a unit in which structure, function, mind and spirit all work together.The therapy aims to pinpoint and treat any problems that are of a mechanical nature. The body's frame consists of the skeleton, muscles, joints and ligaments and all movements or activities such as running, swimming, eating, speaking and walking depend upon it.

A holistic treatment

Still came to believe that it would be safer to encourage the body to heal itself, rather than use the drugs that were then available and that were not always safe. He regarded the body from an engineer's point of view and the combination of this and his medical experience of anatomy, led him to believe that ailments and disorders could occur when the bones or joints no longer functioned in harmony. He believed that manipulation was the cure for the problem. Although his ideas provoked a great deal of opposition from the American medical profession at first, they slowly came to be accepted. The bulk of scientific research has been done in America with a number of medical schools of osteopathy being established. Dr Martin Littlejohn, who was a pupil of Dr Still, brought the practice of osteopathy to the UK around 1900, with the first school being founded in 1917 in London. He emphasized the compassionate care and treatment of the person as a whole, not as a collection of symptoms or unrelated parts.The philosophy and practices of A. T. Still, considered radical in the 1800s, are generally accepted principles of good medicine today.

Injuries and stress

Problems that prevent the body from working correctly or create pain can be due to an injury or stress. This can result in what is known as a tension headache since the stress experienced causes a contraction in muscles. These are situated at the back of the neck at the base of the skull and relief can be obtained by the use of massage. In osteopathy, it is believed that if the basic framework of the body is undamaged, then all physical activities can be accomplished efficiently and without causing any problems. The majority of an osteopath's patients suffer from disorders of the spine, which result in pain in the lower part of the back and the neck. A great deal of pressure is exerted on the spinal column, and especially on the cartilage between the individual vertebrae. This is a constant pressure due to the effects of gravity that occurs merely by standing. If a person stands incorrectly with stooped shoulders, this will exacerbate any problems or perhaps initiate one. The joints and framework of the body are manipulated and massaged where necessary so that the usual action is regained.

Athletes or dancers can receive injuries to muscles or joints such as the ankle, hip, wrist or elbow and they too can benefit from treatment by osteopathy. Pain in the lower back can be experienced by pregnant women who may stand in a different way due to their increasing weight and, if this is the case, osteopathy can often ease matters considerably. To find a fully qualified osteopath, it is advisable to contact the relevant professional body, or the G.P. may be able to help.

The treatment
The first visit

At the first visit to an osteopath, he or she will need to know the complete history of any problems experienced, how they first occurred and what eases or aggravates matters. A patient's case history and any form of therapy that is currently in use will all be of relevance to the practitioner. A thorough examination will then take place observing how the patient sits, stands or lies down and also the manner in which the body is bent to the side, back or front. As each movement takes place, the osteopath is able to take note of the extent and ability of the joint to function. The practitioner will also feel the muscles, soft tissues and ligaments to detect if there is any tension present. Whilst examining the body, the osteopath will note any problems that are present and, as an aid to diagnosis, use may also be made of checking reflexes, such as the knee-jerk reflex. If a patient has been involved in an accident, X-rays can be checked to determine the extent of any problem. It is possible that a disorder would not benefit from treatment by osteopathy and the patient would be advised accordingly. If this is not the case, treatment can commence with the chosen course of therapy.

A solution to tension

There is no set number of consultations necessary, as this will depend upon the nature of the problem and also for how long it has been apparent. It is possible that a severe disorder that has arisen suddenly can be alleviated at once. The osteopath is likely to recommend a number of things so that patients can help themselves between treatments. Techniques such as learning to relax, how to stand and sit correctly and additional exercises can be suggested by the osteopath. Patients generally find that each consultation is quite pleasant and they feel much more relaxed and calm afterwards. The length of each session can vary, but it is generally in the region of half an hour. As the osteopath gently manipulates the joint, it will lessen any tenseness present in the muscles and also improve its ability to work correctly and to its maximum extent. It is this manipulation that can cause a clicking noise to be heard. As well as manipulation, other methods such as massage can be used to good effect. Muscles can be freed from tension if the tissue is massaged and this will also stimulate the flow of blood. In some cases, the patient may experience a temporary deterioration once treatment has commenced, and this is more likely to occur if the ailment has existed for quite some time.

People who have to spend a lot of their life driving are susceptible to a number of problems related to the manner in which they are seated. If their position is incorrect they can suffer from tension headaches, pain in the back and the shoulders and neck can feel stiff. There are a number of ways in which these problems can be remedied such as holding the wheel in the approved manner (at roughly 'ten to two' on the dial of a clock). The arms should not be held out straight and stiff, but should feel relaxed and with the arms bent at the elbow. In order that the driver can maintain a position in which the back and neck feel comfortable, the seat should be moved so that it is tilting backwards a little, although it should not be so far away that the pedals are not easily reached. The legs should not be held straight out, and if the pedals are the correct distance away the knees should be bent a little and feel quite comfortable. It is also important to sit erect and not slump in the seat. The driver's rear should be positioned right at the back of the seat and this should be checked each time before using the vehicle. It is also important that there is adequate vision from the mirror so its position should be altered if necessary. If the driver already has a back problem then it is a simple matter to provide support for the lower part of the back. If this is done it should prevent strain on the shoulders and backbone. Whilst driving, the person should make a conscious effort to ensure that the shoulders are not tensed, but held in a relaxed way. Another point to remember is that the chin should not be stuck out but kept in, otherwise the neck muscles will become tensed and painful. Drivers can perform some beneficial exercises while they are waiting in a queue of traffic. To stretch the neck muscles, put the chin right down on to the chest and then relax. This stretching exercise should be done several times. The following exercise can also be done at the same time as driving and will have a positive effect on the flow of blood to the legs and also will improve how a person is seated. It is simply done by contraction and relaxation of the muscles in the stomach. Another exercise involves raising the shoulders upwards and then moving them backwards in a circular motion. The head should also be inclined forward a little. This should also be done several times to gain the maximum effect.

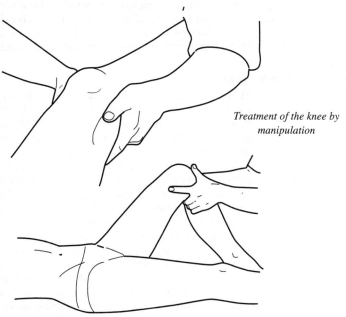

Treatment of the knee by manipulation

The figure above illustrates an example of diagnosis and treatment by manipulation, in which the osteopath examines a knee that has been injured. To determine the extent of the problem, the examination will be detailed and previous accidents or any other relevant details will be requested. If the practitioner concludes that osteopathy will be of benefit to the patient, the joint will be manipulated so that it is able to function correctly and the manipulation will also have the effect of relaxing the muscles that have become tensed due to the injury.

Another form of therapy, which is known as cranial osteopathy, can be used for patients suffering from pain in the face or head. This is effected by the osteopath using slight pressure on these areas including the upper part of the neck. If there is any tautness or tenseness present, the position is maintained while the problem improves. It is now common practice for doctors to recommend some patients to use osteopathy and some general practitioners use the therapy themselves after receiving training. Although its benefits are generally accepted for problems of a mechanical nature, doctors believe it is vital that they first decide upon what is wrong before any possible use can be made of osteopathy.

Polarity Therapy

Introduction

Origins

This is a therapy devised by Dr Randolph Stone (1890–1983) that amalgamates other healing therapies from both east and west. Dr Stone studied many of these therapies, including yoga (*see* page 48) and acupuncture (*see* page 11), and he was also trained to practise osteopathy (*see* page 41) and chiropractic (*see* page 19) among others. He began to search for a cure to the problem that he experienced with some of his patients when, although their disorder had been cured by the use of manipulation, they subsequently became unwell. Through his studies of eastern therapies he accepted the fundamental belief that a form of energy flows along certain channels in the body and that to keep good health the flow must be maintained. In India this energy is referred to as *prana* and in China it was called *chi* or *qi*. The western equivalent of this would probably be called a person's soul or spirit. It is believed that ailments occur when this flow of energy is blocked or is out of balance, and this could happen for different reasons such as tension or stress, disturbances in the mind or unhealthy eating patterns. This energy is purported to be the controlling factor in a person's whole life and therefore affects the mind and body at all levels. It is believed that once the flow of energy has been restored to normal, the ailment will disappear and not recur.

The underlying belief

Dr Stone's polarity therapy states that there are three types of relationships, known as *neutral*, *positive* and *negative*, to be maintained between various areas in the body and five centres of energy. These centres originate from a very old belief held in India, and each centre is held to have an effect on its related part of the body. The centres are known as *ether* (controlling the ears and throat), *earth* (controlling the rectum and bladder), *fire* (controlling the stomach and bowels), *water* (controlling the pelvis and glands), and *air* (controlling the circulation and breathing). The therapy's aim is to maintain a balance and harmony between all these various points, and Dr Stone slowly developed four procedures to do this. They are the use of *diet, stretching exercises, touch and manipulation,* and *mental attitude,* that is, contemplation allied with a positive view of life.

The treatment

Diet

To cleanse the body from a build-up of toxins caused by unhealthy eating and environmental pollution, the person will eat only fresh vegetables, fruit juices and fresh fruit. The length of time for this diet will vary according to the degree of cleansing required, but it is unlikely to be longer than a fortnight. Also available is a special drink that consists of lemon juice, olive oil, garlic and ginger. After the cleansing is complete, there is another diet to be followed that is said to promote and increase health, and finally one to ensure that the body maintains its level of good health.

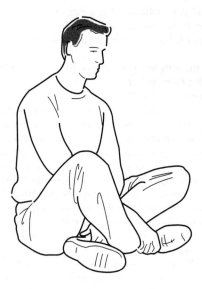

A—crosslegged

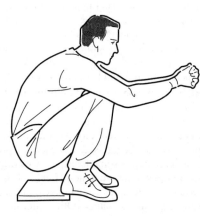

B—squatting

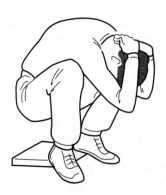

C—squatting

Stretching exercises

Various positions may be adopted for the stretching exercises, such as on the floor with the legs crossed (A) or squatting or sitting with the hands held at the back of the head. It is believed that these exercises free the channels that carry the body's energy and strengthen the sinews, muscles, ligaments and spine. As a way of releasing any stress or tension, the person would be requested to shout out loud at the same time as exercising. For the first exercise, the person can sit on the floor cross-legged with the right hand taking hold of the left ankle and with the left hand holding the right ankle. The eyes should then be shut and the mind relaxed and quiet.

For the squatting exercise, once in this position, clasp the hands out in front for balance and then move backwards and forwards and also in a circular motion. For people unable to balance in this position, a small book or similar item put under the heels should help (B).

For a slight change on the basic squatting position, bend the head forward and place the hands at the back of the neck so that the head and arms are between the knees. Relax the arms a little so that they drop forward slightly and thus the backbone is stretched (C).

Another variation is to hold the hands behind the neck whilst squatting and push the elbows and shoulder blades backwards and inwards. Any tension or stress can be relieved by shouting at the same time as breathing deeply.

Another exercise in which stress can be eased by shouting is known as the *wood chopper*. This is a fairly simple one to perform, and it entails standing with the feet apart and the knees bent. The hands should be clasped above the head as if about to chop some wood and the arms brought down together in a swinging action ending with the arms as far between the legs as possible. As the hands are being swung downwards, the person should shout, so that any tension is relieved. This action can be repeated quite frequently as long as there is no discomfort (D).

Touch and manipulation

Touch and manipulation are used by the therapist to detect any stoppages in the flow of energy along the channels, which are believed to be the reason for disorders. It is said that by the use of pressure, of which there are three sorts, the therapist is able to restore the flow of energy. *Neutral pressure* is gentle and calming and only the tips of the fingers are used. *Positive pressure* is the use of manipulation over the whole of the body with the exception of the head. *Negative pressure* is the use of a firmer and deeper manipulation and touch.

Mental attitude

Mental attitude is the fourth procedure, and basically this encourages people to have a more positive view on all aspects of their lives. This is achieved by talking or

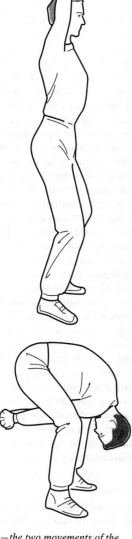

D—the two movements of the woodchopper

counselling sessions, and it is believed that a negative view of things can make a person more susceptible to having an ailment. A positive attitude is regarded as being essential for harmony in the body and mind.

Polarity therapy is claimed to be of some benefit to all people who are ill, although it does not concentrate on a particular set of symptoms but is more concerned with the overall aspect of the patient's health and the achievement of internal harmony and balance. For the therapy to work successfully, each patient has to believe in it completely and be prepared to carry out the practitioner's instructions with regard to diet, exercises, and so on. It is, of course, always advisable to make sure that any therapist is fully qualified before beginning treatment. At the first consultation, the patient will be required to give a complete case history to the therapist, who will then assess the flow of energy through the body and also check on its physical make-up. Reflexes such as the knee-jerk reflex are tested, and any imbalances or blockages in the energy channels are detected by the reflex and pressure point testing. If there is a stoppage or imbalance of the flow, this will be manifested by some physical symptoms. One way in which it is believed a patient can help to speed the restoration of health is by remembering and concentrating on any thoughts, feelings or pictures in the 'mind's eye' that happen while a particular area is being treated. The patient should also have knowledge of the body's ability to heal itself. If a patient is receiving treatment on a painful knee joint, for example, he or she should focus attention on that part of the body whilst being receptive to any feelings that occur. It is believed that if the patient is aware of the overall condition, as a complete person and not just the physical aspect, this will encourage restoration of health. It is possible that a patient will need to keep details of all food consumed to enable the practitioner to detect any harmful effects, and a 'fruit and vegetable' diet may be advised (as described previously). It may be that the patient has some habit, view or manner of life that is not considered conducive to good health. If this is the case, the patient would be able to take advantage of a counselling service in order to help make a change. Other alternative therapies such as the use of herbal medicine may be used to effect a cure.

Polarity therapy has much in common with other eastern remedies that have the common themes of contemplation, exercise, touch or pressure, and diet and that can give much improvement. However, it is recommended that an accurate medical analysis of any condition is found in the first instance.

Yoga

Introduction
Origins

From its Indian origins as far back as 4000 years ago, yoga has been continually practised, but it is only in the present century that its use has become more widespread. Yoga has an effect on the whole person, combining the physical, mental and spiritual sides. The word 'yoga' is derived from a Sanskrit word that means 'yoke' or 'union', and thus reflects on the practices of yoga being total in effect. For many hundreds of years in India only a select few, such as philosophers and like-minded people with their disciples, followed the way of life that yoga dictated. The leaders were known as 'yogis' and it was they who taught their followers by passing on their accumulated knowledge. These small groups of people dwelt in caves or woods, or sometimes a yogi would live like a hermit. Yoga has had quite far-reaching effects over many hundreds of years in India.

The basics of yoga were defined by a yogi called Patanjali who lived about 300 BC. He was a very well-respected teacher and commanded great influence at that time, and his classification is one that is used now. He established the fact of yoga being separated into eight different parts. The first two concern a person's lifestyle, which should be serene with the days spent in contemplation, study, maintaining cleanliness, and living very simply and at peace with others. Anything that involves avarice or greed, etc, or is harmful to others has to be avoided. The third and fourth parts are concerned with physical matters and list a number of exercises designed to promote peace and infuse energy into both the mind and body. The remaining four sections are concerned with the advancement of a person's soul or spirit and mental faculties by being able to isolate himself or herself from outside worries and normal life, contemplation and broadening mental faculties with the ultimate knowledge known as *samadhi*. Mentally, this is a complete change that gives final realization of existence. Much more recently, yoga became available in India to everyone, in complete contrast to centuries ago. Doctors and teachers taught yoga, and it is now the rule that all schoolchildren have lessons in some of the exercises.

Modern practice

Nowadays, the practice of yoga is not restricted to India alone, with millions of people worldwide being followers. There are actually five different types of yoga: *raja*, *jnana*, *karma* and *bakti*, and *hatha*. It is this last system that is known in the west, and it involves the use of exercises and positions. The other methods concentrate on matters such as control over the mind, appreciation and intelligence or a morally correct way of life. These other methods are regarded as being of equal importance by the person completely committed to yoga as a way of life. Although people may have little or no spiritual feeling, the basic belief of yoga is the importance of mental attitudes in establishing the physical improvements from exercise. Because of media coverage of a famous violinist receiving successful treatment to a damaged shoulder by yoga, it became very popular throughout the UK. Prior to the 1960s, it was seldom practised, and only then by people who wanted to learn more of eastern therapies or who had worked and travelled in that area.

It is a belief in yoga that the body's essence of life, or *prana,* is contained in the breath. Through a change in the way of breathing there can be a beneficial effect on the general health. If a person is in a heightened emotional condition, or similar state, this will have an effect on the breathing. Therefore, if the breathing is controlled or altered this should promote joint feelings of peace and calm, both mentally and emotionally. There is a variety of exercises, and each promotes different types of breathing, such as the rib cage, shoulder and diaphragm. Some of the movements and stances in use were originally devised from the observation of animals, since they appeared to be adept at relaxation and moved with minimum effort. These stances, which are maintained for one or two minutes, aim to increase freedom of movement and make the person aware of the various parts of the body and any stress that may be present. It is not intended that they be physically tiring or that the person should 'show off' in front of others. The aim is to concentrate on self-knowledge.

The treatment
The benefits

It is recommended to follow some simple rules when practising yoga. Firstly use a fully qualified therapist, and practise daily if at all possible. It is advisable to check with a G.P. first if a person is undergoing a course of treatment or is on permanent medication, has some sort of infirmity or feels generally unwell. It is always best that yoga is undertaken before mealtimes but if this is not possible then three hours must elapse after a large meal or an hour after a light one. Comfortable clothes are essential and a folded blanket or thick rug should be placed on the ground as the base. Before commencing yoga have a bath or shower and repeat this afterwards to gain the maximum benefit. It is not advisable to do yoga if either the bowels or bladder are full. Should the person have been outside on a hot and sunny day it is not recommended that yoga is practised straight afterwards, as feelings of sickness and dizziness may occur.

Yoga is believed to be of benefit to anyone, providing that they possess determination and patience. If a person has certain physical limitations then these must be taken into account with regard to their expectation, but there is no age barrier. Teachers believe that people suffering from stress and disorder in their lives are in greater need of a time of harmony and peace. Yoga was used in the main to encourage health in the physical and mental states and thereby act as a preventive therapy. Tension or stress was one of the main disorders for which it was used, but nowadays it has been used for differing disorders such as hypertension (high blood pressure), bronchitis, back pain, headaches, asthma, heart disorders, premenstrual tension and an acid stomach. Trials have also been conducted to assess its potential in treating some illnesses such as multiple sclerosis, cerebral palsy, osteoporosis, rheumatoid arthritis and depression experienced after childbirth. Since the effects of tension are often shown by the tightening and contraction of muscles, the stretching exercises performed in yoga are able to release it. Also, being aware of each muscle as it is stretched encourages the person to mentally lose any stress or problems with which they have been beset. Suppleness is developed by the exercises through the use of the bending and twisting actions. This will help to maintain healthy joints, particularly for people who lead rather inactive lives.

There should be no strain felt and after practice some or all of them can be done in order. As mentioned previously, it is best to check with a qualified therapist if the person is an expectant mother, suffers from hypertension, is overweight or is having their monthly period.

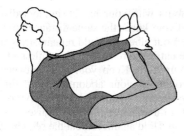

The bow

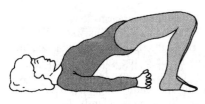

The bridge

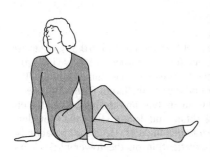

The spinal twist

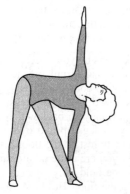

The triangle

The bow

Lie face down on the ground with the knees bent and then raised in the direction of the head. Then hold the ankles and, while inhaling, a pull should be exerted on the ankles so that the chest, head and thighs are raised up away from the floor. To start with it will not be possible to hold the legs together, but this will gradually occur with regular practice. This position should be maintained for up to ten breaths. To complete the bow, exhale and let go of the legs.

The bridge

The bridge is carried out on the floor, starting with the person lying on the back, the knees should be bent, with the legs separated a little and the arms at the side of the body. The person should then inhale and lift the torso and legs, thus forming a bridge. The fingers should then be linked under the body and the arms held straight. The person should then incline the body to each side in turn, ensuring that the shoulders stay underneath. To make the bridge a little bigger, pressure can be exerted by the arms and feet. After inhaling, the position should be maintained for a minimum of one minute and the body returned to a relaxed normal position on the floor.

The spinal twist

The spinal twist entails sitting on the floor with the legs outstretched. The left leg should be bent and placed over the other leg as far as possible. The person should exhale and twist the body to the left. The person's right hand should be moved towards the right foot. The person should have the body supported by placing the left hand on the ground at the back but keeping the back straight. Every time the person exhales the body should be further twisted to the left. The position should be maintained for approximately one minute and then the complete action done again, but this time turning to the right. This is a gentle posture that is easy to perform. Relax.

The spinal twist helps to strengthen the spine, improve posture and promote psychological balance.

The triangle

The triangle commences with the person standing upright with the legs apart and the arms held out at shoulder level. Extend the right foot to the side and, upon exhaling, bend over the right-hand side so that the right hand slips downwards in the direction of the ankle. There should be no forward inclination of the body at this time. As the bending action takes place, the left arm should be lifted upright with the palm of the hand to the front. This stretched position should be kept up for the minimum of a minute, with the person trying to extend the stretch as they exhale. After inhaling, the person should then revert to the beginning of the exercise and do it again but leaning in the opposite direction.

The triangle helps to calm the nerves, acts to remove toxins from the body, and promotes good health in general.

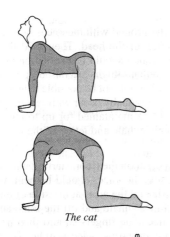

The cat

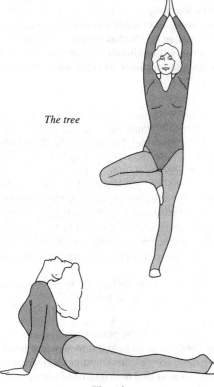

The tree

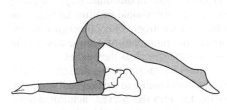

The cobra

The plough

The cat

Kneel on all fours with your hands shoulder-distance apart and your knees the same distance apart as your hands. Your elbows should remain straight throughout the entire exercise. Exhale while arching your back up high. Keep your head between your arms, looking at your abdomen. Hold this pose for a few seconds. Inhale, as you slowly hollow your back to a concave position. Raise your head and look up. Hold again. Repeat the sequence five to ten times, creating a slow flowing movement of the two postures. Relax.

The cat helps to strengthen the spine, improve posture and revitalize the whole body.

The tree

Stand with both feet together, arms loosely by your side. Focus your eyes on an imaginary spot directly ahead of you. Bring the right foot up and place the sole against the inside of the left thigh, as high as possible. When balanced, raise both arms simultaneously, placing the palms together over your head. Hold for 30 seconds. Gently lower your arms. Release your foot from your thigh. Repeat the sequence with the other foot. Relax.

The tree promotes concentration, balance and stability of body and mind.

The cobra

Lie face down. Place the palms on the floor under the shoulders, fingers turned slightly inwards. Slowly lift the forehead, the nose, the chin, and the entire upper body, up to the navel. The weight rests on both hands, the pelvis, and the legs. Keep the elbows slightly bent, and do not allow the shoulders to hunch up towards the ears. Hold for ten seconds, focusing your attention on the lower back. Very slowly lower your trunk to the floor, then the chin, the nose, and the forehead. Relax.

The cobra increases blood supply to the abdominal organs and helps to relieve digestive problems and correct kidney malfunctions.

The plough

Lie on your back, arms by your sides, palms down. Slowly raise your legs and trunk off the floor. Supporting your hips with both hands, bring your legs slightly over your head. Keep your legs as straight as possible. Supporting your back with both hands, continue lifting your legs up and over your head until the toes come to rest on the floor behind your head. Only when you are quite comfortable in the position, release the hold on your back and place your arms flat on the floor. Hold only for ten seconds in the beginning. After your body becomes accustomed to this position, you may hold it longer. Very slowly unroll your body to the starting position. Relax.

The plough helps to reinvigorate the entire nervous system, removing fatigue, listlessness and exhaustion. It is of particular benefit to the pancreas and endocrine glands.

The forward bend

Make sure you are well warmed up before attempting this posture. Sit with your legs stretched out in front of you, knees very straight. Inhale and stretch your arms above your head. Exhale and very slowly and smoothly bend forward from the hips (*not from the waist*) to grasp your toes. If at first this seems difficult, clasp instead your ankles, calves, or knees. It is important that your legs remain straight. Continue to bend forward and down, aiming to touch your knees with your head. Hold for at least ten seconds and observe your breath. Release your hold and very slowly unroll your spine, returning to a sitting position. Repeat twice.

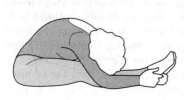

The forward bend

The forward bend slows the respiratory rate to produce a calm and relaxed state of mind. It also increases the suppleness of the spine and improves blood circulation – which helps to regenerate the abdominal organs and improve digestion.

A salute or greeting to the sun

The following twelve stances, known as *a greeting to the sun*, have the aim of relaxing and invigorating the body and mind. This classic exercise coordinates breathing with variations of six yoga poses in a flowing rhythmic way that stretches and relaxes your body and your mind.

As suggested by its name, it was originally done when the sun rose and when it set. Although these stances are quite safe, they should not be done by pregnant women or those having a monthly period, except with expert tuition. If a person has hypertension (high blood pressure), a hernia, clots in the blood or pain in the lower back they are not recommended. Each exercise should follow on smoothly one after the other.

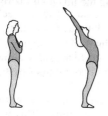

1 Start by facing east, standing up as straight as you can without forcing it, with your feet together. Inhale and visualize the sun just beginning to rise. Exhale and bring the palms of the hands on to your chest as if you were praying.

2 Then inhale and stretch the arms upright with the palms facing the ceiling and lean backwards, pushing the pelvis forward a little, and look up at your hands.

3 Exhale and, keeping the legs straight, place the fingers or palms on to the ground, ideally, your hands are touching the floor in front of or beside your feet. (Don't force this: if you can't reach the floor, let your hands hold on to the lowest part of your legs they can reach.)

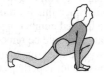

4 Whilst inhaling, bend the knees and place one leg straight out backwards, with the knee touching the ground, in a long, lunging movement. Turn your toes right under and straighten your body from head to heel.

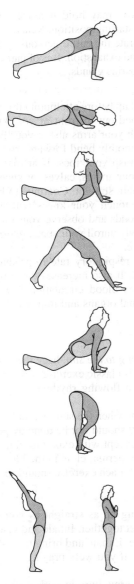

5 With both hands on the ground, raise the head slightly and push the hips to the front. At the same time as holding the breath, stretch the legs out together backwards, and raise the body off the floor supported by the arms.

6 Exhale and fold the body over bent knees so that the head touches the ground with the arms stretched out in front, toes curled, until you are in the classic push-up position.

7 After inhaling and exhaling once, drop your knees to the floor, with your bottom up. Bend the elbows and bring your chest and chin to the floor. Continue breathing out and lower the whole body to the floor, straightening your legs and keeping your toes curled under with the body being supported by the hands at shoulder level and also by the toes. The stomach and hips should not be on the ground.

8 After taking a deep breath, stretch the arms and push the body upwards pushing down on your hands and slowly lifting your head as you straighten the elbows. Arch your back upwards like a snake before it strikes.

9 Exhale and then raise the hips upwards with the feet and hands being kept on the floor so that the body is in an inverted V-shape. The legs and back should be kept straight .

10 Breathe in and lunge forward by bending your right knee and stepping your right foot forward between your hands. When you breathe out, straighten your right leg and bring the left foot next to the right. Lift your buttocks high until you are touching your toes.

11 Inhale and slowly lift the spine, visualizing it unroll one vertebra at a time. Raise your head and look up, bringing your arms straight overhead, and bring the image of the rising sun back to mind.

12 Place the feet together keeping the legs straight. Breathe out and slowly bring your arms back to the sides, allowing the sun to glow brighter and brighter in your mind's eye.

Salute the sun six times at first, gradually increasing the number of repetitions until you are comfortably doing the routine 24 times. This whole sequence of exercises can be performed several times over if wished. If this is the case, it is suggested to alternate the legs used either forwards or backwards in two of the exercises.

As previously mentioned, yoga has recently been used to treat some illnesses such as rheumatoid arthritis, and if a person has such a severe disorder, then a highly skilled and experienced therapist is essential. Since this form of yoga, known as therapeutic yoga, is so new there is only a limited number of suitably experienced therapists available, although this situation should be remedied by the introduction of further training. For those who wish to use yoga to maintain mental and physical health, joining a class with an instructor is perhaps the best way to proceed, so that exercises are performed correctly and any lapses in concentration can be corrected. These classes last usually in the region of an hour and are separated into sessions for beginners and those who are more proficient. Proficiency and progress is achieved by frequent practice, which can be done at home between lessons. One simple exercise that helps reduce stress is quite simple to perform and does not take long. The person should lie on the floor with the arms at the side and the legs together. After inhaling, all the muscles from the toes to the thighs should be tightened in turn. As the person exhales, the muscles in the stomach up to the shoulders should then be tightened, including the hands, which should be clenched. After inhaling again, the chest, throat and face muscles should be tightened, as well as screwing up the face and this should be maintained until the next breath has to be taken. All muscles should then be relaxed, the legs parted and the arms spread out comfortably with the palms facing the ceiling. The person should then totally relax with a sensation of falling through the ground.

The majority of doctors regard yoga as a type of exercise that is beneficial, although some do recommend patients to refer to yoga practitioners. However, if a specific disorder is to be treated, it is very important that the ailment should first be seen by a doctor.

Reflexology

Introduction

Origins

Reflexology is a technique of diagnosis and treatment in which certain areas of the body, particularly the feet, are massaged to alleviate pain or other symptoms in the organs of the body. It is thought to have originated about five thousand years ago in China and was also used by the ancient Egyptians. It was introduced to Western society by Dr William Fitzgerald, who was an ear, nose and throat consultant in America. He applied ten zones (or energy channels) to the surface of the body, hence the term 'zone therapy', and these zones, or channels, were considered to be paths along which flowed a person's vital energy, or 'energy force'. The zones ended at the hands and feet. Thus, when pain was experienced in one part of the body, it could be relieved by applying pressure elsewhere in the body, within the same zone.

Subsequent practitioners of reflexology have concentrated primarily on the feet, although the working of reflexes throughout the body can be employed to beneficial effect.

Massage and energy flow

Reflexology does not use any sort of medication—merely a specific type of massage at the correct locations on the body. The body's energy flow is thought to follow certain routes, connecting every organ and gland with an ending or pressure point on the feet, hands or another part of the body. When the available routes are blocked, and a tenderness on the body points to such a closure, then it indicates some ailment or condition in the body that may be somewhere other than the tender area. The massaging of particular reflex points enables these channels to be cleared, restoring the energy flow and at the same time healing any damage.

The uses of reflexology are numerous, and it is especially effective for the relief of pain (back pain, headaches and toothache), treatment of digestive disorders, stress and tension, colds and influenza, asthma, arthritis, and more. It is also possible to predict a potential illness and either give preventive therapy or suggest that specialist advice be sought. The massaging action of reflexology creates a soothing effect that enhances blood flow, to the overall benefit of the whole body. Reflexology, however, clearly cannot be used to treat conditions that require surgery.

Reflex massage initiates a soothing effect to bring muscular and nervous relief. The pressure of a finger applied to a particular point (or nerve ending) may create a sensation elsewhere in the body, indicating the connection or flow between the two points. This is the basis of reflexology, and although pain may not be alleviated immediately, continued massage over periods of up to one hour will usually have a beneficial effect.

There are certain conditions for which reflexology is inappropriate, including diabetes, some heart disorders, osteoporosis, disorders of the thyroid gland, and phlebitis (inflammation of the veins). It may also not be suitable for pregnant women or anyone suffering from arthritis of the feet.

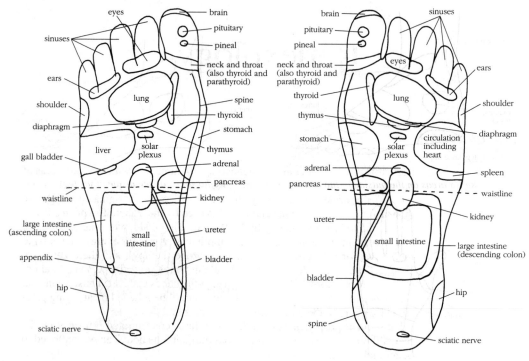

Major reflex points on the sole of the right foot

Major reflex points on the sole of the left foot

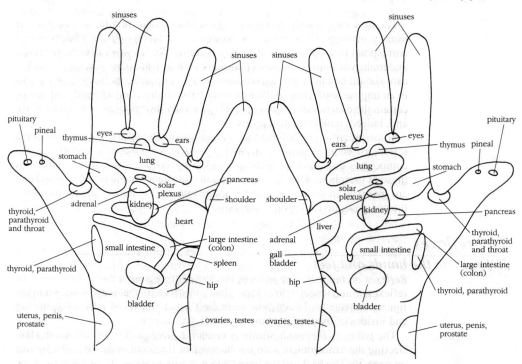

Major reflex points on the palm of the left hand

Major reflex points on the palm of the right hand

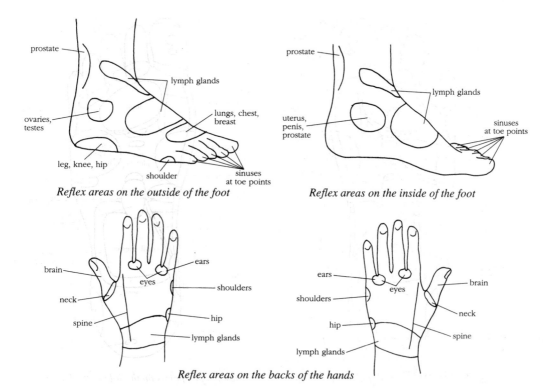

Reflex areas on the outside of the foot

Reflex areas on the inside of the foot

Reflex areas on the backs of the hands

The best way to undergo reflexology is in the hands of a therapist, who will usually massage all reflex areas, concentrating on any tender areas that will correspond to a part of the body that is ailing. Reflexology can, however, be undertaken at home on minor conditions such as back pain, headache, etc, but care should be taken not to over-massage any one reflex point as it may result in an unpleasant feeling. Although there have not been any clinical trials to ascertain the efficacy of reflexology, it is generally thought that it does little harm and, indeed, much benefit may result.

Some practitioners believe that stimulation of the reflex points leads to the release of endorphins (in a manner similar to acupuncture). Endorphins are compounds that occur in the brain and have pain-relieving qualities similar to those of morphine. They are derived from a substance in the pituitary gland and are involved in endocrine control (glands producing hormones, for example, the pancreas, thyroid, ovary and testis).

The reflexes

Reflexes on the hands and feet

Reflexes on the feet—the soles of the feet contain a large number of zones, or reflexes, that connect with organs, glands or nerves in the body, as shown in the figures on page 56. In addition, there are a small number of reflexes on the top and insides of the feet, as shown in the figures above.

The *palms of the hands* similarly contain a large number of reflex areas, reflecting the arrangement seen on the soles of the feet, as shown in the figures on page 56. The backs of the hands again mirror, to some extent, the tops of the feet, containing a smaller number of reflex areas (*see* figures above).

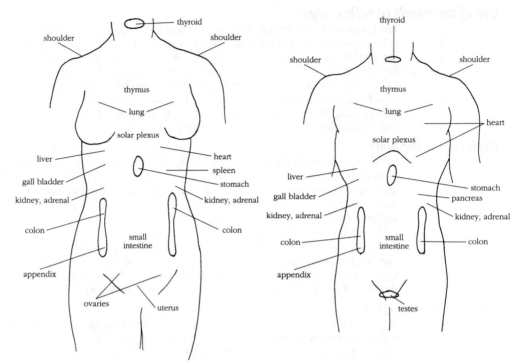

The major reflexes on the body (female)   *The major reflexes on the body (male)*

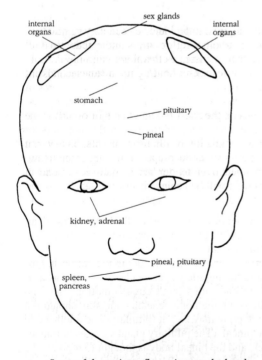

Some of the major reflex points on the head

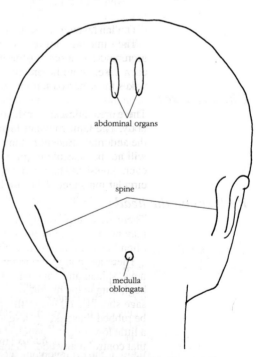

The back of the head showing the medulla oblongata reflex

Use of the hands in reflexology

The hands are considered to have an electrical property, so that the right-hand palm is positive and the left-hand palm is negative. In addition, the right hand has a reinforcing, stimulating effect while the left has a calming, sedative effect. The back of each hand is opposite to the palm, thus the right is negative and the left is positive. This is important when using reflexology because if the object is to revitalize the body and restore the energy flow that has been limited by a blockage then the right hand is likely to be more effective. The left hand, with its calming effect, is best used to stop pain.

Reflexes on the body

Reflexes on the body necessarily differ from those on the feet and hands in that there is less alignment with the ten zones (the figures on page 58 show some of the reflexes on the body). Also, there are a number of reflex points on the body that correspond to several organs or glands. These reflex points are sometimes harder to find accurately and may be more difficult to massage.

The middle finger is thought to have the greatest effect, so this should be used to work the reflex point. Light pressure should be applied to each point, and if pain is felt it means there is a blockage or congestion somewhere. A painful point should be pressed until the discomfort subsides or for a few seconds at a time, a shorter rest being taken in between the applications of pressure.

The abdominal reflex

A general test can be applied by gently pressing into the navel, either with the middle finger or with one or both hands, with the individual lying in a supine position. The presence of a pulse or beat is taken to mean there is a problem in this area. To combat this, the same technique is used, holding for a few seconds (six or seven), releasing slightly, and keeping the fingers in the same area, gently massaging with a circular action. If it is necessary to press quite deep to feel the beat, then heavier massage will be required to provide the necessary stimulation.

The same principle can be applied to other reflex points in the abdominal region, and the absence of a pulse or beat indicates that there is no problem. In each case, should there be a painful response, holding for a few seconds invokes the sedative action.

Chest reflexes

There are a number of reflex points on the chest relating to major organs in the body. The same massage technique can be adopted for these reflex points as for the abdomen. Because many of the points lie over bone or muscle, however, it will not be possible to press in the finger as deeply as for the abdomen. However, pressure should be maintained over tender areas, with a subsequent circular massage, and a similar effect will be achieved.

Reflexes on the head

There are a surprisingly large number of reflex points on the head, although all may not be apparent immediately. With time and experience, such points are often located more by touch than by sight.

There are many important reflexes on the head including the stomach, kidneys, spleen and pancreas. Again, the middle finger can be used for massage, beginning in the middle of the forehead with a gentle circular motion. The massage should go through the skin to rub the bone beneath—the skin should not be rubbed. In so doing, a sensitive point may be felt (pituitary) and another one a little lower down, which is the pineal. (The pituitary gland secretes hormones that control many body functions and the pineal body is thought to regulate the natural variations in the body's activities over a 24-hour period.) This massaging action can be continued to check other parts of the body.

The back of the head also shows a large number of reflexes. However, there are a number of ways of stimulating the body as a whole through the head. These include:
• tapping the head gently with the fists, all over and very quickly for a period of about thirty seconds
• pulling handfuls of hair
• tapping the head gently with a wire brush
Each has a specific result, for example, stimulating the hair, but also enlivening organs and glands over the whole body.

One particularly important reflex point is the medulla oblongata (*see* page 58). The medulla oblongata is the lowest part of the brain stem, which joins to the upper part of the spinal cord. It contains important centres for the control of respiration, swallowing, salivation and the circulation. This reflex point is located at the nape of the neck, towards the base of the skull. Massage of this point opens all channels within the body and generates a vitality, relieving nervous tension and producing almost instant energy. The point should be pressed and massaged to produce the desired effects.

Ear reflexes

The ear has long been used in acupuncture because, in addition to its ease of use, it contains scores of acupoints, which correspond to the reflex points in reflexology. Some of these points are shown in the figure below.

The ear is perhaps the most difficult area of the body to work with because there are so many reflexes in such a small space. It becomes essentially a question of touch, pressing and exploring, and any sore point located can be massaged and worked out. By using a gentle squeeze-and-roll method on the tops of the ears and the ear lobes a number of areas can be stimulated. It has been reported that reflexology can help ear problems such as ringing in the ears, and the condition tinnitus may be alleviated to some extent.

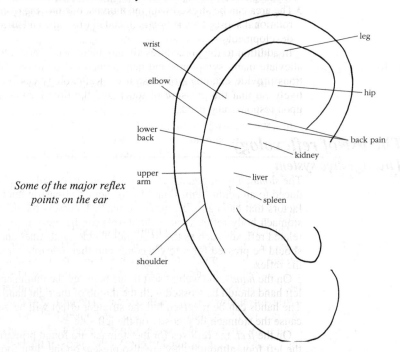

Some of the major reflex points on the ear

Techniques and practice

Some indication of the massaging, manipulative procedures of reflexology have already been mentioned, but a number of general points of guidance can also be made.

The whole process of reflexology is one of calm, gentle movements in a relaxed state. The foot is probably used most in reflexology, in which case shoes and socks and stockings, etc, should be removed. A comfortable position should be adopted on the floor or bed, in a warm, quiet room with the back supported by pillows.

To begin, the whole foot is massaged, indeed both feet should ideally be worked on. However, if working on your own feet it is thought that the right foot should be massaged first (contrary to previous practice). It is considered that the right foot is linked with the past, hence these emotions must be released before the present and future aspects are dealt with in the left foot.

Techniques of massage vary, but a simple method with which to start involves placing the thumb in the middle of the sole of the foot. The thumb then presses with a circular and rocking motion for a few seconds before moving to another reflex. Reference can be made to the diagrams to determine which reflex is being massaged. In all cases, the massage should work beneath the skin, not on the skin. Another method involves starting the massage with the big toe and then moving on to each toe in turn. In using the thumbs to effect the massage, some refinements of motion can be introduced to give slightly different movements.

1 The thumb can be rocked between the tip and the ball, moving forwards over the relevant area. This, along with the circular massage already mentioned, relieves aches and pains.

2 Both thumbs can be used alternately to stroke the skin firmly. This creates a calming effect.

3 The area can be stroked with the thumbs, one moving over the other in a rotational sense. This action is intended to soothe and allow for personal development.

In addition to the procedures already mentioned, reflexology can be used to alleviate many symptoms and help numerous conditions. The following sections provide examples of these uses. Reflexology can be approached intuitively, so that the pressure of touch and the time factor can vary depending upon response and need.

The use of reflexology

The digestive system

The *stomach* is an organ that has thick muscular walls and in which food is reduced to an acidic semi-liquid by the action of gastric juices. There are many factors that can cause an upset stomach. To assess the general condition, the stomach body reflex (above the navel) can be pressed. Around it are several related reflexes such as the liver, gall bladder, intestines and colon. The reflex should be pressed for a few seconds and then released three times to activate the reflex.

On the *hands*, the web of soft tissue between the thumb and forefinger of the left hand should be worked with the thumb of the right hand for a few minutes. The hands can be reversed but the stronger effect will be gained this way, because the stomach lies mostly on the left side.

On the *feet*, the reflexes for the stomach are found primarily on the instep of the left foot, although they are also present on the right foot. These should be massaged, but there are further factors, in addition to the use of reflexology, that will aid digestion. These include eating a sensible diet with a minimum of artificial substances, and not overeating. The use of certain essential oils (aromatherapy) can also be of benefit. In this case peppermint oil can often be particularly effective.

The *colon* is the main part of the large intestine in which water and salts are removed from the food that enters from the small intestine. After extraction of the water, the waste remains are passed on to the rectum as faeces. If this system becomes unbalanced in any way, then the water may not be absorbed or the food remains pass through the colon so quickly that water cannot be absorbed. In such cases, the result is diarrhoea, which can be painful and inconvenient.

Both body and foot reflexes should be massaged for the stomach, intestines, colon and also the liver and kidneys. The thyroid reflex should also be worked to help regulation of the body functions. A useful body reflex is to press and rotate your finger about two inches above the navel for a couple of minutes. This can be repeated numerous times, each time moving the fingers a little clockwise around the navel until a complete circuit has been made.

It is important that the condition be stabilized as soon as possible as continued fluid loss also leads to loss of vital salts and a general nutritional deficiency.

At the outset it is possible to work the colon reflexes on the hand to identify any tender areas. The right thumb should be pressed into the edge of the pad (around the base and side of the thumb) of the left palm and worked around to seek out any tender spots. Any tender reflex should be massaged and pressed for a few seconds. In each case, the tenderness should be worked out. Since there are many reflex points crowded onto the navel, it may not solely be the colon reflex that requires some attention. It is always useful to work the reflex on both sides of the body to ensure a balance is achieved.

A similar approach can be adopted for reflexes on the feet, starting at the centre, or waistline. By applying a rolling pressure, the foot is massaged along to the inner edge and then down the line of the spine and any tender points are worked through pressure and massage. It may be necessary to start with a very light pressure if the area is very tender, and then as the soreness lessens, the pressure can be increased.

Again, diet can be an important factor in maintaining the health of the body and the workings of the colon. Fibre is particularly important in ensuring a healthy digestive system and avoiding ailments such as diverticulitis.

Reflexology can be used for other conditions associated with the digestive system, notably ulcers. A peptic ulcer (in the stomach, duodenum or even the oesophagus) is caused by a break in the mucosal lining. This may be due to the action of acid, bile or enzymes because of unusually high concentrations or a deficiency in the systems that normally protect the mucosa. The result can be a burning sensation, belching and nausea.

To help alleviate the problem, which may often be stress-related, the reflexes in the feet should be massaged, as these are often the most relaxing. Obviously, the important reflexes are the stomach and duodenum, but it is also worthwhile to work on the liver and the endocrine glands (notably the pituitary). If the ulcer is a long-standing problem or if stomach complaints have been experienced for some time, then further medical help is probably needed.

The heart and circulatory system

The heart is obviously a vital organ. This muscular pump is situated between the lungs and slightly left of the midline. It projects forward and lies beneath the fifth rib. Blood returns from the body via the veins and enters the right atrium (the upper chamber), which contracts, forcing the blood into the right ventricle. From there it goes to the lungs where it gains oxygen and releases carbon dioxide before passing to the left atrium and left ventricle. Oxygenated blood then travels throughout the body via the arteries.

By using body reflexes, the heart can be maintained, and conditions can be dealt with by massaging the appropriate reflex points. A useful massage exercise is to work the muscles, rather than the reflex points, of the left arm in a side-to-side movement. This can be followed by the neck muscles and the chest muscles; in each case any tightness or tension should be massaged out. An additional preventive is a good diet, which should be low in fat and food high in cholesterol, but should contain adequate amounts of vitamins, notably the B group, C and E. Exercise is, of course, very important to maintain a good heart and circulation.

There is also a simple test that many reflexologists feel is useful in the diagnosis of possible heart problems. It may also be worth doing if strenuous activity is contemplated in the near future. Pressure is applied to the pad of the left thumb, at the top. The pressure should be quite hard. It is suggested that when this part of the pad hurts, it indicates a constriction in blood vessels, limiting supply. If the bottom of the pad hurts, this is indicative of congested arteries. If the area is too tender to touch (and there is no physical damage to the hand) then there is a possibility of a heart attack. This test thus provides advance warning and enables a medical doctor to be consulted. Should painful areas occur on both hands, this does *not* indicate a heart problem.

Many blood and circulatory disorders will benefit from the same sort of massage. In these cases the foot reflexes for the endocrine glands (hypothalamus, pituitary, pineal, thyroid and parathyroid, thymus, adrenals, pancreas, ovary or testis) should be worked well, as should those for the circulatory system and heart, lungs and lymphatic system.

Conditions that may benefit from such treatment include:

Angina

A suffocating, choking pain usually referring to angina pectoris, which is felt in the chest. It occurs when blood supply to the heart muscle is inadequate and is brought on by exercise and relieved by rest. The coronary arteries may be damaged by atheroma (scarring and build up of fatty deposits). Of particular importance are the heart and circulatory reflexes (veins and arteries) and those of the lymphatic system.

Arteriosclerosis

A general term including atheroma and atherosclerosis (where arteries degenerate and fat deposits reduce blood flow), which results generally in high blood pressure and can lead to angina. Additional reflexes that should be worked include the liver.

Hypertension (high blood pressure)

This may be one of several types, the commonest being *essential* (due to kidney or endocrine disease or an unknown cause) and *malignant* (a serious condition that tends to occur in the younger age groups). In addition to the reflexes for the blood and circulation, those for the shoulders, neck and eyes should be worked, in combination with reflexes for the digestive system and liver.

Palpitations

An irregular heartbeat, often associated with heightened emotions. Also due to heart disease or may be felt during pregnancy. The lung and heart reflexes are particularly important, in addition to those of the circulation.

Some heart conditions are very serious and require immediate hospitalization, e.g. cardiac arrest (when the heart stops) and coronary thrombosis (a coronary artery blockage causing severe chest pain, vomiting, nausea and breathing difficulties. The affected heart muscle dies, a condition known as myocardial infarction). However, massage of appropriate reflexes may help, particularly in less serious cases. These should include the heart and circulation (veins and arteries), lungs, endocrine system and the brain. Each will have some beneficial effect in relieving stress and congestion.

Varicose veins

Veins that have become stretched, twisted and distended, and this often happens to the superficial veins in the legs. The possible causes are numerous and include pregnancy, defective valves, obesity and thrombophlebitis (the inflammation of the wall of a vein with secondary thrombosis). Phlebitis is inflammation of a vein and occurs primarily as a complication of varicose veins. Both these conditions can be treated by massaging the circulatory reflexes and also the leg and liver reflexes. In both cases, resting with the legs in an elevated position is beneficial.

The respiratory system

Asthma is one of the major problems of the respiratory system and its incidence seems to be escalating. The condition is caused by a narrowing of the airways in the lungs. It usually begins in early childhood and may be brought on by exposure to allergens (substances, usually proteins, that cause allergic reactions) exercise or stress.

There are certain body reflexes that can help in this instance. One reflex point is in the lower neck at the base of the V-shape created by the collar bones. Relief may be achieved by pressing the finger into this point with a downward motion for a few seconds. There are additional reflex points on the back, at either side of the spine in the general region of the shoulder blades. These can be worked by someone else with thumb or finger, who should press for a few seconds. Other reflexes that can be worked on the foot include the brain, endocrine glands such as the pineal, pituitary, thymus and thyroid, the lungs, and also the circulatory system. Particular attention should be paid to the lungs, which includes the bronchi and bronchioles, the branching passageways of the lungs where gaseous exchange (oxygen in, carbon dioxide out) takes place. At the point where the instep meets the hard balls of the feet, and along the base of the lung reflex area is the massage point for the diaphragm. Working the whole of this area will help alleviate symptoms of asthma. During an attack of asthma, both thumbs can be placed on the solar plexus reflexes immediately to initiate the soothing process.

The adrenal glands are found one to each kidney, situated on the upper surface of that organ. These are important endocrine glands because they produce hormones such as adrenaline and cortisone. Adrenaline is very important in controlling the rate of respiration and it is used medically in the treatment of bronchial asthma because it relaxes the airways. It is clear therefore, that the adrenal is an important reflex and it is located in the middle of each sole and palm.

Many other respiratory disorders can be helped by using massage of the same reflexes: brain, endocrine glands, lungs and diaphragm, neck and shoulders, augmented by the heart and circulatory system. Conditions responding to this regime include bronchitis, croup, lung disorders and emphysema (distension and thinning, particularly of lung tissue, leading to air-filled spaces that do not contribute to the respiratory process).

Infections of the respiratory tract leading to coughs and colds can also be helped primarily by working the reflexes mentioned above. For colds, the facial reflexes should be massaged, especially that for the nose. However, it is good practice to include the pituitary, and to work the index and middle fingers towards the tip to help alleviate the condition.

With such respiratory problems, there are complementary therapies that can help such as homoeopathy, aromatherapy and Bach flower remedies. There are also many simple actions that can be taken, for example a sore throat may be helped by gargling regularly with a dessertspoon of cider apple vinegar in a glass of water, with just a little being swallowed each time. Honey is also a good substance to take, as are onion and garlic.

The endocrine glands

Summary

Endocrine glands are glands that release hormones directly into the bloodstream, or lymphatic system. Some organs, such as the pancreas, also release secretions via ducts. The major endocrine glands are, in addition to the pancreas, the thyroid, parathyroid, pituitary, pineal, thymus, adrenal and gonads (ovaries and testes).

The endocrine glands are of vital importance in regulating body functions as summarized below:

pituitary	controls growth, gonads, kidneys; known as the master gland
pineal	controls the natural daily rhythms of the body
thyroid	regulates metabolism and growth
parathyroid	controls calcium and phosphorus metabolism
thymus	vital in the immune system, particularly pre-puberty
adrenal	control of heartbeat, respiration and metabolism
gonads	control of reproductive activity
pancreas	control of blood sugar levels

The fact that the endocrine glands are responsible for the very core of body functions means that any imbalance should be corrected immediately to restore the normality. There are some general points relating to massage of these reflex areas. It is good practice to massage the brain reflex first and then the pituitary. This is because the hypothalamus, situated in the forebrain, controls secretions from the pituitary gland. The pituitary gland then follows as this is the most important in the endocrine system. The reflexes should be gently massaged with thumb or finger for a few seconds and then gentle pressure exerted and held for a few seconds before releasing slowly.

The pituitary

An imbalance of pituitary gland secretions, often caused by a benign tumour, can lead to acromegaly (excessive growth of skeletal and soft tissue). Gigantism can result if it occurs during adolescence. There may also be consequent deficiencies in adrenal, gonad and thyroid activity. The brain and endocrine reflexes should be worked in order, supplemented by those for the circulation, liver and digestion. In addition to reflex points on the hands and feet, there is also one on the forehead. If any of these reflex areas is found to be tender, it should be massaged often to maintain the balance necessary for healthy growth.

The pineal

The pineal body, or gland, is situated on the upper part of the mid-brain, although its function is not fully understood. It would seem, however, to be involved in the daily rhythms of the body and may also play a part in controlling sexual activity. The pineal reflex points are found close to those of the pituitary on the big toes, thumbs and on the forehead and upper lip.

The thyroid

The thyroid is located at the base of the neck and it produces two important hormones, thyroxine and triiodothyronine. Under or overactivity of the thyroid leads to specific conditions.

If the thyroid is overactive and secretes too much thyroxine (hyperthyroidism), the condition called thyrotoxicosis develops. It is also known as Grave's disease and is typified by an enlarged gland, protruding eyes and symptoms of excess metabolism such as tremor, hyperactivity, rapid heart rate, breathlessness, etc. The important reflexes on which to concentrate are the brain and solar plexus, endocrine system and also the circulatory and digestive systems. The reflexes are found on the soles and palms and using the thumbs or fingers, the areas should be massaged, but in stages if the area is very tender.

Underactivity of the thyroid, or hypothyroidism, can cause myxoedema producing dry, coarse skin, mental impairment, muscle pain and other symptoms. In children a similar lack causes cretinism, resulting in dwarfism and mental retardation. The reflexes to be worked are essentially those mentioned for hyperthyroidism, and in addition (for both conditions) the liver reflexes on the right sole and palm should benefit from attention.

There are additional thyroid reflexes elsewhere on the body, notably on the neck roughly midway between jaw and collarbone and on either side. These points should be massaged gently with the thumb and fingers on opposite sides of the throat. Using a gentle gyratory motion, the massage can be taken down to the collarbone, the fingers and thumb of the other hand are then used (on opposite sides of the throat) and the procedure repeated.

Goitre is another condition associated with the thyroid and is a swelling of the neck caused by enlargement of the gland, typically due to overactivity of the gland to compensate for an iodine deficiency. The important reflexes to concentrate upon are the brain, solar plexus, endocrine system and circulatory system but working of all body reflexes will help.

The parathyroid

There are four small parathyroid glands located behind or within the thyroid. They control the use of calcium and phosphorus (as phosphate) in the body's metabolism. An imbalance of these vital elements can lead to tetany (muscular spasms), or at the other extreme, calcium may be transferred from the bones to the blood, creating a tendency to bone fractures and breaks.

The reflexes to these glands are found in the same location as those for the thyroid but it will probably be necessary to massage more strongly to achieve an effect. It is a good idea to work on these areas each time reflexology is undertaken as they are vital in maintaining the metabolic equilibrium of the body.

The thymus

The thymus is located in the neck (over the breastbone) and is a vital contributor to the immune system. It is larger in children and is important in the development of the immune response. After puberty it shrinks although seems to become more active later in life. Bone marrow cells mature within the thymus and one group, T-lymphocytes, are dependent upon the presence of the thymus. These are important cells as they produce antibodies.

The commonest disorder associated with the thymus is myasthenia gravis, which lowers the level of acetylcholine (a neurotransmitter) resulting in a weakening of skeletal muscles and those used for breathing, swallowing, etc. The thymus reflexes are found on the soles of the feet and palms of the hand, next to the lung reflexes. The thymus can also be stimulated by tapping with the finger over its position in the middle of the upper chest.

The adrenals

The two adrenals (also known as suprarenals) are situated one above each kidney and consist of an inner medulla and an outer cortex. The medulla produces adrenaline, which increases the rate and depth of respiration, raises the heartbeat and improves muscle performance, with a parallel increase in output of sugar from the liver into the blood.

The cortex of the adrenal glands releases hormones including aldosterone, which controls the balance of electrolytes in the body, and cortisone, which, among other functions, is vital in the response to stress, inflammation and fat deposition in the body.

On both the palms and soles, the adrenal reflexes are located above those for the kidneys and if this area is at all tender, it should be massaged for a few seconds. Because the kidney and adrenal reflexes are close together, the massage should be limited to avoid over-stimulation of the kidney reflexes. Disorders of the adrenal glands should be treated by working the endocrine reflexes starting with the pituitary and including the adrenal reflexes themselves, followed by the reflexes for the circulatory, liver and urinary systems.

Specific disorders include Cushing's syndrome, caused by an overproduction of cortisone, which results in obesity, reddening of the face and neck, growth of body and facial hair, high blood pressure, osteoporosis and possibly mental disturbances, and Addison's disease, which results from damage to the cortex and therefore a deficiency in hormone secretion. The latter was commonly caused by tuberculosis but is now due more to disturbances in the immune system. The symptoms are weakness, wasting, low blood pressure and dark pigmentation of the skin. Both these conditions can be treated by hormone replacement therapy but reflexology can assist, through massage of the endocrine, digestive and liver reflexes.

The gonads

The gonads, or sex glands, comprise the ovaries in women and testes in men. The ovaries produce eggs and also secrete hormones, mainly oestrogen and progesterone. Similarly, the testes produce sperm and the hormone testosterone. Oestrogen controls the female secondary sexual characteristics such as enlargement of the breasts, growth of pubic hair and deposition of body fat. Progesterone is vital in pregnancy as it prepares the uterus for implantation of the egg cell.

The reflexes for these and related organs are found near the ankles on the inside of the feet, just below the angular bone (*see* figure depicting the reflex areas on the inside and outside of the feet on page 57). The same reflex areas are also located on the arms, near the wrist. The ovaries and testes are on the outer edge, while on the opposite, inner edge, are the reflexes for the uterus, penis and prostate.

For any disorders that might involve the ovaries or testes, it is also useful to massage other systems such as the brain, other endocrine glands, the circulation and liver.

The pancreas

This is an important gland with both endocrine and exocrine functions. It is located behind the stomach, between the duodenum and spleen. The exocrine function involves secretion of pancreatic juice via ducts, into the intestine. The endocrine function is vital in balancing blood sugar levels through the secretion of two hormones, insulin and glucagon. Insulin controls the uptake of glucose by body cells and a lack of hormone results in the sugar derived from food being excreted in the urine, the condition known as diabetes mellitus. Glucagon works in the opposite sense to insulin, and increases the supply of blood sugar through the breakdown of glycogen in the liver, to produce glucose.

The primary reflexes for the pancreas are found on the soles and palms, near to the stomach. The thumb should be used, starting on the left foot, working across the reflex area and on to the right foot. If the area is tender, it should be worked until the tenderness goes. Because there are numerous reflexes in this area, there will be stimulation of other organs, to the general wellbeing of the body as a whole.

For other disorders of the pancreas, such as pancreatitis (inflammation of the pancreas) the reflexes associated with digestion should also be worked. Pancreatitis may result from gallstones or alcoholism and, if sufficiently severe, may cause diabetes.

The liver and spleen

The role of the liver

The liver is a very important organ and is critical in regulating metabolic processes. It is the largest gland in the body and is situated in the top right hand part of the abdominal cavity. Among the functions, the liver converts excess glucose to glycogen, which is stored as a food reserve; excess amounts of amino acids are converted into urea for excretion; bile is produced for storage in the gall bladder and some poisons are broken down. The liver also recycles red blood cells to remove the iron when the cells reach the end of their life; it stores vitamins and produces blood clotting substances. Due to its high chemical and biochemical activity, the liver generates a lot of heat and is the major contributor of heat to the body.

The liver reflex points

The reflex area for the liver is a large area, reflecting the size of the organ, on the right palm and right sole, on the outer edge. As a general procedure, the area should be massaged with the left thumb, searching for tender points. More massage may be required for the liver than for other reflexes.

Hepatitis is inflammation of the liver due to viral infection or the presence of toxins. Alcohol abuse commonly causes hepatitis, and it may also be due to drug overdose or drug side effects. Viral infections such as HIV and glandular fever can also cause hepatitis. There are several types of hepatitis, designated A to E, and all may persist in the blood for a long time.

To combat such disorders, after removing the source of any toxins, the reflex for the liver and digestion should be worked and the reflexes for the eyes. Dietary restraint is also important and should involve natural foods with little or no alcohol, caffeine, nicotine and a low intake of fats.

Associated with the liver, anatomically, is the gall bladder. This is a small sac-like organ that stores and concentrates bile. When fats are digested, the gall bladder contracts, sending bile into the duodenum. Sometimes stones form here, and often gallstones can cause severe pain. The gall bladder reflex is found at the foot of the liver on the right palm and foot. On the body there is another reflex just below the ribs on the right-hand side, and below the liver reflex point. A steady pressure should be held around the point, beginning near the navel and working to the right side, maintaining pressure for a few seconds on any tender point.

The role of the spleen

The spleen is situated on the left side of the body behind and below the stomach. The spleen produces leucocytes (white blood cells), lymphocytes (white blood cells involved in the immune system), blood platelets (involved in blood coagulation) and plasma cells. It also acts as a store for red blood cells, which are made available in emergencies (when oxygen demand is greater).

The spleen reflex point

The reflex area for the spleen is found on the left palm or sole, below the reflex for the heart. If a tender point is found in this reflex, it may indicate anaemia and it would then be wise to obtain a blood test.

The kidneys and bladder

The role of the kidneys and bladder

The kidneys are important organs in the body's excretory system. They are responsible for processing the blood continuously to remove nitrogenous wastes (mainly urea) and they also adjust salt concentrations. By testing the reflexes with the thumb, tender areas can be located and worked upon. However, prolonged massage should be avoided—it is better to use shorter periods of 15-20 seconds initially as the system becomes accustomed to the treatment.

It is not surprising, considering the pivotal role of the kidneys in removing body wastes, that any interference with their normal function can lead to serious illnesses. General kidney disorders, kidney stones, nephritis and pyelitis are all best aided by massaging the kidney reflex but also the reflexes for the central nervous system, the endocrine glands (especially the pituitary and adrenal glands), liver, stomach and circulation. Kidney stones are formed by the deposition of solid substances that are naturally found in the urine but which precipitate out for one reason or another. They are commonly salts of calcium, and the alteration in pH of the urine is often a contributory factor. Nephritis is inflammation of the kidney and pyelitis is when part of the kidney, the renal pelvis, becomes inflamed. If the whole kidney becomes affected, it is then called pyelonephritis.

The kidney and bladder reflex points

Disorders associated with the bladder tend to be infections such as cystitis or other physical manifestation of a problem whether through stress or a medical condition. The latter category includes enuresis (bed-wetting) and incontinence. In these cases, the bladder reflex should obviously be worked upon, and the reflexes for the brain, solar plexus and endocrine system.

The reflexes for the kidneys are found just off centre on the palms of both hands and soles of both feet. They are close to the pancreas and stomach. The bladder reflex is towards the base of the palm, near the wrist and on the feet it is found on the inside edge of both soles, towards the heel. There are also body reflexes for both organs.

The body reflexes for the kidneys are at the side of the body, almost at the waistline, between the hip and rib cage. They also occur on the face, just beneath the eyes.

The alleviation of back pain and other skeletal disorders

The reflex points for the spine

Within the working population of most countries, back pain accounts for millions of days in lost production. This is not unexpected as the spine is the primary part of the skeleton, hence any problem with it will inevitably upset the body and its overall wellbeing.

On the soles of the feet, the reflex for the spine is located along the inner edge of both feet running from the base of the big toe almost to the heel. By working this line with the fingers, any tender points can be found and worked upon. The top end of the line, near the toe, is equivalent to the spine at the level of the shoulders.

Treatment of back disorders through reflexology

With back disorders, such as lumbago, additional reflexes should be worked including the brain and endocrine system. Because the body's musculature is a complementary and antagonistic system with the skeleton, creating all the movements of which the body is capable, the muscles are also important when dealing with back pain. It will help therefore to massage muscles, rubbing quite deeply with the fingers, and moving across the muscles.

Back pain can result from a problem elsewhere in the body with posture, tight muscles or even flat feet. It is important to be aware of the possibilities and ensure that the treatment deals with the problem as a whole, and not just in part. Exercise is clearly beneficial and walking can help loosen and strengthen muscles associated with the back. A brisk walk is fine, but jogging is not necessarily the best remedy, as in some cases this can itself prove harmful.

Reflexologists often turn to the muscles in the legs to alleviate back pain, particularly in the area of the lower back. The muscles at the back of the thigh should be massaged with a pressing and pulling action, first with one hand and then the other. The whole of the thigh should be treated, from the top of the leg, to the knee. Massage of both legs in this manner, concentrating on any 'tight' areas, will help improve the overall tone and assist in eliminating causes of back pain.

Study of the diagrams for the feet and hands reveals specific reflex areas for the shoulders, hip and neck. When working on skeletal disorders in general, it is wise to undertake a thorough massage of specific reflex areas such as neck and shoulders, plus those for the brain, solar plexus, the endocrine system, remainder of the skeletal system, endocrine glands, etc. For particular conditions such as bursitis (inflammation of a joint, as in housemaid's knee), general joint pain, stiff neck and similar complaints, a common regime of reflexological massage applies. This should include working the skeletal reflexes along with those for the nervous and endocrine system, digestive and circulatory systems. It is usually the case that the specific complaint will benefit from massage of its reflex area and most of those that comprise a whole body workout. It should always be remembered that there are occasions when surgery may prove essential, e.g. in the case of a hip replacement.

The knee joint can often be the source of pain and discomfort. It may help to apply gentle pressure on either side of the knee, just where the bone ends, using the thumb and middle finger. This should be held for a few seconds, pressing as much as possible (do not press hard if it is too painful) and then the same should be done below the knee.

Relief from arthritis with reflexology

Arthritis can be a crippling disease and many people suffer from it. It is an inflammation of joints or the spine, the symptoms of which are pain and swelling, restriction of movement, redness and warmth of the skin. Two forms of the condition are osteoarthritis and rheumatoid arthritis.

Treatment of osteoarthritis through reflexology

Osteoarthritis involves the cartilage in joints, which then affects the associated bone. What often happens is that the cartilage is lost, to be replaced by osteophytes at the edges of the bones. These are bony projections that occur with the loss of cartilage or with age. The projections affect the joint function, causing pain.

Treatment of rhematoid arthritis through reflexology

Rheumatoid arthritis is the second commonest joint disease after osteoarthritis. It usually affects the feet, ankles, wrists and fingers in which there is a swelling of the joint and inflammation of the synovial membrane (the membraneous envelope around the joint). Then follows erosion and loss of cartilage and loss of bone. At its worst, the condition can be disabling.

Massage of the reflex areas for the affected areas should be worked but, as mentioned previously, it is important to massage the reflexes for the whole body to achieve a complete and balanced approach. The endocrine system is one important system in this respect.

In seeking ways to treat rheumatoid arthritis, the medical profession isolated the glucocorticosteroid hormone, cortisone, from the adrenal glands of cattle. It was found that the use of cortisone had dramatic effects on the symptoms of rheumatoid arthritis. However, the relief was only temporary, and an additional disadvantage was the occurrence of associated side effects, which could be severe, e.g. damage to muscle, bone, stomach ulcers, bleeding and imbalances in the hormonal and nervous systems. The medical use of this compound is therefore very restricted, but it is produced naturally by the adrenal cortex. Being a natural secretion, there are no detrimental side effects. There is a reflex point in the lower back, between the first and second lumbar vertebrae, which can be pressed. Finding this point will be hit and miss initially, but upon locating it (roughly 5 cm up from the coccyx or tailbone), apply gentle pressure, gradually increasing, and hold it for a few seconds. This should be repeated several times. This is helpful for other conditions, in addition to rheumatoid arthritis, such as asthma and bursitis.

As with back disorders, muscle condition is also felt to be important in the treatment of arthritis. The muscles in the area affected by arthritis should be massaged by pressing in with the fingers, either on or near to the area. The massage should be across the muscles, with a deep motion, although it may initially produce discomfort or soreness. Many practitioners regard this as an important supplementary technique in administering reflexology.

Stress and tension

The relaxing effects of reflexology

One of the additional beneficial effects of reflexology when dealing with a particular reflex area or point is that the treatment is very relaxing. If most of the body reflexes are massaged, a feeling of wellbeing is generated, and tension is released. Stress control and relief can be accomplished in a number of ways, some of which happen instinctively, such as deep breathing and, paradoxically, wringing the hands. The latter is an obvious way of working the reflex points, albeit that it is mostly done unconsciously. A related method of calming the nerves is to intertwine the fingers, as in clasping the hands, which enables all the reflexes between the fingers to be pressed. This should be done several times. Deep breathing is a common method of relaxation that ultimately can envelop the whole body, providing that the focus of attention is the attainment of the correct pattern of breathing. Mental attitude is also an important aspect of reflexology. It clearly makes sense, while undergoing massage (with or without a practitioner or partner) to imagine, or listen to, pleasing sounds, rather than worrying about the pressures of modern life. If there is no access to relaxing sounds (bird song, running water, etc) it is perfectly possible to imagine it, and thereby to augment the physical relaxation with mental calm.

Reflex points for treating stress

The *endocrine glands* are considered important in combating stress because they are responsible for the hormonal balance of the body. All reflex areas for these glands, on both soles and palms, should be massaged and special attention given to the thyroid, which controls body temperature and can help restore calm. The adrenal reflex point, almost in the centre of the hand, is also important, and, because it is so near the solar plexus, receives equal attention. (The solar plexus is a network of nerves and ganglia in the sympathetic nervous system concerned with body functions not under conscious control. It is located behind the stomach.)

Quite often stress and tension can result in a sore neck or back. A number of reflex points can be worked to relieve these sorts of complaint. The medulla oblongata is important in this respect as it controls some major body functions such as the circulation. The point on the back of the head (*see* the figure on page 58) should be held with the middle finger for a few seconds and then released, and repeated several times. The reflex points of the spine should also be worked starting at the neck reflex, which is found below the base of the big toe or thumb. By moving down the side of the foot, the whole spine can be covered. To relieve a sore back completely and effectively, other reflexes to be attended to should include the shoulders, hips, and the sciatic nerve. The sciatic nerve is made up of a number of nerve roots from the lower part of the spinal cord, and pain with this origin may be felt in the back of the thigh, buttock and the foot. The reflex point may at first be painful to the touch, but through careful massage it can be worked to assist in promoting relief.

Control of the heart rate is a natural, complementary procedure in promoting stress relief. If a situation, wherever it may be, results in you feeling stressed, massaging the reflex areas for the heart will help, whether on foot or hand.

Sound, restful sleep is refreshing and also contributes to a reduction in stress. Reflexology can also help in this respect through the feeling of relaxation that it induces. The clasping of the hands, mentioned earlier, can be used to combat sleeplessness. The fingers can be clasped on the chest and then worked over each other so that the length of each finger is massaged. The fingers should remain intertwined and simply be released a little to allow each finger over the first knuckle, when the fingers are squeezed together again. This, associated with deep breathing will encourage relaxation.

Reflexology and the reproductive system

Reflex points for the reproductive system

The major reflexes of the reproductive system are those for the uterus, ovary and breast in the female, and the penis, testes and prostate in the male. The ovary reflexes are found on the outer side of the foot, just below the ankle (*see* figures on page 57). On the hand, these are found a little way beyond the wrist (*see* figures on page 57), on the outer edge. On both foot and hand, the breast reflex is found on the outer edge, a little below the base of the little toe or finger. The uterus reflex on the hand occupies a position opposite to the ovaries, i.e. just below the wrist, but on the inner edge of the arm. On the foot, this reflex mirrors that for the ovary, but it is on the inside of the foot, below the ankle.

The male reflexes

The male reflexes occupy the same positions as those of the female, thus the penis reflex is in the same position as that for the uterus and the testes is the same as the ovaries. The prostate gland reflexes are situated with the penis reflex and also at the back of the leg/foot, above the heel, (*see* the figures on page 57).

There are also reflex points on the head for the gonads (*see* sex glands on the diagram of the reflex points on the head on page 58). As well as working the various reflexes for the reproductive system, it is beneficial to pay attention to the endocrine gland reflexes as they have considerable control over the gonads (*see* endocrine glands, page 65). In particular, the pituitary, thyroid and adrenal glands and their hormonal secretions have a large influence on the reproductive system. All these points should be massaged to stimulate activity and ensure that hormone secretion is balanced and gonad activity is normal. The body reflexes can also be used to this end by pressing each point for a few seconds and repeating several times for all endocrine and sex glands.

If any of the endocrine glands are tender, it may be indicating a problem with the sex glands. By working the various reflex points, it is possible to ensure a healthy reproductive system. There are a number of reflexes to the penis and testes that can help in this respect. The sex reflex below the navel should be pressed with fingers or thumb and massaged for a few seconds. Additional reflex points on the legs, about 15 cm above the ankle on the inside of the leg, should also be massaged. Initially, massage here should be for half a minute or so, because any problems will make it tender. However, with further attention it will be possible to work out the soreness. A further point on the leg lies above the knee, in the soft area on the outer edge, above the kneecap. All these reflexes, if worked in turn, will contribute to a healthy system and lead to fewer problems, such as impotence.

Impotence itself can, however, be treated. In addition to undertaking the massage of reflex points and areas mentioned above, there are further techniques that may help. There is a particularly sensitive and stimulating area between the anus and scrotum, which should be pressed gently a number of times. It is also said that if gentle on-off pressure is applied to the scrotum, this will help.

Another problem faced by many men involves the prostate gland. This gland is situated below the bladder and opens into the urethra, which is the duct carrying urine out of the body and which also forms the ejaculatory duct. On ejaculation, the gland secretes an alkaline fluid into the sperm to help sperm motility. In older men particularly, the prostate gland may have become enlarged, causing problems with urination. Working the appropriate reflexes may help this situation as may massaging the base of the penis. However, it is advisable to check with a medical doctor to ensure that there is no other condition present.

The female reflexes

There are a number of female conditions that may be helped by reflexology. In most cases, the reflexes to be worked are very similar and the following complaints are therefore grouped in this way:
- *amenorrhoea* lack of menstruation, other than during pregnancy or pre-puberty
- *endometriosis* the occurrence of endometrial cells, normally found in the womb, elsewhere in the body, e.g. Fallopian tubes or peritoneum, causing pain and bleeding
- *fibroid* a benign tumour of the uterus that may cause pain, bleeding and urine retention
- *leucorrhoea* discharge of white/yellow mucus from the vagina, which may be normal before and after menstruation, but at other times large amounts signify an infection
- *dysmenorrhoea* painful menstruation
- *menorrhagia* excessive blood flow during menstruation

For these and related conditions, the general procedure should be to spend time on the specific female reflex, which in these cases is the uterus. In addition the endocrine gland reflexes should be massaged and to provide a balanced treatment, the reflexes for the other reproductive organs (ovary, etc) should be worked. Further areas to concentrate upon include the urinary and circulatory systems and the central nervous system (brain) with the solar plexus.

Premenstrual tension (or syndrome) is the condition typified by headache, nervousness, irritability, depression and tiredness (in addition to physical symptoms) several days before the start of menstruation. It is advisable, before menstruation starts, to have a thorough massage of the reflexes once or twice per week. Next, the reflexes for the uterus and ovaries should be worked. The uterus reflex is on the inside of the foot in the soft area beneath the ankle. The massage should work all around the ankle, beginning with a gentle pressure, and then working back towards the heel. The other foot should then be dealt with in the same way.

To help overcome depression the endocrine glands are very important to regulate hormones, maintain body rhythms and balance the biochemical functions—all of which have some effect on emotions. Other reflexes to work, in addition to the endocrine glands, include the solar plexus, brain and liver. The liver is very important in this respect and, although the area should not be over-worked, it should not be forgotten.

The *menopause* is the time when a woman's ovaries no longer release an egg cell every month, and child-bearing is no longer possible. This usually occurs between the ages of 45 and 55. It may be preceded by a gradual decline in the frequency of menstruation or there may be an abrupt cessation. There is an imbalance in the sex hormones and this can cause a number of symptoms, including hot flushes, sweats, palpitations, depression and vaginal dryness. Over a longer period there may be a gradual loss of bone (osteoporosis) leading to a greater risk of bone fractures.

In this instance, the endocrine reflexes are once again very important. In conjunction with these, the reflexes for the spine and brain should be worked, the former to promote relaxation. As a general point, the reflexes to the spine can be massaged for any length of time whereas those for organs and glands should be worked periodically and for a few seconds each time.

To help combat hot flushes, the thyroid reflex should be worked since this is the endocrine gland responsible for the control of the metabolic rate. Regulation of breathing through deep breaths will also help.

The breasts are, of course, the mammary glands that produce milk at the appropriate time, but in today's society they have also become important from a cosmetic point of view. Disorders of the breasts can include lumps or cysts, pain or tenderness. Such conditions may be due to an hormonal imbalance but in any event will benefit from a complete treatment of all the reflexes on feet, hands or head. The breast reflex is found on the top of the foot or hand, at the base of the toes or fingers, and this should be worked regularly. Since the endocrine system is of great significance in the reproductive system, all glands reflexes should receive some attention. Reflexological massage can also be used as a general technique to maintain healthy breasts. Essentially the hand should form a cup around the breast with the fingers underneath and the nipple between thumb and forefinger. Using a circular movement the breast is massaged slightly upwards. This should help retain the shape of the breast, and maintain its tone.

Diseases of the immune system

Antibodies and the lymphatic system

The human body resists infection by means of antibodies and white blood cells.

Antibodies are protein substances produced by the lymphoid tissue (spleen, thymus gland and the lymph nodes) that circulate in the blood. They react with their corresponding antigens (foreign bodies that cause antibodies to be formed) and make them harmless. There are a number of immunoglobulins (large protein molecules) that act as antibodies, and each has a particular function. For example, one is responsible for allergic reactions and another is produced to fight bacteria and viruses in the body.

The lymphatic system is also important in the body's immune response. Lymph nodes are swellings that occur at various points in the system. They are found in the neck, groin and armpit, and their main function is to remove foreign particles from the lymph, and to participate in the immune response. In this latter function they become enlarged and produce lymphocytes, a type of white blood cell, which locate and neutralize antigens, or produce antibodies, depending upon their type.

The lymph itself is a colourless, watery fluid. It is derived from blood and is similar to plasma. It contains 95 per cent water, with protein, sugar, salt and lymphocytes. The lymph is circulated by muscular action, and pumped through the lymph nodes for filtering.

It is clear that the lymphatic system, and the immune system overall, are very important in maintaining good health. Any disorder or deficiency in this system will lead to illness, which in some cases may be life-threatening. Reflexology may prove useful in restoring the balance although the need for professional medical advice should always be borne in mind.

Reflex points for the immune system

A number of reflexes to the lymph glands can be worked, on the back of the hands, located over the wrists (*see* the figures on page 57) and on the top of the foot. The spleen is also an important reflex because the spleen itself produces lymphocytes (amongst other things). Associated reflexes that should be worked are those for the endocrine glands, circulation and liver.

In the case of infectious diseases, many of which occur in childhood (such as measles, mumps and chickenpox), the infection will normally run its course and as a result confer immunity to further bouts. To minimize discomfort and aid the recovery, the reflexes for the brain, solar plexus, circulation, endocrine glands and liver should be massaged.

The same applies to most infectious conditions, even autoimmune diseases where the antibodies attack their own body cells. In these cases, the lymph gland reflexes are particularly important.

Reiki

Introduction

A complementary therapy

Reiki is a complementary therapy and one of the many facets of alternative medicine available today. It is a method of natural healing which is centred upon *universal life energy*, the meaning of the Japanese word *reiki*. The therapy was named after Dr Mikao Usui, a Japanese theologist, who rediscovered the art of healing by transferring this universal life energy. Following a prolonged period of meditation, Dr Usui acquired the ability of transferring reiki energy. He was also able to help others to act as channels for this energy.

To benefit fully from the technique, it is preferable to be initiated into the reiki energy. This is done by a reiki master. A number of reiki grand masters brought the practice to the West to allow many people to prepare themselves for self-discovery. Reiki is now used to heal, either the practitioner or others, in meditation and in conjunction with other therapies such as aromatherapy.

In many cases traditional reiki, as generated by Dr Usui, forms the basis of reiki-do, an amplification of the technique which essentially translates into using reiki as a way of life. This aspect of reiki will be discussed more fully in due course.

Reiki energy

Reiki energy is regarded as life energy at its most effective—with the maximum vibration. It is considered to have an almost divine quality and as such includes everything, in a world where problems and disorders are deemed to be due to the feeling of detachment from the world. There is no division of reiki energy into positive and negative forms but when a person undergoes a session of therapy, they allow the energy to be taken into themselves with beneficial effects. Essentially, those receiving reiki energy decide subconsciously just how much of the life energy is taken in.

Those who use reiki regularly often find they are more joyful, lively and their own inbuilt energy is enhanced—almost as if their batteries had been fully charged! Existing conflicts within the person are broken down and there is a greater vitality, leading to relaxation and a stimulation of the body. As this improvement develops, the natural processes of renewal and removal of toxins are enhanced and rendered more effective, ultimately opening up more of the body to the life energy.

Body organs such as the skin, and protective systems such as the immune system are improved providing the individual is prepared regularly to undertake reiki and in the first place to undergo an attunement or initiation into reiki energy. The initiation is merely a means whereby the universal life energy is bestowed through the reiki master. The master acts as a channel and a link with God to release the healing power.

An initiation is not absolutely essential but it allows the individual access to the universal life energy, which is used rather than their own life energy. Also, an initiation conveys a greater capacity for using reiki energy, with no associated tiredness and further, it provides a protective mechanism against any negative manifestations.

The treatment

Effects and limitations

There are several inter-related effects that result from taking in reiki energy:
- it enables the universal life energy to be received;
- it creates a feeling of deep relaxation;
- energy blockages are removed allowing a flow of life energy throughout the body;
- toxins of various sorts are removed; these and other waste products are removed from the system much more quickly.

When the toxins have been removed from the body, more energy can be received and the vital processes and functions become more highly tuned. When the body takes in more and more life energy, it is said that its frequency becomes higher, facilitating contact with the Universal Spirit and generating trust in the universal life energy.

Deep relaxation is central to reiki therapy and this is very much dependent upon the divine quality attributed to the energy. The extent to which reiki can work is defined by the receiver of the energy because only the necessary amount of energy is drawn in. A refusal to accept reiki, whether or not it is made consciously, will result in no energy flowing. This is, in a way, one limitation of reiki, albeit self-imposed. It should also be appreciated that attitude is very important and if someone attempts to use reiki in the wrong way, it will not work. Self-discovery must go hand in hand with everyday experience of real life and it is not possible to hide from the troubles of the real world through misplaced introspection

A qualified therapist in the appropriate discipline must be sought to deal with major problems and difficulties. Of course, adopting reiki in tandem with another therapy will be very beneficial as the reiki will maximise the treatment being received. This applies whether the therapist is a homoeopath, naturopath or medic.

The use of whole-body reiki

Because no one part of the body exists independently, and because a disease or disorder in one area will inevitably affect the whole body, the use of reiki is best applied in a whole-body way, to cleanse and revitalise the complete system.

Many practitioners undertake a particular routine before commencing a regime of whole-body treatment and the main elements are briefly described below.

Preparing for whole-body reiki

It is a good idea to prepare thoroughly for reiki treatment to capitalise fully upon the beneficial effects. The following is a possible routine:

Remove jewellery

Most people wear jewellery of some description, whether stones of a semi-precious or precious nature, metal rings or chains, leather thongs or one of a whole variety of objects. Some metals and stones are believed to attract energies which may interfere with the life energy of reiki. Other items such as watches create a closed circuit which reduces the flow of life energy. In a way, items of jewellery can be seen as objects which create interference in the 'signal' in much the same way that an engine or motor can generate annoying interference in the reception of a radio programme. Earrings can also be a problem because in the case of pierced ears the earrings conflict with the flow of energy—the ear is very important in other therapies such as acupuncture and must therefore be kept unencumbered.

Wash hands

The benefits of washing your hands are twofold. Firstly, there is the physical effect of cleaning which has the additional quality of making the hands pleasant to feel for the recipient of reiki. It is essential that hot, sticky hands are not used in reiki as this would hardly be conducive to the state of relaxation being sought.

The second benefit relates to the aura surrounding the body. This aura may be affected by contact with objects, people, etc over the course of the day and washing removes such influences which could, in sensitive people, have an adverse effect.

Say a prayer

It is helpful at this stage to recite a short prayer asking for healing and to concentrate upon and acknowledge your aims, self-perception and those of the person upon whom your hands will be placed.

Even out the aura

This is a means of gently making contact and starting the therapy, and may be carried out as follows:
• your partner/client/friend should lie down (*see* figure below)
• sitting at their side put your left hand on your sacrum
• with your right hand held about 15–25 cm (6–9 inches) above the body and palm facing down, move your hand along the length of the body from the head to the toes

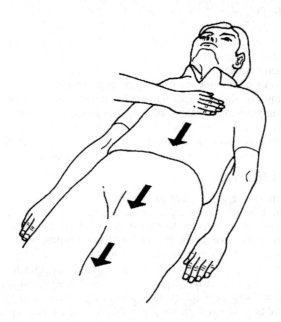

Starting the therapy: the patient lies down

- return the hand to the starting point using a circular motion along the side of the body
- repeat this three or four times

This process can be repeated after the reiki therapy when your left hand can be placed on the sacrum of your partner/client/friend.

Energise

When each reiki therapy session is complete the whole body may be energised via the root chakra (*see* later for chakras). The hand is held vertically above the body and then quickly moved from the pelvis to the head.

These preparatory rituals should only be performed when they are perceived to have some significance. There is little point going through the procedures if you do not see the reason why, but clearly some aspects of the procedure can be understood easily and will be accepted readily by the recipient.

The practicalities of whole-body reiki

Before the treatment

There is great scope for variation in the number and sequence of positions used for whole-body treatment. It will depend greatly upon the practitioner and what is felt to be best for the recipient, but no one sequence can be deemed the best one for all. It is important to be certain that your client/partner is not suffering from any illness or condition that might require the attention of another health professional. Reiki has its particular uses but it is unwise to try to address problems that clearly fall beyond its scope. The client can easily ask advice from their doctor, or other professional, as to whether they should undergo reiki therapy.

When it is clear that therapy can go ahead the next commitment to be made is that of time. It is essential that both parties agree to pledge the time to make the most of the reiki therapy. It is likely that the practitioner will, in acting as a channel for the universal life energy, see their own status develop.

The extent of each session of reiki will vary depending upon circumstances and the individual receiving treatment. Certain positions may be better left out of the sequence or therapy may be focused on a particular area to help relieve blockages or deal with tension. If the recipient is currently on a regime of medication then a shorter session may be appropriate.

Similarly, if dealing with a small child or an elderly or infirm person, it is probably wise to limit the therapy to a session of 15 to 20 minutes. In all cases the reiki practitioner should be sensitive to and aware of the condition, needs and well-being of the recipient.

Positions in reiki therapy

The hands are clearly the 'instruments' of healing in reiki and although the position in which they are placed on the recipient is meaningful, it may not be possible, nor is it essential that the exact position is copied. Just placing the hands on the appropriate part of the body will suffice.

Reiki can be effected through clothing, as the energy will flow just as well, but many people prefer to have no material obstacles to the therapy. In this case, and particularly for partners, the reiki can be undertaken in the nude. If there are any physical blemishes such as a burn or other wound, the hands should be held a few inches above the skin at this area, around the corresponding acupuncture point, or reflex zone.

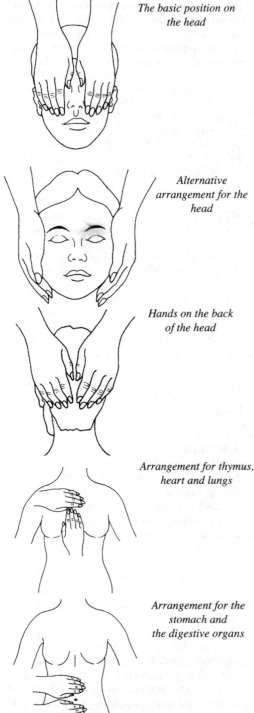

The basic position on the head

Alternative arrangement for the head

Hands on the back of the head

Arrangement for thymus, heart and lungs

Arrangement for the stomach and the digestive organs

The head

On the head, the basic position is shown in the figure below. The hands are placed either side of the nose, with the palms covering the eyes; the thumbs rest by the bridge of the nose and the fingertips cover the cheeks and reach the upper lip. This arrangement covers the sinuses, eyes, pituitary gland, teeth and is useful for dealing with colds, sinusitis, eye complaints, allergies, fatigue and general discontent.

In the second arrangement for the head, the hands are placed over the ears, with the fingertips extending down the jawline to the neck, encompassing the ears of course which includes the semi-circular canals, responsible for balance. The effect also extends to the pharyngeal area. Diseases and problems of these organs — colds, trouble with balance, hearing loss, etc — are dealt with in this arrangement.

If the hands are placed on the back of the head, this helps with conditions such as headaches, colds, asthma and circulatory problems. It generally promotes relaxation.

The chest and abdomen

The next sequence of hand arrangements is for the chest and abdomen. Once again there are many variations, but a selection is presented here.

The arrangement for the thymus, heart and lungs is as follows: one hand is laid across the thymus and the other is at 90° starting just below and between the breasts. The thymus is a bilobed gland in the neck which is an important part of the immune system. This arrangement therefore reinforces the immune system and helps the lymphatics, the heart, lungs and counters any general debility.

The next illustration in the sequence shows the hands placed either side of the navel and slightly to one side. The stomach and digestive organs are the focus of attention here and the conditions/symptoms addressed necessarily have a link with these body systems. As such this will help digestion and the metabolism in general terms, and specifically will combat nausea, heartburn, gastro-intestinal diseases and indigestion. Because the presence of such conditions often results in tension and worry, the relief of symptoms will similarly help relieve anxiety and depression.

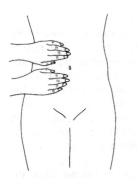

Focus on the gall bladder and liver

Next are two positions in which the hands are placed in a position similar to that shown in the arrangement used to focus on the stomach and digestive organs but further away from the body midline. One version is to approach the body from the right side of the partner/client. The left hand is placed around the base of the ribcage and in this way the gall bladder and liver are the organs to be dealt with. This position is for diseases and conditions of these important organs and associated problems of a metabolic nature. The liver is a vital organ in the process of removing toxins from the body and this arrangement can therefore be very important.

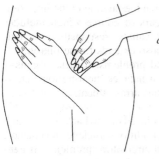

Focus on the appendix, intestines and urogenital organs

The position related to this one is essentially a reflection, where the hands are placed on the left side of the body to encompass the area of the bowels, spleen and some of the pancreas. Accordingly diseases of these organs, indigestion and healthy blood are all dealt with.

The position of the hands where the pelvic bones are covered and meet over the pubic area is for a number of ailments, many associated with the appendix, intestines and urinogenital organs. In addition, this arrangement is considered suitable for allergies, general debility, problems of a sexual nature and related to weight and is appropriate to reinforce the immune system.

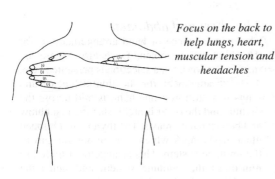

Focus on the back to help lungs, heart, muscular tension and headaches

The back

There are a number of arrangements which can be adopted on the back and lower back. The figure shows one such position with a number of effects but it is likely that by gently experimenting, a slightly different yet equally beneficial arrangement can be found. Here the hands are placed across the shoulder blades at mid to upper point, to influence the intestines, lung, heart and various muscles in the neck and shoulder region. This will help lung and heart diseases, muscular tension, headaches and related conditions.

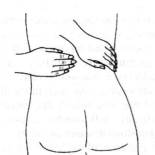

Focus on the lower back to help kidneys and adrenal glands

If the hands are placed lower down the back, around the midriff (on the lower ribs) this position will accommodate the kidneys and adrenal glands. (The adrenal glands are situated one each on the upper surface of each kidney and are important because they manufacture hormones that control a variety of body functions, e.g. adrenaline is one hormone produced).

In addition to these specific positions, there are many other reiki positions to deal with a multitude of complaints and the reader is referred to a more extensive account for greater detail. It must always be remembered that serious conditions or diseases of a particular nature should be dealt with by the appropriate specialist.

The benefits of whole-body reiki

A reinforcing effect

It is believed with reiki, as with many similar forms of therapy, that the body cannot be treated in separate parts or as discrete organs that have little or nothing to do with other parts of the body. There are many conditions and diseases that affect the well-being of the individual as a whole or have a knock-on effect even though the symptoms may be less tangible, such as anxiety or depression.

It is thus important that reiki is used not just to counteract a particular symptom, but to treat the whole body to achieve the relaxation mentioned earlier and with it the removal of blockages in energy flow and the dispersal of toxins.

Long-term whole-body reiki should be adopted in all cases, and in a therapy session of 60 to 90 minutes all parts of the body will be addressed and receive reiki energy. Over a period of time, the general condition of the body is restored and the energy channels are opened to allow the body to deal properly and naturally with both stress and the build-up of toxins.

In cases of recovery from illness, reiki therapy provides the additional energy to bolster recovery and will reinforce the effects of any other method of natural healing. It can be used as a supplementary therapy almost as a general, ongoing policy as it is a truly complementary system of treatment.

Reduction of side-effects

It is well-known that the use of drugs to combat say, an infection may at first seem very effective. However, it is becoming all too obvious that the excessive use of drugs is causing its own problems. In the case of many drugs, uncomfortable, distressing and even threatening side-effects can ensue. With antibiotics, there is now the problem of drug resistance in bacteria, leading to situations where hospital patients are vulnerable to infections from so-called superbugs or killer bugs. This has resulted specifically from the overuse of antibiotics and has reached the point where hospitals now have only one or two very powerful drugs to use in these circumstances.

Reiki therapy can be a very useful adjunct for anyone taking a course of drugs. It can help reduce some side effects and generally aid the body in recovery when the course has been completed. Post-operative recovery will benefit from reiki and it can also help after chemotherapy. In all these cases reiki therapy supplies that extra life energy, enabling the body to bounce back more quickly from the burdens of surgery and chemicals.

In some cases, use of reiki therapy after an operation will lessen pain and the natural healing processes will be accelerated. The key in all these examples is that the reiki therapy must be undertaken on a regular basis. The added benefit of this is that when a person is enjoying good health, the regular therapy increases the body's inbuilt defences which manifests itself as a confidence and outward harmony in dealing with everyday events. It also bestows a greater ability to deal with stressful situations. This very positive outlook can become possible because once the blockages and toxins have been removed from the system, the scope for personal advancement and growth becomes available. In general, the better metabolic functioning afforded by reiki therapy means that benefits and improvements may be experienced in many ways.

Reiki associations

It has already been mentioned that reiki therapy can be undertaken in conjunction with other methods of natural healing. In addition, it can be combined with activities such as meditation and crystal therapy. The following sections consider briefly a few of these combinations which for the present purpose have been called associations.

Reiki and the use of crystals

Crystal therapy is known to many people and involves the use of precious and semi-precious stones. The stones are thought to hold positive energy and they act as a conduit for healing from the practitioner to the recipient. It is also said that the stones generate a healing vibration that acts upon the body. In some cases the stone is placed on the body where treatment is focused, in others it may be positioned on the appropriate acupuncture point. Most therapists use quartz for physical healing, amethyst for spiritual healing and rose quartz to heal emotions. Fluorite may also be used to develop awareness and knowledge of a spiritual nature.

In reiki, three varieties of quartz are commonly used—amethyst, rose quartz and ordinary quartz (or rock crystal). The crystal structure of quartz is often taken to be related to the six chakras and the tip of the crystal to the seventh chakra. Practitioners recommend using rock crystal to avoid feeling overpowered by changes, mounting pressures and the stress of everyday life. Carrying the crystal or wearing it is meant to bring light into your workaday routines.

Rock crystal can also be used in conjunction with reiki meditation (of which see later), being held between, or in, the hands. In this way the energy emanating from the crystal is thought to go into the palms and then the rest of the body via the reflex zones. It is recommended by some in a variety of applications such as relaxation, wound-healing with other therapy and treating particular organs.

Rose quartz, with its soft pink colouration, is used for mending emotional problems. This may be dealing with problematic emotions, such as shutting out certain desires or it may be facing trauma and stress brought about by a separation.

The use of amethyst with reiki is varied. It can help promote the proper function of an organ that has been under treatment; placed on the Third Eye (centre of the forehead) it facilitates clearer vision in one's path through life; and it can reduce tension and fear.

Meditation with reiki

Meditation in its own right is a useful therapy. It needs concentration and time and a will to continue with the practice. Some of the benefits may happen straight away (such as a lowering of the blood pressure) while others require some proficiency. It has been reported that it helps with insomnia, and a high blood pressure can be lowered significantly, enough to allow the dependence on drugs to be reduced. Meditation is undertaken in a quiet room and it must be at least half an hour after consuming food or drink. Sitting comfortably, the mind is then concentrated upon excluding the hustle and bustle, problems, tension and overstimulating thoughts of modern life.

Reiki assists in this concentration, with the flow of energy aiding relaxation. There are some positions that can be adopted in reiki meditation to achieve particular goals. In the first position the legs are drawn up and the soles of the feet put together with the knees falling apart. This can be done while lying down or sitting against a wall or chair. The hands adopt a praying gesture. This is meant to complete the circuit of energy, allowing a flow around the body. The reiki energy removes any blockages and performed regularly, this becomes a power-ful meditation exercise. It can be done for short periods initially, just a couple of minutes, and then built up in small increases.

To achieve complete harmony with your partner, there is a meditation exer-cise which can be done together. Sitting facing each other, the legs are spread, with the knees raised slightly. Moving closer, the legs of one are put over the legs of the partner and palms are put together. This allows a joint circuit of en-ergy which strengthens the harmonious and loving relationship between two people. Done properly, this meditation may take up to half an hour.

Group meditation is also possible with reiki, in which the participants stand in a circle with hands joined.

Aromatherapy blended with reiki

Aromatherapy is covered in greater detail elsewhere in this volume (*see* page 295). It is essentially a healing method that employs essential oils extracted from plants, usually in a neutral oil base (carrier oil). The oils can be used in three ways: by direct application, bathing in water to which a few drops of the appropriate oil have been added, and inhalation.

When used in conjunction with reiki, some oils can be applied directly on particular areas of the body, or their aroma can be made to fill the room using an aroma lamp. Below a few oils are considered and their use compared to their therapeutic value in aromatherapy. It is very likely that someone with a knowl-edge of essential oils will be able to capitalize upon their experience and incor-porate further oils in their reiki therapy.

• *Lavender*—in aromatherapy lavender is a tonic with relaxing effects. It is also antiseptic, antispasmodic and stimulates the appetite. It is a widely-used and versatile oil that is used for minor burns and wounds. Its soothing effects render it helpful for headaches, tension and similar conditions.

In reiki, lavender is associated primarily with patients/recipients who are sensitive and easily hurt, essentially introverts. It can be used in long sessions of reiki when the lavender helps to promote the calm and confidence neces-sary for a period of building and strengthening of the life force energy.

• *Sandalwood*—this oil is used in aromatherapy for its relaxing and antiseptic effects. It forms a very effective oil for application to the skin (especially facial), particularly for dry or sensitive skin.

The use of sandalwood in reiki therapy is quite different. Its benefit seems to be in producing an ambience conducive to the reiki therapy itself because the oil is considered to elicit trust and confidence, between practitioner and recipient.

• *Clary sage*—this is a very useful oil with a number of qualities including tonic, antispasmodic, antidepressant, anti-inflammatory, bactericidal and more. It is also used to treat colds, menstrual problems and its very low toxicity renders it suitable for general use.

In a session of reiki therapy, clary sage has been used to open blocked channels and to enhance sensitivity.

• *Patchouli*—apart from being accredited with some aphrodisiac qualities, patchouli is more commonly used in aromatherapy to treat skin disorders and minor burns because of its anti-inflammatory and antiseptic qualities.

While patchouli is also used in reiki therapy for allergies and impurities of the skin, the fundamental use and aim is to enhance the sensual qualities and aspects of life.

Other reiki associations

Because reiki is very much a positive therapy and benign, it can be undertaken in conjunction with other therapies with no harm. However, there are some beneficial effects of reiki which may affect in some way the activity of other courses of treatment.

- *Prescription drugs*—many reiki therapists believe that reiki can readily affect the way in which such drugs work in the body. It has already been mentioned that side effects of drugs can be lessened through the use of reiki, and in some cases it is reported that the process will be accelerated. In addition, reiki makes the body more receptive and therefore therapy prior to a course of drugs may enhance the effect of the drug. The relaxed state engendered by reiki may also counter, to some extent, the efficacy of an anaesthetic. However, injections such as anaesthetics can more readily and easily be released from the body with the help of reiki.

  Although minor pains can often be remedied through the use of reiki alone, stronger pain killers do not have their effect lessened by reiki. The interaction between reiki and drugs is neither well tested nor documented, but the overall positive effect of the therapy means that it is not likely to cause any problems.

- *Homoeopathy*—in conjunction with this therapy, reiki provides a reinforcing effect by rendering the treatment more effective. Reiki can help avoid strain, improve the removal of toxins and increase the body's sensitivity. After treatment, whole-body reiki will help recovery. *See* page 402 for a full discussion of homoeopathy.

- *Bach remedies*—these are named after Edward Bach, an English doctor, who in the early years of this century gave up his Harley Street practice to concentrate upon finding plants with healing qualities. He identified 38 plants, the flowers of which he floated on clear spring water. This, he believed, transferred medicinal properties to the water which could be given to patients. This practice he developed to mimic the drops of dew on the plant which in the first instance were used. Intended for home self-help, the remedies are meant for treating the whole person. Stock solutions are diluted in water and a few drops taken.

  Typical examples are:

  > *cherry plum* for fear, tension, irrationality
  > *holly* for envy, jealousy and hatred
  > *pine* for guilt and constantly apologizing
  > *sweet chestnut* for despair
  > *wild rose* for apathy

  In common with many other examples, reiki improves the effectiveness of Bach remedies.

Determining the need

Introduction

When undertaking reiki therapy it is often necessary to determine the need for therapy in the client or partner. As therapists work with reiki for longer, they become more sensitive and proficient and are better able to judge problem areas on what is called the subtle plane (the etheric body). Expertise comes only with experience, but it seems that there are certain reactions or feelings detected which may be indicative. Before trying to perceive a person's need, some practitioners 'sensitise' their hands. This involves holding the palms facing, about 40 to 50 cm apart and slowly bringing them together. The movement should be spread out over four or five minutes to allow an attunement and for changes to be perceived.

The following are some possible responses that may be experienced:

- *Attraction*—implies that reiki energy is needed at that point.

- *Repulsion*—suggests a long-established blockage is present which is restricting the flow of energy. This may require a considerable period of therapy to rectify.
- *Flow*—a positive feeling representing the flow of life energy which will be enhanced by further reiki energy, raising the entire system.
- *Heat*—if your hands feel warmer, it signifies a need for life energy. If the whole body produces such a result, reiki energy can be applied anywhere.
- *Cold*—this is probaby due to a blockage in energy flow such that an area of the body has been deprived of energy. Such blockages may also require considerable attention and both whole-body and specific treatment will probably be required.
- *Tingling*—an inflamed area will usually produce a tingling in the hands of the therapist. The strength of the stimulus reflects the severity of the problem and additional help from a medical practitioner may be identified as being necessary.
- *Pain*—this usually represents a build-up of energy in some form. A sharp pain reflects that the energy is beginning to dissipate and in so doing is causing some conflict elsewhere in the system. In this case, whole-body therapy is beneficial before concentrating upon a particular area.

There are other methods to determine need and identify disruptions in the flow of life energy, but these are, in the main, for the more experienced practitioner. However, details can be found in a variety of publications and involve pendulum dowsing, activity of the chakras and the use of systems such as tarot or I Ching. These latter two, however, are not for novices.

When the need is answered

If reiki is practised regularly, it can have a very positive effect and influence. One of the major problems with modern life is the very pace of life itself— every day seems to be hectic, full of demands and pressure which result in stress, discomfort and ragged emotions.

These emotional ups and downs and stressful pressures are smoothed out by reiki. A more balanced approach to life is developed; a greater inner harmony is achieved which means that the quality of life improves and any illnesses or condition become less of a problem, responds more readily to treatment, or is cleared up seemingly of its own accord. The flow of energy from reiki ensures that there is harmony between the Third Eye (which identifies the ideal path for the individual) and the root chakra (or energy centre). (For an explanation of the chakras *see* below).

Introduction to the significance of chakras with reiki

Chakras are a common concept in several disciplines of alternative medicine or traditional Asian medicine. A chakra is a centre of energy, subtle energy in reiki, which has several functions. In addition to being 'representative' of a particular organ or group of organs, a chakra also controls our being on different levels and it links these two representative states.

The chakras

In reiki there is considered to be seven major and a number of minor chakras. The seven major chakras are shown in the figure on page 87. These are from the lowest to the highest: the root chakra, the sexual chakra, the personality chakra, the heart chakra, the expressive chakra, the knowledge chakra, the crown chakra.

The number of major chakras does vary in some instances, e.g. Hindu yoga has six centres, but the greatest variation is in the minor chakras. In some re-

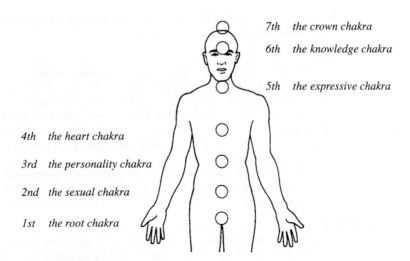

7th   *the crown chakra*

6th   *the knowledge chakra*

5th   *the expressive chakra*

4th   *the heart chakra*

3rd   *the personality chakra*

2nd   *the sexual chakra*

1st   *the root chakra*

gimes of therapy ten minor chakras are identified, and these are interconnected with the major chakras. A typical system could be:
- one in the arch of each foot, connected to the first and third chakras
- one in each knee joint, connected to the fifth and sixth chakras
- one in each palm, connected to the second, third and fourth chakras
- one in each elbow, connected to the second and third chakras
- one below each shoulder, connected to the third and fifth chakras

Brief summaries of the major chakras are given below, followed by an indication of how the chakras interact with reiki.

The root chakra

This is the source of strength and is essential for proper development. The other centres of energy rely upon the root chakra to perform properly. Disorders within the root chakras may result in mental problems (e.g. aggression, confusion) or physical symptoms (e.g. of the intestines, excretory systems, or bones).

The sexual chakra

This is highly influential and governs sensual and sexual factors, the means whereby experiences are felt and registered. Blockages result in a variety of phobias or conditions such as a fear of being touched, a general incomprehension or an obsessive cleanliness. Physical manifestations may include being prone to infections, or problems with the kidneys/bladder or lymphatic system.

The personality chakra

This is also called the solar plexus chakra, this is the power centre and focus of personal freedom or, conversely, feelings of guilt. Mental consequences of a blockage might be anxiety about how others perceive you, envy or selfish greed. Physically there could be digestive disorders, liver and gall bladder problems or disorders of the pancreas.

The heart chakra

This effectively controls self-acceptance and by extension everyone else around us. Blockages may result in attitudes such as selfishness or emotional blackmail. Physical manifestations could be disorders of the lungs and heart, and circulatory problems.

The expressive chakra

The expressive chakra (or throat chakra) controls overall self-expression, whether it is language or gesture. An upset in this centre could well result in an individual who becomes dictatorial while the physical signs could be growth problems, or a muscular tension leading to a lack of vocal control.

The knowledge chakra

Otherwise known as the forehead chakra or Third Eye, this is the focus of intuition, the perception of truth which enables a person to find their own course through life. Accordingly, a blockage of this chakra will culminate in a haphazard approach to life, and probably an inability to settle down to any one task for any length of time.

The crown chakra

It is generally felt that the seventh, crown, chakra is appreciated only by experience and it depends upon the other six for its development.

The practicalities of chakras with reiki

This is quite a complicated aspect of reiki and to develop it as an integral part of a programme of reiki, the reader should seek a more extensive treatment of the subject. Some information is, however, presented here by way of introduction.

Some therapists use the technique of balancing chakras to completely attune the energy on the subtle plane. The chakras are paired, first with sixth, second with fifth and third with fourth by placing the hands on the relevant areas. When it feels through the hands as if the energy is balanced with the first and sixth chakras, then the second and fifth can be balanced in the same way. Other combinations may be used if it is felt that these may be beneficial.

The chakras may suffer a number of problems creating an imbalance and although considerable corrective therapy may be required, a balance can be achieved with reiki. Many practitioners recommend sending reiki energy through a problematic chakra. This involves placing one hand at the front of the body above the chakra, and the other hand at the back of the body. The flow of Universal Life Energy eventually corrects any defects. However, it is important to remember that due to the interconnection of the chakras, defects in one affect the whole system. Therefore the healing cannot be undertaken in isolation. It is always good practice to balance the chakras after a session of specific healing.

Higher levels of reiki

Although it is possible to progress beyond the level of proficiency implied so far, second and third degree reiki are really for the experts. This is particularly so with third degree reiki, the details of which are not written down.

Available power is increased with second degree reiki but should only be accessed by someone working with a reiki master. The greater flow of energy means that the effect of reiki therapy is greater and also its effect on a mental and emotional level is enhanced. Further, it is said that reiki at this level can be transmitted over distances, to one or a number of people. This is, of course, highly specialized and advice should be sought from a reiki master by anyone wishing to pursue this goal.

Reiki-do

In Japanese, *do* means path, hence reiki-do is concerned with a way of life in which reiki figures very prominently. Reiki-do is, of course, founded on the reiki therapy described in the preceding pages and it consists of three aspects which enable personal growth. The three categories of reiki-do are:

- *Inner*—based upon meditation as described earlier, and can be augmented by one of the methods outlined, such as the scents of aromatherapy. It adopts a whole-body system of treatment leading to a greater awareness and vitality.
- *Outer*—the application of reiki energy forms the basis of this part of reiki-do, with the chakras, crystals and other subsidiary therapies.
- *Synergistic*—as the word implies, this is the combination of parts which have, when used together, a greater effect than their combined individual effects; that is a merger of inner and outer reiki-do which exceeds the anticipated combined effect. It is particularly appropriate for anyone who has reasonable experience in this therapy and can appreciate the non-exclusive nature of pleasure and success.

Conclusions

Reiki is a technique of healing available to anyone. It can lead to a more re-laxed approach to life and greater harmony with the total environment. It can also be applied to plants and animals, for example your household pets, and for this and further information about the therapy, the reader is advised to seek more detailed treatments.

Shiatsu

Introduction

Origins

Shiatsu originated in China at least 2000 years ago, when the earliest accounts gave the causes of ailments and the remedies that could be effected through a change of diet and way of life. The use of massage and acupuncture was also recommended. The Japanese also practised this massage, after it had been introduced into their country, and it was known as *anma*. The therapy that is known today as *shiatsu* has gradually evolved with time from anma under influences from both East and West. It is only very recently that it has gained recognition and popularity, with people becoming aware of its existence and benefits.

Although East and West have different viewpoints on health and life, these can complement one another. The Eastern belief is of a primary flow of energy throughout the body, which runs along certain channels known as meridians. It is also believed that this energy exists throughout the universe and that all living creatures are dependent upon it as much as on physical nourishment. The energy is known by three similar names, *ki*, *chi* and *prana* in Japan, China and India respectively. (It should be noted that the term 'energy' in this context is not the same as the physical quantity that is measured in joules or calories.) As in acupuncture, there are certain pressure points on the meridians that relate to certain organs, and these points are known as *tsubos*.

The applications of shiatsu

Shiatsu can be used to treat a variety of minor problems such as insomnia, headaches, anxiety, back pain, etc. Western medicine may be unable to find a physical cause for a problem, and although some pain relief may be provided, the underlying cause of the problem may not be cured. It is possible that one session of shiatsu will be sufficient to remedy the problem by stimulating the flow of energy along the channels. A regime of exercise (possibly a specific routine) with a change in diet and/or lifestyle may also be recommended. Shiatsu can encourage a general feeling of good health in the whole person, not just in the physical sense. After some study or practice, shiatsu can be performed on friends and relatives. There are many benefits for both the giver and the receiver of shiatsu, both on a physical and spiritual level.

Energy or ki

Auras

There are believed to be a number of *auras*, or energy layers, that surround the physical body and can be detected or appreciated (*see* the figure on page 91). The first layer, the *etheric body*, is the most dense and is connected with the body and the way it works. An exercise is described later that enables this layer to be detected. The *astral body* is much wider, is affected by people's feelings and, if viewed by a clairvoyant, is said to change in colour and shape depending on the feelings being experienced. The next aura is the *mental body*, which is involved with the thought processes and intelligence of a person. Similarly,

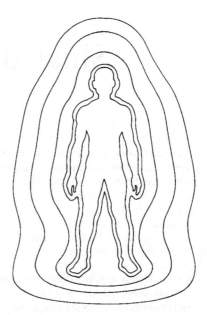

Auras

this can be viewed by a clairvoyant and is said to contain 'pictures' of ideas emanating from the person. These first three auras comprise the personality of a person. The last aura is known as the *causal body*, *soul* or *higher self*. This is concerned more with perceptive feelings and comprehension. It is believed in reincarnation that the first three auras die with the body, but the causal body carries on in its process of development by adopting another personality. As a person grows in maturity and awareness, these different auras are used, and energy is passed from one layer to another. It therefore follows that any alteration in the physical state will, in turn, affect the other layers, and vice versa. (*See also* Aura therapy, page 211 of Treating the Inner Self—Spiritual Healing.)

Seven centres of energy, or chakras

It is believed that there are seven main *chakras* (a chakra being a centre of energy) found in a midline down the body, from the top of the head to the bottom of the torso (*see* figure on page 87 of Reiki) . They are situated along the *sushumna*, or spiritual channel, which runs from the crown of the head to the base of the trunk. Energy enters the channel from both ends. Since the flow is most efficient when the back is straight, this is the ideal posture for meditation or when powers of concentration are required. Each chakra has a component of each aura, and it comprises what is known as a centre of consciousness. Each aura is activated as a person develops, and the same occurs with the chakras, beginning with the lowest (the *base* or *root chakra*) and progressing to the others with time. There is also a change of energy between the *auras* of each chakra.

The *crown chakra* is concerned with the pineal gland, which controls the right eye and upper brain and affects spiritual matters. The *ajna, brow* or *forehead chakra* also known as *the Third Eye*, is linked with the pituitary gland, which controls the left eye, lower brain, nose and nervous system. It has an effect on the intellect, perception, intuition and comprehension. The *throat* or *expressive chakra* is concerned with the thyroid gland and governs the lymphatic system, hands, arms, shoulders, mouth, vocal cords, lungs and throat. It affects

91

communication, creativity and self-expression. The *heart chakra* is concerned with the thymus gland and controls the heart, breasts, vagus nerve and circulatory system, and affects self-awareness, love, humanitarian acts and compassion. The *solar plexus* or *personality chakra* is concerned with the pancreas. It controls the spleen, gall bladder, liver and digestive system and stomach, and has an effect on desire, personal power and the origin of emotions. The *sacral* or *sexual chakra* affects the gonads and controls the lower back, feet, legs and reproductive system. This affects physical, sexual and mental energy, relationships and self-worth. The *base* or *root chakra* is concerned with the adrenal glands. It controls the skeleton, parasympathetic and sympathetic nervous systems, bladder and kidneys, and affects reproduction and the physical will. As an example of this, if a person is suffering from an ailment of the throat, it is possible that he or she may also be unable to voice private thoughts and feelings.

Zang and fu organs

Energy storage and production

According to traditional Eastern therapies, organs have a dual function—their physical one and another that is concerned with the use of energy and might be termed an 'energetic function'. The twelve organs mentioned in the traditional therapies are split into two groups known as *zang* and *fu*, and each is described below.

Zang organs are for energy storage, and the fu organs produce energy from sustenance and drink and also control excretion. The organs can be listed in pairs, each zang matched by a fu with a similar function. Although the pancreas is not specifically mentioned, it is usually included with the spleen. The same applies to the 'triple heater' or 'triple burner', which is connected with the solar plexus, lower abdomen and the thorax. The lungs are a zang organ and are concerned with assimilation of energy, or ki, from the air, which with energy from food ensures the complete body is fed and that mental alertness and a positive attitude are maintained. This is paired with the fu organ of the large intestine, which takes sustenance from the small intestine, absorbs necessary liquids and excretes waste material via the faeces. It is also concerned with self-confidence. The spleen is a zang organ and changes energy or ki from food into energy that is needed by the body. It is concerned with the mental functions of concentration, thinking and analysing. This is paired with the fu organ of the stomach, which prepares food so that nutrients can be extracted and also any energy, or ki, can be taken. It also provides 'food for thought'. The zang organ of the heart assists blood formation from ki and controls the flow of blood and the blood vessels. It is where the mind is housed and therefore affects awareness, belief, long-term memory and feelings. This is paired with the fu organ of the small intestine, which divides food into necessary and unnecessary parts, the latter passing to the large intestine. It is also concerned with the making of decisions. The kidneys are a zang organ and they produce basic energy, or ki, for the other five paired organs and also for reproduction, birth, development and maturity. They also sustain the skeleton and brain and provide willpower and 'get up and go'. They are paired with the fu organ of the bladder, which stores waste fluids until they are passed as urine and also gives strength or courage. The zang organ of the 'heart governor' is concerned with the flow of blood throughout the body. It is a protector and help for the heart and has a bearing on relationships with other people (although there is no organ known as the 'heart governor' it is connected with the heart and its functions). This is paired with the 'triple heater' or 'burner', which passes ki around the body and

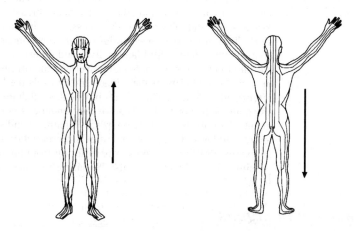

The flow of energy along the meridians

allows an emotional exchange with others. The liver is the sixth zang organ, and it assists with a regular flow of ki to achieve the most favourable physiological effects and emotional calmness. Positive feelings, humour, planning and creativity are also connected with it. The gall bladder is the sixth fu organ, with which the liver is paired, and this keeps bile from the liver and passes it to the intestines. It concerns decision-making and forward thinking.

The meridian system

The meridians, as previously mentioned, are a system of invisible channels on the back and front of the body along which energy, or ki, flows. There are twelve principal meridians plus two additional ones, which are called *the governing vessel* and the *conception* or *directing vessel*. Each meridian passes partly through the body and partly along the skin, joining various chakras and organs (the organs as recognized in traditional Eastern medicine). One end of every meridian is beneath the skin while the other is on the surface of the skin on the feet or hands. Along each meridian are acupressure or acupuncture points, which in shiatsu are called *tsubos*. These points allow the flow of energy along the meridian to be altered if necessary (*see* the figures above). The meridians receive energy from the chakras and organs (as described previously), from the meridians with ends located on the feet and hands and also via the pressure points, or tsubos. Energy, or ki, can pass from one meridian into another as there is a 'pathway' linking each meridian to two others. The energy passes in a continuous cycle or flow and in a set order from one meridian to another. By working on the meridians, and particularly the pressure points, a number of beneficial effects can be achieved with problems such as muscle tension, backache and headache. Since the flow of energy is stimulated by working on the meridians this will in turn affect the joints, muscles and skin and thereby ease these complaints. Since a person's mental state, feelings and moods are also altered by the flow of energy, this can induce a more positive frame of mind.

A person in good health should have a constant flow of ki, with no concentrations or imbalances in any part of the body. It is believed that the greater the amount of ki there is within a person's body, the greater the vitality, mental alertness and overall awareness that person will possess.

Feeling ki

It is possible for a person to 'feel' ki, and the following exercise helps demonstrate what it is like. Stand upright with the feet apart and the arms stretched upwards. Rub the hands together as if they were very cold, so that a feeling of warmth is generated. The backs of the hands, wrists and forearms should also be rubbed. The arms should be put down at the side of the body and shaken vigorously. This should then be repeated from the beginning, with the arms above the head and concluding with the shaking. Then hold the hands out to the front—they should have a pleasant feeling of warmth and vitality, which is due to the circulation of blood and energy that has been generated. The hands should be placed to the sides, then after inhaling deeply concentrate on relaxing as you exhale. This procedure should be done several times, and then it should be possible to feel the ki. The hands should be placed about 1 m (3 feet) apart, with the palms of the hands facing inwards. After relaxation, concentrate your thoughts on the gap between your hands and then gradually reduce the space between them—but they must not touch. It is likely that when the hands come quite close, about 15-30 cm (6-12 inches), a feeling of tingling or warmth may be felt, or the sensation that there is something between the hands. This will be when the auras that surround the hands touch. To reinforce the sensation, the hands should be taken apart again and then closed together so that the feeling is experienced again and becomes more familiar.

The following exercise also enables ki to be felt, but this time it is the etheric aura around another person's head and shoulders. The previous procedure to generate ki should be repeated, but this time the hand should be placed near to another person's head, within 60 centimetres-1 metre (2-3 feet). This person should be sitting upright on the floor or on a chair. The hand should be moved gradually nearer to the seated person's head, concentrating attention on the gap between your hand and his or her head. If no sensation is felt, the hand should be moved back to its original position and the process should be repeated.

Feeling ki

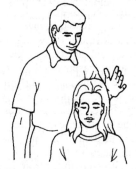

Again, a feeling of tingling or warmth will probably be experienced as the person's aura is felt. When this has been achieved, the hand can progress round the head and down to the shoulders, noting the edge of the aura at the same time. If the person has no success in experiencing the aura, it is likely that the mind is not clear of other thoughts, so relaxation is suggested prior to any further attempt.

It is also possible for a person, by concentrating his or her thoughts and by a slight change of position, to alter the flow of ki in the body. This will have the effect of either making him or her feel a lot heavier or lighter, depending on which is desired. Taken to extremes, someone who is skilled at the control of ki will prove too heavy to be lifted by four people.

Basic rules

There are some basic rules that should be followed before the practice of shiatsu. Clothing should be comfortable, loose-fitting and made of natural fibres since this will help with the flow of energy or ki. The room should be warm, quiet, have adequate space and be neat and clean. If not, this can have an adverse effect on the flow of ki. The person receiving the therapy should ideally lie on a futon (a quilted Japanese mattress) or similar mat on the floor. If necessary, pillows or cushions should be ready to hand if the person does not feel comfortable. Shiatsu should not be given or received by someone who has just eaten a large meal—it is advisable to delay for several hours. No pressure should be exerted on varicose veins or injuries such as cuts or breaks in bones. Although shiatsu can be of benefit to women while pregnant, there are four areas that should be avoided and these are the stomach, any part of the legs from the knees downwards, the fleshy web of skin between the forefinger and thumb, and an area on the shoulders at each side of the neck. Ensure that the person is calm and relaxed. It is generally not advisable to practise shiatsu on people who have serious illnesses such as heart disorders, multiple sclerosis or cancer. An experienced practitioner may be able to help, but a detailed and accurate diagnosis and course of treatment is essential. A verbal check on the person's overall health is important and also to ascertain if a woman is pregnant. If there is any worry or doubt about proceeding, then the safest option is not to go ahead.

Although the general feeling after receiving shiatsu is one of wellbeing and relaxation, there are occasionally unpleasant results, such as coughing, generation of mucus or symptoms of a cold; a feeling of tiredness; a headache or other pains and aches; or feeling emotional. The coughing and production of mucus is due to the body being encouraged to rid itself of its surplus foods (such as sugars and fats) in this form. A cold can sometimes develop when the mucus is produced, usually when the cells of the body are not healthy. Tiredness can occur, frequently with a person who suffers from nervous tension. After therapy has removed this stress or tension, then the body's need for sleep and rest becomes apparent. A short-lived headache or other pain may also develop, for which there are two main reasons. Since shiatsu redresses the balance of ki in the body, this means that blockages in the flow of energy are released and the ki can rush around the body, causing a temporary imbalance in one part and resulting in an ache or pain. It is also possible that too much time or pressure may have been applied to a particular area. The amount needed varies considerably from one person to another. If a pain or headache is still present after a few days, however, it is sensible to obtain qualified medical help. Emotional feelings can occur while the energy is being stimulated to flow and balance is regained. The feelings may be connected with something from the past that has been suppressed and so, when these emotions resurface, it is best for them to be expressed in a way that is beneficial, such as crying. There may, of course, be no reaction at all. Some people are completely 'out of touch' with their bodies and are aware only that all is not well when pain is felt. If this is so, then any beneficial effects from shiatsu may not register. Because of a modern diet that contains an abundance of animal fats, people become overweight through the deposition of fat below the skin and around the internal organs. The body is unable to 'burn off' this fat, and this layer forms a barrier to ki. The flow is stopped, and overweight people do not tend to benefit as much because of the difficulty in stimulating the flow of ki in the body.

Exercises and the three main centres

The body is divided into three main centres—the *head*, the *heart*, and the *abdominal* centres. The head centre is concerned with activities of a mental nature, such as imaginative and intellectual thought processes, and is concerned with the brow chakra. The heart centre is concerned with interactions among people and to the world in general, including the natural world. It is related to the chakra of the throat and heart. The abdominal centre is related to the base, sacral and solar plexus chakras and is concerned with the practical aspects of life and physical activity. Ideally, energy should be divided equally among the three but because of a number of factors, such as activity, education, diet, culture, etc, this is frequently not so. In shiatsu, more importance is attached to the abdominal centre, known as the *hara*. The following exercise uses abdominal breathing and, by so doing, not only is oxygen inhaled but also ki is taken into the hara where it increases a person's vitality. Once the technique is mastered, it can be practised virtually anywhere and will restore composure and calmness.

Sit on the floor with the back straight and, if possible, in the position known in Japan as *seiza* (*see* figure below). The hands should be placed loosely together in the lap and the mind and body should become relaxed after some deep breathing. One hand should be put on the stomach, below the navel, and the other on the chest. When inhaling, this should not be done with the chest but with the abdomen, which should increase in size. As the person exhales the abdomen should contract, and this procedure should be practised for a few minutes. After a rest it should be repeated, inhaling quite deeply but still the chest should not be allowed to rise. Some people may not find this exercise at all difficult while others may need more practice. It may be that there is stress or tension in the diaphragm. Once the technique has been mastered and the hands do not need to be placed on the chest and abdomen, imagine that ki is being inhaled down into the hara. Sit in the same position and inhale slowly via the nose and imagine the ki descending (*see* figure below). (It may aid concentration if the eyes are closed.) The breath should be held for about four seconds and concentration should be centred on the ki. Then exhale gradually through the mouth and repeat the process for a few minutes.

The next exercise is known as a centred movement, which practises movement of the ki, since it is one person's ki that should have an effect on another. After practising shiatsu on a partner, you should not feel tired but refreshed and exhilarated. This is a benefit of the extra ki in the body. The exercise should be begun on hands and knees (a body width apart), and it is most important that you are relaxed and comfortable with no tension. This position is the basis for

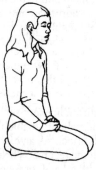

Seiza

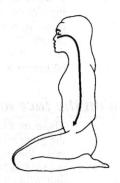

Inhaling through the nose

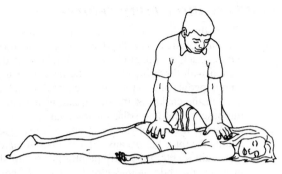

A centred movement

other movements that are practised on others. While the position is maintained, begin to move the body backwards and forwards so that you are conscious of the transfer of weight, either on to the hands or knees. The body should then be moved slowly in a circular way, again being aware of the shift of weight from the hands, to hands and knees, to knees, etc, returning to the original position. You should also realize that as the whole body is moved, the abdomen is its 'centre of gravity'. Practise maintaining a position for about five seconds, registering the increase in weight on the hands when you move forwards and the reduction when you rock backwards. Then return to the original position. It is important that the body weight is always used at right angles to the receiver as this will have the maximum effect on the flow of ki. The reason for holding a particular position is that this has the effect of making the person's ki move.

The centred movement previously described can be practised on a partner in exactly the same way, following the same rules. The right hand should be placed on the sacrum, which is between the hips, and the left hand midway between the shoulder blades. As before, you should rock forwards and hold the position for about five seconds and then repeat after rocking backwards on to the knees (*see* figure above). This basic procedure can be repeated about twelve times, and if you are not sure whether too much or too little pressure is being used, check with your partner. You will eventually acquire the skill of knowing what amount is right for a particular person.

To summarize, there are some basic rules to be followed when practising shiatsu. A person should make use of body weight and not muscular strength, and there should be no effort involved. At all times a calm and relaxed state should be maintained, and the weight of the body should be at right angles in relation to the receiver's body. The person's whole body should be moved when altering weight on to the receiver, maintaining the hara as the centre. Any weight or pressure held should be for a short time only and both hands should be used equally. It is best to maintain a regular pattern of movement while giving shiatsu, and always keep in physical contact with the receiver by keeping a hand on him or her throughout the therapy.

Shiatsu on the face and head

There are a large number of different exercises and techniques, but at each time the giver must be relaxed and calm to enable the flow of ki to occur and thus make the shiatsu work to full effect. As an example, the following exercise on the face and head begins with the receiver's head being held firmly in one hand and, using the thumb of the other hand, pressing upwards in a straight line between the eyebrows towards the hairline. Each movement should only be quite

Shiatsu on the face and head

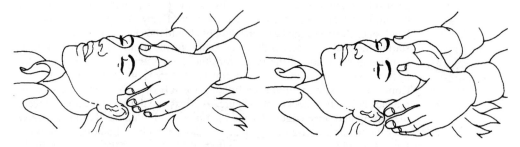

A—press between the eyebrows towards the hairline

B—press from the eyebrows across the brow

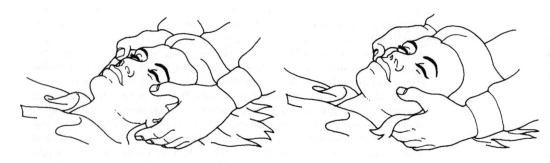

C—work the thumbs across the bone below the eyes

D—press across the face below the cheekbones

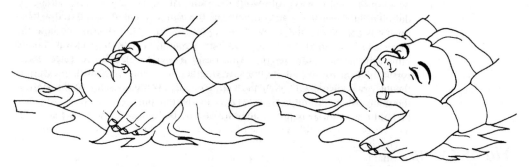

E—press the area between the nose and upper lip

F—press with thumbs outwards over the upper jaw

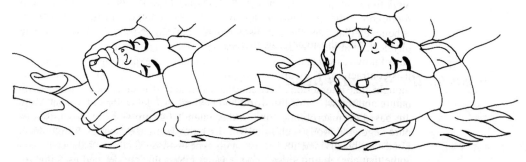

G—press outwards over the lower part of the jaw

H—place fingers beneath the jaw and lean back

small, about 12 millimetres (0.5 inch). The fingers should then be placed on each side of the head and both thumbs used to press from the inner end of the eyebrows towards the hairline (*see* page 98, figure A). Again, holding the hands at each side of the head, the thumbs should then be used to press from the start of the eyebrows across the brow to the outside (figure B). With the fingers in place at each side of the face, work the thumbs across the bone below the eyes, moving approximately 6 millimetres (0.25 inch) at a time (figure C). Commencing with the thumbs a little to one side of each nostril, press across the face below the cheekbones (figure D). Press one thumb in the area between the top lip and nose (figure E) and then press with both the thumbs outwards over the upper jaw (figure F). Next, press one thumb in the hollow below the lower lip and then press outwards with both thumbs over the lower part of the jaw (figure G). The giver then puts all fingers of the hands beneath the lower jaw and then leans backwards so that pressure is exerted (figure H).

Kyo and jitsu energy

As a person progresses in the study of shiatsu and comes to understand the needs and requirements of others, he or she will gradually be able to give beneficial therapy. It is believed that energy, as previously defined, is the basis for all life, and it is divided into two types known as *kyo* and *jitsu*. If the energy is low or deficient, it is known as kyo, and if there is an excess or the energy is high, it is known as jitsu. These two factors will therefore affect the type of shiatsu that is given and, with practice, it should be possible to assess visually and also by touch what type a person is. A few general guidelines as to how a person can vary his or her shiatsu to suit either kyo or jitsu types are given below. As the person progresses, however, it is likely that an intuitive awareness will develop of what is most suitable for a particular person. For kyo types (low or deficient in energy), a gentle and sensitive touch is required, and any stretched positions can be maintained for a longer time as this will bring more energy to that part of the body. Pressure, held by the thumb or palm, can also be maintained for an increased length of time, approximately 10-15 seconds. For jitsu types (high or excess energy), the stretches can be done quite quickly so that the energy is dispersed, and also shaking or rocking areas of the body can have the same effect. The pressure that is exerted by the thumbs or palms should also be held for a shorter length of time, so that excess energy is dispelled.

Yin and yang

As previously mentioned, a change in diet may also be recommended by a shiatsu practitioner. From the viewpoint of traditional Oriental medicine, food can be defined in an 'energetic' way. This differs from the Western definition of foods consisting of protein, minerals, fats, carbohydrates, fibre and vitamins. It is believed that, according to its 'energetic' definition, food will have differing physical, mental, spiritual and emotional effects. This energy is split into two parts known as *yin* and *yang*. Yin is where energy is expanding and yang where it is contracting. They are thus opposites and, from traditional beliefs, it was thought that interactions between them formed all manner of occurrences in nature and the whole of the world and beyond. All definitions of yin and yang are based on macrobiotic food (a diet intended to prolong life, comprised of pure vegetable foods such as brown rice), this being the most usual reference. Food can be divided into three main types—those that are 'balanced', and some that are yin and some that are yang. Foods that are defined as being yin are milk, alcohol, honey, sugar, oil, fruit juices, spices, stimulants, most drugs (such as aspirin, etc), tropical vegetables and fruits, refined foods, and most food additives of a chemical nature. Yang foods are poultry, seafood, eggs, meat, salt, fish, miso and cheese. Balanced foods are seeds, nuts, vegetables, cereal grains, beans, sea vegetables and temperate fruits (such as apples and pears).

The balance between yin and yang is very important to the body, for example, in the production of hormones such as oestrogen and progesterone, and glycogen and insulin and the expansion and contraction of the lungs, etc. A 'balanced' way of eating, mainly from the grains, beans, seeds, nuts and vegetables, etc, is important as this will help to achieve the energy balance in the meridians, organs and chakras, as defined previously. When these two opposing forces of yin and yang are in harmony and balanced, physical and mental health will result.

Body reading

It is possible for practitioners of shiatsu, as they become increasingly experienced, to assess a person's physical and mental state of health by observing the body and forming accurate observations. If the traditional ways of Eastern diagnosis are studied, this can assist greatly. The Eastern methods were based on the senses of hearing, seeing, smelling and touching and also by questioning people to obtain information leading to an overall diagnosis. This is known as body reading.

Makko-ho exercises

Makko-ho exercises are six stretching exercises, each of which affects one pair of the meridians by stimulating its flow of energy. If the complete set of exercises is performed, all the body's meridians will have been stimulated in turn, which should result in increased vigour and an absence of tiredness. Before

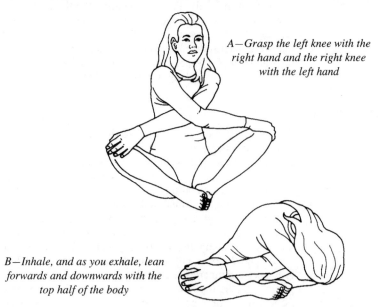

A—Grasp the left knee with the right hand and the right knee with the left hand

B—Inhale, and as you exhale, lean forwards and downwards with the top half of the body

beginning the exercises, you should feel calm and relaxed. It may prove beneficial to perform some abdominal breathing first (as previously described). One example is the triple heater and heart governor meridian stretch. Sit on the ground with either the feet together or crossed. The right hand should grasp the left knee and the left hand the right knee, both quite firmly (*see* figure A on page 100). Then inhale and, as you exhale, lean forwards and downwards with the top half of the body so that the knees are pushed apart (*see* figure B on page 100). Hold this position for approximately 30 seconds while breathing normally, and then, after inhaling, return to the upright position. After completion of all exercises, lie flat on the ground for several minutes and relax.

2

TREATING THE INNER SELF

The last section concentrated on the physical therapies that treat the body in order to make body, mind and spirit healthier. This section concentrates on how we might heal ourselves from within—whether that be through a psychologically based theory, spiritual healing, stress management or through a change in outlook and lifestyle.

Explore your Inner Self

A state of confusion

The last 100 years have seen a great many radical changes, that have had a dramatic effect on our way of life. Many of these changes were for the better in that today more people had a comfortable lifestyle than they ever did at the beginning of the twentieth century. Some of the effects, however, were not so good. People began to feel stressed and confused, to the extent that they began to question their whole way of life and even their own identity.

'Who exactly am I and why on earth am I doing this?' became a common *cri de coeur*, if not actually spoken then at least thought. Some who felt a desire to know more about themselves toyed with the idea for a bit, but set it aside and got on with their rat-race lives to the best of their ability. Others again felt that 'Know thyself' was a good maxim for the remainder of their lives and set about putting the knowing of themselves into action.

Exploring one's inner self is obviously no mean task. Even thinking of a way to approach the task is daunting. Different people find different courses of action helpful, and differences in situation can affect the nature of the approach. This section describes some of the ways that people explore in order to get a clearer picture of themselves.

Today stress and speed are key words, and many feel that they are on a kind of relentless treadmill from which it is impossible to escape. Everything is in a state of hurry and hassle, and there is no time to stand and stare—let alone to think.

It is understandable that this sort of pressure causes some people to have what are known to the lay person as nervous breakdowns. In the case of others, it is their physical health that breaks down. In yet other cases, it proves to be marriages and relationships that cannot stand the strain. In less dramatic cases, some people simply opt out of what they have previously been doing.

People speak of experiencing a personal crisis— a moment of truth when some kind of decision about their lives has to be made. Others speak of requiring space. Many simply want to get off the roundabout of life, which they feel is somehow hurtling round almost out of control, and to stand still for a while.

Certainly the last decade has found many people feeling lost, as though they have completely strayed from the way on which they had intended to set out. It is a set of circumstances very likely to induce people to try to seek inner strength and inner knowledge in an attempt to improve their lot in some way, and many are doing just that.

It is often something specific that triggers off such a response, some circumstance or life event that makes someone stop in his or her tracks and think. What exactly the crisis point is, of course, differs from person to person and from circumstance to circumstance.

People who have suffered from mental breakdowns, or who have suffered from severe reactive clinical depression in response to some form of life crisis, often begin to explore their inner selves as they begin to recover. Having been seriously ill, they often take a new look at life and at themselves, and sometimes alter their entire lifestyles. Those who have been seriously physically ill, such as those who have had a near-death experience during a heart attack, often have a similar response.

It is not always something obviously tragic or unfortunate that leads people to embark on a journey of self-discovery. Sometimes it is a particular age, often the age of forty in men, that triggers it. Sometimes it seems to be nothing in particular that acts as a trigger, just a sudden realization that life is going nowhere and some reappraisal is necessary.

Even a happy event can lead people to try to explore their inner selves. The birth of a baby to a high-powered woman executive might find her suddenly wondering what she really wants out of life and who she really is. Likewise, the marriage of a daughter might find a mother wondering about her role in the family and looking within herself to find out to what extent she has done what she really wanted to do.

The reasons why people embark on a journey of self-discovery are many and varied. The ways in which they set out to explore their inner selves are also many and varied. The following sections deal with these various ways.

A helping hand

It may seem something of a contradiction in terms to speak of seeking another's help when one sets out to discover one's inner self. Surely only the person involved can bring about such a personal revelation?

To some extent this is true, but some people need a little help, at least to get started on their journey of discovery. Whether or not they do need some assistance will depend partly on the personality of the individual concerned and perhaps partly on the set of the circumstances that led him or her to look at the inner self.

Dealing with depression

Some life changes are too difficult to make without the help of others, although the wish to change must come from within the person his or herself. Clinical depression, or what is popularly known as a nervous breakdown, is too serious a condition to be treated without some form of medical treatment.

The nature of the medical treatment will vary according to the severity of the illness. If, for example, clinical depression is diagnosed early on it can be treated by the patient's general practitioner, but it is the nature of the disorder that, even today, when a great deal more is known about the condition, it is frequently not identified until it has become quite severe, when psychiatric treatment and sometimes hospitalization become necessary.

Drug treatment is often extremely effective in the treatment of clinical depression, and there is a variety of drugs available today. It is recognized, however, that depression is a condition where the person suffering from it needs to talk to someone, to discuss the life event, such as bereavement or divorce, that led to the onset of the condition or the set of circumstances that led the person to be a depressive personality. Psychiatrists are skilled in the art of drawing people out to talk about themselves and by so doing can obtain some idea of what has led to their mental health problems.

In the course of their talks with their psychiatrists, often when they are in a stage of recovery and so more appreciative of what is going on, patients frequently feel that they have learned much more about themselves. While trying to explain their concerns and reactions to their doctors, and to set these in the context of the background to their illness, they have given themselves an insight into their true selves.

Some people continue with their self-exploration as a do-it-yourself exercise after having been discharged by their psychiatrists. After they have been shown the way, they feel confident about continuing on their journey of self-discovery on their own. Frequently, self-knowledge acquired in this way leads people to change their lives, or at least to appreciate certain aspects of life more. Some realize, for example, that it was their high-pressure, low-satisfaction jobs that were at the heart of their breakdowns, and they look for a career more in line with what they now see as their true personalities, or indeed decide to opt out of the career structure altogether. Perhaps they are country people at heart, who have been forced to live in a hectic urban environment, and they now revert to type.

It is an unfortunate feature of very severe clinical depression that it can lead to patients suffering from suicidal tendencies. When they have been cured of the feelings of black despair that induce such tendencies, they begin to feel that life is worth living again, and their newly discovered selves begin to think about what is best for them. Nothing much has changed about the world, or about their place in it, but their illness has been a learning experience that has made them see both themselves and the world in a different light.

Psychotherapy

Therapy involving discussion between therapist and client need not be organized by a doctor specializing in mental illness, and the client undergoing the therapy need not be mentally ill. He or she may just feel that there is something wrong with life and be seeking help, or someone who knows the person well may have recommended such a course of action. The person in charge of the therapy programme will not be a psychiatrist but a psychoanalyst or psychotherapist.

Many people find psychotherapy a very useful and rewarding step on their way to self-discovery. At the very least they have talked about things that they would never have dreamt of speaking about before and have learned to face up to them. They have been helped to come to terms with the past and have been able to achieve some understanding of how the past, with its suppressed fears and emotions, had affected the present and prevented them living life to the full. In a very real sense, many people discover who they really are through psychotherapy. Now they are ready to build a future.

There are some who see drawbacks in psychotherapy. The process of psychotherapy, as we have seen, aims to release blocked and negative emotions by getting clients to talk about things that had happened in their lives but had been subconsciously blocked out by them. Some sceptics are afraid that some of the psychotherapists' clients are talking not only about terrible things that had happened in their lives but about terrible things that had not happened at all but are the products of the clients' imagination.

This phenomenon, the existence of which is denied by many, is known as 'false memory'. Cited examples of it include people who suddenly claim that they were abused in some way, often sexually abused, when this seems highly unlikely in the light of evidence put forward by parents, other family members, neighbours, and so on. There are stories of parents being completely rejected by their grown-up children after therapy, when previously they had seemed to enjoy a very happy relationship—although it has to be borne in mind that only two people need to know the truth about abuse, onlookers being often ignorant of the truth.

Not enough is yet known about 'false memory', although the argument about it rages on. What is the case is that more and more people are turning to psychotherapy. People nowadays are considerably better informed, and they have a much better idea of when to seek help and where to find it. Many know the importance of being put in touch with themselves and with their own feelings, and many choose to do so by means of psychotherapy.

Counselling

If people have a particular problem that is having a harmful effect on their lives, they may care to seek help not from a psychiatrist or a psychotherapist but from a counsellor. Counselling has become a very important part of our lives today, although it is quite a recent phenomenon.

Counselling tends to seek to help someone deal with a particular experience rather than delve into the subconscious, as psychotherapy does, but the simple fact of talking to someone about a specific problem can have a wider therapeutic effect. We have become increasingly aware of the trauma, both long-term and short-term, that can be caused by some life events, and counselling is very often recommended to someone who has just experienced such an event.

Talking about a problem to someone and working our way through it can make us start thinking more closely about our emotions and thoughts generally. The net result is often that we find we have gone through a learning experience that has left us wanting to know more about ourselves.

Counselling is appropriate in a wide range of life events such as bereavement and post-traumatic stress. For example, someone who has been involved in a car accident in which others have been killed may be advised to seek counselling. Couples who have suffered a miscarriage and are having difficulty in coming to terms with the situation may be advised to seek counselling to try to deal with the potential long-term effects of such bereavement.

Public bodies are also becoming aware of the need for counselling for people who have potentially traumatising jobs, such as the police, paramedics and those in the fire service. Before, it was assumed that coping with traumas was part of the job. Now, for example, police officers who have watched a colleague being shot to death, or a firefighter who has failed to rescue a child from a blazing building, may well be offered counselling, and it has been suggested that this also be offered to soldiers who have experienced trauma in battle. People who undergo trauma and who do not receive counselling are thought to be in danger of what is known as post-traumatic stress syndrome or disorder.

Schools often offer counselling to schoolchildren if one of their number is suddenly killed. It is recognized now that the other children in the school need to be able to grieve and so are offered counselling to try to obviate any ill effects in later life.

When someone seeks counselling about a problem, he or she will be put in touch with a professional who will discuss the situation from a sympathetic point of view and often offer practical advice. Frequently the object of counselling is to talk through the problem in such a way that the discussion will enable the person seeking counselling to discover for himself or herself the solution to the problem. It is often this working-through process that puts the person concerned in control of his or her own life again.

There are some extremely effective counsellors around, some of them attached to a particular body or organization. As is the case with psychotherapists, however, there are some counsellors practising who have minimal skills and minimum training, partly because it very rapidly became rather a trendy profession with no very obvious basic qualifications. Again it is wise to seek guidance from your general practitioner or hospital, or from a friend with some experience of the field of counselling.

Hypnotherapy

Some people, in an effort to help themselves sort out their problems, turn to a hypnotherapist. These problems range from trying to break an addiction, such as smoking, to trying to slim by receiving help in controlling the appetite, from trying to increase one's level of confidence, to trying not to be so self-conscious, or to trying to help solve some emotional problems.

We will see later in this section how hypnotherapy can be used in several ways, such as helping people to stop smoking. Hypnosis can, however, be used specifically to get us to be more in touch with ourselves. Sometimes called hypnoanalysis in this context, it was used by Freud before he went on to practise psychoanalysis. By means of hypnotic suggestion, the person seeking help through hypnosis can move backwards in time, in a kind of regression, and relive memories that would not be recoverable by ordinary memory or an act of will. This can add to our self-knowledge in a similar way to psychoanalysis. However, many people prefer psychoanalysis or psychotherapy to hypnoanalysis since they feel that they are more in control, although this might not be the case. There is sometimes a vague feeling among people in general that to undergo hypnosis is to put oneself entirely in someone else's power, although this is not in fact true.

There is another way that hypnosis can help us on our journey of self-discovery. If cure by hypnosis is effective in cases of addiction, it helps to put the addict back in charge of his or her life instead of being under the control of the addictive substance. Addiction often results in alienation from one's self. By the same token, breaking free from addiction frees the self and is instrumental in allowing former addicts to get to know their real selves.

Self-help groups for addicts

This section is dealing with people who can help others on a journey of self-discovery, usually by helping them cope with some problem or disorder that is having an effect on their lives. It may seem like a contradiction in terms, therefore, to mention self-help groups, such groups being a set of people who have the same kind of problem and who meet together to work through this, and to offer advice and support to each other.These groups are included in this section, simply because, as is the case with counselling, someone has to point the person seeking help in the right direction, and the other members of the group have to give any new member a great deal of support. Only then can he or she learn to begin to cope with the problem involved and begin to contribute effectively within the group.

The first self-help groups began in the United States in the 1930s to help people suffering from alcoholism to cure themselves. Alcoholics Anonymous was the first well-known self-help group, and it is probably still the best known. They hold regular meetings to help members face up to their drink problem, to help them break the habit, and to help them fight the temptation to start again. The meetings provide a forum where you can share your problem with others, knowing that they too have first-hand experience of the problem. People who are trying to break free of their addiction know that they are in no danger of being patronized by do-gooders or of being in receipt of contempt or condemnation. They are among their own.

A similar group is Gamblers Anonymous, which provides the help for those addicted to gambling that Alcoholics Anonymous does for those addicted to alcohol. The extent of gambling addiction in this country has increased greatly in recent years, partly because the potential for gambling has increased so much. Formerly it was only betting on horses that was the problem, but there is concern, particularly with reference to the young, about addiction to fruit machines, and now there are worries that the National Lottery, particularly in its scratch-card versions, will add to gambling tendencies, especially in people who are too poor to indulge such tendencies with equanimity. Those of us who buy the occasional lottery ticket have no idea of the forces that are at work in someone spending the week's housekeeping on scratch-cards. It is all too easy to condemn without appreciating the problem. At Gamblers Anonymous this ready condemnation is unheard of.

Self-help groups for those with some form of addiction are extremely important because they not only help addicts to keep away from their particular form of addiction but they also help them to rebuild their lives and give them back their self-esteem and self-control. Addicts are never in control of their own lives until they can relinquish their addiction, because to be addicted to something is to be controlled by it. Thus it is that alcohol, gambling, or whatever form the addiction takes, rules the addicts, and they themselves are virtually powerless.

The source of the addiction alienates addicts from their true selves. While they are in its grip they cannot really know themselves, as their true selves have become submerged and subjugated. Coming to terms with addiction and ceasing to be the slave of the addictive substance means that the former addicts can come terms with themselves and embark on what is a very important journey of self-discovery, to find the lost self.

The self-help groups for addicts that have so far been mentioned have been large groups designed either for people suffering from alcohol abuse or from gambling addiction. There are, of course, other addictions—one very obvious and very serious one being that of drug abuse—and there are self-help groups for some of these, some local groups and some branches of larger groups.

Addicts need all the help they can get, although of course they first have to want to break free from the addiction. It is frequently maintained that addicts are never really cured, that the most that they can hope for is that they will stay away from the addictive substance or habit, although that is in fact a major achievement. Being able not actually to involve themselves with the addiction to a large extent puts them in charge of themselves again, although many of them need the support of the self-help group for life.

Self-help groups for non-addicts

Self-help groups do not exist simply for addicts. They have proved of enormous help to many others and deal with a wide range of problems or experiences. For example, parents whose children have been the victims of cot death often find great comfort from being with people who have been in the same terrible situation. They realize that they are not alone and that they are in no way to blame for the tragedy, although some of them will have been torturing themselves with this thought.

Another well-known self-help group is Al-Anon, which provides help and understanding for the members of the family of someone who is suffering from alcohol abuse. This is a particularly useful group since alcohol destroys not only individuals but whole families, coming, as it often does, accompanied by violence, poverty and loss of self-esteem. Often family members feel, usually quite wrongly, a sense of blame and a sense of failure if they have been unable to get the alcoholic to stop drinking.

Other self-help groups include those formed by people who have been raped, suffered sexual abuse, people who are suffering from Aids or who are HIV-positive, people who are part of the adoption triangle and people who suffer from depression. Obviously, the nature of the groups will vary, but they have in common the fact that the members all know what other members are going through, and they know exactly what to do to help. Being part of a group takes away the terrible sense of isolation that is often felt by people who are suffering in some way. 'Why me?' they often ask, and it is something of a comfort that God or fate has not selected them alone to undergo tragedy or disorder.

We have seen how self-help groups for people fighting an addiction can help the members lose their sense of alienation and discover more about themselves while helping them to fight the addiction. Whatever traumatic experience members of other groups are recovering from, it will have left its mark. The help and support that they receive from fellow group members will enable them to recover enough from the trauma to be able to stop and think, and to use the learning experience in a positive way so that it may well in some way enrich their lives. The whole experience will certainly tell them a good deal about themselves, their strengths and weaknesses, and will be a major stage in any journey of self-discovery.

Women's self-help groups

There are some organizations that aim to encourage self-help among women with particular needs. Such organizations, of which Women's Aid is a well-known example, provide refuges for battered wives and encourage the women to take charge of their lives. The location of the refuges is kept strictly secret so that husbands who have acted violently towards their wives will not be able to track them down and attempt to take them back.

As has been indicated, the aim of these women's organizations is to get women who have suffered at the hands of violent partners to take charge of their own lives and to try to make new and independent lives for themselves away from the tyranny of violence. To some extent, however, the self-help is the second part of this aim. First the women have to feel assured that there is somewhere safe to go before they take the huge step of leaving their home and partner. Organizations like Women's Aid provide such assurance, with their refuges and staff providing backup support and advice on benefits, childcare, job opportunities and many other areas of concern.

Women, particularly women with children, never leave violent partners lightly. Most of them keep hoping for some form of miraculous change in the man concerned, who may ordinarily be very charming. When they eventually face the fact that this is not going to happen, when they start to become terrified for their children as well as for themselves, indeed when they begin to fear for their very lives, they often still hesitate before leaving, even if they know about the work of the women's organizations and the refuges.

The recurrent violence, which will often have been accompanied by verbal abuse, will very likely have left the women with very low self-esteem. They have probably been told repeatedly that they are useless, and they have begun to believe what has been said. Worse, they frequently feel that they are responsible for what is happening to them. A woman may feel that if her partner is so charming to everyone else then it must be something in her that is inviting the blows.

A woman who leaves her partner and then returns to him feels even less self-esteem, since she has tried and failed. The failure may well have been no fault of her own, but she will not see it that way. Many battered women go to their parents or other family members and return because the partner turned up at their house, made a scene and offered violence to her family. They sometimes return because their families do not have the space to accommodate them and the children, or the money to support them, or sometimes are not willing to offer them either financial or emotional support. Sadly, they frequently return when their violent partners tell them that they will take the children from them if they do not return.

The woman who has heard about one of the agencies that help battered wives — such agencies, fortunately, are now much better known than they were formerly — and decides that there is no hope other than to leave and seek their help, has already embarked on a journey of self-discovery as well as one of self-help. When she leaves she realizes that she has more strength than she thought she had — the sheer act of leaving is testament to this. After she has received help and advice she will realize that she has far greater potential than she felt she ever had before, and this will in turn lead to greater self-confidence. When she has been out on her own for a bit, and coping with children and home on her own, she may well begin to take stock and really begin to discover even greater depths in herself.

For some women their new-found liberation from violence and their new independence will have been part of a journey of self-discovery, but for others it may be a part of a journey of rediscovery. They may have been quite different people, when they married, from the frightened, shivering, worthless-feeling wrecks that they became. The incidence of domestic violence is not related to class, education or money, and some women might have had quite good jobs before marrying jealous men and giving up their jobs. As she re-establishes her life independently of her violent husband she will probably also end up on a journey of discovery as she reflects on how far she can come and on how far she can go.

Thus we have seen how some people who have been rendered vulnerable in some way, or who have suffered some form of trauma, can achieve some degree of self-discovery in the course of seeking help with their problems.

There can be benefits from the experience of trauma, and these benefits are enhanced by the help given in the various ways described above. Thus psychiatry, psychotherapy, counselling and self-help groups can not only help people towards a greater sense of wellbeing and a greater sense of being at peace with themselves, but they can also help them to have a greater understanding of their inner selves.

Religious support

In a way, the professionals involved in the processes described in this chapter so far are the priests of the modern world. In earlier centuries, or even in the earlier decades of the 20th century, people with some of the problems described above would seek the help of a priest or minister of the church. Particularly in the second part of the 20th century, however, the number of people taking part in organized traditional religions diminished considerably, and so this was no longer an option for them.

Of course the priest or minister would not have the range of professional expertise of some of today's advisers. In earlier times, the kind of trauma and emotional problems that are now generally acknowledged as affecting the lives of people were simply not known or not recognized as such. Problems were seen in more simplistic terms, and members of the clergy were expected to be able to deal with these.

Things were often seen in moral or ethical terms, and clergymen were judged to be eminently qualified to deal with such issues. Spiritual issues, such as crises of faith, were obviously also adjudged to be part of their remit, and many more issues than were strictly relevant to the spiritual topic were included under its umbrella. There may well have been objections to this kind of blanket coverage of problems by the clergy, but there was little alternative.

At least in the case of families whose members had tended to stay much in the same place for some time, the relevant clergymen had a background to go on when offering advice. He probably had a very real idea of the weaknesses and strengths of the various family members, and this might well have proved useful when trying to show someone the way forward to a greater contact with his or her inner self. No one exists in a vacuum, and the past often has a very powerful influence on the present and even on the future.

So much for the influence of the clergy on the family, which in time waned dramatically as it became no longer the norm in Britain for people to attend church regularly, whether or not they were members of the Church of England, the Roman Catholic Church, the Church of Scotland, the Methodist Church, the Baptist Church or any of the others. There are still some people who do not attend church regularly but who still opt to get married, to be buried and to have their children baptised under the auspices of the church—some may even feel a nostalgic desire to attend church at Christmas and Easter.

On the other hand, secular arrangements for the major events in life are becoming more and more common in Britain all the time. More and more people are choosing to be married in registry offices, and efforts are being made to make civil wedding ceremonies more civilized, welcoming and considerably less bleak. In any case, more and more couples are opting to live together instead of getting married, some for part of the time that they are together, some for all of the time that they are together, even after they have children. The net result is that many couples are relinquishing even the tenuous connection that they had with the church. Even so there are still brides who think that a church is a better backdrop for their wedding photographs than a registry office.

Even people who declared themselves to be agnostics or even atheists in life used to be buried under the auspices of the church. In recent years, it has become common for the burial service to be a cremation service, churchyards and cemeteries being no longer able to cope with the sheer volume of corpses and cremation becoming a more compact acceptable alternative. For a long time the cremation ceremony was still very much a 'service'. Although the ceremony would take place in a crematorium rather than a church, the person who usually officiated at such a ceremony was a minister or priest of the church.

Gradually the secular impression created by the often rather bleak crematorium got people used to dissociating the idea of interment and the church. Frequently the relatives of the person being cremated had to make a lot of enquiries in order to find a minister or priest to officiate, and even then the cleric had a great deal of difficulty finding something complimentary and truthful to say about someone whom he or she had hardly known—if at all. Many people began to feel that the whole thing was becoming a bit hypocritical and sought to make the whole cremation ceremony more secular. This has become particularly easy to organize if the person who has died was a member of the Humanist Society, as they will provide for someone to officiate at a secular ceremony.

For many, the church baptismal service has long been something that does not reflect the beliefs of those participating. Either godparents or parents, or both, are required to promise to bring the child up according to the dictates of the church and to be responsible for his or her spiritual and moral welfare. This many of them have done—and never been near a church after the baptismal service or seen to it that the child has. Gradually the secularization of marriage and burial ceremonies has spilled over into baptismal ceremonies. Formerly, there was a general feeling that children were not quite legally registered if they were not baptised in church, there being some confusion between civil registration of the birth, compulsory by law, at the local registry office, and baptism in church. In time more people became aware that the civil registration was enough.

Certainly, by the very late decades of the 20th century, the church had ceased to play a major part in many people's lives. If births, marriages and deaths could be officially recognized without benefit of clergy then many people had little use for the church. Of course this is by way of being a generalization. Many people, particularly those of an older generation, have gone on attending church regularly, and some others have gone on paying lip-service to the church by using it for family marriages, births and deaths, and perhaps have graced it occasionally at Christmas and Easter. Another point worth making is that many of the churches have tried valiantly to modernize themselves, indeed have even made themselves trendy, in an effort to attract more people, particularly younger people, back to the church. Alas, in many cases the effort has not been totally successful. Perhaps one could say in all charity that the efforts were a classic case of too little, too late.

What has been missing for some considerable time is the emphasis placed on pastoral care by the clergy in the average community. Many families would feel extremely embarrassed, and even encroached upon, if a member of the clergy called, even if the family was going through a bereavement or other family crisis, and even if its members were still technically members of the church. On the other side of the clerical fence, so to speak, the clergy, although coping with fewer church members, are probably also trying to cope with larger workloads, fewer clerical colleagues and an ageing church membership, which makes more demands on their time, not least in terms of bereavement. They may have very little time to experience the embarrassment they might encounter if they enter a house of church membership, but not of churchgoers, or even a house of agnostics or atheists that happens to be situated in their parish.

This represents a complete turnaround. There was a time in the relatively recent past when pastoral care was of major importance in the community. If something major went wrong in the life of a member of the family, the local minister or priest was likely to be among the first to be consulted. Thus, if a husband died, or a child was stillborn, or a daughter became pregnant while unmarried, or a son ran away from home, then both spiritual comfort and practical help would be sought from the relevant local cleric. Before the advent of a higher general standard of education and while literacy levels were quite low, the local clergyman was also the person to whom people turned if some kind of official letter had to be written or even read.

The standing of the clergy in the average community has fallen drastically, although the extent of this falling-off has obviously differed from church to church, area to area, and even person to person. With this reduction of importance of church and clergy in the average family's life has come an inevitable decrease in pastoral care. When the family members could no longer turn to the parish minister or priest for help or comfort, then they had to look elsewhere — to psychotherapists, counsellors and self-help groups in fact.

The fact that a great many people have abandoned the church as a source of solace, and even of self-discovery, does not mean that this is true for everyone. There is still a significant number of people in Britain who are staunch members of the church and who regard religion as a spiritual quest and thus a journey of self-discovery.

Furthermore, there are many people who were not brought up in the ways of organized religion but who seek membership of a church to help them find a faith, often in an attempt to help them find themselves, or at least to help them come to terms with themselves. Some of these speak of suddenly seeing the light, as though their lives up to the point of their conversion to religion had been deep in darkness. Such people may be seen as being against the trend, but there are others who, to some extent, might be seen in the same context.

These include people who, in their early years, were brought up to be regular churchgoers and believers in religion but who somehow let such habits and such beliefs lapse, only to find that at the point of some crisis in their lives they felt a need to revert to these and began to attend church regularly, and to consult priests and ministers of religion. They frequently feel that they have somehow lost themselves along life's way and have a deep conviction that the only way to get back in touch with themselves is through the church. Some of these turn to a church other than the one in which they were brought up. For example, a member of the Church of England might feel that he or she wishes to join the Roman Catholic Church.

Often people who either join the church or revert to regular churchgoing are seeking help, sometimes consciously, sometimes unconsciously, with a problem, whether this be an emotional, mental or spiritual one. Whatever the problem, they are probably also seeking to find spiritual enlightenment or fulfilment, and by so doing to extend their knowledge of themselves.

They see their parish minister or priest as a source of help, support and enlightenment, someone to whom they can entrust their deepest thoughts and feelings without fear of these being passed on without consultation. Often by talking these through with the cleric, the problem-ridden people can find their own answers to what is bothering them, while at the same time adding a spiritual dimension to their lives that enriches and extends them.

This is all very well for people who have a religious faith or for people who are working their way towards a religious faith. They have someone trustworthy on hand to whom they can confide their innermost secrets and thoughts, and by so doing they can explore their inner selves. People without religious faith and without a church connection do not have such an outlet. That is why they seek help from other sources, which take on the mantle of a religious confessor and confidant and which can help them on their path to greater self-knowledge. Thus the need for psychotherapists, counsellors and self-help groups.

In our multicultural society it is not uncommon for people to seek solace in one of the eastern religions, although they were not born into one of these. At school many people learn something about other religions as well as Christianity, and some feel drawn to these. The eastern influence on some people's religious feelings was very prominent in the 1960s, when a good many people, particularly young people, went off to India in search of spiritual fulfilment and often in search of a guru, a spiritual teacher, who would bring them such fulfilment. The guru took the place that a clergyman would once have held in their lives but had the advantage of being considerably more exotic in their eyes. This trend towards eastern religions was increased by the interest of the Beatles, the British pop group that leapt to extraordinary fame in the 1960s. John Lennon in particular was drawn towards the East and influenced other young people.

For many young people, looking towards the East for spiritual satisfaction was an attempt to get in touch with their inner selves, the guru being a guide to show the way. It was also an attempt to give expression to their dissatisfaction with the materialistic way of life of the West, often the way of life of their middle-class or upper-class relatives. This dissatisfaction was also displayed by people who embraced the Hippie culture in the 1960s and later by people who embraced the New Age philosophy in the late 1980s and 1990s. These movements are treated in greater detail in the next section.

Of course not everyone who felt drawn towards the religions and philosophies of the East went to India in search of a guru—neither did they all seek out one of the gurus who came to the West. Indeed, many more people than embraced the whole panoply of a religion such as Hinduism or Buddhism simply adopted parts of these. Thus they came to be drawn towards meditation and yoga, and these activities often took the place that Christian prayer would once have done in their lives.

As has been mentioned, many people in the 1960s felt drawn to gurus in the hope that they would give them spiritual leadership and help them to a greater realization of their inner selves. Later in the 20th century there was an increased tendency for people to join religious cults and to look towards the cult leader for the same kind of guidance that some had looked for in gurus in the 1960s, and countless others had looked for in clergymen throughout the centuries. Cult members were often looking for some kind of inner fulfilment or realization and looked to the cult leader to help them in their journey towards this. Religious cults were more common in the United States than in Britain, but in both countries fears were expressed that members of the cults were being brainwashed, although there is often a danger that someone vulnerable, seeking emotional or spiritual help, will form too great an attachment to the person seeking to provide such help.

There is a very real need in many of us to find spiritual fulfilment, whether or not we would categorize the need as such, and in order to do this we often feel that we have to find ourselves or to reach a clearer understanding of ourselves. This often involves seeking help from someone professionally concerned in some way with this kind of work, and such a person is personally central to the success of the other person's search for self. Such help has been described in this section, but there is also help to be provided in a less central, more peripheral way, by other people. This kind of help, together with the kind of help that people embarking on a journey of self-discovery might provide for themselves, is described in the next section.

Self-help

The previous section dealt with situations in which other people, at least at first, play a major part in our attempts to seek out our inner selves. This sectionexplores the attempts made by people themselves to undertake a journey of self-discovery. Although again they may receive help and encouragement from other people, the other people do not play such a major role as, for example, a psychotherapist.

There are many different ways in which people seek to become more in touch with themselves and to find out more about themselves. Some people find a method that suits them right away, although the actual self-exploration might take a considerable time. Others try various methods before hitting on the one that contributes to their self-discovery.

Solitary self-exploration

Some seek solitude in which to create the right kind of atmosphere for communing with themselves. This can be quite informal and might take the form of a quiet holiday in which the person on a journey of self-exploration goes off alone, often somewhere solitary, such as a remote cottage, to find time and space to think and reflect, and to provide an opportunity for self-analysis. People who opt out of their usual worlds in this way, whether for a short or long time, often do so to give themselves the opportunity to look at their lives and to consider the past, present and what seems to be the likely future. Some go back refreshed by such self-analysis and others, on the basis of it, decide to change their whole lifestyles.

They may, for example, have been pressurized by their parents to follow some formally-structured career while they themselves would rather have done something quite different, such as write poetry or paint pictures. At this point in their lives, having taken time to find out more about themselves, and their thoughts and feelings, they may decide to be true to themselves and their personal aspirations and turn their backs on their careers to do something that will bring them more fulfilment.

Some decide not only to leave the work they have been doing but the whole environment in which they have been living. Reflection on their lives has brought them a realization of the futility of their existence and a dislike of the materialism that has brought so much stress into their lives. They feel a need not only to get back to themselves but to get back to nature and a simpler way of life.

It is in such circumstances that, for example, a London stockbroker, used to a highly paid job and an affluent city lifestyle, might abandon his way of life and buy a croft in some remote part of Scotland with a view to living off the land and leading a virtually self-sufficient life. Of course, such dramatic changes do not always work out, and it is likely that he would discover that the whole thing was a wild romantic dream, hastily selling up the croft to return to the affluence of Surrey. Still, at least he would have learnt something about his true self, even although it might have proved an expensive venture.

New Age travelling

The desire to lead a simple, non-materialistic life does not necessarily involve a solitary life. The later decades of the 20th century saw the evolvement of the New Age travellers. These are people who seek a less materialistic, simpler, more golden age, but they wish to do so in the company of others who share their philosophy. There are often various other aspects to their philosophy, such as a concern for the environment and animal rights, a preference for natural remedies rather than formal medicine, and a leaning towards more ancient religions. New Age travellers are also intent on finding themselves, but they choose to do so in a communal, peripatetic way, moving on in vans and caravans from place to place and in so doing frequently falling foul of landowners or the police. Their desire to shake off the shackles of materialism and to lead a freer, less restricted life has something in common with the Hippies of the 1960s.

Retreats

Of course, not everyone who feels the need to take time out changes an entire lifestyle, whether to go off alone or as part of a group. As we have seen, many people simply want to be alone for a while to sort themselves out. This can be done in quite a structured, formal way as well as in the informal way described above. One example of this more formal way of taking time for reflection and self-exploration is the retreat; a place, as the name suggests, where one can get away from it all.

Retreats vary quite a bit. Some are extremely Spartan, encouraging one to concentrate on the mind, soul and spirit, rather than on the needs and delights of the body. Others are less basic, providing at least a minimum standard of comfort, although one should obviously not expect pampered luxury from a retreat. Some retreats are more organized and structured than others and provide lectures, discussions and workshops on various subjects for those who wish to attend. Others leave people more to their own devices, leaving them to meditate or pray and reflect as they wish.

Many retreats are religious in nature. Some of these relate to one of the Christian denominations, and people attend them to spend time in prayer and Bible study as well as to spend time in reflection. Other retreats of a religious nature relate to one of the Eastern religious movements rather than to Christianity. In such retreats people tend to spend a good deal of time in meditation.

Yet other retreats of a religious nature may be based on the teachings of one of the sects that have become popular in trecent years. Retreats may differ widely in their nature, but they have one important thing in common—they provide the opportunity for people to get out of the world for a while, to have time for self-exploration and perhaps to achieve a degree of spiritual and mental refreshment.

For some people a short time spent at a retreat proves not to be enough. They feel the need to get out of the world for a longer time in order to spend time communing with themselves, and often with God. Such people sometimes choose to join religious communities for a time in order to find themselves and come to terms with themselves.

Personal growth and women's groups

Some people feel that they might be more inclined to initiate an exploration of their inner self, and to persist with it, if they had some support from a group. In particular the last couple of decades have seen a rise in a number of what are known as personal growth societies, which are in many ways a later form of the consciousness-raising groups popular in the 1970s.

Such societies often attract people who feel that they have not achieved what they should have achieved in life. They feel stunted in some way or feel that they have taken a wrong direction somewhere along the path of their lives. The members of such societies, in their efforts to achieve their aims, often begin with an attempt to get to know their true selves and to find out how they have become what they are. Until they do so they feel that they cannot come to terms with themselves or maximize their potential by finding out their true capabilities.

There are groups, other than personal growth societies, that people join in order to find out more about themselves. We have seen in the previous section that many people join self-help groups, but these tend to be people who have a particular problem for which they seek the help of group-members. Other people, for example, might join a women's group.

Such groups became very popular in the later decades of the 20th century with the rise of feminism and the interest in the Women's Movement. The initial aim of a women's group is not specifically to enable the members to explore their inner selves. Many are formed with the aim of discussing issues that are important to women which are many and varied. They include such issues as equal opportunities in the workplace, equal pay, health issues, such as screening for breast cancer, childcare and domestic violence. Several such groups were formed initially simply to discuss women's literature.

Although women's groups were not necessarily started with the intention of leading their members to explore their inner consciousness, they often have this effect. When women begin to discuss the role of women in society and how it has changed in recent years, it often leads them to begin to think about their own individual roles in society and within the family, and to reassess themselves, their achievements and aspirations. They have, in fact, begun a journey to find their inner selves, although the original journey was designed to explore the standing and potential of women in the world.

For hundreds of years women were totally underestimated, and the struggle to assert themselves and to establish even a relatively fair position for themselves in society has been an extremely hard one. The fact that they had to put up a joint fight in order to achieve this, however, brought them together in a spirit of sisterhood and raised their consciousness of what it means to be a woman and the problems that this can bring. This encouraged the habit of joint discussion over women's issues.

Men's groups

In the early years of the 21st century things are beginning to change with re-spect to men's group. More men are beginning to feel the need to meet to dis-cuss joint issues with other men and to receive support. These issues are often very specific ones. For example, men who are single parents sometimes form groups, or men who are separated or divorced and feel the need to fight for their rights as fathers sometimes do likewise. In addition, men are beginning to become aware of health problems that are specific to the male sex, and it is ex-tremely feasible that this concern may give rise to the formation of more spe-cifically male groups.

Another reason why men are beginning to group together in a way that has been common in women for some time relates to their concern for their rights and for their standing in society, the very issues that first drew women together. Because of women's success in the workplace, and because of the lack of em-ployment opportunities generally, men have begun to feel threatened and to think that the assertion of women's rights has gone too far at the expense of their own.

More men are beginning to feel the need to discuss joint issues with other men and receive support. These issues are often very specific ones, divorce, being a single parent, the rights of fathers and men's health problems. If the formation of purely male groups continues to increase, it will certainly encour-age individual men to explore their inner selves simply because such groups will set them thinking about their individual lives and roles in the same way that they set women thinking about theirs.

Thus, some people find the way to self-exploration through membership of some kind of discussion group, whether or not they had that specific intention when they became members. Others feel that self-exploration is a more solitary pursuit.

Relaxation

Another and increasingly common method of getting in touch with one's inner self using one's own resources is through meditation. Mention has been made in the preceding section of how an interest in Eastern religions and spiritual movements arose in the West in the 1960s. This in turn inspired an interest in meditation, which is often an essential part of such religions, even among peo-ple who do not embrace the whole religion.

An essential part of meditation is relaxation. Some people begin with relaxa-tion and move on to meditation. Others find that relaxation alone fulfils their needs. They find that through relaxation they can unwind totally and free them-selves from a buildup of stress. By devoting time and space to completely re-laxing themselves and to making their minds completely free of the accumula-tion of thoughts and worries that usually occupy our 21st-century minds, they feel that through relaxation alone they can commune with themselves and so explore their inner selves. In screening out the world, they give themselves the chance of looking into their subconscious, in the way that other people achieve through meditation.

Of course, there are degrees of relaxation, and some people use relaxation techniques simply to de-stress themselves. It represents a therapeutic pause in an overcrowded life. Others, again, see it as an opportunity to make time for themselves, to clear the mind of all the impediments that have built up there, and to unleash emotions and memories. For this second group, relaxation is a stage on a journey of exploration, even a final stage.

Relaxation techniques vary with the preference of the individual, and it is important for everyone who is interested in relaxation to find the method that is right for him or her. Some people, even if they lead highly stressed lives, find it easy to relax. Others find it extremely difficult, often thinking that they have no time for such a pursuit and often imagining that they will find it boring since they assume, quite wrongly, that deep relaxation is essentially a zombie-like state in which your level of consciousness is markedly dimmed.

It is usually the case that to relax, people like to find a comfortable position, although not a position that induces sleep. This applies especially to those who are just begining to learn relaxation techniques. Such a position varies from person to person. For example, some like to lie on the floor and others prefer to lean back in a comfortable chair. As long as you are comfortable, but not too comfortable, it really does not matter. People who have mastered the art of relaxation after much practice can go into their relaxation routine anywhere, but there is no point in putting obstacles in your way to begin with.

Comfort should also be considered when choosing clothes for relaxation sessions. Loose and comfortable clothing is considerably more conducive to relaxation than the rather tight suit that you may have worn to the office. If you are trying to slough off the worries of the day, you are less likely to achieve your aim if you are constantly aware of the tightness of your waistband.

It is important deliberately to set aside some time each day for your relaxation session. We all know how easy it is to have good intentions but somehow never find the time to carry these out. A little self-discipline is necessary to make some time for oneself, and it is easier to do this on a regular basis, rather than simply snatch a few minutes at a different time each day, at least until your relaxation session becomes a central part of your life. Again, people who are experienced in relaxation techniques can snatch a few minutes anywhere to go into their routine and relieve their stress, but it takes some considerable time to achieve such expertise.

If you are just embarking on a relaxation programme, it is also important to provide yourself with somewhere quiet and private to set about the process. Until you have learnt something about the art of switching off, it is not fair to yourself to try out your relaxation technique in busy or noisy surroundings. It is all too easy to become distracted and then to assume that you are not a suitable candidate for relaxation. In time you may become one of those lucky people who can go into a relaxation programme anywhere, no matter how noisy or stressful your surroundings are, but it is rather foolish to assume that you will be able to do this right away.

Physical considerations must be thought of if you are contemplating a relaxation programme. Not only do clothing, place and time have to be considered but also the state of one's stomach. If you have just eaten a very heavy meal and go into your relaxation technique, you are very likely to fall asleep. On the other hand, if you have not eaten all day and are absolutely ravenous, you will very likely find it difficult to take your mind off your hunger long enough to concentrate on your relaxation technique.

Time, space, clothing and the state of the stomach are important to the person embarking on a relaxation programme, but there are other things that will help would-be relaxers to achieve their aim. One of these is a concentration on breathing techniques. Most of us, although we are probably unaware of the fact, have a shallow, erratic breathing pattern, in keeping with our busy, erratic lives. Controlled, regular breathing, however, is important both in relaxation and meditation. Apart from anything else, it induces a sense of calm that is central to both of these.

In order to master the breathing techniques used in relaxation and meditation programmes, it is worth becoming aware of the timing of the four-second breath, which is the basis of many breathing techniques. You breathe in to a count of four and breathe out to a count of four, often holding the breath at the top of the lungs to a count of two in between breathing in and breathing out, and holding the lungs empty to the count of two in between breathing out and breathing in again. If you practise this a few times by the clock, you will learn to judge the timing without recourse to a clock or watch and will be able to perform automatically the breathing techniques based on the four-second sequence.

Concentration on breathing directs one's thoughts away from the day's concerns and problems and enables one to concentrate purely on oneself. Perhaps the best-known example of using breathing techniques to induce relaxation and to divert concentration from problems, or in this particular case pain, is its use in natural childbirth. Expectant mothers are taught a series of regular breathing techniques at antenatal classes so that they might put these into practice during labour and so decrease their pain levels and the levels of drugs that are otherwise necessary.

Breathing techniques are thus an important part of thought-control or concentration-direction. Another effective way to accomplish this is by muscular relaxation techniques. This involves concentration on parts of the body in turn, for example, on the legs, and on how to recognize tension and relaxation in the muscles related to these. Total relaxation occurs when you are able to concentrate on the whole body part by part, getting each part to relax. More information on relaxation of body parts is given further on in the chapter in the discussion on meditation. As with concentration on breathing, concentration on relaxed muscles or parts of the body helps to direct one's concentration away from the problems and pressures of one's life.

Obviously, there is more to advanced relaxation and meditation techniques than are described here. For anyone interested in the subject, however, there is a great deal of help available. There are various books on the subject obtainable either from your public libraries—although these are so popular now that you may have to reserve them—or from bookshops. Also there are various classes and courses run throughout the country so that people can acquire the essential techniques of relaxation that they can then practise by themselves.

Whether or not you join a class is a matter of personal preference. Some people find that it helps them to get started on something if they make the commitment to join a class. Others find it more difficult to follow written instructions given in a book than spoken instructions given by a teacher or class leader. Both such groups will obviously opt for a class, but many others are quite happy to follow written instructions at home at their own pace, perhaps seeking the advice of a friend with some knowledge of the subject.

Some people who opt for the home-based situation find that relaxation tapes are extremely helpful. These are readily available, and many of them talk would-be relaxers through relaxation techniques or a whole relaxation programme. A degree of self-discipline and concentration is required to get started on such a tape scheme. As with most things in life, the tapes tend to vary in quality.

Ordinary music tapes are often just as helpful in a relaxation programme. Such tapes should not be too stimulating, or they will defeat the purpose, or too soporific, or they will send the would-be relaxer to sleep. Something reasonably quiet and repetitive is usually what is required, but choice of music is very much a matter of personal taste and preference.

Massage

Other people associate relaxation with massage. Although to some extent this can be self-administered in that one can massage those areas of the body that one can reach with ease, such as the legs, arms and feet, it is one area in this section where a little outside help should be used to augment the self-help. Massage by a friend or family member, or by a professional, is more common and probably more relaxing.

See also Massage page 29.

Aromatherapy

Some people performing—or receiving—massage prefer to use some form of lubricant, although this is not an essential part of massage. Recently massage with aromatherapy oils became extremely popular, and aromatherapy generally became associated with relaxation and the removal of the effects of stress as well as with natural healing and alternative medicine. Aromatherapy is a kind of holistic therapy that uses essential oils. It aims not only to achieve relaxation and healing but also to achieve and maintain physical and mental equilibrium. The use of aromatic oils in healing is an ancient one. They were used in ancient Egypt almost 3000 years before Christ for medicinal as well as cosmetic purposes and for embalming their dead. The Greeks also made use of plants and herbs in medicine, as did the Arab physicians later. Knights who had taken part in the Crusades brought back from the East to Europe perfumes and the knowledge of how to distil them. The Europeans did not have many of the aromatic, gum-yielding trees that were common in the East, but they used the aromatic shrubs that were native to the Mediterranean, such as lavender, rosemary and thyme, together with other herbs and plants.

Many forms of plant medicine were used in Europe throughout the Middle Ages and during the Tudor era. By the 17th century, however, chemical compounds were beginning to replace the use of plants in medicine, although many of the active ingredients of medicinal plants, such as quinine, morphine and atropine, found a place in the new medicine. The plant-based substances, especially in the 20th century, began to be replaced by synthetic drugs.

Then, in the last few decades, there came a movement towards natural things generally and a movement towards natural things in medicine in particular. There was a reaction against formal medicine, and various forms of alternative medicine began to be popular. These included acupuncture, homoeopathy, herbal medicine, hypnosis, and so on, and particular attention was placed on holistic medicine, to treating the body and the mind as a whole.

As part of the movement towards natural, non-drug-based forms of medicine, aromatherapy has become very popular, and the essential oils have become generally available, although these tend to vary in quality.

Not everyone uses aromatherapy to cure or relieve medical disorders. Others use it because it gives them a sense of wellbeing, and many use it for purposes of relaxation. It is now common for people to combine massage and aromatherapy to help them relax by having a massage with essential oils either from a friend or family member or from a professional masseur or masseuse. When combined with base oils to dilute them, the essential oils are very readily absorbed through the skin, and so they make the ideal massage oil. The person applying the massage will choose a blend of oils to suit the particular client, and a great deal of skill is required to get this right. Essential oils should not be used neat.

People who regularly have massage sessions with a blend of oils especially designed to relax them often indicate that they are left after the massage sessions with a great sense of calm and peace, which is an excellent frame of mind for exploring one's deeper self. The essential oils, however, need not be used just as a massage lubricant to achieve relaxation. Many people use a few drops of essential oils in a bath to rid themselves of stress and become more relaxed. Others prefer to use them as an inhalation. In both these cases, as with massage, it is important to find out about the properties and uses of the various essential oils because by no means all of them make you feel relaxed, some having the effect of stimulating you.

As has been indicated above, the extent to which relaxation helps people to explore their inner selves depends to a great extent on the degree of relaxation achieved. The deeper the degree of relaxation, the more likely it is that you will be able to get more in touch with yourself.

See also Aromatherapy, page 295.

Yoga

Many people either add a yoga component to their relaxation programme or take up yoga as a regular pursuit to increase the degree of their relaxation. There are several forms of yoga, the word being a general term for various spiritual disciplines followed by devotees of Hinduism to attain a higher consciousness, and also the name of one of the six orthodox systems of Indian philosophy. It is an integral part of Hinduism, and its name derives from the 'yoke' that binds the individual self and universal self together. A common form practised in the West is Hatha yoga, which emphasizes physical control and postures.

Yoga is now very popular in this country. It is based on a system of physical exercises and postures and of controlled breathing. You will find many classes on yoga throughout the country, but many of them do not concentrate on the spiritual aspect of yoga. Of course, this is by no means always the case, and you may well be fortunate enough to find a teacher who will bring this extra dimension to the class.

Whether or not you are looking for a teacher who will be able to impart the Hindu principles of yoga, or whether you are simply looking to it as a potential aid to relaxation or to reduce your stress levels, you should spend some time taking advice so that you may find someone competent. As with other areas of alternative therapy and medicine, where there are few hard and fast qualifications required, not everyone who has set up as a yoga teacher is truly competent. It is important to be taught by someone with training and experience, if only so that you may adopt the relevant postures without in any way injuring yourself. Yoga is certainly one method of relaxation that needs to be taught, although after you have mastered the basic techniques you can practise them alone at home

Even if the spiritual content is either missing or not very strongly emphasized, yoga is for many people an excellent way of achieving relaxation and a sense of wellbeing and peace. Partly because of the degree of concentration involved, many people also find yoga a good way of blocking out the world, bringing them calm and inner peace and giving them the opportunity and means of exploring their inner selves.

See also Yoga, page 48.

Meditation

Meditation is yet another way in which people set out to rid themselves of stress and perhaps embark on a journey of self-discovery. As we have seen above, relaxation is one of the components of this, and many people who successfully establish a relaxation programme for themselves go no further, seeing relaxation as an end in itself. Others, however, go on to master, or to try to master, the art of meditation. Although meditation is the cornerstone of many religions and cults, and in many cases corresponds to prayer, people who decide to practise meditation do not necessarily adopt the other aspects of the religion or cult.

The verb 'to meditate' can mean simply to think deeply about something, but meditation in its true meaning is more than just deep thought. Like thought, meditation is a mental discipline, but it requires even more concentration than our usual thought processes. It is a state of mind in which all thoughts are concentrated on a single point or subject. Such concentration is very difficult to achieve and takes time, patience and persistence. Our minds have a tendency to wander from subject to subject, and concentration on one point has to be worked at.

Many people give up on meditation at an early stage since they lack the patience and commitment to come anywhere near achieving the degree of concentration that is necessary to reap its benefits. People who do persist with the practice of meditation, however, often say that the benefits that meditation has brought to them have been very great indeed, one of the most important being that it has brought them inner peace and inner knowledge, which has in turn brought self-realization, central to any journey of self-discovery.

Some people say that they meditate to bring the mind into a state of calmness and concentration so that it can explore its consciousness. Others view it as a way of achieving a greater clarity of perception, or of finding a new way of perceiving the world and of relating to it. Others again feel that through it they can come into contact with their very soul or even with God. This sounds extremely interesting, but how do you set about meditating? As has already been pointed out, the physical conditions that are conducive to deep relaxation tend also to be conducive to meditation.

One of the purposes of meditation is to make space in our minds, leaving room for higher thoughts and for communication with one's inner or higher self. If the desire to know yourself has been one of the reasons why you have taken up meditation, then you can use this as the focus of your meditation, starting with a phrase such as 'Know yourself' and the meaning and implications of that. You can then move on to focus on different aspects of your being, using your memories of the different stages of your life, the different emotional states you have known, and so on. You might even consider using the phrase 'Who am I?' as a starting point for one of your meditation sessions, hoping that in the course of the meditation you will find your true self.

This kind of meditation, performed in a structured way, has been called 'self-inquiry' by Ramana Maharishi. If this form of meditation is carried out on a strictly structured question-and-answer basis it is said to be very difficult to achieve and to require several months of practise in other structured forms of meditation.

There are people who are cynical about meditation, and most of us are very ill-informed about it. It is quite common, for example, to think of people who are meditating as rather weird people who go into self-imposed hypnotic trances. People who have been successfully meditating for some time, however, often speak of the inner knowledge that meditation has brought to them, and so, clearly, someone interested in exploring the inner self should try to master the techniques of it.

What must be remembered is that meditation is a rigorous discipline of the mind, which requires practice, time and steady, regular hard work. Anyone seriously thinking of taking up meditation should be prepared for this and should be prepared for setbacks. It is not an easy path to sudden enlightenment.

See also Meditation page 130.

Dance movement therapy

Dance movement therapy is aimed at helping people to resolve deep-seated problems by communicating with, and relating to others through the medium of physical movements and dance. The ability to express deep inner feelings in 'body language' and physical movements is innate in human beings. Young children express themselves freely in this way and without inhibition, and dancing would appear to be common to all past and present races and tribes. However, in modern industrial societies, many people find themselves unable to communicate their problems and fears either verbally or physically and may repress them to such an extent that they become ill. Dance movement therapy aims to help people to explore, recognize and come to terms with feelings and problems that they usually repress, and to communicate them to others. This therapy can help emotional, psychological and stress-related disorders, anxiety and depression, addiction, problems related to physical or sexual abuse, and learning disabilities. Children with behavioural or intellectual problems, autism or other mental and physical disabilities are often very responsive to this therapy.

People of any age can take part in dance movement therapy as the aim is to explore gently physical movements that are within each person's capabilities. The therapist may suggest movements, but hopes to encourage patients to learn to take the initiative. Eventually some groups learn to talk over feelings and problems that have emerged through taking part and are better able to resolve them.

Dance therapy sessions are organized in some hospitals and 'drop-in' and day-care centres.

Music therapy

Making music has always been important in all cultures and societies, as a means of self-expression and communication. Many people have experienced the powerful effects of music, which may stimulate feelings of excitement, tranquillity, sadness or joy. Music therapy consists of creating music, using a range of different instruments and the human voice, as a means of helping people to communicate their innermost thoughts, fears and feelings.

Music therapy can help people with a variety of different disorders. It is especially valuable in helping people with intellectual impairment or learning difficulties. However, those who are physically disabled in some way may also benefit, especially people who need to improve their breathing or extend their range of movements. The sessions are conducted by a trained therapist who has a qualification in music, and the treatment may be available at some hospitals. Many therapists work in residential homes and schools and the demand for the service greatly exceeds the number of people working in this field. The approach taken depends upon the nature of the patient's problems. If the person is a child who is intellectually impaired and who perhaps cannot talk, the therapist builds up a relationship using instruments, vocal sounds and the shared experience of music-making. With a patient who is physically disabled or who has psychological or emotional problems, a different approach with more discussion is likely to be adopted.

Since most people react in some way to music and enjoy the experience of music-making, this form of therapy is usually highly beneficial and successful. Anyone can benefit and the person need not have any previous musical ability, knowledge or experience. Music therapy is especially helpful for children with intellectual and/or physical disabilities.

These then are some of the ways by which people might help themselves towards a greater understanding of themselves. Some of these ways may depend, at least initially, on the help and guidance of others, but the onus is on the person seeking this understanding to make the time and effort—often considerable—to enable this to come about. Many have found that the effort and time involved were a small price to pay for the self-knowledge that they were able to uncover.

Hypnotherapy

Introduction

Origins

The word hypnotherapy is based on the term hypnosis, which is derived from the Greek word *hypnos* meaning 'sleep'. The word hypnosis was invented in the 19th century by James Braid, a Scottish surgeon, who sometimes used the technique of mesmerism while performing operations. He was not the only doctor to practise hypnotism at that time. In India, James Esdaile used it as the sole anaesthetic for many operations. This was in complete contravention to medical opinion at that time, since for over 50 years the practice and theory of mesmerism had been condemned.

Mesmerism

Mesmerism originated with Dr Franz Mesmer (1734–1815) who became convinced, from his research into the power and use of magnets, that magnetism existed as an unseen fluid that passed through and joined everything in the world. Magnets and powers of hypnosis seem to have been used for centuries whether in ancient Greece, by medicine men and witch doctors or by priests. Mesmer believed that illness was precipitated when this force did not flow freely and that to cure ailments, the use of magnets was necessary to correct the flow. For a time his popularity increased in his practice in Vienna, but when unsuccessful cases occurred, he was criticized by the University and forced to leave the city. After moving to Paris in 1778 he again found fame by having a clientele who came for the theatrical atmosphere and effects as well as to be cured. His patients were put into a trance by the combination of soft lights and music as they stood holding on to a container that held iron filings and water. Dr Mesmer maintained that they then received the effects of the 'magnetism' while he held a rod made of iron. It is now thought that his strong personality, charisma and powers of suggestion were the source of any cures, with his patients actually being 'mesmerised'. After investigation by the French medical profession and establishment, no scientific basis to his practice was found. They also did not approve of the methods he used and were aware of the scandal connected with his name. As a result his methods faded into obscurity.

Approval and application

With the advent of new anaesthetics such as chloroform and ether, the technique of hypnotherapy fell out of use, although it was obvious that it could successfully deaden pain. Around the 1900s, hypnotism was again investigated by the British Medical Association, but approval was not forthcoming. It has only recently regained some popularity with hypnotherapists viewing the trance as a condition in which body and mind can be calm and serene. While in this state, alterations can be made that are not achievable while the patient is completely conscious. The state of being neither fully awake nor fully asleep can be compared to when a person is 'miles away', i.e. daydreaming, or to a person who is sleepwalking. Whilst in a trance a person can function correctly and carry out tasks, converse sensibly and carry out requests. Unlike a sleep-walker, a person in a trance is open to requests or suggestions from the therapist. Both mental or physical changes can be effected, such as the lessening of pain, healing disorders and encouraging relaxation. Sometimes, a patient may have a problem that originates with an event that happened some time ago, e.g. in their childhood. If this is the case, and the patient can be helped to accept what has happened in the past through the use of hypnotherapy, this can also boost morale and self-confidence.

The aim of hypnotherapy is that the patient and therapist work together to achieve a cure. There is a variety of disorders that have been treated with success, such as migraine, irritable bowel syndrome, ulcers and skin disorders along with other problems caused by stress and anxiety. Illnesses known as hysterical illness are a relatively common problem that hypnotherapists treat. They include phobias (a fear of flying, heights, etc), insomnia and asthma. The pain of childbirth can also be relieved.

To ensure that any hypnotherapist is fully trained, it is advisable to contact the relevant professional organization. As well as the hypnotherapist being fully trained, a patient must feel that they can trust and talk openly to their therapist on personal matters, if need be. The nature and character of the therapist is therefore also extremely important so that the two can work together to alleviate the problem. The cost of private sessions, and the number needed can vary considerably although on average five to ten sessions will be required, depending on the condition being treated. Consultations may differ in manner from one therapist to another but detailed case notes will be taken including all relevant treatments, both past and current, and any other information that it is felt might be relevant to the problem. Each session will last from approximately 30 minutes to 1 hour. It is not usual for hypnosis to be used at the first consultation although a patient's reaction to it may be assessed. The patient should also be fully informed as to the content of each session and should be prepared to cooperate with the therapist in any discussion as to the aim of the treatment.

Reputation

Hypnotherapy often receives a bad press. It is frequently associated in people's minds with stage or television shows where people are sometimes made to look extremely foolish when hypnotized. The impression created is that the subject, usually someone from the audience who has been foolish enough to volunteer, is completely under the control of the hypnotist. Lots of stories, many of them doubtless apocryphal, circulate about how people injured themselves or were even killed or died while under hypnosis.

There may be a few charlatans in hypnosis, but then so there are in most areas of life, including therapy and healing. There are a great many skilled hypnotists as well, however, using their skills for therapeutic purposes, and many members of the medical and dental professions recognize that hypnosis can play an important role in mental and physical health.

The trance state

Many people think that when one is in a hypnotic state one is actually asleep, but this is not the case. Hypnosis is not sleep. It is more a state where one withdraws from the normal state of consciousness but yet does not reach the unconscious state. It is like a borderline state between consciousness and unconsciousness, which acts as a link between the two states. When in a hypnotic state, one remains, to some extent, aware and deeply absorbed but open to hypnotic suggestion.

Some people are easier to put under hypnosis than others. It is quite important that the intended subject has some belief in hypnosis, and is prepared to let go and be totally relaxed. The person bringing about a hypnotic state in someone usually adopts a fairly unobtrusive manner and a quiet, monotonous tone of voice. He or she frequently fixes the person about to be hypnotized with a steady, fixed gaze and the patient is asked to concentrate their attention on a fixed object or something that is moving slowly. This encourages the patient to become drowsy. Often the process begins with the patient closing his or her eyes and the therapist asking him or her to think relaxing thoughts. Often the person is asked to imagine a beautiful scene. As the therapist's soothing voice guides the patient down a path of deeper and deeper relaxation, the patient gradually becomes totally focused on the picture he or she sees in the mind— mirroring what happens when the patient is engrossed in a book or a daydream. All outside images and thoughts disappear.

In this state of focused concentration, the patient becomes suggestible. The therapist may then ask the patient to concentrate on his or her own breathing and other sensations inside the body. At this point, the therapist suggests ways that patients can accomplish individual goals. The therapist is able to encourage the patient to view any problem more positively, to realize what they can achieve and also to understand any events in their past history and how they might be likely to react in the future. It is quite unusual for a patient to actually go to sleep after they have been in a trance. Should this happen it only demonstrates that the person has not had sufficient sleep and is merely tired. It is quite commonplace for a patient to use hypnosis on themselves after the ailment or problem, such as insomnia or asthma, has been resolved. With a little daily practice, they will be able to help themselves considerably should the need arise for further or frequent treatment. To assist the patient, a therapist might provide a pre-recorded tape of the known commencement of each session, which leads up to the trance.

Practical application

The following example shows how a person could overcome a fear of flying. At the first visit to the hypnotherapist, once in a trance, the patient was told to imagine travelling and arriving at an airport. At the second and subsequent visits, the person gradually imagined the stages of boarding an aeroplane, going on a very short flight and finally travelling to a different country. To help the patient afterwards, a recording of the consultations had been made and these could be played in the home whenever required. The treatment proved to be completely successful with the patient being able to fly overseas frequently.

It is considered advisable to consult a hypnotherapist who is qualified as a general practitioner too, since should there be any specific disease present it will be recognized as such. Not all doctors are convinced that there is a scientific foundation for hypnosis, but for those who are also qualified hypnotherapists, the practice is incorporated with conventional treatments. Once a person is in a trance and past events have been brought to mind, other bodily functions such as brain activity and the pulse rate will react as if the event was actually happening. When a person in a trance imagines themselves to be a very young baby and the foot is stroked gently underneath, the reflex action is for the toes to curl upwards. This is the reflex response of a baby under six months old, after which the toes no longer curl upwards but downwards. This demonstrates how the person actually regresses to being very young and with the reflex actions applicable to that age.

Although aware of the existence of this sort of evidence, doubt has been expressed by some doctors that people are actually put into a trance. They tend to believe that there are different sorts of consciousness, with the level related to reality ceasing to work and another level taking control that is associated more with the imaginative and perceptive part of the mind. When fully conscious, the normal reaction would be to reject any thoughts or suggestions placed whilst under the influence of hypnosis. Concern has been expressed that a patient's memories of past events have been slightly modified or altered in some way to become what the patient or therapist would want them to be. Although these uncertainties about the trance state do exist, it is still recognized that hypnotherapy provides relief from pain without the use of drugs and is valuable in the treatment of various psychosomatic disorders.

Increasing numbers of medical and mental health professionals now use hypnosis to overcome the pain of chronic headaches, backaches, childbirth, cancer, severe burns, dental phobias, and more. Some psychologists use hypnosis to help patients overcome bad habits, anxiety, phobias, and depression, even to help patients recall past events—although the accuracy of this recall is controversial. Family doctors have begun using hypnosis to treat psychosomatic illness, to control appetite, and to reduce the need for medication, or lower its dosage, in chronic illness.

As is the case if you are seeking a psychotherapist, you should be very careful when seeking a hypnotist, simply because of the difficulty of imposing a standard of training and skill in such a discipline. Again it is worth starting with your general practitioner or your local health centre, or perhaps with a friend who has undergone hypnosis and found it useful. There are some people who have mastered the art of self-hypnosis, but it is important to seek professional advice and to do quite a lot of research on the subject before you actually try this. You do not want to become involved in something that you find you cannot handle.

Meditation

Introduction

Wellbeing, passive alertness and inner calm

'Select a clean spot, neither too high nor too low, and seat yourself firmly on a cloth, a deerskin, or kusha grass. Then, once seated, strive to still your thoughts. Make your mind one-pointed in meditation and your heart will be purified . . .'

These words come from the *Bhagavad Gita,* the best known and most influential of the Hindu scriptures. The book devotes an entire section to the practice of meditation, which is central to the Hindu way of life. It is also an integral part of the other great oriental religions, Buddhism and its close cousin Zen.

But while meditation, in the minds of many, is married to the East, it also has its place in Sufism, Christianity and Judaism. (That said, meditation does not require adherence to any of the faiths and religions that advocate it.)

Many people view meditation as peaceful but ineffectual self-centredness; in the words of one cynic, 'a form of self-indulgent passive introversion'. They are wrong—the benefits to be gained from meditation in any of its various forms are many. Those who meditate regularly believe that it leads to a significant lowering of tension and negative emotions while at the same time increasing efficiency at work and deepening the sense of inner calm.

This feeling of wellbeing brings physical benefits, for regular meditation eliminates or reduces stress, and who in the helter-skelter days of the early 21st century is not stressed at some time or other? In reducing stress, meditation can ease migraine and tension headaches, reduce blood pressure, benefit the heart and reduce the pain of menstrual cramps.

Through meditation we seek to achieve a state of passive alertness that transcends the everyday level of thought and distraction. Achieving this 'higher level' of consciousness may at first seem a difficult proposition, but with practice and effort it is something all of us can do. Some people are put off by the image of meditation as something steeped in impenetrable Eastern mysticism, but meditators don't have to submerge themselves in religious or spiritual teaching to gain from this art. Meditation is really a very simple way of lightening the mind, forgetting about everyday stresses and concentrating solely on mental relaxation

What is meditation?

In its simplest form, meditation is nothing more than allowing the mind to be lulled by a simple repetitive sensation—waves lapping on the beach, the tinkling of a fountain, repeating a word or sound over and over again, even something as mundane as the sound of machinery. Any of these, and countless others, can be used as something onto which the mind focuses so strongly that problems and anxieties are crowded out. In its more refined, mystical guise, it is a means to total self-fulfilment, being completely at one with the universe.

Meditation is neither a time-consuming process (twenty minutes a day are all that is needed), nor is it, as many suspect, a form of self-hypnosis. Practised properly, it is a life-enhancing voyage during which preconceived opinions and ideas fade, the senses and the intellect are refined, and the ability to concentrate is increased.

Its benefits quickly become apparent, and those who practise it often say that the day they first took to meditation on a regular basis was a watershed in their lives.

Meditation and contemplation

Confusion sometimes arises when the words 'meditation' and 'contemplation' are used interchangeably. A working distinction between the two is that meditation can be considered a preparatory step and contributory to the achievement of contemplation.

Meditation involves concentration, narrowing the focus of attention to a single theme, catechism or doctrine while remaining cognitive and intellectual. Contemplation is a direct intuitive seeing, using spiritual facilities that are beyond discursive thought. In the words of Richard of Saint-Victor, a 12th-century theologian, 'Meditation investigates, contemplation wonders.'

The need for a teacher

No one in their right mind would sit down at a piano and expect to play a Chopin nocturne if they had never played before. So why should someone who is about to meditate for the first time expect to sit down and expect to lose themselves in meditation right away? Like all things worth doing, the best way to learn meditation is to study with someone who has already mastered it. If we are to compare the mind with a piano in order to create beautiful music, we need to study with an expert who is familiar with the instrument and who can help us gain a mastery over it.

A good teacher must be qualified, compassionate, expert, patient, sincere and sympathetic, someone in whom the pupil may have complete confidence — but where to find such a paragon? Some novices are lucky and find the right 'guru' straightaway. Others may take months, even years before they meet the one that is right for them. Those who fall into the latter category should not be disheartened: they should carry on practising basic meditation techniques, trying different teachers and following their own judgement until, eventually, they find someone who can help them to get the most out of meditation.

Some people, unable to find a suitable teacher, turn to one or other of the many audio tapes on the market aimed at the increasing numbers of people who are turning to meditation either for health or spiritual reasons. Before committing yourself to the expense of buying one, enquire at your local library to find out if it has an audio section. If there is such a tape on its shelves, borrow it for a few days to find out if it helps you.

Keeping a level head

Where you meditate and when you meditate is up to you, but a word of advice — don't be tempted to adopt a holier-than-thou attitude among friends and colleagues. They may, after some weeks or months, realize that you appear to be calmer and more relaxed and that you have subtly changed in some way or other that they cannot put their finger on. They may ask you what has brought about the change. Then by all means tell them that you have taken up meditating but broadcasting your experiences can defeat the object of the exercise!

Caveat!

Meditation is not suitable for everyone. Anyone who is suffering from clinical depression or any mild form of mental illness should first consult their doctor.

It should never be used as a substitute for medical treatment, and anyone on any form of medication, should likewise consult their doctor.

Meditation creates an altered state of consciousness. Newcomers have no way of knowing how they will respond to it, so it is best to limit the first few sessions to ten minutes at most. Finally, meditation should not be seen as a panacea. It should be seen as a means to an end, not as the end in itself.

Crossing the bridge

In his book *Complete Meditation*, American guru Steve Kravette wrote, 'By practising meditation and being completely who you are, you will become more than you are now. You will be able to cross the next evolutionary bridge and begin to develop the full potential of your creaturehood.'

Meditation is a journey, enjoy it.

The effects on the body

Although meditation has existed for several thousands of years, it was only during the 1960s that it became popular in Western culture. Today many thousands of people benefit greatly from regularly sitting in a quiet place and focusing their attention on an object for a short period of time. Meditation has several effects on the body. As well as slowing down the heart rate, it can significantly reduce the oxygen consumption and carbon dioxide production. Within a few minutes of starting to meditate these can fall up to 20 per cent below normal levels. Meditation also raises levels of skin resistance to pain or an electrical current, which tends to fall when we are stressed and anxious. This indicates an increase of muscle relaxation and can account for phenomena such as walking through fire or lying on a bed of nails.

During meditation there is also a reduction of activity in the nervous system. The branch responsible for calming us down, the parasympathetic branch of the autonomic nervous system, dominates. Lactate, manufactured by the metabolism of the skeletal muscles, is also significantly reduced. While meditating, blood lactate levels decrease about four times faster than they do when the body is in a normal state of rest. The most likely reason for this decrease is that the blood circulation increases, thereby increasing the delivery of oxygen to the muscles and inhibiting the production of lactate. During meditation the body achieves what is called a hypometabolic state. This is a different state from that experienced during sleep or while under hypnosis and can best be described as deep and prolonged relaxation.

Meditation has also been shown to have a significant effect on the way the brain works. During meditation the brain manufactures a balanced pattern of alpha and theta brain-wave rhythms. Recent research suggests that this may indicate that while in a state of deep relaxation the brain is better able to find a balance between its logical and rational and its creative and imaginative sides. The result of this improved functionality is healthier, more productive and fulfilled individuals. Practised regularly, therefore, meditation helps fight depression, reduce hypertension and relieve anxiety, migraine and psychosomatic illness. Research also shows that concentration, memory and creativity are improved through regular sessions of meditation.

Regular meditation is also of great benefit for those who suffer from low energy and who have difficulty sleeping. The quality of sleep improves when meditation is practised regularly, and most meditators testify to feeling less tired throughout the day, needing less sleep at night and waking up feeling more refreshed. Meditators in training centres in Burma and Thailand can reach the point where they need only four hours of sleep a night.

When starting to meditate it is important to find a quiet, peaceful area and to use the same place regularly. The familiarity of a sympathetic environment will help you to slide into meditation mode. Soft background music, incense or low lights are the tools some people use to create a conducive atmosphere. Environmental music, featuring the sound of waterfalls, rain or birdsong is proving increasingly popular with meditators. Practised meditators, however, are eventually able to meditate in busy, crowded places such as bus stations and offices.

Try to meditate for around 20 to 30 minutes each day. There are two stages involved in the process of meditation. First comes physical relaxation, where the focus of attention is on the body and tension build-up is tackled. Once the body is relaxed, the clarifying and emptying of the mind can begin. Given practice, the first stage will become easier to complete and a greater proportion of the time used for meditation can be given to calming the mind.

Meditation in the world's religions

Buddhism

Meditation lies at the very centre of Buddhism, the term used in the West to describe the teachings of an Indian prince, Guatama Siddhartha, who lived from c.563 BC to 483 BC. Siddhartha's wealthy father did everything he could to protect his son from the evils of the world, and it was not until the young man was in his late twenties that he saw a beggar, a sick man, a decrepit old man and a corpse for the first time and realized just how privileged he was. When he asked a wandering monk about sickness and suffering, the mendicant told him that misery and pain were part and parcel of everyday life. Inspired by the monk's example, Siddhartha left his wife and family and turned his back on wealth and self-indulgence.

At first he looked to Hinduism for answers to the problems of suffering, but finding no answers in the faith of his ancestors, he began to conduct his own search for the truth and meaning of life.

Six years later, sitting deep in thought in the shade of a bo tree on the banks of the Neranjari River he achieved enlightenment, and seeing it as his duty to help others along the path he had trodden for so long, he began to preach his message.

At the heart of Buddhism lie the Four Noble Truths:

- all life is suffering
- suffering is caused by selfish desires
- putting an end to these desires stops suffering
- the way to end suffering is to follow the Eightfold Path.

This path demands that those who seek enlightenment must trust in the Four Noble Truths until they can see them for themselves. They must have the right values, the right speech, conduct themselves in the right manner and have the right means of livelihood. They must endeavour in the right way, have right control of their minds and have the right kind of meditation.

One of the major disciplines of the Buddhist meditator is to attain 'unification of the mind' by eliminating all distractions. As the practitioner learns to meditate for long periods, agitation, scepticism and doubt disappear and are replaced by a feeling of bliss. The meditator becomes absorbed in thought (a process known as *jhana*) and moves deeper and deeper until he or she finally acquires an awareness of infinite space.

Many Buddhists regard the pursuit of various *jhana* levels as secondary to the 'Path of Mindfulness', which in the end leads to *nirvana*. The meditator learns to break out of stereotyped thought and comes to perceive every moment of everyday reality as if it were a new event. The ego shrinks in importance; the universe is seen to be in a state of total and ever-changing flux. This realization leads to a sense of detachment from the world of experience, an abandonment of all desires, the abolition of self-interest and, ultimately, the ego itself.

Meditation can take place anywhere, for Buddhism is essentially a religion for the individual. Meditation is not a communal act. Even within organized Buddhist communities, the way one meditates is a matter for the individual and not for the community. There is no prescribed pattern of worship for Buddhists. They may, if they so wish, visit pagodas, temples and shrines and focus on something there while meditating. But it is equally proper for them to meditate in their own homes, sitting in whichever position they choose (usually cross-legged) on the floor.

Some Buddhist families may have a statue of the Buddha in a specially built shrine in their homes; some burn incense and use prayer beads to help them concentrate the mind; some use mantras and mandalas, while others simply adopt their usual meditative position and quickly lose themselves in meditation.

It is estimated that more than 300 million people around the world practise Buddhism, and it is an interesting comment on early 21st-century life that more and more young people in the West are treading the same path and that Buddhism is one of the fastest-growing religions in the Western world.

Zen Buddhism

According to legend, in AD 520 the Indian thinker Bodhidharma (the first patriarch of Zen Buddhism) journeyed from India to China, where he presented himself at the court of the Emperor Wu, a devout Buddhist. When the emperor asked Bodhidharma what merit he, the emperor, had gained on the Path to Enlightenment by building temples and assiduously copying holy writings, the Indian incurred his wrath by telling him that there was no merit in such deeds as they showed worldly attachment. True merit was only to be found in acts of absolute wisdom, beyond the realm of rational thought. Truth, said Bodhidharma, is emptiness, and holiness for holiness' sake has nothing to recommend it.

Wu was so furious with Bodhidharma's doctrine that the Indian left court and spent several years in a monastery contemplating a wall. He later communicated his thoughts and teachings—the *Visuddhimagga,* or Path to Purification, which describes the meditative approach from the Buddhist point of view—to Hui-k'o who thus became the second patriarch of Zen Buddhism.

Meditation has always been a keystone of Buddhism. Zen teaches that it is everything. Its followers do not believe in rituals or reading the Buddha's sermons *(sutras)*. In Zen, meditation is more total and more intense than in any other Buddhist sect. The Buddhist who follows the Zen path must strive to avoid all conscious thought except the point on which he or she is meditating.

There is a famous story of a man who went to a Zen master and asked to be taught Zen. The master said nothing but poured the seeker a cup of tea, using a cup that was already full, and kept pouring until the pot was empty. Then he spoke. 'You are like this cup,' he said. 'You are full. How can I pour Zen into you? Empty yourself and come back.'

Christianity

Modern Christianity stresses the importance of doing good deeds, loving one's neighbour and avoiding sin; the mystical side of the religion has largely been swept aside. But Christianity is essentially a mystical religion, for the true Christian seeks to be united with God through following the way of Christ, who said, 'I am the way, the truth and the light. No one comes to the Father except through me.'

Meditation should play an important part in Christian worship, and it is interesting to note in this respect the volume of music that has been composed down the centuries to encourage meditation. Traditional Christian teaching advocates meditation as a means of getting closer to God. St Teresa of Avila, for example, recommended the *via positiva*—concentrating the mind on God's love and absolute goodness in order to acquire some sense of His magnitude.

It is through such contemplation that the Christian meditator strives to overcome the limitations of conscious thought and achieve a state of ecstasy in the perfect union with God in love and adoration.

Meditation is still widely practised in monasteries, convents and other religious communities, and more and more Christians are spending time 'in retreat', sometimes for a day or two, sometimes for longer, in quiet contemplation.

Christian meditation usually concentrates on the life of Jesus, Mary and the saints, and the most common aid to meditation is probably the Crucifix, although some Christians find that their concentration is heightened if they repeat the name of Jesus or Mary or recite short prayers while they meditate (*see* Mantra page 146).

Hinduism

It is probably with yoga that most Westerners associate meditation. A few years ago the mention of the word would conjure up images of scraggy men, dressed in loincloths, sitting in a meditative trance, and stories of yogis who had been in such a state for so long that birds had nested on their heads were widely circulated to general amusement. Westerners who 'did yoga' were regarded at best as cranks, but today, with more and more people in the West taking it up and with an awakening interest in oriental religion generally, if someone confesses to trying yoga, the reaction is generally one of interest and an expressed desire to know more.

The watershed for the increased interest in yoga meditation probably came in the 1960s with the huge publicity given to the pop groups who travelled to India and returned extolling the virtues of transcendental meditation. But what was new to the West has been practised for thousands of years in the subcontinent.

There is no formal creed in Hinduism, rather a number of religious concepts have developed and have been elaborated since it was founded, probably about 3000 years ago. These ideas were centred on the aim of every Hindu, which is to attain ultimate freedom, or *moksha,* to be free of the endless cycle of rebirths and to be at one with Brahman—the one ultimate reality. Humans learn through yoga (the word derives from the Sanskrit *yuj,* meaning 'to bind together') to achieve this union.

Yoga, the means of gaining liberation from the senses, is one of the four main concepts that underlie Hindu spiritual philosophy. The others are *karma,* the law of causality that links mankind to the universe, *maya,* the illusion of the manifest world, and *nirvana,* the absolute reality that lies beyond illusion.

Yoga encourages the practitioner to see things as they are rather than as they seem. All bodily and mental tensions must cease to be if this is to be so, and, accordingly, one of the basic yoga techniques is meditation as this turns consciousness towards inner calm and finally transcendence.

Judaism

When a man strips away the material aspect which envelops him, he will depict in his mind only the divine energy, so that its light will be of infinite greatness.' The words of Rabbi Dov Baer underline the importance of meditation in Jewish mysticism, which has its roots in the Kabbalah, the movement that combines a complex system of philosophy with specific techniques for increasing spiritual awareness.

Kabbalistic teaching holds that everything in the universe is derived from one source and that the purpose of our existence is to recognize our identity with God and all of creation through meditation and other spiritual practices.

Kabbalistic Jews most often practise visual meditation (*see* page 150), focusing their thoughts on the Tree of Life or the characters of the Jewish alphabet, each of which is said to contain an aspect of the creative energy. Jews who follow the meditative path claim that they are open to a state of awareness that transcends their normal level of consciousness. They hold that their physical health also benefits. This is in line with the teaching of early Jewish mystics, who recognized the relationship between a person's state of mind and his or her physical wellbeing.

Sufism

Some say that Sufism (the word comes from 'sufi' and was originally applied to someone who wore *suf*, or undyed wool) developed from Islam. Others believe that it developed as a reaction against it. Whatever its origins, most Sufis are Muslim, although the latter is not a prerequisite of the former, and non-Islamic Sufi groups are found in many parts of the world.

Sufis base their beliefs on certain passages of the Koran, and some early Christian ideas. Their aim is to transcend everyday thought processes and to achieve a mystical union of the physical, the spiritual and the mental. The Sufist way of life involves fasting, storytelling, dancing and meditation.

There are many different types of meditation. Perhaps the strangest is one practised by a particular group of Sufists—the whirling dervishes who achieve a state of meditative ecstasy by spinning round and round at an ever-increasing rate, hoping to empty the mind of everything apart from communicating with God. Most forms of meditation can be easily practised at home—this one should not.

Posture

Having decided that meditation is something you would like to try, maybe for relaxation, maybe from more mystical motives, what is the next move? Before going on to look at meditation techniques, there are some basics that should first be considered.

Posture is very important in meditation. In Eastern cultures the condition of the body is thought to reflect the health of the mind and spirit, so successful meditation requires that the spine be kept straight. This is thought to assist the channelling of energy from the mind through the body. During meditation you should feel relaxed but not sleepy, and maintaining an upright position helps this. It is not necessary to use one of the Eastern cross-legged postures—lying on your back can be very effective—but they are worth mastering. The traditional meditation postures ensure that the body is stable, symmetrical and immobile, and there is also an easy passage for the circulation of blood in the brain, spine and abdomen. The centre of gravity is established below the navel. The Japanese call this area the *tanden*, or 'vital centre'.

It is essential to adopt the correct position, not necessarily a sitting one, when meditating. Many practitioners of the art consider that the centuries-old seven-point posture is the best for helping to achieve a calm, clear state of mind and has yet to be bettered.

Others recommend the Siddhasana, while many beginners opt for a simple cross-legged position (the easy posture), sitting in a chair (Egyptian posture) or kneeling with the buttocks on the ankles (Japanese posture).

Cupping the hands

Some teachers recommend that the hands be cupped if the pupil is in a posture where it is appropriate to do so. Right-handed people who decide to do this should cup the left hand over the right and, similarly, left-handed pupils should cup the right hand over the left, the point being to immobilize the dominant hand.

Easy posture

The easy posture is one of the best cross-legged postures for beginners. The knees are kept low and the ankles are crossed sailor-fashion, with the back and head sitting straight. With the muscles of the lower back bearing the weight of the body and with the head, neck and trunk in line, the centre of gravity passes from the base of the spine right through the top of the head. The back should not be tense and the stomach muscles relaxed. The hands can either be resting lightly on the knees or held in the lap, either one on top of the other or cupped lightly in the lap.

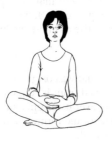

Easy posture

Siddhasana

Sitting on the floor with the back straight, stretch the legs out in front of you. Bend the left knee and, grasping the left foot with both hands, draw it towards the body until the heel is resting against the part of the lower body that lies between the anus and genitalia. Now draw the right foot towards the body until the heel is on the pubic bone. Tuck the toes of the right foot between the calf and the thigh of the left leg. Rest the hands, palms upwards on the knees. Siddhasana is sometimes called the perfect posture.

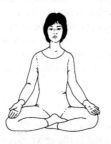

Siddhasana

The Egyptian posture

The Egyptian posture involves sitting in a straight-backed chair. The meditator sits firmly and rocks back and forward slightly until his or her weight finds a point of balance. The hands are cupped in the lap, with the left over the right—if right-handed.

Older people, or those with back problems who are unable to sit on the floor, can sit on a chair or on a low bench and lose themselves in meditation just as effectively as the more supple.

The ideal chair is one specially designed to encourage good posture: the chair is backless and has a slanted seat and knee rest. A straight-backed chair can also be used, in which case, sit on the front part of the seat with the feet flat on the floor and the legs slightly apart, the lower legs perpendicular to the floor.

It is inadvisable to meditate while sitting in an armchair or on the edge of a bed as the upholstery encourages you to slouch and become drowsy.

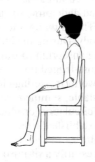

The Egyptian posture

The Japanese posture

In this posture, also called the thunderbolt posture, the meditator sits on his or her knees, keeping them together. Again the back is kept erect, and the meditator rests on the back of the heels. The palms of the hand are rested on the corresponding thighs or can be cupped in the centre of the lap. Popular in Japan, this position also features heavily in Indian yoga.

Some people find this a convenient and comfortable position for meditation as it is easy to keep the spine straight.

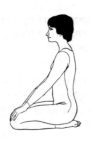

The Japanese posture

Lying flat

This position is called *shavasanaor,* the corpse position. Lie flat on the floor on a carpet, blanket or hard mattress. Part the

137

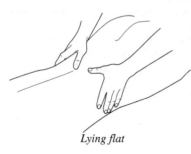

Lying flat

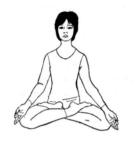

Lotus posture

legs a little and let the feet flop to the side. The arms should be slightly away from the body, hands on the floor, palms up.

Some teachers encourage their pupils to take up this position and relax for a short time before assuming one of the other positions for the meditation session. Relaxing like this prepares the mind for the meditation proper. When you are in the corpse position, starting with the toes and working upwards to the brow, flex each muscle and shake each joint and then relax it before moving on to the next. When you have flexed the face muscles, go back to the beginning and tell each muscle to relax.

At first, some people feel self-conscious lying on their back and saying aloud, 'Toes relax!', 'Feet relax!' and so on. Their self-consciousness soon evaporates when they realize that the method works. When you are completely relaxed lie still for a few minutes, simply concentrating on your breathing before starting the meditation proper or assuming one of the other positions.

Lotus posture

The lotus posture is one of the most advanced postures to master. For the beginner it is often better to try the half-lotus position, where just one foot is upturned on the opposite thigh, before attempting the full lotus. This posture results in classic symmetry. In full position both feet are upturned on corresponding thighs. The knees must both rest on the mat. Again, the wrists can be rested on the thighs or cupped in the lap.

Seven simple exercises

Before trying to assume the lotus position, try these floor exercises to loosen the joints affected. Try to maintain a straight back and fixed head position throughout each exercise.

1 Stretch the legs straight out in front of you. Bend your right knee so that you can grasp the right ankle with both hands and put it on the left leg just above the knee so that the right foot is extending beyond the left leg. Keeping a firm grip on the ankle with the right hand, use the left hand to rotate the foot ten times in one direction and ten times in the other. Repeat the exercise with the left ankle and foot on the right leg.

2 Sitting in the same position as for the first exercise, put the right knee on the left leg as before and with both hands grasping the right ankle, lift it above the leg and shake the foot for twenty seconds. Repeat with the other leg.

3 Place the right foot on the left leg as before. Holding the foot in the left hand and wrapping the right hand around the leg at the ankle, lift the right leg as high as you can and make a large circle with the foot, drawing it close to the body at the top of the circle and pushing it away at the bottom. Repeat ten times before doing the same with the other leg.

4 With the palms of the hands flat on the floor behind and beyond the buttocks, bend the right knee and place the right foot as high up the left thigh as you can comfortably get it with the right knee as close to the ground as possible. Hold this position for a minute and then repeat with the other leg.

5 Supporting the body with the left hand flat on the floor in the same position as for the last exercise, put the right foot as high up the left thigh as possible, place the right hand on the right knee and gently bounce for a count of ten. Repeat with the left leg.

6 Stretch the legs out in front of you and then slowly bend the knees outwards

and draw the soles of the feet together. With the soles touching each other, bring the heels as close to the groin as possible and then, holding the toes with both hands, bounce the knees ten times, keeping them as close to the floor as possible. Hold for a count of ten.

7 Do the same as for the last exercise, but when the heels are as close to the groin as you can get them, put the hands on the knees and press them as far down to the floor as you can. Again, hold for a count of ten.

Seven-point posture

1 If possible, try to sit with the legs crossed in the lotus position, or *varja,* with each foot placed sole upwards on the thigh of the opposite leg. To get into the lotus position loosen up with the seven simple exercises on page 138 and then sit on the floor, legs stretched out in front of you. Now bend the right knee and, grasping the right foot with both hands, place it on top of the left thigh, heel pressing into the abdomen. Repeat the process with the left foot. The soles should be turned up, with both knees on the ground.

If you cannot get into the full lotus position, try the half-lotus. Do the same seven exercises before stretching the legs out in front of you. Bend the left knee and put the left foot beneath the right thigh, as close to the buttock as you can get it. Now bend the right knee and put the right foot, sole up, on top of the left thigh. Keep both knees on the ground and the back straight. When you find that you can maintain this position comfortably throughout the session over a period of four or five weeks, you will be able to start trying the full lotus.

Sitting on a hard cushion will encourage you to keep the back straight and help you to sit for longer without getting irritating pins and needles in the legs and feet.

2 The hands should be held loosely on the lap about one centimetre below the navel, right hand on top of left, palms upwards, fingers aligned. Both hands should be slightly cupped so that the tips of the thumbs meet to form a triangle. The shoulders and arms should be relaxed. Never be tempted to press the arms against the body—they should be held a few centimetres away to allow the air to circulate which helps prevent feelings of drowsiness.

3 The back must be straight but relaxed. Try to imagine the spinal vertebrae as a pile of two-pence pieces, delicately balanced one on top of the other, which will crash to the ground if it is disturbed. A straight back encourages the energy to flow freely, and you will be able to meditate for longer and longer periods.

4 Many newcomers to meditation find it easier to concentrate with the eyes fully closed. This is not wrong, but it is better to gaze downwards through slightly open eyes. Closed eyes encourage sleepiness and dreamlike images that mar meditation.

5 The jaw and mouth should both be relaxed, the teeth slightly apart, the lips lightly together.

6 Keep the tongue touching the palate just behind the upper teeth to reduce the flow of saliva and thus the need to swallow.

7 Bend the neck forward so that your gaze is directed to the floor in front of you. Don't drop it too low: this encourages sleepiness.

The seven point position keeps the body and mind comfortable and free of tension. Beginners should not expect to be able to adopt it right away; it takes time to master.

The meditation session

Once you are sitting comfortably in the seven-point posture, *Siddhasana,* or whichever of the other recommended positions suits you best, spend a minute or two settling your body and mind, deciding which meditation you will do and how long you will meditate.

Some meditators prostrate themselves three times before settling down to meditate, believing that this counteracts pride, which is a barrier to effective meditation.

Now run through your thoughts. Set your goals. Why are you about to meditate? What do you hope to achieve by it? The more motivated you are and the clearer your goal, the more successful the meditation is likely to be.

Many people take up meditation simply to relax, but the more experienced they become, the more far-reaching are their aims, and they feel themselves drawn to the more mystical side of meditation—the search for an understanding of the nature of reality. The deeper they search, the calmer, happier and more satisfied they become. Some go too far! They assume a smug, self-satisfied attitude that is not just off-putting to others but defeats the whole object of the exercise.

Which technique?

There are many different methods of meditation. Some have been handed down from generation to generation for thousands of years and remain in their pure form. Others have been adapted to suit current circumstances. Deciding which of them is right for you can be quite bewildering, but bear in mind that the techniques are not ends in themselves: they are the motorway on which the journey to meditation moves.

The best technique for you is the one with which you feel most comfortable.

Experiment

Start perhaps with breath-awareness techniques, which are the simplest. Many people go no further. Others experiment with different techniques until they find another method they prefer or they come back to breath awareness. Despite the extravagant claims made by the followers of their own particular favourite, there is no technique that is better than any of the others.

Try not to decide on a method after just one session. Give it a trial run over a week or two, jotting down the frame of mind you were in before you went into meditation and how you felt when you came out of it. At the end of the trial period, try and see if that particular method has improved the quality of your life. If it has, and you feel comfortable with it, stick to it, for by using a method that suits you and making it part of your life you will make much faster progress than if you dabble in one and then move on to another just for experiment's sake.

Proper breathing

This is vital to proper meditation. Generally, you should breathe in at your normal rate through the nose. Don't be tempted to force yourself to breathe more deeply or more slowly than usual. You will probably find that the deeper you meditate, the slower and more deeply you will breathe.

A technique called bellows breathing, or *bhastrika pranayama,* is recommended by experienced meditators to quieten the mind before meditation proper begins. The practice involves breathing in and out rapidly by forcing the abdominal muscles to expand and contract rapidly. It takes a great deal of practice to breathe properly in this way, and even those who have mastered the technique should never try it until at least three hours after eating, and they should eat nothing for at least half an hour afterwards.

It should be noted that breathing in this way can produce dizziness and nausea and should never be practised by pregnant women, anyone with hyper- or hypotension or with heart or lung problems. It is best learned from a teacher rather than from the pages of a book such as this.

The time . . .

There are no set rules as to how often you should meditate—some people meditate every day, others find just once a week suits them. It doesn't matter, as long as you meditate regularly, but remember that if you let too long a period elapse between sessions you will be as out of shape, meditatively speaking, as ballet dancers would be if they didn't go to a class regularly. There will certainly be days when you are due to meditate when it is the last thing you want to do, but try anyway, even if only for a few minutes. It is best not to meditate for at least two hours after eating a meal.

. . . and the place

If you have a large house, reserve a room specially for meditation, but if space is a problem, set aside a corner of a suitable room. Put a mat on the floor close to a table or bench for books you may need for your meditation, or for the picture or image on which you are going to focus your thoughts.

Make sure the area is clean, quiet and as pleasing as you can make it so that it is somewhere you will look forward to being in. Make sure, too, that you tell your family you don't want to be disturbed while you are meditating.

Some people burn candles and incense sticks. If you think they will help you to meditate or make the room more conducive to meditation by all means follow their example. Remember that to meditate effectively you must be as relaxed as possible.

The meditation object

This is something on which the attention can focus and on which it may rest, ideally for the full session, although in practice this rarely happens as even experienced meditators may find their attention wandering at some time or other (*see* below), but the meditation object is always there to come back to.

The object may be something to look at—a flower, a candle, a religious icon or a *mandala* or *yantra,* symbols specially designed for meditation. It may be something you can listen to—a cassette recording the sound of the sea or a running river or birdsong, for example. It can be as everyday as the ticking of the clock or as esoteric as the tinkling of temple bells.

Many meditators use a *mantra,* a word or phrase repeated again and again either out loud or mentally.

The meditation object can even be your own breath.

These are all discussed in more detail on subsequent pages.

Problems

Even the most practised meditators may experience difficulties, so beginners should not be put off if they find it hard to get into a meditative state of mind or to maintain concentration.

One of the most common problems is mental excitement. The mind becomes restless and the attention is continually distracted. Sometimes we are unable to banish nagging problems from our thoughts—for example, job security, paying household bills, health worries. If we are in a particularly good frame of mind, we may unintentionally recall things that have made us smile—a new friendship, an enjoyable conversation, even a television programme we have enjoyed.

In our everyday lives we let our minds jump from thought to thought, from worry to worry, so mental wandering is a deeply ingrained habit and, like any habit, is difficult to give up. One popular way of overcoming it is to concentrate on breathing, which has a very calming effect on one's state of mind.

Be patient. It takes time and constant practice to learn how to slow down and control the mind. Don't give up. Even an experienced meditator such as St Teresa of Avila experienced difficulties. When she overheard a novice at her convent remark that it must be wonderful to 'be like Sister Teresa' and not be bothered by distractions during her prayers and meditations, she surprised the girl by saying, 'What do you think I am, a saint?'

Another common problem is drowsiness. When we are in a completely relaxed frame of mind, it is all too easy to drop off. If you start to feel sleepy while meditating, make sure that you are sitting up straight and your head is not bent too far forward. If you are meditating with your eyes closed, open them and meditate with the gaze directed at the floor just in front of you. If you are meditating in a centrally heated room, turn down the heating or open a window to freshen the air. Increasing the amount of light in the room can also help you to stay awake.

Physical tension

Any physical discomfort makes effective meditation difficult. Often such discomfort is a physical manifestation of mental turmoil—it could be an unresolved problem or worry, or something that has made you angry. So if your meditation is disrupted by physical discomfort for no obvious reason, then try to recognize any such problems and settle it in meditation.

One way of getting rid of physical tension is to focus your attention for a moment on each part of the body in turn, starting with the head and working downwards, making a conscious effort to make it relax. You can do this at the start of the session or during it if need be.

Deep, slow breathing can also help. Concentrate as hard as you can, and as you breathe out, try to imagine the pain or tension evaporating.

Long-term benefits

Try not to expect too much too quickly. Don't think that because you have been meditating every day for a week or two and feel absolutely no benefit, meditation is not working for you. It can take months, sometimes years, for positive changes to manifest themselves, and even when they do, they can happen over such an extended period you may not be aware of the difference regular meditation is making to you. Others, however, will certainly realize that something about you has changed for the better.

Breaking the spell

Avoid coming out of meditation too quickly, for if you do, most of the benefits you have achieved will be lost. Once you have finished meditating remain in your meditative position for a minute or two and then slowly stretch, catlike, quietly reflecting on how good you now feel—calmer and better equipped to cope with everyday living. Instead of acting impulsively or emotionally, you will be more thoughtful and better equipped to deal with life's problems.

Breathing meditations

Awareness of breath

Correct abdominal breathing lies at the heart of all kinds of meditation. In 'awareness of breath' meditation, breathing itself is the object of the meditation. Such meditation is held in the highest regard among Buddhists, Hindus and Taoists, all of whom believe in it not just as a means of inducing peace of mind but also of encouraging physical and mental health.

Breathing awareness can also be used as a prelude to another form of meditation. If this is to be the case, five minutes or so will calm the nerves and focus and still the mind, putting it in a receptive mood for the session proper.

Awareness of breath meditation techniques are ideal for the novice meditator because they are entirely natural and most people feel quite comfortable with them. The techniques simply involve being aware of the breath as it enters and leaves the body.

Sit motionless in any of the postures you find comfortable, remembering to keep the back, head and neck in perfect balance, and begin to think about your breathing, becoming aware of each intake of breath, the pause, the expulsion of stale air from the lungs, the pause, the next breath. Your attention will wander. Don't be put off; bring it back to the object of your meditation and start again on the next inhalation.

It is not unusual for the pattern of breathing to change during meditation. At first, when you may be feeling a little self-conscious, you may find that you are holding each breath for longer than usual, but as the meditation proceeds you should find that breathing becomes smoother and deeper, or it may become shallow and slow. Don't be concerned by this. As you concentrate on your breathing and lose yourself in the meditation, the body establishes a rate of breathing that is right for that particular time.

There are several methods for encouraging attention to focus on the breath. None of them is better than any of the others. Try them all, and if you are happier with one over the rest, stick with it. Naturally they all require you to adopt a suitable posture and choose an appropriate place. One newcomer to breath awareness meditation decided to try it in a stuffy underground train. He closed his eyes, put his thoughts in order, began to breathe in and out as he had learned . . . and was woken by the guard when the train reached the terminus many stops past his own.

The simplest methods

Take up a comfortable posture. You may shut your eyes to aid concentration, but it is better to keep them half open. Breathe as naturally as you can, counting either each inhalation or exhalation up to ten, and repeat this for 20 minutes. Counting is an aid to concentration and helps to prevent the mind from wandering.

Some people find it helps if they focus their attention on the tip of the nose or the inside of the nostrils as the breath enters and leaves the body. Others use the movement of the abdomen as the focus of their attention.

Mindfulness of breathing meditation

'A monk having gone to the forest, to the foot of a tree, or to an empty place, sits down cross-legged, keeps his body erect and his mindfulness alert. Just mindful he breathes in and mindful he breathes out.'

Thus did the Suddha advocate to his followers mindfulness of breathing meditation, also called 'following the breath'.

According to this widely practised method of meditation, the abdomen or nose is the focus of attention, which is a development of basic awareness of breath meditation which many people find unsatisfying after a month or two.

There is no counting in mindfulness of breath meditation, rather it is the flow of breath in and out on which the mind is concentrated. To practise it, sit comfortably in any of the prescribed positions with the eyes closed and breathe in and out quite naturally, focusing the attention either on the abdomen or the nose.

If it's the abdomen, become aware of the pause in breathing at the limit of each sea-swell-like rise and fall of the abdomen. If it's the nose, concentrate on the nostrils where the flow of inhaled and exhaled air can be felt.

You are certain to find at first that your attention wanders even if you have been successfully practising counting the breath meditation for some time. When you realize that your attention has meandered, simply return it to the abdomen or nose and continue the meditation.

As you give in to the seductive rhythm of your abdomen as it rises and falls or your sensation of the inflow or outflow of air in the nostrils, your breathing will become smoother and much quieter as the meditation deepens.

Try to avoid controlling your breathing in any way. This can be difficult. Watching the breath without trying to interfere with it seems simple, but it takes some practice for the mind to become used to the fact that you are trying to surrender yourself completely to the spontaneous flow of the breath. Beginners usually find that their breathing becomes uneven, quickening and slowing for no apparent reason. They should not worry, for in time the breath settles to its own rhythm.

Many of those who practise following the breath meditation find it helps if they make themselves aware of the journey of each breath from the moment it enters the nostril to the moment it is expelled. Others picture an aura of energy and light just in front of the forehead. With each breath some of the power is taken into the body and the meditator focuses on its journey deep into the body.

Most of the faiths or religions that advocate breathing meditation have their own techniques. Zen Buddhists, for example, sometimes imagine that a ball of lead drops slowly through the body with each breath-making the stale deoxygenized air fall out.

Many have their own methods of dealing with the inevitable distractions. Some Buddhist teachers encourage their pupils to use the distractions themselves as the objects of meditation for a moment before they are dissolved and following the breath can be resumed.

Active meditation

The Sufi circle

Most meditations are done on one's own or with a teacher. Movement meditation as practised by some Sufis (best known for their dramatic whirling dancing) is done by groups of five to fifteen people and involves chanting as well.

Form a circle with your companions, standing with feet apart some distance from each other but not so far that you have to stretch your arms as you join hands. Now, very slowly lean backwards raising your face to the ceiling (or sky if you are doing this outdoors) and bring the hands up. When everyone is comfortably looking as straight up as they can, say the words 'Ya Hai' loudly in unison. Now all the people in the group bring their arms down and their heads and bodies forward, until they are facing downwards. Now say in the sane ringing, triumphant tone, 'Ya Huk', and return to the 'Ya Hai' position and repeat again and again, establishing a speed and a rhythm comfortable to everyone. Seen from above, the group looks like a blossom opening and closing in perfect harmony.

The point of this meditation is total involvement of awareness of the movement and the accompanying sounds, and each person must be conscious of the physical condition of each of the others in the group. If someone finds that he or she is having to push himself or herself to keep up with the group as it establishes its rhythm, that person steps back and brings the hands of the people on either side together so that the circle remains intact. There must be complete freedom to do this. No one should feel compelled to keep up: if so, the whole point of the meditation is lost.

The aim is to go beyond fatigue to the point where exhaustion is forgotten and all are so lost in the movement and chanting that they become unaware of everything apart from the awareness of self and universe being in total harmony which is the point of all meditation.

Most groups start with 10- to 15-minute sessions to establish harmony and a rate at which everyone is comfortable, and when this is achieved, extend the sessions to half an hour.

Sensory awareness meditation

Movement is also a part of this sensory awareness meditation in which it is combined with breathing awareness.

Begin by lying on your back on a rug or mat. Your legs can be fully extended or drawn in towards the buttocks with the feet flat on the floor. When you are comfortable, close your eyes and concentrate for a few minutes on letting each part of the body in turn sink more deeply into the floor, starting with the feet and moving upwards through the calves, knees, thighs, pelvis, ribcage, chest, hands, lower arms, elbows, upper arms and neck to the head. Concentrate not just on the surfaces that are in contact with the floor but with the sides and top too.

Now, concentrating on each exhalation of breath, try to feel your whole body sink deeply into the floor.

After about 15 minutes, lay the hands on the diaphragm, keeping the upper arms and elbows firmly on the floor. After the diaphragm has moved the hands up and down, up and down for a minute or two, they will feel as if they have been incorporated into the breathing process. Very slowly raise them a little from the body, concentrating all the time on your breathing, then return them to the diaphragm, allowing them once again to become part of the breathing process.

Repeat this for 10 minutes or so, gradually increasing the distance the hands are moved away from the body each time until they eventually come to land on the floor. Slowly you will come to think that the whole cycle is happening by itself with absolutely no effort on your part, and you will find yourself at one with the world.

Tai Chi Ch'uan

Although it is not meditation in the accepted meaning of the word, the aim of Tai Chi (the 'Ch'uan' is usually dropped) is to combine motion, unity and dance so that those who practise its art surrender to the natural flow of the universe and become one with it—exactly the aim of more passive meditation.

Tai Chi is a means of exploring the processes of mind and body through creative movement and reflects the I Ching belief that nature is always in motion. It is said to have originated with the meditation of a Taoist monk, Chang Sanfeng, who one day saw a magpie trying to attack a snake. The reptile teased the bird by writhing and curling in a spiral motion, always remaining just out of the bird's reach. Similar movements are now an integral part of Tai Chi.

In Tai Chi, the image of water symbolizes the flow of energy. It represents the way the flow of energy yields to the form of its container. Earth is seen as a link between person and planet. The use of circular forms of expression shows unity and containment.

It is not possible to learn Tai Chi from the pages of a book. Traditionally the practice was handed down from master to pupil. Today most large towns offer Tai Chi classes, and anyone wishing to learn its ways and mysteries should join a group.

The classes always begin with a period of meditative stillness, and then the pupils step forward on the right foot—an energy step, with fire being visualized shooting from the palms of the hands. Then the energy is pulled back into the body and the weight transferred to the left foot, everyone now visualizing water cascading over him or her. With the body turning to the left, the palms are rotated and curved back to the right. The body continues to turn to the right with both feet firmly fixed to the floor, then the left foot is brought round, returning the body to the centre.

Tai Chi is a process of self-discovery and, like yoga (*see* page 48), demonstrates the link between body, movement and posture, and contemplative states of being. In the words of one expert, Al Huang, who wrote the classic *Embrace Tiger, Return to Mountain,* 'Tai Chi is to help you get acquainted with your own sense of personal growth, the creative process of just being you.'

Attention to life meditation

This is not meditation in the strictest sense of the word, and it is not a method to be used in daily or twice-daily sessions. Rather, it is part of everyday activity, its object being to focus consciously all your attention on the particular movement, activity or task you are performing to the exclusion of everything else.

Take something as mundane as dishwashing. As you wash each dish, close your eyes and concentrate on feeling each sensation—the warmth of the water, the texture of the plate, the soapiness of the lather, the smell of the detergent. Focus on each part of the activity. To do so, consciously relax all the muscles not essential to the task and work the muscles actually being used as sparingly as possible.

In focusing your thinking on the task in hand in as concentrated a manner as possible, you are actually meditating, albeit for a very short time, but it is surprising how effective such short-span meditation can be, especially in helping to remove feelings of stress.

Meditation on the run

Many long-distance runners hit a point, usually about three-quarters of an hour into a run, when they experience what is commonly called a 'high'. This is remarkably similar to what happens during mantra or chanting meditation, with the rhythmic repetition of the word or phrase being replaced by the rhythm of the run. The runner's conscious mind shuts down, allowing other areas of consciousness to open up.

So, if you enjoy a jog, use it not just to make the body fit, but to put your mind in better shape too.

Don't try to compete with other runners in the park or against the clock to beat your own personal best time. If you do, you are shutting your mind to the possibility of meditation.

Run easily, establishing a regular rhythm, and focus your attention on your breathing, your pulse and heartbeat, and after a while you will reach a point where you will be as perfectly in tune with the world as a Buddhist monk sitting hour after hour in contemplative meditation.

Mantra

Repeating a word or phrase—a mantra—over and over again is probably the most practised and widespread path to meditation and one of the oldest. Mantra yoga is mentioned in the *Vedas,* the oldest of the world's scriptures. The mantra may be chanted aloud or repeated silently. The repetition of the mantra is known in India as *japa,* and according to the traditions of that country there are fourteen different kinds of *japa.* Today, in the West, only two of them are in common use—voiced repetition and mental repetition.

The power of the mantra is the power of sound to affect people and alter their state of mind. If you doubt that sound can do this, pause for a moment and consider how irritated you get if someone is playing music too loudly or if you are sitting next to someone who is plugged into a personal stereo and the music is almost audible to you. If sound can irritate, then surely the converse is true — sound can make you feel tranquil, and to focus on a mantra during meditation can lead to some of the deepest and most profound sessions you are likely to experience.

Sound is energy produced by a vibrating object. It is transmitted by waves of different frequencies. Followers of mantra meditation believe that different sounds resonate with different energy centres in the body and that these sounds can be combined in the form of the mantra.

Most of the major religions have their own mantra, and a selection of these are at the end of this section. For those who wish to use a mantra in their meditation but who want to avoid religion, any word or phrase, no matter how meaningless, will do.

In India, until the 11th century, it was usual for gurus to devise personal mantras for each of their pupils. Each pupil treasured his mantra and refused to divulge it to his fellows for he had been warned that in doing so the power of the mantra would be weakened. In the 11th century, Ramanuja, a leading figure in the history of Indian yoga and one suspicious of the almost mystical power of the gurus, shouted his mantra from the roof of a temple so that all could share it. The practice of secret mantras now only survives, generally speaking, in the school of Transcendental Meditation (TM) practised by the Maharishi Mahesh.

Those who are suspicious of any religious aspects associated with mantra can do little better than choose their mantra by the method recommended by Lawrence LeShant, a leading expert in the subject. He advocates the 'La-de' method of mantra selection: simply opening a telephone directory at random and blindly letting the forefinger fall on the page. The first syllable of that name becomes the first syllable of the mantra. Repeat the process, linking the second syllable selected at random with the first and — hey presto! — you have a mantra.

To practise meditation with a mantra, begin, as usual, by taking up the position that you find most comfortable and breathe gently and rhythmically through the nostrils, taking the breath deep into the abdomen. Then repeat the mantra, either aloud or silently inward, focusing your concentration on it as completely as you can. When your mind has become still, it is no longer necessary to continue repeating the mantra, but, as with other forms of meditation, when you become aware that your thoughts have wandered, start repeating the mantra again, concentrating your conscious thoughts on it.

Once you have chosen a mantra with which you are comfortable, stick with it. It's amazing how in times of stress, repeating your mantra a few times silently to yourself restores calm and helps you to put things into proper perspective.

Many mantra meditators repeat the mantra in rhythm with their breathing, saying it once or twice on inhalation and once or twice on breathing out. They are usually repeated silently, but some teachers encourage their pupils to say them aloud, especially if they are leading a group meditation.

Om

Om, a Sanskrit word pronounced to rhyme with 'Rome' is one of the most widely used mantras. According to Hindu belief, om is the primal sound and it is accorded the highest value as an object of meditation and one well worth trying. Breathe in gently, and as you exhale recite the word as three sounds, 'a' (as in father), 'oo' (as in room) and 'mmm'. Try to feel the sounds vibrating in your body. The 'a' will feel as if it is ringing in your belly, the 'oo' will resonate in your chest and the 'mmm' will positively resound in the bones of your skull. Link the sounds to your breathing rhythm, keeping it slow and calm and avoiding deepening it in any way.

After saying *om* aloud for ten breaths, soften the voice until you are saying the word under your breath, then lower it even further, keeping your attention firmly focused on it. It won't be long before your lips stop moving and the syllables lose their shape, leaving you with just an idea that clings to your mind. Banish any intrusive thoughts by imagining them as puffs of smoke and watch them being blown away by a gentle breeze.

The Jesus prayer

Some Christians use the name of Jesus as their mantra, others use short prayers, one of the most popular of which is the Jesus prayer which was probably devised by Orthodox monks. It has two forms, either 'Lord Jesus Christ, son of God, have mercy on me', or 'Lord Jesus Christ, have mercy on me'. The prayer follows the advice of a seventh-century mystic who is reputed to have written, 'If many words are used in prayer, all sorts of distracting pictures hover in the mind, but worship is lost. If little is said . . . the mind remains concentrated.' His words could be paraphrased to define mantra—a few words to concentrate the mind.

The rosary

You do not have to be Roman Catholic to meditate on the rosary; any Christian can use the beads as a focus for their meditation. With your eyes closed, pass the beads slowly through the fingers, noticing how the smaller beads are periodically punctuated by large ones. Each time you finger a small bead repeat the words of the Hail Mary:

Hail Mary, full of grace,
The Lord is with thee.
Blessed art thou among women
And blessed is the fruit of thy womb, Jesus.
Hail Mary, Mother of God,
Pray for us sinners now
And at the hour of our death.
Amen

Move on to the next bead: if it is small, repeat the Hail Mary, if it is one of the larger beads, say the Lord's Prayer. The meditation should last for the usual twenty minutes.

Humming like a bee

While not a mantra in the true sense of the word, there are many people who hum while meditating. If you would like to try this, take up your usual position but close your right nostril with your right thumb and inhale through the left nostril, holding your breath as deep and as low in the abdomen as you can. Now exhale and as you do so make a humming noise deep in your throat, focusing your thoughts on the sound.

Do this five times and repeat the exercise with the right nostril, then alternate five times with each nostril for the full twenty-minute meditation.

Transcendental Meditation

This form of mantra meditation was introduced to the West in 1959 by the Maharishi Mahesh and became popular in the 1960s when several influential young men and women, pop stars prominent amongst them, claiming they

were disillusioned with Western values, turned to the East for spiritual fulfilment. Its central feature is contemplation on and repetition of a Sanskrit mantra
personally bestowed on each follower by his or her guru, originally Mahesh
himself.

In the Maharishi's own words, in TM '. . . the attention comes from outside to
the inside, to the source of thought, and then the conscious mind . . . gains that
transcendent pure awareness which is bliss consciousness. It is just thinking,
but thinking in a manner so that awareness goes deep within and gains that inner being of pure consciousness.'

Those who follow TM meditate for 40 minutes a day in two periods of 20
minutes, repeating their mantra inwardly without moving the lips. The two periods of meditation must be separated by at least six hours of normal activity.
Unlike many other Indian schools of meditation, TM demands no conscious
changes in lifestyle. The Maharishi claims that such changes will happen spontaneously as the meditation sessions progress.

A great deal of research was conducted on TM, and it emerged that it did create significant psychological changes associated with relaxation. Sceptics,
however, queried the methodology of much of the research, and their constant
barracking weakened the validity of some of the findings. Those who follow
TM insist on the mantra being chosen with much ceremony and in secrecy by
the master teacher, but this practice has not been shown to be any more effective than one that uses simple words.

Who says what

Faith	Mantra	Meaning
Buddhism*	Gate, Gate, Pargate, Paramsagate, Bodhi Svahag	*Gone, gone, gone to the other shore, safely passed to that other shore, Enlightened One*
	Namo Buddya, Namo Dharmaya, Namo Sanghaya	*I go to the Buddha for refuge, I go to the Dharma for refuge, I go to the Sangha for refuge*
	Bhagavan Sarva Tathagatha, Tathagatha	*Blessed be all your Buddhas*
	Om Tare Tutare Ture Swaha	*Hail to Tara*
	Namo Amitabha	*I go to the Buddha for light*
	Om Mani Padme Hum	*Hail to the Jewel in the Lotus*

*Buddhist mantras are associated with mandalas—images of the cosmos,
prayer wheels and beads and counters. It is common among Buddhists to repeat
the mantra 108 times because of the numbers: 1 = the absolute; 0 is the cosmos;
and 8 is the infinite.

Sikh	Eck Ong Kar Sat Nam Siri Wha Guru	*The Supreme is one, His names are many*
Hindu	Tat Tuam Asi	*Thou art that*
	So ham	*That I am*
	Hare Krishna	*Hail to Krishna*
	Hare Rama	*Hail to Rama*

| | Om Namah Sivaya, Shanti, Shanti | *Om reverence to Shiva, peace peace* |

The following mantras have particular healing associations for Hindus:

Hrim *(throat and liver)*

Hrum *(liver and spleen)*

Hraim *(kidneys)*

Hra *(heart and chest)*

Islam	Allah, Allah, La Ilaha Illa'llah	*God, God, there is no God but one God*
	Insha Allah	*If God wills*
	Ya-Salaam	*God, the source of peace*
	An-Nur	*God, the light*
Judaism	Adonai	*Lord*
	Shalom	*Peace*
	Ehyeh Asher Ehyeh	*I am that I am*
	Quadosh, Quadosh, Quadosh Adonai Tzeba'oth	*Holy, Holy, Holy Lord of Hosts*
	Eli, Eli, Eli	*My God, My God, My God*
	Barukh Ata Adonai	*Blessed is the Lord*
Christian	Lord Jesus Christ, Son of God, Have Mercy on us	
	Kyrie Eleison, Christe Eleison, Kyrie Eleison	*Lord have mercy, Christ have mercy, God have mercy*
	Laudamus	*We praise thee*
	Alleluia	
	Holy, Holy, Holy	
	En Emoi Christus	*Christ in me*
	Ave Maria	*Hail Mary*
Sufism	Hu-E-Haiy	*God the living*
	He-La	*The word is the mirror wherein the Divine reverberates outwardly. Through sound the world will be reabsorbed. The word is both sound and light, for light is the meaning of the word*

Visual meditation

Visual meditation uses our natural capacity to think in pictures and our ability to create images in what is often called the mind's eye. It may be practised with the eyes open or shut or by opening and shutting them for alternate periods, concentrating on the after-image that remains in our mind when the eyes are closed. The latter method is most usually recommended for beginners.

Place the object of your meditation (on which more later) at eye level between a metre and two metres from your face. If you decide to use a mandala or yantra (*see* page 152) the central point should be level with the eyes. Assume whichever meditation position you favour, and in as relaxed a way as possible, gaze at the image, focusing your attention on it, trying to become *absorbed* in what you are looking at rather than just thinking about it. After two or three minutes or as soon as you feel any sign of eye strain, close your eyes and visualize the object for as long as you can, still trying to be part of it. Open the eyes again and continue alternating open-eyed and closed-eyed meditation for the full session.

Initially it will be difficult to retain the image in your mind's eye for long when your eyes are closed: don't worry. When the image starts to fade, open the eyes and gaze at the object again. As you become more practised in the art, you will find that you can retain the image for longer and longer.

Meditating on a candle

Many of those who come to visual meditation for the first time find that a lighted candle in a darkened room is the ideal object of focus. One method recommended for beginners is to light a candle in a darkened, draught-free room, draught-free so that the flame burns as steadily as possible. To meditate on a candle, sit as motionless as you can in any of the recommended positions and gaze at the flame so that it holds your attention completely. Let the image fill your mind for a minute before quickly closing the eyes. Notice how the candle has imprinted itself on the darkness. Hold it in your mind's eye, not worrying about any change of colour. If it slips to the side, bring it back to the centre and keep concentrating until the image fades completely. Now open the eyes and resume gazing at the candle. Continue in this way for ten minutes at first, gradually increasing the time until you can sit comfortably for a full twenty-minutes.

A flower or a bowl

Some people begin their visualizing techniques with a flower. One expert tells his novice pupils to gaze at a patterned china bowl, taking it all in at first, then allowing the eyes to travel over it, tracing its lines and colours, the pattern that decorates it, the way it catches the light. Only when his pupils come to experience the bowl's visual qualities for the first time, does he move on to telling them to close their eyes and try to focus on the image of the bowl held in the mind.

It takes practice

At first, it is hard to hold a mental picture of the object, but with practice it becomes easier and easier until the point is reached when the actual object can be abandoned completely and you can meditate on the mental image with no external visual stimulus being used. This can be extremely difficult, and if you have been successful with the alternating method but have had problems when you have tried to meditate holding a mental image in your mind for the entire session, you have probably been trying too hard or expecting too much. It can take years of practice before you can see the image clearly. Think of the mind as a musical instrument that has to be tuned with patience and sensitivity before it can be used to produce beautiful music.

Some who practise visual meditation find it helps to train the mind by closing the eyes and picturing a friend, concentrating on each feature in turn, the colour of the skin and hair, the shape and colour of the eyes, and so on, and then returning to the complete face, holding on to the image for as long as they can, and when it starts to blur, focusing again on the separate features.

Many different symbols

Roman Catholics and Anglicans have long used the image of Christ on the cross as a symbol in visualization meditation. Christians who belong to the 'low' Churches often meditate on the empty cross, while many people who belong to the Orthodox Church use small painted panels bearing an image of Christ or the Virgin Mary or any of the saints as visualization symbols.

Buddhists may meditate on a mental image of Buddha himself or one of the other Buddhas, especially Tara, the liberator, the mother of all Buddhas. They see her as the manifestation of all that is positive. Bathed in radiant emerald-green light, swathed in silk and bedecked with jewels, she smiles lovingly at those who focus their meditations on her.

Jewish meditators might visualize the Tree of Life that represents the *Sefirot,* or ten divine energies.

The *Visuddhimagga,* a fourth-century Buddhist text, lists ten different subjects for visual meditation. These are known as *kasinas* and comprise air, earth, fire and water (the four elements), blue, yellow, red and green (the four colours of nature), light and space. To meditate on any of the elements, the meditator simply stares at an appropriate object, a pot filled with earth, for example, or a bowl of water. To visualize any of the four colours, simply gaze at an object of that colour—a flower, a piece of fabric, anything at all. To meditate on light, focus the attention on the light cast by a lightbulb, and any empty container can be used as a focus when meditating on space.

Buddhists, in common with Hindus, also use *mandalas*, the most famous of which is probably the Buddhist wheel of life, and Hindus commonly meditate on *yantras* (*see* below).

Chinese meditators often use the famous yin-yang symbol. It looks like a white tadpole with a black eye and a black tadpole with a white eye, curled up against each other, their outline forming a perfect circle representing tai chi (supreme ultimate).

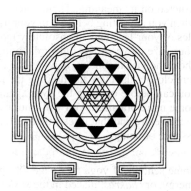

This is an example of a mandala

Yantras and mandalas

To scholars of Sanskrit, *yantra* is a word meaning 'instrument', and *mandala* is a word that means 'circle'—the supreme universal symbol. To the meditator, a yantra is a diagram that possesses the power to transform the consciousness of those who have been introduced to knowledge of what the yantras represent.

A mandala is essentially a type of yantra, the yantra being more specific to a particular deity, the mandala being more general. Both are diagrammatic in form, designed so that the focus of the meditator comes to rest on a central focal point, the *bindu,* which is said to represent the essence of being.

They can be astonishingly beautiful to look at, especially those of Tibetan Tantric Buddhists whose richly symbolic and gloriously designed mandalas have come to be prized by collectors as works of art.

(There is another aspect of Tantric Buddhism that westerners find fascinating, mistaking it more often than not as an indulgence of the sexual appetites rather than a tool for meditation—*maithuna,* or ritual sexual intercourse. Those who practise it claim that it is a potent means of allowing *kundalini* energy—the force awakened by meditation on the chakras (*see* below)—to be released, allowing the yogi to move on to meditating a higher chakra. Before performing *maithuna,* the yogi performs certain rituals and recites the mantra given to him by his guru as well as other mantras that are part of the rituals. Maithuna must be carried out in the prescribed manner, the yogi having been taught exactly where and how he may touch his partner's body. It is the female who is active during maithuna, since its aim is the arousal of energy rather than the climax, at which moment the yogi consecrates his semen as a sacrificial offering.)

The lotus blossom, the symbol of enlightenment, is widely used as part of the patterns, symbolizing the unfolding of creation. According to Hindu mythology, Brahma stood at the centre of a thousand-petalled lotus before creating the universe, and Buddhists believe that at the birth of the Buddha, a large lotus sprang from the earth, and Buddha stepped into its centre. From there he gazed into the ten directions of space, once along each of the eight petals, once upwards and once downwards.

Mandalas and yantras may be drawn, painted or carved in stone. Some eastern mystics even meditate on yantras that they draw for themselves in the sand or earth. Such temporary ones often serve as teaching aids between master and pupils.

Meditating with a mandala or yantra

Before you can meditate with a mandala or yantra you will have to be instructed on its meaning. Then, place it so that the central point is at eye level when you are sitting before it in your usual meditating position. Relax the muscles of your face and sit absolutely motionless, gazing at the centre point. Let your gaze move slowly outwards to the edge, taking in but trying not to think about the visual content. Now let the gaze move slowly back to the centre before closing the eyes and holding the image in your mind's eye for as long as you can before opening the eyes again and repeating the process. As you become more practised, you will find that your eye will automatically be drawn to the centre and that it rests there effortlessly on the point that symbolizes the essence of being.

Chakras

Some schools of yoga (*see* page 48), believe that there are centres of psychic energy, or *chakras,* placed in the *sushumna,* the central canal of the astral body roughly corresponding to the spinal column in the physical body. The chakras sit at various points between the base of the spine and the top of the head. Two schools of yoga, Tantric and Kundalini, practise meditation on each of them in turn.

Each chakra has its own yantra and its own mantra (apart from the topmost one). Starting with the lowest of them, the *muladhara,* situated between the anus and genitals, the meditator visualizes its yantra while repeating its mantra, either inwardly or aloud, until ready to move on.

As the meditation works its way through the chakra, the latent energy of each one is released, imbuing the meditator with stronger and stronger sensations of warmth and light at the centre until, when the final meditation is completed, the physical will have merged with the spiritual—the meditator's consciousness merges with the universe.

Each chakra is adorned with its own number of lotus petals, governed by the number of the body channels that conjoin at that point in the astral body. The muladhara is adorned with four such petals and its mantra is '*lam*'. In ascending order the chakras are the six-petalled *svadhishtana*: its mantra is '*vam*'. The *manipura* has ten petals and its mantra is '*ram*'. Next comes the *anahata*,with twelve petals and the mantra '*yam*'. Then, with sixteen petals and the mantra '*ham*', is the *vishuddha* chakra. The *ajna* chakra, with its two petals and the mantra '*om*' is next, followed by the topmost, the *sahasrara*, or thousand-petal chakra, which has no mantra.

Anyone wishing to practise this form of meditation needs detailed instruction from an experienced teacher over a long period of time, but the following meditation may give you just a flavour of the full effect.

The space between the eyebrows meditation

This space corresponds to the ajna chakra. Sit, kneel or lie in your usual position with your eyes closed. Gently swivel your eyeballs upwards and try to visualize them as focused on the space between your eyebrows. See how close this space is to the brain—feel its central position, visualize viewing it from the outside: now visualize it from the inside. The space between the eyebrows is a part of you. As the meditation deepens feel yourself becoming a part of that space. If unwanted thoughts intrude, mentally blow them away and return your focus to the space between the eyebrows.

It is not possible here to describe the whys and wherefores of every type of visual meditation. But the ones described below have all been used successfully by meditators the world over.

Colour visualizing

There are many methods of using colour as a means of reaching the meditative state. The two given here are among the simplest.

For the first, sit in whichever position you favour and begin to breathe deeply. As usual, don't force the breath, but let it find its own pace and depth. When it has settled to a slow, rhythmic rate, begin to visualize the colours red, orange and yellow, flowing upwards into your solar plexus, visualizing each colour one at a time as a gently flowing river.

Spend a minute or so on each colour and then picture a stream of green flowing into the solar plexus from directly in front of you. After a minute or so, follow the green with blue, indigo and violet, each in turn flowing into you from the same source as the green.

Once the spectrum is completed, imagine yourself bathed in a blue light before ending the meditation by opening your eyes.

Don't be put off if at first you find it difficult to visualize a colour: with practice this becomes easier.

The second method is to sit with eyes closed before focusing the thoughts on any colour you wish. Fill your mind with that colour to the exclusion of everything else and refuse to be frustrated by other thoughts that may come to mind. Wrap them slowly in the colour so that they are enveloped in it. It sometimes helps to imagine an object of your chosen shade—a field of yellow corn perhaps—and gradually concentrate your thoughts on it until the field becomes totally unimportant and your mind is a canvas of yellow. (Some people who practise colour meditation, in fact, begin each session by picturing an easel on which rests a blank canvas that stroke by stroke fills up with the chosen colour.)

Body of light visualizing

This is an advanced meditation. Sit comfortably with your back straight, breathing naturally. When your mind is clear and calm, visualize the space above your head as a sphere of white light slightly smaller in size than your head. Try to see it as pure and transparent, and spend several minutes concentrating on it.

See the sphere of light as representing goodness, wisdom and love—as the fulfilment of your own highest potential. Then visualize that it is getting smaller and smaller until it is about two centimetres in diameter and that slowly it begins to descend through your head towards your heart, then begins to expand once more until it spreads to every part of your body. As it does so, see it dissolve all the organs and solid parts of your body until they too become pure, formless white light.

Concentrate on the perception of your body as a mass of light and believe all your problems, negative emotions and the things that hold you back have vanished. Let any thoughts or distractions dissolve in the light, and with practice you will achieve a joyful serenity and reach a state of wholeness and perfection.

Purification visualizing

Purification is a recurring theme in Buddhist meditation. When we see ourselves as impure or negative, that is what we become. With our self-esteem at a low ebb we feel limited and inadequate and don't give ourselves a chance to change. Believing we are pure in essence is the first step to becoming pure in practice.

This simple meditation contains the essence of purification, banishing problems and mistakes, trying to see them as temporary instructions, not as part of our nature.

Begin by settling comfortably into a suitable position, then concentrate on breathing normally and observing how long each exhalation and inhalation lasts. After a minute or two, imagine that all your negative energy, the mistakes you have made in the past, the things that are holding you back are leaving your body in a cloud of black smoke each time you breathe out. When you inhale, visualize that everything positive in the universe is entering your body in a stream of white light, as radiant as it is pure. Visualize it flowing to every part of your body, bathing it in its intensity.

Banish distractions by seeing them as black smoke and exhale them along with the other negative aspects of your experience.

Bubbles of thought meditation

Sitting in a comfortable position, visualize your mind as the smooth, calm surface of a pond. As thoughts enter your mind, see them as bubbles rising from the depths of the pond. They should be observed, not pursued, so that the conscious and deliberate following through of each thought is avoided and you become detached from it as you watch it bubble to the surface. Note the thought and then gently return to contemplating the smooth, rippleless surface of the pond.

As time passes and you pass into deeper layers of consciousness, see yourself sinking under the surface of the pond, becoming one with it.

After about 10 minutes, refocus your mind on your surroundings to bring the meditation to an end.

Inner heat meditation

This is an extremely advanced meditation requiring sophisticated breathing techniques as well as visualization. It is included here as an example of the most demanding meditation techniques. It was developed by a Tibetan Buddhist who believed that mental energy flows through the body within an invisible psychic nervous system made up of thousands of thin, transparent channels. The principal ones—the central, right and left channels—run parallel to and just in front of the spinal column. Pure mental energy can function within the central channel whereas diluted (deluded) energy flows through the others.

In our normal state, the central channel is blocked by knots of nervous energy at the various chakras discussed above. This energy blocks pure energy from the mind, making it unable to function properly.

Inner heat meditation is an excellent method for transforming powerful negative energy, helping us to develop spontaneous control over all actions of body, speech and mind.

Begin by adopting your usual meditation posture, settle your thoughts and your breathing, and visualize the central channel as a transparent, hollow tube, about the same diameter as your forefinger, running straight down the centre of the body just in front of the spinal column, from the crown of your head to the base of your spine.

Now visualize the left and right channels, slightly thinner than the central one, starting from the left and right nostril respectively, reaching up to the top of the head then curving to run downwards on either side of the central channel before curving inwards to join the central channel about a hand's breadth below the navel.

Take your time. There is no hurry whatsoever, and once the visualization (some people say it helps to see it as a very simple central heating system) is firmly fixed, imagine a red-hot ember the size of a seed inside the central channel level with the navel. If it helps to strengthen this visualization, see yourself reaching into a fire and taking out a small ember that you put in place.

When you really feel the intense heat, gently contract the lower pelvic muscles and see air energy rising from the lowest chakra up to the ember. Now breathe deeply through both nostrils, seeing the air travelling down the left and right channels round into the central channel, where it joins with the heat and air energy brought up from below.

When you have inhaled, swallow and push down gently with the diaphragm, compressing the energy brought down from above: the air energy is locked in, trapped from above and below.

Now hold the breath as long as possible without forcing it and concentrate on the glowing ember in the navel area, its heat now spreading through the compressed air energy.

When you breathe out, visualize the warm air rising through the central channel, seeing it burn away the negative energies blocking each of the chakras.

Repeat the cycle seven times, intensifying the heat with each breath. By the time you breathe out for the seventh time, visualize the ember bursting into flames, shooting up the central channel and burning out the remaining negative energy in the chakras. When the flames reach the crown of the head, they melt into wonderful, almost sensual, energy that rushes down the now pure central channel, intensifying in pleasure as it passes each chakra, finally engulfing the remains of the ember and making it explode in a blissful heat that reaches every cell of your body, filling you with happiness.

If you ever succeed in this meditation, don't try to analyse the bliss, just accept it, relax, enjoy and concentrate on it calmly and in a controlled manner. It is, as we said, extremely complex, but those who have mastered it believe it is, the best of all visual meditation techniques.

Visual meditation and health

Although the following is not meditation in the true sense of the word, visualization is required, and we demonstrate how it can be used to treat two specific health problems. Space precludes us from dealing with more ailments and how they may be treated, but if you try the ones discussed below, perhaps you may be tempted to look further into this area: it can be extremely rewarding.

Assume your usual meditation posture unless your malady prevents it, in which case, make yourself as comfortable as you can with the back as straight as you can get it and the head in perfect alignment. Concentrate on your breathing for a moment or two until it becomes settled and regular.

For *painful joints,* picture the affected area in your mind and visualize the blood vessels leading to and from it congested with dark red blood. Notice how taut the muscles are and how tangled the nerves. With this image firmly fixed, see a tide of pink, oxygen-full blood enriched with healing white cells flood through the veins and arteries. Observe how the muscles relax and your nerves untangle. Hold this image in your mind and then visualize the whole area again free from congestion, the muscles working smoothly, the nerves strands of polished wire. Let the image fade from view and, hopefully, the pain will have eased.

For *bronchial problems,* visualize your lungs clogged with dark yellow mucus. Now see the colour lighten, starting from the bottom of each lung until the mucous membranes are producing just enough mucus to keep the lungs properly lubricated and there is a ball of mucus being pushed up your throat and coughed out. You should be breathing much more easily at the end of this visualization.

Similar techniques, where the affected area is visualized first in its stricken state then as being cleansed before being seen in perfect working order, can be applied to a whole host of complaints. When all else fails, why not try them?

Other techniques to try

Tactile meditation

Before you begin, choose an object to hold while you are meditating—something light, for if it is too heavy its weight will affect your concentration and hence your focus. It need not be soft, but it should not be sharp. Now close your eyes and concentrate on the texture of the object in your hand, focusing on how it feels rather than what it is.

Another method of using touch to help reach the meditative state requires either a set of worry beads or four or five pebbles. Relax in your favourite position, holding the beads or pebbles in the open palm of one hand and with the other move them rhythmically and methodically between your fingers, counting them one at a time.

Feel each bead or pebble as you count, focusing all your attention on the slow, repetitive movement.

Music and meditation

The relevance of music as an aid to meditation is a personal one. Its effect depends on facilitating your meditations, and that in turn depends on your own instincts and intuitions.

Percussion instruments have long been used in meditation, especially where it is practised by atavists. The music they produce symbolizes rhythm and vitality.

Gongs and bells are said to purify the surrounding atmosphere making it more conducive to meditation. Many religions use peals of bells to help their adherents regather wandering thoughts. If you want to use bells as an aid to meditation, focus your thoughts on the sound, trying to experience it beyond audibility.

Harps have long been associated with meditation. In China the *cheng* and other zither-like instruments are widely used, while in India, the sitar and the vina accompany meditative chanting.

The gentle tinkling of the Aeolian harp can create a perfectly calm state of mind as you approach your meditations, and help you to focus your thought.

To meditate to music, take up your usual position, close your eyes and listen to a favourite piece, immersing yourself in it completely. Try to become one with the sound, letting the sound encompass you, and if your thoughts are invaded by memories associated with the piece you have selected, imagine them as musical notes floating off into the distance.

Transcendental meditation

Transcendental meditation, or TM, involves concentrating on a particular sound, or mantra. Many instructors make a point of issuing each person with a mantra to suit his or her individual nervous system, but there is no scientific data to prove that this in any way increases the benefits of meditation. There is, however, much to be said about choosing one word or syllable and using it as a mantra. One word or sound can have very personal connotations, and repeating it can quieten the mind and aid concentration, becoming in the process a channel for the flow of peacefulness and strength throughout the body.

If meditation is new to you, experiment with postures, background sounds, mantras, etc, until you find what suits you. It is important that you make an effort every day, even if only for five minutes at first, and stick at it. It may take some time before you find a routine that works for you, but if you are willing to spend that time on yourself then eventually you will reap the rewards.

Zen meditation

The word 'Zen' derives from the Sanskrit *dhyana,* meaning 'meditation'. With its roots in the Yisuddhimagga tradition, it is widely practised in Japan, having arrived there through the Ch'an meditation school of China.

Zen's main practice is *zazen,* or sitting on a cushion facing a wall, and is done daily by those who practise it, usually adopting the full lotus position. Meditation sessions are quite lengthy, hence, in zazen, great stress is placed on correct posture. The body is held upright, and it should be theoretically possible to draw a line from the centre of the forehead down through the nose, chin, throat, navel into the coccyx at the tail of the spine. Every part of the body must be in balance: if it is not, incorrect balance in one part of the body will cause strain in another and ruin the meditation.

The left hand rests within the right, the middle joints of the middle fingers touching, with the thumbs, also lightly touching each other, held at the navel and the arms slightly away from the rest of the body.

Apart from the fact that novices to Zen are sometimes advised to count their breaths, from one to ten, and the use of *koan (see* below), zazen uses no mantra, mandala or other object of meditation. In zazen, thoughts are allowed to come and go without being banished by the meditator, who remains attentive and alert throughout the meditation, concentrating on sitting as still as possible in a state of quiet awareness.

Zen masters often ask their pupils impenetrable questions, known as koan, an unanswerable puzzle designed to precipitate awakening by breaking through the limited confines of consciousness. A common one is 'What was your face before you were born?' From then on, whenever the koan comes to mind, the pupil banishes all other thoughts and concentrates on his *koan.* As he comes to realize that there is no answer *per se*, he reaches a state that has been described by those who have achieved it as 'feverish concentration', from which arises 'supreme frustration', and with conscious thought transcended, the pupil attains *samadhi,* the state of total concentration.

The first koan is said to have arisen when the great Zen master Hui-neng was attacked by robbers. He begged them to be silent for a moment and then said to them, 'When you are thinking of neither good nor evil, what is at that moment your original face?' The assailants were so astonished that they begged Hui for an explanation. The master sent them on their way, and the men found that the question came to dominate their thoughts to such an extent that when something else came to mind, they banished it and resumed their meditation on the question until they found they had arrived at samadhi.

Yoga

Yoga is a technique of self-awareness that integrates the mind and the body. The word derives from the Sanskrit *yuj* meaning 'to bind together', and through practising yoga, the yogi tries to bind himself with the universal process of being.

Yoga recognizes the interrelatedness of mind and body. Hatha yoga teaches techniques of physical control of the body through postures known as *asanas* and breathing techniques called *pranayama*. The asanas make the body supple and benefit the neuromuscular system, each posture combining mental acuity with breathing techniques and a specific body movement. Pranayama builds up the body's energy.

Yoga is a means of seeing things as they really are rather than as they seem. In Yoga, all body and mental tensions have to cease if this end is to be achieved. Accordingly, one of the basic yoga techniques is meditation, which turns our consciousness towards the inner calm helping us to achieve *samadhi,* or pure consciousness.

The dharanas

Yoga is perhaps the only discipline that encourages meditation on sex. Such meditation is found in the *Vijnanabhairava,* an ancient book on yoga that is essentially a dialogue between Shiva and his enlightened consort. When she asks Shiva how the supreme state can be realized, Shiva suggests 112 *dharanas* or centring techniques, that enable those who practise them to attain divine consciousness. Among the dharanas is one that suggests meditating on the delights of a remembered intensely pleasurable sexual experience. In practice, the meditator must turn his or her attention away from the actual experience and trace the pleasure back to its source—the inner self.

The *Vijnanabhairava* also promotes the Hamsah meditation technique. By it, the meditator watches the breath going in and coming out, making a *ha* sound with each inhalation and a *sah* sound to accompany each exhalation. The *m* is inserted between the two other sounds. Hamsah is often called 'the universal mantra'.

See also Hinduism page 135; and Yoga, page 48.

Grabbing the moment meditation

Once you gain experience in meditating, it is possible to go into meditative mode for short periods whenever you need to. All it takes to meditate in this way is a few seconds of concentrated focus, and you will find yourself refreshed and ready to cope with stress. We have used the right hand in some of the meditations described below: if you are left-handed, use the thumb and two fingers of the left hand instead.

The wedding ring meditation

To meditate on your wedding ring, simply inhale deeply and bring the tip of the thumb on whichever hand you wear your wedding ring into contact with the first two fingers so that the ring finger is slightly raised. As you exhale slowly, focus your eyes on the ring, gazing at a glint that catches the light. Repeat four or five times.

The red light meditation

Next time you are held up at traffic lights, stare at the red light with both eyes, willing yourself into it. Breathe in and out slowly as many times as you can until the lights change, and you will take off in a better frame of mind than before.

Meditation at work

Most people have jobs that involve doing the same thing day after day, be it something as active as waiting tables in a restaurant or as sedentary as working in an office in front of a computer. Most people at some time or other during their working day find themselves drifting off into their own thoughts: use this time to improve your work efficiency by meditating. The moment you first realize you are lost in thought, visualize a blank screen and then picture yourself on that screen, seeing yourself work faster and more productively, more safely and more creatively, than you have ever worked before. Try to hold this image for a moment or two, and in time you should find yourself working more efficiently and getting more out of the job too.

Spot meditation

Breathe in deeply and touch the tip of the first two fingers of your right hand with your right thumb. As you breathe out focus your attention on the first thing that catches your eyes and maintain the focus for four or five more breathing cycles.

Pain relief meditation

If you suddenly feel pain, for instance if you stand up too quickly and find you have an agonizing pain in the back, focus your thoughts on the part of the body that is aching. Again join the thumb and first two fingers of the right hand and breathe deeply taking the breath right into the pain. As you breathe out, see the pain being carried away on your expired breath.

Countdown to calmness

For a brief meditation that brings instant calm, breathe in, once more touching the tip of the thumb with the tips of the first two fingers of the right hand. Breathe out slowly, counting down from ten to zero as you do so and visualizing each number in turn in your mind's eye, watching one fade as it is replaced by the next. When you reach zero, you will be infused with a feeling of serenity you thought out of reach a few moments before.

Back to the future

Find an old photograph of yourself and focus your attention on it. Project the image you are looking at forward to the present and try to see if the person is still you. Then let him or her fade back into the photograph. After the meditation try and work out if the boy or girl in the photograph would be happy with what he or she has become. If so, good for you: if not, by taking up meditation you have at least taken a step in the right direction.

Postscript

Once you have learned to meditate, it is a skill that you will have for the rest of your life, but while it will give you a sense of inner serenity it does not mean that you are free of pressures and disturbing emotions. Meditation is not an escape from these problems: it enables you to see them as something you can deal with.

Once you have become used to meditation, you will find you can practise it anywhere—on a train, in an aeroplane, at your office desk during the course of a working day.

And remember there is no right way to meditate and no wrong way to meditate. The only right way is the one that you are most comfortable with, the one that enables you to get out of meditation whatever it is you want.

Psychotherapy

Resolving problems in the mind

Professional therapy

Psychotherapy involves exploring and seeking to resolve problems by talking to a professionally trained person who is skilled at helping people to find a way forward through their difficulties. There are many different forms and approaches in psychotherapy, and most involve the person having to delve into his or her inner thoughts and feelings in a process of self-discovery. The psychotherapist guides the person through this process, helping the patient to bring problems to the surface so that they can be examined and resolved. In many cases, there may be deep-seated fears and problems that the patient has suppressed for many years. These may be the cause of the feelings and worries that the person is currently experiencing.

Sessions of treatment in psychotherapy may be on a short or long-term basis depending upon the nature of the patient's problems. Some forms of psychotherapy concentrate on resolving one particular problem with the patient following advice given by the therapist. Usually, these are shorter forms of therapy although it is not unusual for deeper problems to emerge that require further and more lengthy exploration. In all forms of psychotherapy it is important that a good relationship of mutual trust and confidence is built up between patient and therapist. It may be necessary for the patient to consult more than one therapist in the first instance, to find the one with whom he or she feels most at ease.

Therapy involving discussion between therapist and client need not be organized by a doctor specializing in mental illness, and the client undergoing the therapy need not be mentally ill. He or she may just feel that there is something wrong with life and be seeking help, or someone who knows the person may well have recommended such a course of action. The person in charge of the therapy programme will not be a psychiatrist but a psychoanalyst or psychotherapist.

A word of warning is necessary here for anyone contemplating this kind of therapy. Psychiatrists are qualified doctors, usually attached to a hospital, and people are usually referred to them by a general practitioner. You can have confidence, therefore, in his or her training, even if you do not get on with the actual person. This is not the case, however, with all psychotherapists.

Many psychotherapists hold a suitable professional qualification, such as a degree in psychology, and some may even be medical doctors, but there is nothing to prevent anyone setting up in business without such qualifications. Some people would argue that it is the skills of the therapist, not the qualifications, that count, but it is as well to check up on the nature of these skills first.

Many general practitioners will be able to make a recommendation. Failing this, do try to get hold of a personal recommendation from someone who has previously attended, and been satisfied with the psychotherapist. An attempt has been made to set up a register for therapists, and you could probably obtain details of this from your local library. You must feel that you can trust the person to whom you are entrusting your mind.

To some extent the skills required by the psychotherapist are those required by the successful psychiatrist. For a start, they must have good listening skills and have the ability to get people to talk about themselves, without revealing any reaction of condemnation or shock. Both need skill in interpreting what they hear from the client.

Resolving problems

Often the problems that the clients of a psychotherapist have are not too dissimilar from those of the patients of a psychiatrist. Sometimes the difference is only one of degree. For example, two different people might feel that something is not right in their lives and might put this fact down to a bad relationship with a parent—sometimes physical or sexual abuse might be involved—but it is the extent to which this has affected the individual and what he or she decides to do about it that makes the difference.

One may become completely obsessed with the problem—something like the death of a parent, or the birth of a child may set this off. His or her mind ceases to be able to function in the way it normally does, and he or she becomes mentally ill. Medical help has to be sought, and the general practitioner recommends referral to a psychiatrist.

Another person who has much the same problem may not be mentally affected by it to nearly the same extent but may be conscious of the effect it is having on his or her life—perhaps he or she is having difficulties in forming lasting relationships. The person realizes that help must be sought and thinks of psychotherapy.

Psychoanalysis

The basis of modern psychoanalysis and psychotherapy goes back to the Austrian psychiatrist Sigmund Freud, the originator of psychoanalysis. The disciplines seek to tap into the subconscious of the individual undergoing analysis or therapy and to release any hidden fears and to unblock any repressed emotions. By these means, people seek to discover more about themselves.

The major difference between psychoanalysis and psychotherapy is that, as the name suggests, the latter seeks to heal. The suppressed fears and emotions that emerge from analysis are not an end in themselves but a means by which the healing process may begin. By unblocking the subconscious, the therapist tries to help the client towards a better understanding of himself or herself and to help him or her cope more effectively with life in the light of this understanding.

The psychoanalytic technique originated at the start of the 20th century with Freud's treatment of hysteria . With his collaborator, Austrian neurologist Josef Breuer, he hypnotised his patients to analyse their subconscious minds. Later on, in collaboration with Jean Martin Charcot he was able to access the subconscious in the normal waking state through a method called *free association*, where the patient was allowed to say whatever came into his or her mind, sometimes giving important clues to painful and poignant memories, through *resistance*—the points at which he or she changed the topic or forgot what they were trying to say.

Freud theorised that neuroses are caused by repressed sexual urges and these could be interpreted through the analysis of dream symbols. The symbol itself is the *manifest content*, what the symbol really represents is known as the *latent content*, and it is this latent content that the dream interpreter seeks to find.

Genuine self-discovery can only be achieved when the patient rids him or herself of the repressive forces that keep emotional insights locked safely away. Freud had the theory of *catharsis*—the recovery of certain repressed memories bringing with them a host of associated strong emotions. But the benefits of such retrieval of emotions in such a manner was thought to have dubious benefits and such emotional releases are thought to have only a temporary therapeutic effect.

Modern versions of psychoananlysis still use tecniques that originated with Freud at least in part, with rather less emphasis on the psychosexual element that dominates Freud's theories.

The psychotherapist

The role of the psychotherapist is to listen and interpret what the client is saying. Some people feel that simply talking to a complete stranger is, in fact, therapeutic. Friends and members of the family may be too involved, overemotional, or even condemnatory or judgmental, and are often too busy to really listen. The psychotherapist is someone who is totally uninvolved and detached, whose good opinion or otherwise does not matter, and who has time to listen. Furthermore—and this is an important part of psychotherapy—the talking can go on over a longish period of time, often quite a few months, so that there is no sense of rush. There is plenty of time to explore past experiences and relationships. The person with a problem feels that at last there is someone there to listen and help.

The basic aim of analysis and therapy may not vary from one therapist to another, but the method of approach does. Some of them are closer to the techniques of Freud than others and advocate that clients say anything that comes into their heads, using a kind of free association as a means of unblocking the unconscious. Other therapists may prompt the client with a few gentle leading questions, especially as a means of getting each session started.

Some adopt a more formal, traditional approach than others and ask the client to lie on a sofa in such a way that he or she is unable to see the therapist. External stimuli are reduced to a minimum in an effort to get the client to concentrate as much as possible on his or her own thoughts. Others regard this as being too rigid an approach and choose to talk to their clients in a less formal setting, although the therapists themselves are never intrusive.

Many people find psychotherapy a very useful and rewarding therapy. At the very least they can talk about things they have never dreamt of speaking about before and can learn to face up to them. They can learn to come to terms with the past and be able to reach some understanding of how the past, with its suppressed fears and emotions, has effected their present and prevented them living life to the full. People can feel much more comfortable with themselves, and be able to go forward in a much more relaxed and confident way to build a future.

Behaviour therapy

Behaviour therapy deals with the modification of abnormal behaviour, e.g. phobias or obsessional behaviour, and involves systems of gradual densensitization and counter-conditioning to promote a more normal response to the stimuli. The patient constructs a list of scenes he or she would not find at all stressful working up to a scene which provokes unbearable anxiety. A patient with a life-long snake phobia might, for example, have to imagine and talk about drawings of snakes and snake-like things, then progress to photographs of earth-worms, then perhaps handling earth-worms and so on until the patient can imagine the most fear-arousing scene—an encounter with a real snake with the normal amount of anxiety expected.

For patients coping with an addiction (e.g. to drugs, alcohol or food), aversive therapy links the subtance they desire with unpleasant feelings. An alcoholic may be forced to drink some alcohol after he has been given a nausea-inducing drug. Outside the therapist's office, however, this therapy probably has very little effect.

Behaviour therapy also includes those therapies which seek to socially educate the patient, such as through step-by-step training in assertiveness, or through role-paying

Humanistic therapies

The humanistic approach is more patient-centred, that is, encouraging the patient to help himself through non-directive techniques that never advise the patient but reiterate what the patient has seemed to express his or herself. One exponent of this system was Carl Rogers in the early 1940s. This technique holds that personality development is like growth but that sometimes this growth is stunted because the patient is out of touch with his or her own feelings. It is the therapist's role to create a relationship between therapist and client that allows the feelings to be released and for growth to resume. Humanistic therapists have to have an empathic role, unconditionally accepting patients to show them that they are held in esteem and so that they in turn may feel their own self worth.

Visualization Therapy

The positive effects of a content state of mind

It is now widely accepted that the mind exerts a great deal of influence on the health of the body. People with a cheerful, optimistic outlook on life often experience better health than those who are gloomy and pessimistic. In the case of some serious illnesses such as cancer, it is recognized that people who maintain a positive and determined attitude often do better than those who are passive or fatalistic. In these instances, life in both its extent and quality appear to be affected by the person's state of mind. In visualization therapy it is recognized that the pictures created by the mind (as well as thoughts), can have powerful positive or negative effects on the health of the body. Those using this technique believe that it not only helps people suffering from stress and psychological and emotional problems, but also patients with physical illnesses and symptoms. These include cancer, rheumatic and arthritic disorders and other painful conditions.

In visualization therapy, the patient is first taught the technique of creating a mental image. A person suffering from an emotional or psychological problem is asked to create a picture that is connected with his or her difficulty. The feelings created by the image are explored and discussed with the therapist and changes are made to the picture that, with time, help to resolve the problem. This is how visualization differs from visual meditation. In visual meditation the visual image way well be a symbolic one, but it's only purpose is to empty the mind of all other distraction.

For people with physical illnesses, the image created is often aimed at helping to relieve and ease pain by creating an image of the diseased or painful area and make adjustments to it with the aim of reducing the impact of the symptoms, though its benefits in the treatment of physical disorders remain controversial.

This form of treatment is normally used with other techniques. It is beneficial for people suffering from stress and emotional problems. Children often respond well to visualization therapy as they are naturally imaginative and find it easy to create mental pictures.

Whatever we create in our lives, whether it is an omelette or a multinational corporation or a love affair, begins as an image in our minds. Inner images that we may have formed long ago, and are now outside our conscious awareness, shape and often limit our ability to make creative life choices and changes. Through image work—or visualization—it is possible to tap into, explore, and change these inner programmes that guide our lives, and to identify and bring about the future that is really right for us.

Visualization promotes relaxation and relaxation promotes visualization. Each session should start with a simple programme as follows.

Progressive relaxation

Clear a space

Take a moment to give yourself permission to rest. Mentally or physically clear a space, which is your personal territory and is not to be intruded on by worry, phone calls, or other internal or external demands. If there is anything you feel worried about, settle your mind by simply writing it down to look at later.

Begin to relax

Sit quietly and focus on your breathing for a moment. Give a few long, loud sighs, feeling that each sigh starts at the top of your head and travels down through you, coming out of the soles of your feet. Whether your eyes are open or closed, roll your eyeballs up toward the ceiling, then let them drop. Notice any tension in your body and then let go of it. Imagine that you are sending a breath of peace to every part of your body. Remind yourself that you have nothing to do, and no place to go, and nothing you need worry about just now.

Relax body and mind

Focus on each part of your body in turn, starting with your feet. First be aware of how they feel. Now tense them, and then let them relax, sending the breath of peace there. Say to yourself, 'My foot is heavy and relaxed, and as it relaxes I feel a deep sense of peace through me.' Or simply repeat, 'Heavy and warm, warm and relaxed.' Move up your body in this way, until your whole body is included in the itinerary: 'My shoulders relaxed and peaceful, my torso and legs relaxed and peaceful, my feet warm, relaxed and peaceful. . . .' When you reach your face and head, include your scalp, the muscles round your eyes, your lips, tongue and throat.

Let the relaxation enter your mind. Imagine that there is a little person in your head, sweeping out all the thoughts and worries. Then he paints the inside of your brain with a white light.

Allow dark heaviness to descend and lightness to rise

If your eyes are not already closed, let them close, and imagine that your eyelids are dark, heavy blinds that are impossible to raise. Imagine that you have a dark, heavy blind at the top of your head, and pull this blind down through your body, letting the heaviness sink into the ground. Allow a feeling of lightness to emerge from the ground through your body and into your mind. Let your mind or spirit feel light, and float up, as if through a hole in the top of your head, and float out and away, like a kite in a summer sky.

Invite an image to deepen relaxation

Think of a time when you were completely relaxed and feeling good about yourself. You may have been listening to music, or doing something active like swimming in the sea. When you have conjured up this picture, step into the picture, and match your breathing to that of the relaxed you in the picture.

Alternatively, in your mind travel to a place where you have been, or could be, very happy. This can be a real place or an imagined one. In this place, there is a feeling of deep peace. Creating an inner sanctuary like this can be valuable for future visualization sessions, when you can return to your own personal haven.

Countdown to deeper relaxation

Say to yourself, 'I am going to count down from ten to one, and with each number I will feel more and more relaxed and more in touch with my inner self.'

Create a relaxation cue

When you feel completely at peace, allow an image—or a word—to arise that sums up this feeling, and touch together the thumb and forefinger of either hand. Say to yourself, 'As I repeat this image or word and touch, I feel more and more relaxed and at peace, and each time I use it in the future it will bring back this wonderful feeling, and the more I use it, the better it will work.'

Now practise your visualization—emerge

When you have finished your visualization session, and want to emerge from your deeply relaxed state, suggest to yourself, 'I am going to count up from one to five and with each number I will feel more and more awake, but still relaxed. When I reach five, I will open my eyes feeling relaxed and alert, as if I have woken from a long, refreshing sleep.'

The image as metaphor

The most basic use of visualization involves inviting an image to emerge in response to a question, and then working with the image. The images that come in this way have the powerful ability to sum up with a telling metaphor the basic structure of whatever it is you are asking about. The metaphor tends to be so accurate that the more you explore it, the more it can seem to correspond on every level and in every detail, not only with the specific problem but with your life as a whole. Suddenly the implicit becomes explicit and a resolution emerges.

Begin by encouraging an image to emerge, and then study it from a number of perspectives. Then enter the image, and deepen the exploration from inside it. Finally, look back and get a sense of what led up to the present situation, and look forward to what is the next step for you. Try out this step in your mind.

Begin by clearing a space and relaxing, as described above. Now invite an image to emerge. Say: 'I would like to allow an image to emerge of an animal, plant or object that somehow represents who I am or what I need to know at this moment in my life: the first image that comes to mind, whether as a word, a picture, a sound or a fleeting sense. This image is now sitting in the chair opposite.'

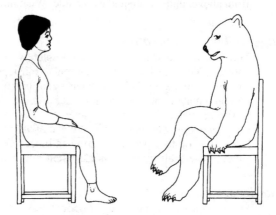

When the image emerges, say, 'Thank you, Unconscious. I appreciate the gift.'

If nothing happens, try the following strategies until something emerges:
• Looking back over the past few days, remembering everything I have seen, I notice one memory image that seems to draw my attention. That image is now in the chair opposite me.

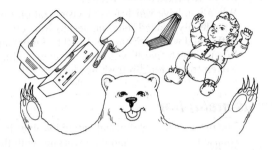

- I imagine that my unconscious is like a wonderful rich sea full of treasures, and floating up out of this sea is an image that represents who I am or what I need to know at this moment in my life. This image is now sitting opposite me.
- Take felt-tip pens and paper and suggest, 'I would like to allow an image to emerge on this paper of an animal, a plant, or an object, etc [as above].'

  If nothing emerges, try, 'Unconscious, I thank you for your efforts to protect me, but I would like to explore these images. Please help me to do so in a safe and natural way . . . .'

  As a last resort, take the 'nothingness' or the blankness of not having an image to be your image, and explore that.

Study the image

Allow the image to become clearer. What does it look like? What colour is it? Does it make a sound? Does it have a smell? Does it move, and if so, how? What is its relationship to the environment?

Imagine that your mind or spirit is free to study it from every perspective — from above, underneath and every side. What more do you notice?

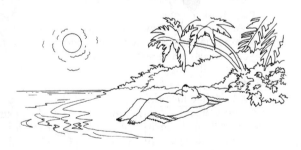

Become the image

Step into the image. Get up and sit in the chair where you saw the image, or just step into the image in your mind. Feel it absolutely, for example, the wind blowing through your wings if you are a bird, or the earth around your roots if you are a plant. Now return to your own seat and question the image. Change seats when you are the image, answering the questions. As you tune into the image, questions relevant to your own situation will arise, but here are some suggestions:

- Tell me about yourself.
- What is the essence of being you—the 'boatness' of the boat, the 'bearness' of the bear, or whatever the image is.
- Where are you? What can you see and feel around you?
- How does it feel to be you?
- What is the best thing about your life and what is the worst thing?
- What do you hope for and what do you fear?
- Do you feel at home in the world around you or at conflict with it?
- Is there a problem that needs solving?
- What else do you notice about being you at this moment in your life?

Get a sense of the history

Ask the image about the background of the present situation:

- What led up to your present situation?
- Was there a time when things were different?
- When? How were they different? How and when did the change take place?

Get a sense of the possibilities

Ask:

- What's next? What do you need to do to make your life better or to feel more complete?
- What seems right? What should happen?
- If you could wave a magic wand over your life, how would you like it to be?

It is now x time later (x can be ten minutes, a day, a year, or whatever period you like) and you feel good about your life. What is happening now? What did you do?

If an answer emerges, imagine it and enjoy it. If you get stuck without an answer at this stage, ask:

- What's stopping you from moving forward?
- What do you fear will happen?
- What feels useful about the seemingly negative aspects of the way you are now?

Let your mind float up from your body and look down, studying the image from above. If you could tell it something from this perspective that would help it, what would it be?

As soon as an answer emerges to these questions, follow through by suggestion, 'do it, and enjoy it,' and continue to ask, 'What happens next?' until you reach a natural resting point.

Appreciate and emerge

Tune back into the original image. What is happening now? Is there a change? How do you feel about the future? Review the pictures and feelings you have just been through, and notice the best picture/feeling in all that. Allow yourself to feel/be that again, and notice exactly what it is like, both physically and emotionally, so that you can recognize that state of mind and body in future.

Reflect

Using your conscious resources, spend a few moments reflecting on what you have just been through, and also keep the image in the back of your mind over the next few days and continue this process. Ask yourself:

'How does this image reflect my life as it is and has been? What do I feel good about as I look at this clarification of my underlying programme? What do I feel uneasy about? How does the image fit in with previous images I have had of myself?'

Look forward

Ask yourself: What are the practical implications of all this? What does it really mean to make this change? What do I need to do to take the next step?'

'If I had already made this change, suggested by the image, how would I deal differently with this problem and with life in general? What would a day in my life be like if I had this new image in the background? How does it differ from a typical day now? What could stop me from making this change? How do I usually sabotage myself?'

Emerge

When you are ready to emerge from this deeply relaxed state, suggest the following: 'I'm going to count up from one to five and when I say five, I will open my eyes, feeling relaxed and alert, feeling better than before, as if I've had a long refreshing sleep, and bringing back with me the best feelings, pictures, and insights from my explorations. One, two—coming up to the surface, eyelids lightening; three—alert but still relaxed; four, five—eyes open.'

At various moments during the next few days or weeks, ask yourself how you might experience things differently if you were the image-being at its best. Or ask it for advice: 'What do you think I should do now?'

Every now and then, tune in to the image-being to see what state it is in. Is the bear feeling friendly, or is it running around in a confused way, or is it hiding in fright? This is a good indication of your present state of mind.

My future self

This exercise can be used for any time period in the future. It is useful to start by imagining your eighty-year-old self, so as to get a sense of your long-term goals. Then choose whatever shorter time period feels most relevant to you.

Clear a space and relax, as above. Suggest to yourself: 'I am on a spaceship zooming off the face of the earth. I return to earth at age eighty (or six months/ five years/ten years later—whatever period you want to work with) and I discover my future self—completely happy with my life.'

Explore the image of your future self, in the given period of the future. Make the image as vivid and concrete as possible: what are you wearing? How do you feel in your body, mind and spirit? Ask yourself: 'What is the good feeling I have? What was the most important thing I did or experienced to reach this good feeling? Looking back at the younger me, what do I notice? What do I want to whisper that would make life easier for him or her?'

Having established a clear image, ask it specific questions:
• How have my relationships—with friends, family and colleagues—been?
• What did I accomplish or create and how exactly did I go about it?
• How was my self-esteem and how did I take care of myself physically?
• How do I feel about the way life has treated me? What did I learn about life itself?
• What do I feel best about? What could I tell the younger me that would help him or her?

This exercise can also be done from the negative point of view:

It's x time from now and I feel absolutely terrible. What is this terrible feeling? What is the most important thing I did to make it happen? Reviewing my personal and professional life, where did I go wrong? What could I tell the younger me that will help him or her not to end up like this? Finally, before and after emerging, reflect on what all this means and what the implications are. Decide on specific and practical ways in which you can use these new insights to improve your life now.

Quick visualization

This is a very useful technique when you want to relax—before an interview, a party, or any stressful situation.

Simply say to yourself: 'It's the end of this event and I feel really good about it. What is this good feeling? What did I do to bring it about?'

Or: 'It's the end of this event and I feel really bad about it. What is this awful feeling? What did I do to bring it about? With this hindsight, what steps can I take to avoid it?'

If you have decided on a life change or goal that you want to achieve, a useful exercise is:

The Cinema Exercise
Clear a space and relax, as above.

Now imagine that you are in your own private cinema. You are sitting in the middle of the cinema, with the screen in front of you.

Allow a picture to emerge on the screen as you are now, before you have achieved the goal. Examine the picture. How do you feel about the person? Allow yourself to accept and support him or her, even if you do not completely approve of his or her behaviour. Recognize they are doing their best at the moment, until they are able, with your help, to move on. Now let the picture move off the screen, to the left, into the past. This is how you were, but no longer are.

Now allow a picture of yourself to emerge as you will be, after you have achieved your goal or made this life change. Look at this new picture. How is it different from the old picture? In your imagination, leave your seat, walk up to the screen and step into the picture. How does it feel to be this person? How is it different from the other person you were? Become clear how you act and what it is that makes this form of action so successful. Spend a day as this person, noticing all the details of your life, from how you get up, through the day of work and leisure, to going to bed.

Still living as the new person, imagine that you have two helpers, who may be real or imaginary people. One is a supporter, who cheers you on, and one is an expert at what you are doing who can advise you. Who are they? Ask them whatever you like and see what they say. Step into their image, to experience the feeling of operating expertly, and of loving and supporting the new person you have become.

Look back and see what led up to this point. Look at the person you were before. What steps did you take to become this new person?

Now step out of the screen and go back to your seat. Look at the person on the screen and realize that this is really as you could be and will be. Make a decision that this goal is possible, desirable and one to which you have a right. Decide that you will put all your energy and intentions into becoming that person.

Put the image on the screen into a bubble and say to yourself, 'I fully intend for this to happen, and I release it.' Send the balloon off, out of sight.

Before and after emerging, reflect on the concrete implications of what you have learned, and look forward to see what you intend to do in a practical sense to make your vision come true. Spend some time every day practising being the person you will be after having made the life change.

When you want to do something that has been weighing on your mind, and about which you have been procrastinating, allow an image of yourself doing it to emerge on the screen, put the image in a bubble, and intend and release. This cuts down anxiety and gets the problem out of your mind and into the area of potentials waiting to be actualized.

Spiritual Healing

Introduction

Technology in the 21st century

Today's society stands as a multimedia monument to the scientific and technological triumphs of the past century. The radio crackled into life, man walked on the moon, and diseases that previously ravaged entire populations, such as tuberculosis and smallpox, were virtually eradicated overnight. Nowadays we can communicate through cyberspace, genetically engineer outsize fruit, and line up to be treated with the latest wonder-drug.

There is no denying that the advancements of science have made our lives infinitely easier, longer and more comfortable. We wonder how past generations can have possibly survived without mobile phones and watches that can withstand the pressure of thousands of fathoms of water.

Somewhere down the line science replaced religion and philosophy as the perceived source of infinite knowledge. Even the mysteries of creation, previously the domain of the divine, could be explained away in scientific terms.

In recent years, however, society has begun to doubt the omnipotence of science, realizing that it cannot provide answers for some of the most fundamental questions of existence. From this realization a new spirituality has emerged, which is heralding a gradual shift in attitude. The materialism and high-powered competitiveness of the 1980s has given way to a slightly more relaxed, positive and intuitive mood.

In no other arena has this generational shift been more apparent than in attitudes towards health. More and more people, doctors and patients alike, are adopting a more holistic approach to health, acknowledging the importance of lifestyle, proper diet and regular exercise in the upkeep of a healthy body. Even more importantly, people are beginning to recognize and understand the significance of the state of their mental, spiritual and emotional wellbeing on their physical health.

In reality, we have always known how strongly our emotions affect our physical being—think how many times dealing with someone difficult and demanding has brought on a headache. Even without realizing it, we connect the idea of wellness with the idea of emotion when we say that we do not 'feel well', when we do not know specifically what is wrong with us. We also acknowledge our spiritual nature when we claim to be in 'high' or 'low' spirits.

It is in this atmosphere of renewed enthusiasm for the holistic ideal, however, that such concepts have been widely accepted into our collective consciousness. This in itself has paved the way for numerous alternative therapies, some of which have been practised for centuries either in other cultures or our own, to be adopted further into mainstream society. A whole world of esoteric therapies has become more socially acceptable as well as more readily available. Faith healing is just one of these therapies.

Some people feel uneasy about the term 'faith healing'. To many it positively smacks of jiggery-pokery, probably because of recent publicity about fraudulent American television evangelists, as well as a deeper-rooted fear and suspicion of anything that sounds vaguely occultist.

In fact, faith healing is one of the most conservative and respectable of all the battery of so-called alternative therapies, being wholeheartedly welcomed into institutions such as churches and hospitals, as it is.

We should perhaps attempt at the outset to fashion some working definition of faith healing. This may be an elusive task because the term is such a wide one, offering itself to various differing schools. It should be pointed out that faith healing has become an umbrella term for the diverse strands of healing that fall within its range. In its purest meaning, faith healing is the belief in 'right' thinking, practised within a religious system. Christian faith healers believe that all healing comes from God.

The term is really unsatisfactory because it implies that faith is the obligatory prerequisite to being helped by the healing forces. This excludes many nonbelievers, who have been some of the most startling subjects and benefactors of healing. Another problem for some people with the term 'faith healing' is that it places the source of healing in a person's faith, not in Christ or a divinity. Apart from belittling the role of God in healing, this definition is also potentially harmful for those who do not experience any alleviation of symptoms following healing, leading them to believe that it is their fault for not having enough faith, which can result in a spiritual crisis.

A more flexible definition of faith healing is that of a therapy based on something other than current scientific knowledge. The term 'spiritual healing' is employed by those who are reluctant to be emphatic as to the origins of healing, be it from God or some other universal source. In this book the terms 'faith' and 'spiritual' healing are somewhat interchangeable.

The word 'healing' comes from the Anglo-Saxon word 'healan', which connotes both the body and the spiritual element of the human being as the thing to be healed.

At this point, it would be politic to draw attention to the difference between healing and curing because they are *not* the same thing. Although it is true that miraculous cures do take place following faith healing, this is not the premise of the therapy. Healing could involve the temporary or permanent alleviation of symptoms, or it could mean reaching a state of wellbeing. On the other hand, the healing could just be arriving at a point of acceptance.

Redefining healing also means changing attitudes towards disease. It has been suggested that perhaps all diseases are psychologically rooted or stress-related. Some healers believe that all symptoms of disease are the result of some deeper spiritual disorder, and that the patient must subsequently look at his or her life and assess what it is that is making him or her unwell. For example, stress, over-work and unexpressed anger are widely recognized as contributing factors in the emergence of many medical conditions, ranging from migraines to cancer. This kind of direct cause and effect approach can be harmful, however, as it may suggest to the patient that he or she is somehow responsible for the illness. This could induce feelings of guilt and shame, both extremely negative emotions, which would become another barrier to wellbeing. By all means analyse your lifestyle in order to understand the possible origins of an ailment, just do not hold yourself to account.

It should also be emphasized that faith healing is a complementary therapy intended to be employed in conjunction with orthodox medicine, *not* to replace it.

The proof of the effectiveness of this type of healing is anecdotal rather than scientific, which invites scepticism. In any analysis of faith healing we must accept that there are things in life that defy scientific explanation. As Shakespeare says through Hamlet, 'There are more things in heaven and earth, [Horatio], than are dreamt of in your philosophy'. Surely it is not beyond us to admit that our own knowledge may be flawed and imperfect.

It would be a tragedy indeed if we allowed our fear and mistrust of the unknown to deter us from embracing all that faith healing has to offer. With this in mind let us explore spiritual healing and its many possibilities.

The healing tradition

History

Whence came faith healing? The practice has been prevalent in virtually all cultures and religious customs through the ages. Primitive peoples required a shaman, or medicine man, to cure their ills. The Ancient Greeks and Romans erected temples to Asclepius, the god of medicine. In the Judaic scriptures paranormal cures such as the answer to Abraham's prayer against barrenness and those of leprosy by Elisha and Moses are much in evidence.

Unorthodox healing—that is, the cure or assuagement of bodily or mental ills by supplication or religious rituals, which may either augment or replace medical care—includes fringe medicine, faith healing, spiritual healing and miracle cures. Along with this diversity of schools, there is a correspondent diversity of opinions expressed about it. To its detractors it is merely superstition and quackery, practised by metaphysical 'wide boys' out for a fast buck. To its adherents it is an alternative perspective on the way we think of illness, the basic truth of which has yet to be accepted or assimilated into medical practice. Faith healing can also boast a rich and fascinating history, one replete with spirit and humour. It would be a mean soul that could not laugh at the enterprising Edinburgh quack James Graham, selling his celestial bed in a valiant attempt to emulate the great Cagliostro, a charlatan who practised alchemy and mysticism as the means to realize cures at the time of Louis XVI. Graham sold beds that he professed could provide painless childbirth, along with chairs that alleviated rheumatism, and for the noblemen that could pay for it, he could provide the elixir of life. Then there is the sheer romanticism and lust for life of a figure like Grigori Rasputin, leaving his wife and children to roam rural Russia as a faith healer after a strange religious revelation.

The revival of interest in faith healing is no doubt due in some part to the New Age movement. This theorizes that humankind is entering the Age of Aquarius and that we are due for a worldwide spiritual renewal. Part of the agenda of New Ageism is a preoccupation with complementary medicine, green issues, and interest in occultist and spiritualist practices. What is important to remember, however, is that this resurgence of interest in complementary therapy is nothing new—it occurs at regular intervals, a healthy antidote to the almost totalitarian stranglehold that the established medical world has on the way we perceive the concept of health and therapy. It will be no shock to learn that pre-Civil War America was just as infatuated with complementary medicine, albeit in a slightly different incarnation, as modern America is today. Perhaps the last British wave of this occurred in Georgian England, among fashionable society. No doubt New Ageism will not be the last of these flirtations with underground medicine.

New Age healing

The resurgence of interest in healing at present must be due in some part to the New Age movement, although the kind of healing prescribed by New Agers has more in common with Jungian psychology than with healing practised down the centuries. New Age healing consists of what is termed 'healing of the memories', 'healing emotional hurts', or 'soul healing'. The main idea behind this is that what is to be healed are negative past experiences rather than the physical body. These ideas were developed principally by Agnes Sanford and

Morton Kelsey, although the influence of both Jungian and Freudian psychology hang heavily over the proceedings. The movement borrows heavily from Freud's idea of depth psychology, whereby one's childhood experiences are plundered for traumas and upset, which must then be confronted and healed. Jungian psychology is also utilized, in that New Age healing encourages you to visualize Jesus accompanying you during the traumatic event of the past. This visualization of the past with Jesus as a companion also extends to visualizing the desired state you wish to reach in the healing process. The effect this has on the subconscious is supposedly meant to bring about what is wished for. Like Christian Science, many of its doctrines oppose and eschew Christian ideas.

Of course, there is the darker side of faith healing, or rather the abuse of faith healing. There can be no whitewash of this in any respectable assessment of the topic. The excesses of the Eddy movement are unrelated to the issue of the validity of healing. We will not elaborate on the moral bankruptcy of the Elmer Gantry breed of televangelist faith healer, not because it as insignificant but because it deflects us again from asking the real questions—the question of the validity or otherwise of healing in the war on disease.

Before we can proceed, we have to accept that there really is something to be studied, abandon our prejudices and preconceptions, and set out with an open mind, something that is harder to do than we would often care to admit.

Healers and healing past and present

We shall endeavour here to provide a brief potted history of the history and personalities of faith healing through the centuries, with an awareness that we will ultimately fail because of the huge expanse of the subject. What we do hope to provide is an entertaining jaunt through the history of healing without being too dry or scholastic.

Faith healing was the dominant form of treatment five hundred years before Christ, concurrent with the time that hygienic therapy began among the Greeks. (Hygienic therapy advocates manipulation of the environment that sufferers inhabit, to help them recover. Rest, fresh air and diet are its principal weapons against disease.)

Gradually drug cures became popular, and this was integrated into the usual faith healing practices. When Christianity began to make its influence felt, these drug cures were forced out, and once again pure faith healing became predominant and maintained its ascendancy for thirteen centuries. At the time of the Renaissance, faith healing began to lose its virtual monopoly on medical therapy but still had purchase in non-medical cults.

Pythagoras

Pythagoras, the sixth century BC astronomer, mathematician and physician, considered healing to be the most elevated of pursuits and saw it as an integral part of his deliberation on ethics, mind and soul. He called the healing energy pneuma, which he theorized arose from a fire at the core of the universe, which gave human beings their animation and immortal soul. His adherents believed this *pneuma* could be perceptible in a lucent body and that this light was capable of curing illness. They believed that all matter is comprised of opposites that are in conflict and have to be in equilibrium in order to be in harmony.

Hippocrates

Hippocrates (460–377 BC) was born on the Greek Island of Kos into a family of priests and physicians. He was educated at a famous school in Kos and received medical training from his father and other medical practitioners. By the time he had moved to Athens he had acquired outstanding proficiency in the diagnosis, prognosis and treatment of disease. He kept detailed accounts of mumps, epilepsy, hysteria, arthritis and tuberculosis. Hippocrates argued that all illness, both mental and physical, was caused by natural factors, such as organic injury or an imbalance of body fluids. The Greeks, beginning with Thales, had a tendency to replace magico-religious explanations for things with naturalistic explanations.

Hippocrates is held to be the father of modern medicine, although Alcmaeon and Empodocles had challenged medical practices based on superstition and magic before him. Hippocrates laid the basis of modern scientific medicine in his writings, called the *Hippocratic Corpus*. He also created the basis of medical ethics embodied in the Hippocratic Oath.

Hippocrates believed that the body had self-healing mechanisms, and it was the physician's duty to aid these natural processes. The cures of Hippocrates involved proper diet, rest and fresh air.

Hippocrates recognized that the alleviation of some symptoms by the so-called 'laying on of hands' was accompanied by a sensation of warmth and tingling. He described the healing energy: 'the heat that oozes out of the hand, being applied to the sick, is highly salutary'. He postulated that just as 'health may be implanted in the sick by certain gestures, and by contact, as some diseases may be communicated from one to the other'.

He postulated his own notion of the 'healing energy', or pneuma, and called it the *vis medicae naturae*. He believed that the proper flow of the pneuma could be disrupted by malign influences, which disturbed the relationship between the individual and the cosmos.

Unlike Pythagoras, Hippocrates advanced the view that mind and body were separate. The Hippocratic system was codified by Galen in the second century AD, although Galen himself suspected that the efficacy of the healing temples that were employed in Ancient Rome relied on some form of mental manipulation.

The idea that mind and body were separate became the orthodoxy to hold sway for many centuries afterwards. A few lone voices, such as Plato's, spoke out against this idea: 'The great error of our day,' he wrote, 'is that physicians separate the soul from the body.'

Asclepius

Perhaps the cult of Asclepius, the Greek god of healing, demonstrates that in the early Graeco-Roman tradition, magic and medicine ran side by side in the battle against illness. It is not really clear whether Asclepius was a real historical figure or a mythical one. Outside the stream of early rational medicine was a widespread popular belief in the powers of early miracle-working wizards such as Serapis and Apollonius of Tyana. It was also believed that to sleep with the fourth book of the Iliad under one's pillow at night ensured a cure for the quartan ague!

The Asclepeion at Pergamum is one of the finest preserved and best-known medical establishments of the Graeco-Roman era, being founded in the first half of the fourth century BC by Archias, who had been healed by Asclepius at Epidaurus. Archias had suffered a sprain while out hunting and had met a fast cure under the management of Asclepius. Archias was so impressed by the treatment he had received that he 'brought the God to Pergamum' in the founding of a temple there. The oracle at Delphi had already proclaimed that Asclepius was a healer of diseases. The tale of the growth of the cult of Asclepius in Rome in the year 292 BC is told by Livy.

Classical civilization entrusted its patients to the incubation cure, a treatment that arose from the cult of Asclepius. The patient would pass a night in the 'incubation temple' in the belief that the gods would cure them in a dream. After ritual purification, suppliants for aid slept in the basement, or *adyton*, of the temple at the end of a long tunnel. Here they hoped to dream the dreams on whose interpretation by the priests depended their future treatment and welfare. The playwright Aristophanes (408–388 BC) makes reference to this ritual cult in his play *Plutus*.

Cures at Pergamum

Nicanor, a lame man, was sitting by the temple when a young boy ran up to him and snatched away his crutches. Nicanor chased after the boy in hot pursuit and was cured. There is also the story of two women who became pregnant after their visit to the temple. Andromache, the wife of King Arybbas of Epirus, 'for the sake of offspring', slept in the temple and saw in a dream a handsome youth who uncovered and disrobed her, the god touched her with his hand, whereupon a child was born to her. The second lady, Agameda of Ceoa, was also infertile and went to sleep in the temple whereupon she dreamt of a serpent lying on her belly. Five children were later born to her.'

The plausibility of the cures at Pergamun are striking, especially the cures of psychologically-induced ailments, although the cures administered at other health centres, such as Epidaurus, are no less striking. One patient remained sceptical, however. 'When parchance my penis was hurt . . . I feared the surgeon's hands. I was reluctant to entrust my membrum virile to the care and the very great gods such as Phoebus and the son of Phoebus.'

Much of Greek thinking on medicine was appropriated by the Romans, and it was the Romans who developed the idea of a public hospital system. But after the collapse of the Roman Empire there was a virtually complete return to magic and mysticism.

Paracelsus

Practising in the 16th century, Philippus Paracelsus (1493–1541) is regarded as the father of modern therapeutics. Leaving his native Switzerland after becoming unhappy with the means of procuring wisdom in his indigenous country, he travelled around Europe. Something of an unorthodox healer, during his travels he became acquainted with physic not in common use among doctors of medicine and accomplished many miraculous cures, acquiring a great reputation in the process.

Paracelsus developed the idea that human beings were an integral part of nature, suggesting that they were continuous with nature and reflected internally the broader cosmos in the external world. He claimed that healing energies existed and radiated in and around humans. He called this force *Archaeus*. This force was an ambivalent one because it could cause as well as cure disease. It was also contained, he argued, in stars and also in magnets. The notion of magnetism, as expounded by Mesmer, has its roots in Paracelsus. He also believed that negative thoughts could block the flow of *Archaeus* and result in illness. For most of his life he was regarded as a charlatan, but he massively enriched science in the course of his life, primarily in the fields of chemistry and medicine. He died at the hospital of St Sebastian at Salzburg in 1541.

Valentine Greatrakes and 'the king's evil'

'The king's evil' was the name sometimes given to tuberculosis involvement of the lymph glands, formerly called scrofula. In fact, the term 'king's evil' came to be used for ailments other than scrofula, including a wide variety of complaints affecting the head, neck and eyes, especially swollen lips, tumours, sores and blisters. The disease had hideously disfiguring effects on the face and the body, and was widespread in the 17th century. It was so called because it was believed that the monarch had special powers of healing this disease, provided by the doctrine of the divine right of kings, a practice that began with the Anglo-Saxon king, Edward the Confessor, in the tenth century. The healing ability was called 'thaumaturgic', or miraculous. Under the Plantagenets, the royal touch swiftly became a vital attribute of kingship. Edward I (1272–1307) touched over a thousand people a year for the king's evil, and the practice was equally popular with his successors, Edward II and Edward III.

The healing benediction

Under the Tudors and Stuarts, the royal touch became increasingly popular, and elaborate ceremony was associated with it. After prayer, the king would touch the sufferer with his hand and then give him a coin. Originally, this coin would be silver, but by the time of Henry VII it had been replaced by gold. By the time of Charles I the coins themselves were thought to have healing powers.

We even have Shakespeare in social historian mode to describe the royal touch in *Macbeth*. The laying on of hands is referred to in these lines spoken by Malcolm, who is here describing the act of touching to combat the king's evil:

> How he solicits heaven,
> Himself best knows; but strangely visited people,
> All swoln and ulcerous, pitiful to the eye,
> The mere despair of surgery, he cures,
> Hanging a golden stamp about their necks,
> Put on with holy prayers; and 'tis spoken,
> To the succeeding royalty he leaves
> The healing benediction.
>
> (Act 4, scene 3, line 149)

The practice of royal healing reached its height at the end of the 17th century. In France, Louis XVI gave the touch to a crowd approaching two thousand strong on one Easter Sunday. In England at around the same time, Charles II was giving the royal touch to five thousand sufferers a year.

The rise of the Stroker

Some may feel that there is an inherent irony in the idea of a Puritan faith healer, as the Puritan regards the physical body to be junk. But so it was that perhaps the greatest British healer of all arose from the ranks of the New Model Army.

Valentine Greatrakes was born in 1628 of English parentage and was thirty-four before he felt the impulse, the 'strange persuasion', that he had healing powers. At the beginning of the Irish Rebellion in 1641, he joined Cromwell's army as a cavalry lieutenant in Ireland. He was a wealthy man with an estate in Lismore, County Waterford. Cromwell banished Charles I, refusing to countenance his kingship or the purported power of the royal touch.

Because the royal touch was not available during the Commonwealth interregnum (Cromwell had tried and failed to administer it himself), Greatrakes was seized with the conviction that God had ordained that it was he who was blessed with the gift of 'curing the King's Evil, which for the extra ordinariness thereof, I thought fit to conceal for some time'. Greatrakes, or the 'Stroker' as he came to be known (Greatrakes moved his hands in a stroking motion without actually touching the sufferer's body), was called a 'charlatan' in contemporary accounts, and even his own wife was deeply sceptical of his healing powers, calling them the result of 'idle imagination'. His wife's job was in the charitable dispensing of medicine to the poor, and this gave him the perfect opportunity to test his powers, imaginary or not.

An ecclesiastic who witnessed Greatrakes at work ventured that what was happening was 'more than ordinary' but that it was 'not miraculous'. Some of the alleged 'healings' would last as long as six weeks. The charge of charlatan was perhaps unfair because Greatrakes himself was as mystified by his own success rate as everybody else. All he would offer was an intimation that some form of exorcism was involved. He was also a man of independent means and did not attempt to charge his patients. Neither did he claim to be infallible; there were those that claimed that their pains returned after their supposed cures. One of his most famous failures was that of the first royal astronomer of England, John Flamsteed.

Greatrakes would originally treat maladies connected with the bones, and after a period of success that lasted two years he had developed enough confidence to believe that he could also treat agues, an intermittent fever with hot and cold sweats. The extension of his services was fuelled by the coming of various dreams, the import of which was that he should begin and then extend his ministry. His method was to direct the ailment by squeezing it to an extremity of the body where it could be isolated and then ejected. His fame and success were so great that he was forced to build an extension to his house to accommodate sufferers awaiting treatment. His fame spread to London, causing huge shiploads of sufferers to cross the Irish sea in the hope of an audience with the Stroker.

In 1666 Greatrakes travelled to London, where he exhibited his healing powers and met the famous of the day, who included the poet Andrew Marvell and the chemist Robert Boyle. Boyle was to investigate Greatrakes's powers and find in favour of them. In 1667 Greatrakes's powers began to recede to nothing. Fewer and fewer patients came to visit him, his curative powers were no longer news, and the Stroker went into retirement.

Johann Joseph Gassner

Born in Austria, Gassner (1727–79) had a Jesuit education and was ordained as a Roman Catholic priest. He was the victim of illnesses such as headaches, gastric complaints and chest pains, illnesses that he would feel intensify as he gave Mass. He concluded that this was indeed none other than the devil trying to take possession of him.

His answer to this was to style a form of self-exorcism by which he found he could successfully alleviate these aches and pains. From the success of his self-diagnosis and treatment he began to shape the idea that a large proportion of human illness—with some exceptions—was due to diabolic influence.

When Gassner was nearing fifty he started to experiment, using his techniques on others who were suffering mental disturbance. This was so successful that as many as two thousand people a month were administered to at one of Gassner's mass healing ceremonies. Gassner employed a truncated form of exorcism, which departed from the standard ritual of bell, book and candle, a methodology that was to scandalize the church of the day. He had a powerful patron in the Bishop of Regensburg, yet this did not prevent the church's usual perfunctory dismissal of the Austrian healer. With Gassner's growing success, the demand for a convincing rebuttal of his practices from the established church became great. The church was also disgruntled by his eclectic approach to the healing ceremony. At one mass meeting at Ellwangen, Gassner amalgamated Roman Catholic ritual with evangelical showmanship and a personal idiosyncratic lingo of possession. It was witnessed that he would give a command in Latin to a patient to fall to the ground, and this would be followed, even though the patient knew no Latin. His patients would be seen to weep, become belligerent, and fall into trances.

Although his ability to achieve a form of mass hysteria is well documented, his ability to cure permanently was not so solid. The only certain cures he could convincingly claim were cures of rheumatic complaints. Eventually the end of Gassner's ministry came when the church forbade him to practise.

Maximillian Hehl was professor of astronomy at Vienna University and assigned himself the task of attempting to explain the cures and hysteria that Gassner had brought about. In doing so he came into contact and influenced the next key figure in healing—Friedrich Anton Mesmer.

Franz Mesmer

Friedrich Anton Mesmer (1734–1815) appeared in Vienna at the end of the 18th century. He was born near Lake Konstanz, at Iznang in Swabia, a gamekeeper's son. Unusually for a healer, he qualified as a physician and gained four doctorates. In Vienna, he met a Jesuit priest called Maximillian Hehl, the same eccentric astronomer with an interest in the paranormal who had tried to study the method of Gassner. Through him Mesmer developed his interest in astronomy. Hehl told Mesmer of the cures he had brought about using a magnet. Mesmer himself then copied this method to try to cure one of his patients, where all other forms of treatment had failed. Tellingly, the success of the treatment on this and further patients always involved Mesmer telling his patient what exactly was expected to occur.

He developed a large practice, married a wealthy widow and lived in an impressive house on the Danube. His salon was frequented by such illustrious company as Haydn, Mozart and Gluck.

It was at this point that he began to develop his ideas on what he chose to call 'animal magnetism'. It was Mesmer who managed to draw attention to the notion of mental healing as distinct from religion. He substituted the notion of animal magnetism for religion in his practices, and after studying the techniques of Gassner, as Hehl had done before him, Mesmer came to the conclusion that he had stumbled on the same method that Gassner had utilized. He demonstrated his use of magnetic passes around the body in the treatment of illness. The passes first of all provoked a crisis: 'An attempt by nature to resist the illness' in Mesmer's words. This would manifest itself as hysteria in the patient. This technique is now better known as catharsis, a technique appropriated later by Sigmund Freud and Bleule. Mesmer at first employed magnets to this end, but later he discovered that his treatment was just as effective without their use. The person whose repute or personal charisma can induce the mental condition of concentration, obeisance, and positive expectation can presently disregard the application of passes and magnets and oil, as Mesmer did.

When magnetic therapy became popular, Hehl claimed to have been the first to use it. This led to a dispute between Hehl and Mesmer, which Mesmer won, perhaps unfairly.

He postulated that he injected a magnetic fluid into the patient. He inspired a faithful coterie but failed to be accepted by the medical establishment. He also advanced the idea that a psychic ether pervades space. This ether is then subject to tides that are caused by heavenly bodies. These tides run through all organic bodies, i.e. humankind. The free passage of these tides in the body is responsible for good health. Conversely, their blockage leads to ill health.

Although his salon was popular among the rich and fashion-conscious Viennese, an eighteen-year-old patient of Mesmer's, called Maria Paradies, managed to provoke a scandal by claiming to have fallen in love with him after he allegedly restored her sight. Mesmer was forced to leave Vienna, ostensibly because he was a fraud. Mesmer's arrival in Paris in 1778 caused a sensation. Waving his hands over his patients' faces and gazing deeply into their eyes, he would 'mesmerize' them with an iron rod and put them into a deep trance. He had now taken to administering his treatment to groups rather than lone individuals, realizing the power of collective psychology that could be activated in his treatments. Indeed, he called this the 'contagion effect'. He would also increase the use of ritual in his treatment, placing his patients in a dimly lit room and entering wearing a lilac cloak and waving a yellow wand.

He was also to find a receptive audience in Paris with Empress Marie Theresa of Austria's daughter, Marie Antoinette, who became a disciple and Mesmer's patron. She offered Mesmer a chateau and a lifetime pension if he would disclose the secrets of his success. He declined. What Mesmer really wanted was acceptance from the medical profession.

Mesmer offered to submit his powers to the tests of the medical profession but was rebuffed. Eventually, a commission was set up in August 1784 in France to study Mesmer's success, which took an unenthusiastic view of his abilities and thereby marginalized him. The commission concluded that while many of Mesmer's abilities could be well substantiated, his success was due not to animal magnetism but to the suggestibility of his patients. The commission branded Mesmer a fanatic and a mystic, and admittedly some of his patients were observed to be badly affected by Mesmer's methods. Yet he still managed to make a considerable fortune from his practices. He died at the age of eighty in Switzerland.

Emil Coue

In Nancy, France, in the 1880s, the French healer Emil Coue studied mesmerism and became intrigued with the idea that a mysterious energy called animal magnetism flowed between the healer and the patient. Coue was a chemist, a man of science, and cynical about healing, so much so that he began to conduct experiments that attempted to unseat the popular belief in mesmerism. These experiments were conducted by selecting a group of patients being treated conventionally and dispensing to them bottles of coloured water of no medicinal value. The patients believed that this water was a new wonder-drug. He found that those who were given the coloured water recovered more successfully than those who followed the doctor's prescribed course of drugs. Coue concluded that it was not mesmerism but suggestion that had cured them.

He developed from this his theory of autosuggestion, which entailed that all his patients had to do was to believe that their illnesses could be counteracted simply by believing with all their heart that the illness they suffered would vanish. He implored his patients to say to themselves the slogan, 'Every day, in every way, I get better and better.'

Zouave Jacob

A Frenchman born in 1828, Jacob served as a trombonist in the military band of the Zouaves. His gift of healing was first noticed when he served in the Crimea and Algeria, but it first came to public attention when a national paper published articles on his healing ability while he was serving in Châlons. When his fame began to grow, the public would flood to his tent and disrupt the work he was allotted. A transfer to Versailles landed him a rich patron in Paris. Jacob was discharged from the army at the age of thirty-nine, when the same crowds that had pursued him in Châlons followed him to Paris. Like Greatrakes, Jacob had no explanation for his abilities and was not an especially religious person. He believed that his powers were not supernatural in origin. He claimed that he could cure 'all kinds of diseases' but that he was not regularly victorious over any one disease. Also in his favour was the refusal to accept money for his abilities, even when it was stipulated it should go to the poor. One friend described him as 'a most intractable, disagreeable fellow'. Jacob was no charmer, so any idea that his popularity spread because of personal charisma can be dismissed at once.

After one healing session, a group of the healed moved to thank him for his attention, but Jacob was seen to dismiss them 'brutally', as one commentator observed.

His methodology included touch and command as well as staring deep into the patient's eyes — a journalist described his 'trancelike carriage' and the intensity of his eyes, from which 'intense light shot out'. He would also stipulate that the patient should be in his presence. Sometimes his command to walk would be punctuated by him stamping his foot on the floor with 'rude violence'. Jacob could diagnose the ailment of a patient almost immediately on sight and was, as far as we can tell, always right. At the height of his powers, he could bring a roomful of cripples to walk with the command 'arise and be well'.

Eventually the combined antagonism from both the clerical and medical professions led to a falling off in popularity for Jacob. He continued to heal up to his death in 1914, but his glory days were gone.

Grigori Rasputin

The most notorious faith healer in Russian history was the debauchee Grigori Rasputin. Born in an obscure Siberian village, he was the third and last child of Efim Akovlevich, a well-to-do farmer. As well as the gift of healing, he was reputed to be blessed with clairvoyance, as a child being able to detect any missing object in the house and to sniff out the local thieves in his community. As a child he would also hear the stories of the pilgrims that passed through his town, exciting him and imbuing him with a sense of the religious at an early age. At twenty, he married a local girl, Praskovia Feodorovna, and fathered four children.

According to his daughter, a chance frolic with three Siberian peasant girls in a lake led to a religious revelation, and soon afterwards, in approximately 1900, he joined a maverick religious sect, called the Khlist, who openly advocated sexual indulgence in their philosophy. They were flagellants who believed that man must at first sin in order to be redeemed later, so Rasputin set about sinning in his own inimitable way. Rasputin proved to have such a natural aptitude for this that he was exiled from his own village by the local priests and so began an odyssey of itinerant wandering through rustic Russia, performing cures and initiating thousands of women into flagellation. Rasputin had an uncanny ability to calm the troubled minds of those who surrounded him. As well as this, he had a virtually unerring ability to assess the strengths and weaknesses of character in his contemporaries, an ability that was eventually to be utilized by the Tsarina herself.

By 1905 he had settled in St Petersburg, where tales of his amazing healing powers had reached the ear of both Tsar Nicholas II and Tsarina Alexandra. One of the most famous healings that Rasputin administered was to one of his own disciples, Olga Lokhtina. Olga was to be the first of Grigori's upper-class friends. Rasputin purportedly cured her of a nervous stomach disorder, called neurasthenia, that she had been plagued with for five years. In this cure Rasputin used both impassioned prayer and hypnotic suggestion, convincing Olga that he was in league with the Almighty in assuaging the illness.

He rose to become a close familiar of Tsarina Alexandra, mainly because of his ability through hypnosis to help her sick son, Alexis, who was afflicted with haemophilia. The child of Lili Dehn, the Tsarina's lady in waiting, was also cured of a fever by Rasputin after heartfelt prayer. By the end of 1906 he had established a firm reputation as a healer.

Rasputin also gave the Tsar and his wife a feeling of being in touch with the real Russia of the peasants. The notion that true faith was more likely to be found among the people was common, and no doubt this contributed to the allure Rasputin held for the Tsarina. He would assure them that Russia loved the Tsar. Correspondingly, the Assyrian healer Mrs Davitashvili has been quick to emulate this asset and pretend to a oneness with the people. She has said: 'It is every citizen's duty to inform the president of the people's views.' Rasputin used the Tsarina's favour to protect himself and broaden his influence, even though his wild sexual antics were scandalizing the whole of St Petersburg. In 1916, a gang of conservative noblemen, led by Felix Yusopov, assassinated him.

Felix Kersten: faith healing and the Third Reich

That the Nazi movement was deeply interested in the occult is no big surprise to anyone nowadays. Yet fewer people are aware that the presence of healing fell on the Third Reich. That a death cult should embrace a life cult is strange enough, but one of the strangest stories of all faith healing is that of the relationship between Heinrich Himmler and his personal healer, Felix Kersten. Kersten was born in 1898 in Finland, but spent most of his early life in the Netherlands and came to regard himself as Dutch. He became adept at massage, and extended his powers after meeting a mysterious oriental occultist called Ko. Through the tutelage of Ko, Kersten developed a method that allowed him to be able to diagnose ailments by means of that ancient technique, the laying on of hands. He could also, he discovered, transfer some of his own energy into the body of the recipient, in the manner of a spiritual healer. When he laid hands on the body of a patient he could feel his whole being flowing through the tips of his fingers into the patient. His ability to relieve pain began to be nothing short of miraculous, and even after the departure of Ko, his amazing powers remained.

His reputation began to grow, his practice prospered, and eventually he rose to such a pre-eminent position that he became the personal doctor of the Dutch royal family. This sudden rise to fame was not without its drawbacks, however. In 1938 he was asked to contact the head of the SS and high priest of the Nazi movement, Heinrich Himmler, with a view to assisting his stomach ailments.

Since Himmler's appointment as head of the SS, the stomach cramps from which he had periodically suffered from the beginning of the Nazi years had become so bad and unremitting that he was in a state of almost constant pain. The visits of doctors and the ministrations of orthodox medicine had done nothing to alleviate these pains, yet after a period of five minutes with Kersten, on his first timorous meeting with the head of the most feared organization in the world, the pains had gone. Himmler was suitably impressed, and Kersten was appointed as personal doctor. Kersten then became so invaluable to Himmler that the head of the SS could barely countenance the idea of being apart from him. Himmler was probably aware that Kersten's sympathies lay with the Jews but was too dependent on him to care.

After his appointment Kersten used his influence subtly to attempt to dissuade Himmler from his maniacal barbarities against the Jews. His first success was with his own native land. Himmler, in July 1942, travelled to Finland to demand that the Finnish Jews be handed over to Germany and the political power of the Third Reich. In Finland Kersten made contact with the Finnish foreign minister and hit on a plan to stall the Nazi plans. He persuaded Himmler that the Jewish question was far too important to be decided by anything less than parliament, which did not meet for another four months, in November. It was December before Himmler raised the issue again, only to be dissuaded again by Kersten. The Finnish Jews were saved.

This was only the first of many successes for Kersten. He also managed, among other things, to mastermind the release of concentration camp prisoners to Sweden. His only failure was his attempt to persuade Himmler to make peace with the Western Allies, after the attempted deposing of Hitler.

Jose de Freitas—Arigo

Jose de Freitas, or 'Arigo' as he was affectionately known to his followers, astounded Brazil through the 1950s by his use of so-called 'psychic surgery'. He operated in completely insanitary conditions and his tools were highly unorthodox—table knives and scissors.

His ministry was begun with perhaps the strangest initiation rites in the history of faith healing. He was present at the bedside of a dying woman, who happened to be the wife of an acquaintance. Suddenly, this unlettered ex-miner from Conghonhas do Campo, with no instruction in medicine, moved to grasp a nearby kitchen knife and then, without further ado, plunged it straight into the stomach of the woman. He then managed to extract a huge tumour from the stomach, only nearly to collapse after the realization of what he had done hit him. Later, a doctor found the tumour to have been a uterine tumour. Arigo claimed no memory of the incident. The patient, who had been considered near death, made a full recovery and claimed to have felt no pain during the involuntary operation.

A yet more bizarre twist in the story was to follow. In a trance Arigo revealed that a German doctor, Adolphus Fritz (whose identity still remains unconfirmed), guided him in these unique operations by speaking into his right ear while the operations were conducted. Stranger still, Arigo claimed Fritz had died in Estonia in 1918. To compound this, Arigo once broke into fluent German when speaking to the German husband of a patient, under the influence of Fritz.

Twice jailed by the Brazilian authorities despite the avowal and support of his devoted followers, first in 1956 and again in 1964, Arigo's fame spread, and the sick flooded to his small house in Conghonhas do Campo. In 1968 a team of doctors saw him treat over a thousand patients. They were led by the doctor Andrija Puharich, who was stirred by what he witnessed. He would watch Arigo stare solemnly at the patient and then make an impromptu diagnosis of his or her illness. This diagnosis would then invariably be found to be accurate by the team on investigation. After having told his friends that they would not see him again, he was found dead in a car crash.

Djuna Davitashvili

The former Soviet Union's best-known healer, Djuna Davitashvili, began her career as a qualified medical researcher before developing her 'information-energy interaction with living organisms', coupled with 'contact and non-contact' massage. Possessed of penetrating and hypnotic eyes, her amazing success rate has allowed her to build up her own busy clinic in Moscow.

At the time of the inception of this book, President Boris Yeltsin was reported to be consulting Davitashvili, who chanced to be the selfsame faith healer used by one of his predecessors, Leonid Brezhnev. The illness of Yeltsin now dictates that foreign observers adopt a wait and see approach rather than give willing assistance to reform. Yeltsin's use of the powers of Djuna Davitashvili was rich with irony, as Yeltsin was part of the team of Gorbachev supporters that mocked, for political ends, Brezhnev's use of faith healing.

Davitashvili calls herself a 'chaneller of bioenergy'. Davitashvili is Assyrian and a Russian monarchist—her love of nobility has lead her to emulate them, as she is known to be fond of giving out 'titles' to believers in her mystical powers. Djuna Davitashvili claims to be a regular visitor to the Soviet leader, boosting his 'bioenergy' and alleviating the weight of office with her technique of 'contactless massage'.

Djuna Davitashvili is also famed for her powers of diagnosis. She participated in tests for the Washington Research Centre, which established that she could diagnose the various complaints of a group of forty-three subjects with a 97 per cent accuracy. She even went so far as to diagnose hitherto undetected complaints in the study group that were later substantiated by examination.

Perhaps we should not be so shocked at the use of healers by the Soviet premier as both Yeltsin and Brezhnev spent their formative years in an atmosphere of profound superstition and belief in folk medicine. It was the old Russia that retained its belief in faith cure and folk medicine long after the dominance of such practices weakened in Europe. It was only just over a century ago that every Russian village had a wizard, almost as a matter of course, and witches were hardly less prevalent. And of course one of the most famous faith healers of all time, and a creature of this very culture, Rasputin, died within living memory.

Faith healing and the Church

'And great multitudes came unto him, having with them those that were lame, blind, dumb, maimed, and many others, and cast them down at Jesus's feet; and he healed them; Insomuch that the multitude wondered, when they saw the dumb to speak, the maimed to be whole, the lame to walk, and the blind to see; and they glorified the God of Israel.'

(Matthew 15:30)

Healing was one of the most important ministries of a youthful church, which was fervent to evangelize and extend the Gospel of Jesus Christ. The notion of healing, for instance, is deeply embedded in the Catholic liturgy. The sacraments of penance and the anointing of the sick place healing firmly in the middle of the liturgical life of the church. In the Maundy Thursday service, for instance, when the priest blesses the oil of the sick he says: 'May your blessing come upon all who are anointed with this oil that they may be freed from pain, illness and disease and made well again in body, mind and soul.' It is clear from this that originally the anointing was intended as a curative ritual, but this metamorphosed in the Dark Ages into 'extreme unction', with the accent on spiritual readiness for death because it had proved so ineffective. Yet in the modern age the logical implications of what really lies behind these words is tactfully ignored. In Old English texts, the word 'healand' could be used in place of the word 'Jesus'.

For reasons we shall explore, however, the place of healing has been torn from the heart of its teaching and bulldozed to the sidelines. Eventually healing became a perfunctory practice within the church, and this has remained the case up to the present day.

The Christian religion has been systematically denatured. There are millions of people in the world at this very moment who are needlessly suffering because the church has not adequately brought the healing message of Christ's ministry into the lives of its believers, and, indeed, its nonbelievers. How did this happen?

During the apostolic era of the church, healing was a common activity of the church, and this goes some way to explain the remarkable growth in popularity of what was, after all, a sect among sects. Some commentators have pointed out that the immense success of Christianity over other religious sects that were competing with it at the time of its inception was due to the fact that it was commonly believed that the early Christian church was the most capable and successful sect at the practice of healing. This means that the practice of faith healing is one of the cornerstones of our civilization, as Western culture is a mixture of Christian and Hellenistic influences. The successful practice by the early Christians ensured that Christianity waxed while other religious sects waned. Healing was looked upon as one of the most significant vocations of a nascent church that was ardent to convert with the Gospel of Jesus Christ. Thus it truly could be said that it was under the aegis of faith healing that Christianity rose to prominence.

The healing ministry of Jesus

His reputation continued to grow, and large crowds would gather to hear him and to have their sickness cured, but he would always go off to some place where he could be alone and pray.'

(Luke 5:15–16)

Perhaps some readers may be offended to hear Jesus discussed solely as a faith healer, with the implication that he can be equated with a huge panoply of faith healers, many of whom were charlatans. Although it cannot be denied that Jesus was the archetypal healer-priest figure embodied in the earlier traditions of Greece and Egypt, it is instead our intention to show that faith healing held a deeper significance to Christ's ministry and was used as a symbolic tool by Jesus in a way that no other faith healer has ever approached or contemplated. This is why we devote an entire section to the faith healing career of Christ.

The concept of healing someone for the Hebrews entailed healing all that they were, and this attitude would have been shared by Christ himself. In fact, this is evidenced by Jesus's remark to a man who was lame. Jesus pointedly asked of him: 'Do you want to get well?' (John 5:6, NIV). His question was concerned with the mental attitude of his patient as well as his physical condition. When Christ healed the paralytic, he first healed his soul, and then his body (Matthew 9:2–7). Neither soul nor body was prioritized.

Even a rudimentary scan of the Bible reveals that the ministry of Christ and faith healing are concepts that are inextricably linked. Christ is said to be responsible for fifty paranormal occurrences recorded in the Gospels, although many of them would be viewed as the casting out of spirits rather than faith healing.

Jesus faced opposition virtually as soon as he began his public ministry. After healing the sick and casting out many evil spirits, his family were scandalized enough that they went to take charge of him, for they said 'He is out of his mind' (Mark 3:21). Even his mother Mary went to Capernaum to take charge of Jesus.

Jesus employed healing by touch: 'Then he touched their eyes, saying "According to your faith be it unto you". And their eyes were opened.' This was the origin of the practice of kings to touch the afflicted to ward off the king's evil. Sometimes this theme was varied by using spittle. Jesus himself employed this method, part of the lore of the time.

Sometimes an order was employed by Jesus in the healing process: 'Rise, take up thy bed and walk.' Jesus was also aware of the cathartic effect of the removal of unconscious guilt feelings: 'Your sins are forgiven you.' According to the New Testament, Jesus Christ sometimes brought about physical cures through the forgiveness of sin (Matthew 9:2–7). The early Christians followed his example and prayed for the healing of the sick (James 5:14–16). A sacrament of healing, the anointing of the sick, developed in the Catholic tradition, and faith healing services have been part of the Protestant tradition also.

The example of Jesus turning around in the crowd in the book of Mark is interesting:

> 'Who touched my clothes?'
> You see the people crowding against you,' his
> disciples answered, 'and yet you can ask, "Who
> touched me?"'
> But Jesus kept looking around to see who had done it.
>
> (Mark 5:30–32 NIV)

Jesus also seemed to be able to radiate a healing power about him, as when the woman suffering with a continual menstrual flow and thus ceremonially unclean touched Jesus's garment unobserved, only to find him turn around and demand: 'Who touched my garment?' Jesus had felt the healing power be drawn from him, even though his attention was focused elsewhere. The story makes clear that it is her faith that cures her and not the magic of Jesus' robe, although at the time it was a widespread belief that cures could be brought about by touching a healer.

Christ would heal hundreds of sufferers until too exhausted to carry on. He also said that others were endowed with this ability: 'He who believes in me will also do the works that I do.'

More individual healings occur in the New Testament than in the Old. At the beginning of his public ministry, Jesus announced that the Kingdom of God was near (Mark 1:15) and immediately began healing the sick and casting out demons. Of the 3,774 verses in the four Gospels, 484 relate specifically to the healing of physical and mental illness and the resurrection of the dead. Of the 1,257 narrative verses in the Gospels, 484 verses are devoted to describing Jesus's healing miracles. The last miracle that Christ wrought before the crucifixion, as documented in St Luke, was perhaps also one of the most wonderful and awe-inspiring:

> 'And a certain one of them smote the servant of the
> high priest and struck off his right ear. But Jesus
> answered and said, "Suffer ye thus far." And he
> touched his ear and healed him.'
>
> (Luke 22:50)

The ability to heal was given to the seventy-two disciples:

> Cure those who are sick and say, 'The Kingdom of
> God is very near to you'.
>
> (Luke 10:9–10).

> Jesus promised to everyone who believed in him that
> he will perform the same works as I do myself.
>
> (John 14:12).

> It was expected that in the early church the apostolate
> of healing would intensify. It is written that 'these
> will be the signs that will be associated with believers;
> they will lay their hands on the sick who will recover'
>
> (Mark 16:16–18)

If a layman was found to have the gift of healing it was considered to be a qualification for ordination.

In the first miracle after the Pentecost, Peter gave strength to a man of whom it was said that he had been 'lame from his mother's womb'. The apostle Paul saw a man at Lystra, who was thought to be 'a cripple from his mother's womb'. Paul implored the man in a loud voice to 'stand upright on thy feet', and thus the man rose to his feet. When Eutychus fell from the third storey and was 'taken up dead', Paul restored him to life again. Paul, when visiting the island of Melita, appeared to the people of the island holding a viper. When the people saw that Paul came to no harm in spite of this, they came to the conclusion that he was a god. Paul is then credited with healing the diseases of the whole island. Healing, then, came to occupy the centre of the early church's activities, with successful cures being carried out by St Jerome.

The decline of healing

After the apostolic era of the church, a change in emphasis on the significance of suffering occurred. Suffering began to be viewed as such a blessing that it was wrong to seek healing. One could perfectly imitate Christ by subjecting oneself to his suffering. Instead of healing, the church began to highlight almost exclusively the spiritual significance, and even worthiness, of suffering. Suffering became a sign of predestination and immediate entry into heaven, because it was conjectured that the sick did their suffering on earth. The notion that suffering has an ultimate redemptive value is still with us today.

In his early writings St Augustine argued that healing was meant for the early church but Christians should not look for a continuance of healing. Eventually he came to change his mind in his book *Retractions*, and declared in it that he was wrong. What had made him change his mind was his experience as bishop of Hippo (*c.* 420 AD):

> ' . . . I realized how many miracles were occurring in
> our own day and which were so like the miracles of
> old . . . how wrong it would be to allow the memory
> of these marvels of divine power to perish from
> among our people . . .'

As the church began to consolidate its power, it became antagonistic towards pagan healing traditions until, by the Middle Ages, healing had become a renegade practice and the Catholic church warned its congregations that lay healers were in league with the devil. By the 16th century, in virtually all of Europe healing was banned.

Priests had been free to practise medicine right up to the 13th century, when a papal decree had disallowed the practice. The result of this was that religion and medicine went their separate ways. The church would attend to one's soul and the physician to one's body.

Philosophy played a prominent part in the fall of healing. As well as Descartes' divorcing of the mind and body, Spinoza (1632–77) managed comprehensively to unseat the church's belief in the miraculous by suggesting that God was the cause of everything and he acted in accordance with rigid inviolable laws. Rationalism was systematically to undermine the belief in the supernatural and, by extension, the reality of healing.

Healing in Britain

The position on healing in England in the 16th century was ambivalent. Healing was easily equated with witchcraft because of its mystery and invisible processes, but protection was offered to herbalists and other folk medicine practices. In the England of the 16th and 17th century, the customary reaction to illness was to probe one's individual soul for moral misdemeanours. Physical sickness was a theological issue, and this is clear in the Elizabethan Prayer Book's command to clergymen visiting the sick to remind their patients that the illness that had befallen them was of God's decree. The ancient link between the Christian view of illness as a curse from God exists in the names of certain illnesses—St Vitus dance and St Anthony's fire (Sydenham's chorea and ergotism respectively) are two examples.

In the England of the 18th century, healing was losing ground rapidly. Thomas Hobbes (1588–1679), the author of *Leviathan*, argued that the miracles enumerated in the Old Testament could not be given credence because if they had actually happened they would have automatically brought about a world-wide wholesale belief in the Christian religion.

The Age of Enlightenment brought about perhaps the severest critic of healing, David Hume. In his 1748 essay on miracles he argues that they are a 'violation of the laws of nature'. These laws were fixed and inviolable, and he would not tolerate the suggestion that they could be transcended.

In recent history a growing awareness of literary forms in the Bible by scripture scholars and theologians has led to some quarters questioning whether or not we should take the miracles of Christ in a literal way. Today people are more interested in the historical truth of the miracles, so that the miracle stories are interpreted as having a symbolic meaning rather than a literal one. There was admittedly an inclination to embellish healing stories and inflate the numbers involved. For instance, Mark (10:46) has one blind man whereas Matthew has two (20:30). It has also been observed that some miracles resemble Rabbinic stories and older legends. Furthermore, there is a description of Vespasian healing a blind man using saliva, and a myth in the cult of Dionysus describing water being turned into wine. The healing miracles in the Bible also follow the template of other miracle stories in the Gentile miracle story tradition.

Christian existentialists such as Husserl and Kierkegaard denied the supernatural as a reality. The German Lutheran theologian Rudolf Bultmann was also to deny the objective reality of Jesus's healings.

The only form of healing accepted by many churches is so-called 'spiritual' healing. If genuine physical healing takes place, it is regarded as a problem; the Catholic church tends to distance itself from healers who claim divine inspiration in case these healers should turn out to be charlatans. While this approach is no doubt politic, it tends to undermine the place of healing in religious life. As well as this, many Christians believe that the 'well of healing' dried up with the early church and limit the healing ministry of Christ to three short years of his life.

While it may be fashionable to query the literal truth of the healings of Jesus, whether we accept the healing miracles or not, we have to see the healing ministry of Christ as central to the life of Jesus Christ and his message. Healing was Christ's symbolic way of saying to his people that he understood their problems, and was not unaware of them.

Christ's whole existence was full of suffering, his death on the cross being only the culmination of his sufferings. The Hebrews whom Jesus dwelt amongst, and indeed ministered to, saw people in a holistic sense—that is, as a person with a body, a soul, feelings and a personal history. All these things had to be integrated into a harmonious unity of absolute concord in the healing process. Illness is not just a meaningless event but to a large extent the child of a person's fears, aspirations and actions. This is a central tenet of the philosophy of holism. Holism is a philosophy that may appear new but clearly is linked to the older tradition of Plato, the Hebrews and the Chinese, along with the Yogis.

Lourdes

A place of healing?

In previous parts of this section we have tended to concentrate on the personalities who have become well known as a result of their alleged powers of spiritual healing. Any account of faith healing, however, would not be complete without an examination of the places where many people claim to have been cured of debilitating illnesses after visiting the supposed place of healing. Medjugorje in Bosnia-Herzogovina, the Portuguese village of Fatima, and Knock in the Irish Republic are regarded as nothing less than holy shrines by thousands of people (Catholics and non-Catholics alike) who make their annual pilgrimage to these places. It is Lourdes, however, a small town in the French Pyrenees, which, more than any other shrine has become synonymous with faith healing. We will examine how Lourdes became the place of worship that it is today, and whether any authenticity can be attached to the many recorded cases of miracle cures.

The story of St Bernadette

The story of Lourdes began in February 1858 when a fourteen-year-old peasant girl named Bernadette Soubirous looked upwards and saw what she considered to be an apparition of the Virgin Mary. Bernadette claimed that she beheld the apparition a further seventeen times. Considering that Lourdes today is held in such reverence by so many pilgrims, it may surprise many that Bernadette's claim to have seen the Virgin Mary was initially met with great suspicion by many people, including her parish priest, who went so far as to accuse her of lying. Others more tolerantly regarded her as a young girl with a fertile imagination who craved attention, while others were so hostile towards her that they physically attacked her. Bernadette began to refer to the vision as 'Aquero', which in local dialect meant 'that one'. It was when Bernadette found the courage to talk to the vision that she was told by the mysterious 'lady in white': 'I cannot promise happiness to you in this world, only in the next.' During the ninth apparition, Bernadette was told to search in a muddy grotto, and it was here that she came across a spring, the story quickly spreading throughout the village that the water that flowed from it would provide a miracle cure to people who were afflicted by illness if they drank it. If indeed Bernadette was a young girl who merely craved attention, then she was certainly getting it by now, with thousands of people from the village and beyond gathering at the site of the alleged miracle, hopeful that they would behold the Virgin Mary in front of them. Nonetheless, the whole spectacle was still viewed with deep suspicion and hostility by many. Her parish priest was as sceptical as he was when she told him about the first vision, and the commissioner of police regarded her as a nuisance, warning her not to make any more visits to the spring. She was interviewed by several people in authority, who were becoming increasingly concerned about the amount of people who were congregating at the spring. During one of the last apparitions to take place, the figure told her that a shrine should be built at the place where the sightings occurred. The parish priest, when told of this by Bernadette, retorted that he would only believe such a story if a miracle occurred that could be witnessed by the mass of people gathered there, not just Bernadette. But although such an event would take place later, something happened that made the Roman Catholic authorities treat the matter seriously for the first time. On another visit to the spring, the white figure appeared to Bernadette again and told her that she was 'the Immaculate Conception'.

A week later, Bernadette went to the same spot where, by this time, crowds would regularly be gathering to pay homage. She carried a solitary candle and looked awestruck at what many now considered to be the Virgin Mary. Astonishingly, she felt no pain as the flame on the candle burnt downwards and dropped searing wax on her hands. Even more astonishing was the fact that there were no burn marks on her hands. These two occurrences finally convinced the parish priest that Bernadette was speaking the truth.

By now, pilgrims were arriving from all over the world, finally convinced that the apparition that appeared before Bernadette so many times was the Virgin Mary, and that it was her miraculous powers that caused the water to flow from the spring. Bernadette, now unable to lead a normal life, found sanctuary in the local nunnery, where she remained until her death in 1879 at the age of thirty-five. Bernadette was beatified in 1925 and canonized eight years later.

One final footnote is worth mentioning. Before her sanctification, the court of canonization set up a commission, which entailed opening the sarcophagus, followed by exhumation and examination of the body. Considering that more than forty years had passed since Bernadette's death, the physicians were stunned at what they saw. Franz Werfel, in his book *The Song of Bernadette*, wrote that: 'Bernadette's girlish body showed no signs of corruption. It was almost unchanged. Face, hands and arms were white and their flesh soft. The mouth was a little open, as though breathing, so that the shimmer of the teeth was visible. The body itself was rigid and so firm that the nuns of Nevers, who witnessed the official exhumation, were able to lift it and deposit it unharmed in a new coffin, like that of one just dead.'

Miracles happen—don't they?

There have been so many recorded cases of alleged miracle cures at Lourdes that it is extremely difficult to ascertain how many of these cases are fallacies and how many are genuine. (Or at least how many pilgrims genuinely felt that their illnesses and disabilities were cured as a direct result of their visiting the shrine, even though their return to health may have been brought about by circumstances that owed nothing to divine intervention.)

It should be emphasized here that of the many thousands of pilgrims who have claimed that the healing powers of Lourdes have had a beneficial effect on them, fewer than a hundred have actually been recognized by the Roman Catholic church as being miraculous. This does not mean, however, that the Vatican has always been unerringly correct in its assumptions that miraculous healing powers have occurred or otherwise. The criteria for the authentication of supposed miracles have become increasingly stringent with the advancement of science and technology. This stringency has meant that there are doubtless several cases that, although regarded as genuine one hundred years ago, would not be viewed as such in the late 20th century.

Before discussing whether the incidents of people being cured of illness and disease at Lourdes can really be assumed to be the result of miraculous and unearthly powers, we will recount some of the more well-known tales of pilgrims who have claimed that divine intervention has been largely responsible for them to lead a life free of illness.

John Traynor

The story of John Traynor, an Irishman born in 1883, is one of the most famous cases to be associated with Lourdes and its supposed healing powers. After being drafted into the Royal Navy in 1914, the ship on which he sailed was posted to Egypt, where he had at least two head wounds inflicted upon him. Furthermore, he suffered bullet wounds in his chest, with one bullet becoming lodged close to vital nerves in his shoulder, which rendered his right arm completely paralysed. Traynor refused to heed the advice of surgeons, who urged him to agree to have his right arm amputated. Worse was to follow, however. He began to suffer epileptic fits, was unable to control his bodily functions, and by 1923 was a virtual paraplegic.

During this year, it came to his attention that an excursion was planned to Lourdes by the Liverpool diocese and, ignoring pleas from people who thought that the strain of the journey would kill him, he travelled with the rest of the pilgrims to France. It soon became apparent that the concern that his fellow travellers had displayed at the outset of the journey were being realized, for his condition deteriorated and he suffered another epileptic fit, and after being admitted to a Lourdes hospital, his epilepsy and paraplegia were officially recorded. It was only two days later that Traynor was taken down to the baths and afterwards to the ceremony of the Blessed Sacrament. It was here that he felt a tingling sensation in his right arm, and he eventually realized that he could at last move the limb that had been paralysed for the previous eight years. Later that day he could walk seven steps, and he began to feel his reflexes returning. Little by little, Traynor began to feel his limbs returning to normal use, and the following morning he rose from his bed unaided and ran outside for about a half a mile. Shortly after this remarkable occurrence, the pilgrims with whom he had travelled were due to return to Liverpool, but before their departure doctors conducted another examination on Traynor. They were amazed at the extraordinary transformation of his physical condition. Having recovered the use of his lower limbs, he could now walk quite normally, and his right arm had been restored to the condition it had been in prior to the wounds that had been inflicted. Moreover, his epilepsy appeared to have been cured, and doctors also recorded that a hole in his skull that had troubled him for years had all but disappeared. What was equally surprising was the fact that Traynor initially found it very difficult to recall any details of the crippling illness that had beset him for so long. Further examinations were carried out on Traynor on his return to Liverpool, which only confirmed what the medical team at Lourdes already knew. With the evident freedom of movement that he now enjoyed, Traynor was able to work again and, as if to prove once and for all that he had been cured, he set up his own business, occasionally carrying huge sacks of coal with his previously paralysed arm. Because the Government had classed Traynor as 'an incurable and powerless epileptic', he was entitled to a 100 per cent state pension. Evidently, however, Traynor was anything but 'incurable' and 'powerless', and he wrote to the Ministry of Pensions to inform it of his recovery. He was told that he would continue to receive his pension because his 'condition' was such that he would never regain the health that he had once enjoyed.

Traynor continued to make the pilgrimage to Lourdes almost every year until he died in 1943 at the age of sixty.

Delizia Cirollie

The tale of John Traynor has been told countless times since its occurrence in the 1920s. It is interesting to note, however, that the Roman Catholic hierarchy did not proclaim his recovery as being literally miraculous in origin. One such case that the Vatican did consider to be an example of a miracle was the case of Delizia Cirollie. Her experience at Lourdes, and her subsequent cure, is one of the most recent incidents at the shrine to be approved by the Vatican as being the result of heavenly intervention.

Delizia was a twelve-year-old girl who lived in a small village near Mount Etna in Sicily when in 1976 her right knee began causing her severe pain. She was referred to a specialist clinic at the University of Catania, where an X-ray and biopsy revealed a huge protuberance of bone. It was a far worse condition than had been thought. Because Delizia was a minor, the decision rested with her parents as to what the next course of action should be, and they refused to heed the advice of the medical team, who informed them that amputation would be the most humane method of combating such a crippling disease.

Delizia's parents were able to afford a visit to Lourdes in August of that year as a result of the sympathy and generosity of her family, friends and neighbours, although initially it seemed that the pilgrimage would have no beneficial effect whatsoever, with no signs of any miraculous healing process on her afflicted knee, despite the daily rituals that she so faithfully performed. In fact, the growth on her knee began to protrude even more, and, despite the continued prayers for her recovery and her daily intake of water from the spring, most people, including Delizia herself, were sadly accepting that the young girl had very little time left to live.

Then, in December of that year, the miracle happened. She was able to walk again, albeit a short distance at first, but soon she was able to walk for long periods of time without feeling any pain. Her convalescence was finally complete when the protuberance on her knee disappeared. The medical experts at Lourdes held differing views on the precise nature of the growth, and it was not until several years later that it was diagnosed that Delizia had been suffering from a rare form of cancer known as Ewing's tumour—a disease that nobody before Delizia had recovered from.

Divine intervention or rational explanation?

'It is our judgement that Mary, the Immaculate Mother of God, did really appear to Bernadette Soubirous in February 1858 and on certain subsequent days—to the number of eighteen times in all—in the grotto of Massabielle, near the town of Lourdes; that this Apparition bears every mark of truth and that the faithful are justified in believing it as certain.'

(Extract from a report on a special commission set up by the Bishop of Tarbes.)

The Roman Catholic church has often been criticized for its unflinchingly dogmatic views on certain subjects. It is only fair to state, however, that the authorities in the Vatican do not hold a rigid dogma relating to the many instances of faith healing at Lourdes. The complex doctrine of the Immaculate Conception was approved in Rome in 1854, only four years before the vision appeared before Bernadette and declared herself to be the Mother of Jesus. The extraordinary events in Lourdes could have prompted the Roman Catholic church to declare that a belief in the doctrine of the Immaculate Conception and a belief that the visions that Bernadette beheld were the Virgin Mary were inextricably linked, but the Church has never stated that the apparitions constitute an article of faith, although some would simply regard this standpoint as an example of the inherent conservatism of the Catholic hierarchy. It must not be assumed, therefore, that the church has a fixed attitude regarding alleged miracle cures at the shrine. We need only remind ourselves of the tiny minority of cures that the Church has officially proclaimed as miraculous to realize that this is not the case. The criteria for deciding whether a miracle could have brought about a restoration of health to a person previously afflicted was issued by Pope Benedict XIV in the 18th century. Seven conditions had to be met:

1 The disability or disease must be exceedingly difficult or even impossible to cure, as well as being an illness of a very serious nature.
2 The possibility of the invalid making a recovery from such an illness must be nonexistent.
3 If the person had received previous medical treatment, this treatment must be proved to have had no beneficial effect.
4 The cure must occur almost at once.
5 The cure must be complete.
6 It must be proved that the cure did not arise from natural causes.
7 There must be no relapse of the illness from which the invalid has recovered.

These guidelines are strictly applied, and as a direct result many alleged cases of miracle cures are rejected as non-miraculous. The panel of doctors who study the cases are chosen for their objectivity. The argument for cures arising directly as a result of divine intervention seems strong, but this has not prevented the cynics from attempting to debunk many purported cures.

One of the most notable sceptics was Dr D. J. West, a former President of the Society for Psychical Research, a man thought to have an open mind on matters relating to psychic phenomena. He found much of the evidence for cures self-contradictory. His report, *Eleven Lourdes Miracles*, was published in 1957 after visiting Lourdes and painstakingly examining the medical records relating to miracle cures. Dr West found that the details of many cases were not as scrupulously kept as had previously been thought. He began to doubt that the original diagnosis of the doctors of particular illnesses were 100 per cent accurate.

He also found that in some cases the doctors could not offer conclusive proof that the patients had not already started to recover before they made the pilgrimage to Lourdes. Furthermore, he found that no proof could be offered that the patients whose cases he examined were suffering from incurable illnesses or disease.

Also, in several of the cases that he chose to study, there were disagreements between members of the medical team, who were unable to decide whether or not the cures defied scientific or medical explanation.

In fairness to Dr West, his report did not actually state that miraculous events did not actually take place at Lourdes, only that the evidence that appeared to lend credibility to the miraculous eradication of illnesses was not as conclusive as it was originally thought to be.

Dr West's report came in for severe criticism from Professor David Morrell, who worked at St Thomas's Hospital in London. He stated correctly that of the eleven cases studied by Dr West, none had proved to have been recoveries that came about as a result of natural causes. Professor Morrell pointed out that *Eleven Lourdes Miracles* concentrated on cases from the 1930s and 1940s, when medical tests were much more reliant on clinical findings for the diagnosis of illness. Moreover, he argued that there could obviously be no way of knowing whether an invalid would be miraculously cured following a visit to Lourdes. If it had been known, then previous medical records would undoubtedly have been more carefully kept, he argued. Professor Morrell was particularly condemnatory of Dr West's assertion that hysteria, neurosis and suggestibility were present in some of the cases that he studied. As Professor Morrell said:

> 'If I see a paralysed patient with contraction flex or spasms and gross neurological signs suddenly cured, I find this difficult to explain irrespective of the diagnosis. The startling thing to me about these cases is that desperately ill patients got suddenly better and stayed better. This is hardly typical of hysterical or functional illness . . .'

We must not overlook the fact that the great majority of visitors to Lourdes are not people suffering from incurable illnesses, but tourists who arrive there simply to satisfy their curiosity and generally enjoy their holiday. This is worth mentioning because it is easy for the sick to get carried away by the sheer atmosphere that Lourdes engenders, which could leave some of them open to suggestibility. This was doubtless the case when Princess Grace of Monaco arrived at Lourdes with a pilgrimage from her country. One of the pilgrims claimed that a wound on her leg had suddenly disappeared, and many were quick to proclaim this as a miracle. It soon became clear, however, that the wound, which was sustained in a serious road accident, would have disappeared anyway. It was merely a coincidence that the wound began to heal when she visited Lourdes. Of course, stories like this do nothing to explain the mystery of miracle cures, which are presently beyond the realms of scientific explanation.

Many believers in the healing powers of Lourdes often claim that the doctors of some patients have refused to cooperate and have been reluctant to take part in the investigative process. This is cited as one of the reasons why, in some cases, subsequent examinations did not result in the cures being called miraculous. This is not as fanciful as it may sound at first. Nowadays the medical profession has a more open-minded approach to the Lourdes phenomenon, but it was not always so. Such was the degree of scepticism with which the profession viewed events at Lourdes that a doctor who was brave enough to put forward the view that a miracle may have occurred risked being laughed out of his job. Little wonder that so few doctors were willing to cooperate.

This hostility is perhaps best typified by the story of Alexis Carrell in 1902. A young French doctor and an eventual Nobel Prize winner, Carrell went on a pilgrimage to Lourdes, more out of curiosity than anything else. He became aware that one of the sick pilgrims was in such a bad condition that she was spitting blood. Her pulse rate was alarmingly high and her face had turned blue. Carrell concluded that she was suffering from tuberculosis. He was amazed to observe that once the girl had felt the bath water and taken part in the blessed sacrament procession, she was cured of her illness. In Carrell's book, *Journey to Lourdes*, he defied the scepticism of his profession by stating that many events at Lourdes 'prove the reality of certain links between psychological and organic processes. They prove the objective value of spiritual activity which has been ignored by doctors, teachers and sociologists.'

It was opinions such as these that only increased the hostility of his colleagues at the university in Lyons where he lectured, and he was forced to leave. What aggrieved Carrell was the fact that his colleagues were so willing to dismiss events he had seen take place in front of his own eyes.

To conclude, we are forced to admit that we are not much nearer to unravelling the mystery of Lourdes than we were when the apparitions first appeared to Bernadette in 1858. Tests have shown that the water at the spring at Lourdes is no more remarkable than the water that we use in everyday life. What is remarkable, of course, is that many people have made recoveries after having come into contact with the water. Until such time as advances in science and medicine can settle these arguments, however, the mystery of Lourdes will remain unsolved.

The variability of disease

In this book we would hope to avoid slobbering over the slippers of faith healing and present the subject fairly. This entails telling a few truths about the nature of disease. Anyone who would advocate the use of faith healing or a visit to a shrine should consider the following points carefully.

With every disease that has a fatal outcome, there are some patients who fare better than the average. For example, in one study, 2 per cent of patients with widespread liver metastases from colorectal cancer survived for five years. These survivors could not ascribe their good fortune to effective treatment, for none was available to them. Instead they demonstrate the natural variability of disease.

In many diseases, such as cancer and multiple sclerosis, a patient's progress follows an oscillating route but a route that is generally moving downwards. Many patients will find that their condition suddenly alleviates and plateaus for a time, even although the general trend is downwards. Many doctors and healers in contact with the sufferer will take the credit for this apparent return to health, playing on the ignorance of the sufferer. Yet it is a rudimentary of logic that because C follows B, we cannot therefore say that B caused C. B here, of course, is the visit to the healer or conventional doctor and C the remission of the illness. All that has happened is a plateauing stage in a downward spiral. The later deterioration to a condition worse than before is frequently out of the public eye and conveniently disregarded.

The respected American cancer researcher Emil J Freireich codified this phenomenon into the 'Freireich Experimental Plan', which demonstrated that any treatment administered to an illness could be proved to have been effective.

Neurotic patients can often experience rapid fluctuations in the progress of their illness. Unexpected improvements can and do occur over a given length of time, and it is such an event that problematizes the work of the healer. This phenomenon is usually known as 'spontaneous remission'. Clearly, a cold will eventually go away no matter what you do, even if you do nothing at all.

Most visitors to a faith healer will be at their lowest ebb. For them the only way is up—and although not to deny the therapeutic value of the healer, it is likely that in cases where patients enjoyed a sudden improvement, they were on an upward surge that would have happened anyway.

Faith healers also have the dice loaded in their favour because the majority of people who will come to them for treatment will be fairly well educated when it comes to medicine, at least educated enough to be aware of the possibilities of healing and complementary therapy. What occurs is a form of medicinal natural selection; extremely disturbed patients, such as sexual deviants and alcoholics, will probably be unaware of the potential of complementary therapy or not regard it as a possible line of enquiry.

Another problem is that the healer has a vested interest in declaring his or her treatment a success and may assess events accordingly. The patients of faith healers themselves are scarcely any more objective. The typical account of a healing will run something like this:

> I believe with all my heart that on February 19— I witnessed a healing, a healing that cannot be adequately explained by the normal dictates of medicine. My daughter Sally has been rescued from the jaws of death, and I wish to proclaim God's work through your journal.
>
> My daughter was born with a closed pylorus, the sphincter that connects the stomach with the bowel. Consequently Sally could not retain even a thimbleful of milk or a Farley's rusk, and without such nourishment, the child grew alarmingly weak, and her body grew smaller and smaller until everyone concluded that she was on the verge of death.
>
> We first sent for a priest, who bent down and kneeled at the foot of the bed. We earnestly hoped for some upturn, and watched her day and night. Yet it seemed our prayers were not answered and we began to fear the worst.
>
> One evening, during this critical period, a friend of the family happened to mention that she was friendly with a member of the local Christian Science network. Having been ushered into the house in an atmosphere of hope and trepidation, the practitioner confidently went to work. By morning Sally was able to take a full glass of milk and retain it. We thank the Lord for saving our daughter, and we are now firm Christian Scientists.

A passage like this inevitably plays to our emotions, indeed, it is an appeal to our emotionalism. It would be a hard heart indeed that queried the truth of it. There is probably something very deep within human beings that wants to believe in stories like this and that healers can make a difference to the sorry lot of ordinary men and women who are unfortunate enough to be plagued by illness. The truth is that humankind, to all intents and purposes, is powerless against the onslaught of disease. This is a truth that few of us would not find hard to stomach.

Disease is still mysterious to us. One day, a cell becomes cancerous. It begins to eat away at the other cells that surround it, forming a colony. This colony is detected and then destroyed, but colonies of the same cancer begin to appear elsewhere. Still no one can adequately explain why this happens.

Another prime example of the enigma of illness is disseminated sclerosis, a disease in which degeneration occurs in the myelin sheath of the nerve fibres of the brain and spinal cord. The cause of the disease is unknown, and there is no known cure. Death usually results from pneumonia or chronic urinary infection. The tendency to spontaneous improvement is a remarkable feature of the early stages of the disease and can make diagnosis and acceptance of diagnosis and supposed cure problematic for all concerned. The function of the doctor is to administer the palliative use of drugs, the inverse of the homeopathic art of healing.

Healing and hysteria

A highly charged religious atmosphere surrounding the place of pilgrimage, such as Lourdes, or a healing session can sometimes influence a patient and imbue him or her with a desire to combat the illness that once they had regarded as a fait accompli. Urged on by the atmosphere of excitement and by dramatic renderings from the platform, cripples elatedly throw away their crutches and the once blind claim their sight has been miraculously restored. There is known to be a form of hysteria observable at mass healing gatherings in which the illness of the patient is temporarily cast aside, and he or she can confidently walk up and down the stage and appear to have been healed. Such phenomena are usually ephemeral and the patients return to their former state once the show is over. An instance of this occurred when the American faith healer Maurice Cerullo visited Britain in 1992. He staged a mass healing during which a young girl, called Natalia Barned, who was confined to a wheelchair was seen to walk across his stage unaided. What had happened was probably a triumph of will on the part of the young girl. What is key here is the emotional state of the sufferer—it is known that during periods of religious ecstasy the symptoms of quite serious illnesses can be temporarily alleviated.

These factors—the variability of illness, the short-termism of many healing cures and our own emotionalism, considered together—should all be kept in mind when assessing the validity of healing. But we should also bear in mind that none of this necessarily negates the practice of healing, as cures do occur that cannot be refuted by these factors.

Christian Science

Origins—Mary Baker Eddy

Socially, politically and economically, early 19th-century America was experiencing a great deal of changes. This was soon to be intensified by the Civil War (1861–65). The mood of stern Calvinism was gradually changing, and new quasi-scientific movements began to appear. New England and New York had become hotbeds of interest in all things connected with unconventional medicine. The 19th century can fairly be described as the golden age of the quack doctor. Mass education had brought with it the popular press with a large un-critical readership ready to swallow any miracle as long as it was framed in pseudo-scientific language. Doctors were thin on the ground and science had caught the popular imagination and added a new irresistible frisson to the an-cient practice of quackery, which had previously had to rely on folklore and superstition for its credibility.

The 1890s saw the rise to prominence of Mary Morse Baker, better known as Mary Baker Eddy (1821–1910). Mark Twain called her 'the most daring and masculine woman that has appeared on the earth in centuries'. It was this New Hampshire mystagogue who founded the Christian Science movement.

Formative years

Her upbringing was pervaded by a claustrophobic Calvinism provided by her father, Mark Baker. Her mother's death in childbirth in 1849, when Mary was a teenager, profoundly affected her. It would be the first of many deaths of peo-ple that were close to her in her life. Throughout her childhood she was given to temper tantrums, usually brought about by arguments with her father. These tantrums graduated to hysteria and even visions in her adolescent years. Once she claimed to hear voices calling her 'three times in ascending scale', a story that echoes the Biblical story of Samuel. She was also given to extended bouts of dieting, which would bring her to an almost emaciated state. When the trau-mas of adolescence became too much she could be restored to equanimity only by being rocked like a child in the arms of her father, a fact that more than one psychologist has seized on in search of the illuminating principle of her life.

At twenty-two she married George Washington Glover, a building contractor eleven years her senior. His death from yellow fever the following year, 1844, left Baker with a son, her only child, and financially virtually penniless. Her child was eventually fostered, and they would enjoy an ambivalent relationship for the rest of their lives.

Phineas Parkhurst Quimby

Her next husband, a dentist by the name of Patterson, eventually left her, but by this point she had met the figure who would dictate the future course of her life, Phineas Parkhurst Quimby (1802–66). Baker, on hearing of the miraculous cures being administered by Quimby, decided to travel to Maine from Boston in order to gain an audience with this Swedenborgian. She and Quimby first met at the International Hotel in Portland, Maine, in October 1862. Baker was immediately taken by his ideas and his personal magnetism. He was a healer who denied the efficacy of medicine and proposed instead that the only real curative force was that of the patient's belief in the healer and his ability to heal. Quimby possessed a strong personal magnetism, and although he was poorly educated, he managed to mould his experiences into a philosophy; he founded the anti-materialist Swedenborgian school of New Thought, whose following included at least a dozen other American healers. Quimby claimed disarmingly that his cures were not due to any paranormal force but instead merely to the faith that his various patients had in him, and this alone. Quimby opined: 'I tell the patient his troubles, and what he thinks is his disease, and my explanation is the cure.'

His results were obtained by placing his hand on the patient's head and abdo-men in order to let the healing magnetic forces take hold. In this he believed that he had rediscovered the very method that Jesus had employed in healing. He would eventually discard his mesmerism for a metaphysical form of faith healing. Quimby was significant in the history of faith healing because he forged a link between the use of the hypnotic and the wholly suggestive ap-proaches, as he progressed from the former to the latter in his career.

Quimby urged that we 'think good, not evil'. If the mind could be cleared of negative thoughts, then this would lead to a healthy body. Baker told Quimby that she had been suffering from 'spinal inflammation'. The cure administered by Quimby began to be effective before their consultation—her anticipation built up to such an extent that she felt better even before he ministered to her. His treatment ensured that she could walk normally and climb stairs again. Eventually she succumbed to invalidity and gastric pains once more, but she had become a firm believer in Quimby's ideas, although prior to meeting Quimby she had written 'If I believe I am sick, I am sick . . . all disease is in the mind.' She spent the next two years adapting Quimby's philosophy to her own ideas and would one day dismiss him as an 'illiterate mesmerist' and deride his mesmerism as a 'big bubble', an idea she had long been disabused of.

In October 1865, Eddy's father died. Quimby himself met with illness. He had resisted orthodox medicine in the treatment of his illness, a stomach ulcer, and instead insisted that his illness could be brought to heel by the power of his own 'active will'. He died in January 1866.

In February 1866 came the formative moment, when Baker slipped on an icy patch in the street and was knocked unconscious. She claimed her miraculous recovery was accountable to her reliance on the Bible. From being an incurable invalid, she recovered enough to be able to walk around unaided. Some commentators have speculated that Baker's illness was the result of a neurotic depressive reaction. As the Christian Science movement gained ground her health continued to fluctuate wildly, depending on her mood and situation.

This single-minded child of the Calvinist gloom appropriated a mixture of the ideas of Quimby and German metaphysics in the development of her movement. Some observers describe Christian Science as an amalgam of a metaphysical system that relies on an obsolete theory of logical monism adjusted from the German Idealists, a Christian sect and a method of therapy.

Publication of Science and Health

Her ideas (Quimby had already used the term 'Christian Science' in describing his philosophy) were formally enunciated in her magnum opus, *Science and Health*. Her hypothesis was that 'the only realities are the divine mind and its ideas . . . . Rightly understood, instead of possessing sentient matter, we have sensationless bodies . . . . Whence came to me this conviction in antagonism to the testimony of the human senses? From the self-evident fact that matter has no sensation; from the common human experience of the falsity of all material things; from the obvious fact that mortal mind is what suffers, feels, sees: since matter cannot suffer.'

Baker also wrote: 'I cannot be supermodest in my estimation of the Christian Science textbook'. This perhaps unconsciously ironic appraisal of the bible of the Christian Science movement comes from the *Christian Science Journal* of 1901. In writing the book she had 'borrowed' verbatim thirty-three pages of a work by the scholar Francis Lieber, which dealt with the work of the German philosopher Hegel. Another hundred pages of Lieber's work she simply reworded. This reworking of ideas already extant was, in truth, completely appropriate to the spirit of all the other competing forms of Christian healing at the time, which were all variations on a theme compounded of contemporary religious ideas, occult practices and metaphysics, with the leaders of these various sects all drawing from the same well.

Other aspects of the movement were probably appropriated from other sects; for example, her advocacy of silent prayer was taken from Quakerism. It is ironic that one of her former students, called Arens, was sued by her for infringing her copyright on Christian Science ideas in his book *Old Theology in its Application to the Healing of the Sick.* She was renowned for the swift repression of any potential rivalry for the leadership of the movement.

In 1877 she married for a third time, aged fifty-six, to a forty-five-year-old agent for a sewing machine manufacturer, called Asa Gilbert Eddy. Like her, he also suffered from poor health. A passive recipient of his wife's doctrines, he was the first acolyte to become a public convert to the Church of Christ, Scientist, which she founded in Boston in 1879. Although supposedly cured of assorted abdominal and chest pains by his wife, Asa's pains returned after a short interval. Like Quimby before him, he insisted that he could control the pains himself. Eddy claimed that her husband was being 'mentally murdered' by means of animal magnetism employed by her enemies. This streak of paranoia became marked in her later years. For instance, she ascribed her public maligning and ridicule, as well as her personal misfortune, to the result of an unseen baleful influence, what she called 'animal magnetism'. Eventually they resorted to orthodox medicine for treatment. Organic heart disease was diagnosed and later confirmed at Asa's autopsy. Eddy refused to accept this diagnosis and insisted that an unseen psychic Mafia had murdered her husband.

Eddy's wealth

Mary Baker Eddy eventually left Boston and retired to Concord, visiting the centre of Christian Science in Boston only another four times in her life, although still maintaining a strong grip on the movement and its organization to the end of her life. She founded a college and a newspaper and lectured continuously until she died of pneumonia in 1910. Like Mesmer, she managed to accumulate a fortune from her religious healing work. Membership of the Christian Science movement rose to a peak in the 1930s with an estimated 300,000 members. Since then membership has drastically fallen as Christian Science has had to compete in the marketplace with other sects.

Although the name of Christ appears in the movement's title, Eddy did write: 'If there had never existed such a Galilean prophet (Jesus) it would make no difference to me.' (*Science and Health*). And the movement's denial of the role of the physician goes against the use of the physician advocated in the Bible, specifically in Ecclesiastes:

> 'The Lord hath created medicines out of the earth;
> and he that is wise will not abhor them . . . . Give
> place to the physician, for the Lord hath created him;
> let him not go from thee, for thou hast need of him.
> There is a time when in their hands there is good
> success.'

It is difficult to assess the Christian Science movement. There is little attention to charity, no interest in any supernatural power, and health and wealth are promised to its followers, who are and were mainly middle class. Christian Science could happily deny the reality of matter but did not so easily deny the value of money. At the end of her life, Eddy had become a wealthy woman, with a fortune estimated at upwards of four million dollars. To take a short course at her 'metaphysical college' cost 300 dollars alone.

The Christian Science movement's views on healing can appear to be inconsistent. Some members will employ the use of dentists, doctors, opticians and doctors, if need be. Indeed, Eddy herself used drugs, especially morphine to dull pain, on numerous occasions towards the end of her life. Beyond this, there are ethical problems with the philosophy of the group. Treating all pain as delusional instead of as a warning sign that demands enquiry into the cause is obviously foolish, as is risking the aggravation of a depression in a patient, brought about by telling him or her that his or her illness is both delusional and equivalent to sin and, by extension, the fault of the patient. For instance, Eddy denied that food promulgated life—she was given to making remarks such as 'we have no evidence of food sustaining life, except false evidence'.

Eddy's teaching on the unreality of matter, sin and suffering seems to conflict with the Biblical doctrines of the Creation, Fall and Redemption. It should also be remembered that Jesus himself said no word that could reasonably be interpreted as hostile to the physical medicine of his time.

Christian Science also has its own individual slant on healing, although the movement is not primarily curative in aim. The distinction between the Christian Scientist and that of the standard faith healer on the matter of healing is that, while the latter holds that pain and disease are actually illusions of the imagination, the faith healer admits their existence but affirms the possibility of their removal by non-scientific means.

Eddy's personal philosophy could be strange. On the health of infants, she advises: 'The condition of the stomach, bowels, food, clothing, etc, is of no serious importance to your child.' The Christian Scientist is happy if his patient knows little or nothing, because 'a patient thoroughly booked in on medical theories has less sense of the divine power, and is more difficult to heal through Mind, than an aboriginal Indian who never bowed the knee to the Baal of civilization.'

As well as reality and food, the idea that procreation was what produced life came in for some heavy criticism: 'Until it is learned that generation rests on no sexual basis, let marriage continue . . . . The suggestion that life germinates in eggs is shown by divine metaphysics to be a mistake' (quoted in Godwin).

Some passages of *Christian Science* are just plain confused: 'The nothingness of nothing is plain; but we need to understand that error is nothing, and that its nothingness is not saved, but must be demonstrated in order to prove the somethingness . . . of Truth.'

She claimed to have administered one cure by preaching to a horse. Perhaps it should be said that to mock the ideas of Christian Science is taking an easy target. We should remember that Eddy's time was not our own before we rush to judge her approach to healing. It would be the turn of the century before Sigmund Freud and Carl Jung stated that certain illnesses could reside in the unconscious mind.

Eddy's philosophies

'In less than three weeks from the time of us turning to Christian Science treatment, Kristen's burn was completely covered with fresh skin. There was no need for a bandage any more, and the visible signs of the burn were fading. Kristen was back in her Kindergarten class shortly thereafter. Christian Science treatment was continued and she now walks and runs normally . . . .'

So speaks another happy customer of the Christian Science approach. Yet Kristen's burn would no doubt have healed substantially after the space of three weeks given no treatment whatsoever. As Disraeli once said, 'Time is the great physician'. Note we are told that this 'three weeks' is only the three weeks since the Christian Science treatment began, not since the burn was incurred. One has to ask precisely what would constitute failure for Christian Science treatment in the light of this. We should bear in mind that 80 to 90 per cent of illnesses recover under any treatment or with absolutely no treatment.

Medical training and registration were still in a rudimentary state in Eddy's time, so her self-awarded title of 'doctor' would have been honorary. In England the Apothecaries Act of 1815 stopped unqualified doctors from practising medicine. Yet we cannot deny this able commander her due, which resided in her tremendous organizational ability. Her youthful girlish appearance was a great asset, presenting both a physically attractive woman with dark brooding eyes but at the same time a 'safe' mother figure, which appealed to the many insecure and neurotic males who attended her. Other competing contemporary religious movements, such as Andrew Jackson Davis's doctrines of life health and cures, failed to show the staying power of Eddy's movement, even though during the 1840s his movement was as big as Christian Science in terms of popularity. Jackson simply did not have the drive and ambition and sheer blind energy of Eddy. In her favour, Mrs Eddy's positive encouraging nature must have consoled the many who felt forsaken by conventional medicine.

As was once said of Oscar Wilde, Eddy stood in direct symbolic relation to her time. Virtually all her adult life was spent during the reign of Queen Victoria, which also coincided with the emergence of the emancipation for women movement and the fight for female suffrage. Mrs Eddy and her followers were a great boost to the female cause as it was highly unusual at the time for a woman to be giving lectures and addressing public meetings.

Another means by which she captured the zeitgeist was by grasping, either consciously or unconsciously, the need for a movement that would alleviate religious insecurities by reconciling the old Christian orthodoxy with the unknown element of the new emergent science—although, of course, there was very little or nothing about the movement that could be called truly scientific—nevertheless, she intimately understood what was needed to massage and reassure the psychological hurts and uncertainties that lay deep in the American psyche. She anticipated the mood of the middle classes and catered to it. Christian Science's advocacy of 'healthy-mindedness', as William James put it, coupled with an open and receptive attitude to materialism, told the middle classes exactly what they wanted to hear. Mrs Eddy's receptivity to her public was truly awe-inspiring. No doubt she would have made an excellent politician in another time. She also anticipated many of the practices of modern medicine. The modern psychological approach to chronic pain is based on the relief of anxiety, distraction and suggestion, which is strikingly similar to the approach advocated by Eddy. In a sense, Eddy's hypothesis is correct—unhappiness and suffering do indeed only exist in the mind; it is her contention that illness and disease do not have objective existence that one has to refute.

In the various photographs taken of Eddy we see a wistful melancholic face—a face remarkably similar to that of Greatrakes—with black hair framing eyes brimming with soulful intensity. In the two most commonly printed photographs of her she appears to be quietly amused at some inward joke to herself. Perhaps the joke was on us.

Spiritual healing therapies

Outside the realm of the evangelist and the healing ministries of the church, there is a whole different movement that embraces the healing ethic while not wishing to limit itself to the confines of a particular religious doctrine. The spiritual healer seeks to provide for the large sections of society that do not subscribe to any given religious system but do acknowledge the spiritual dimension of their existence.

In addition, spiritual healers reject the term 'faith healing' because, apart from suggesting a required religious belief, it implies that the patient must at least have faith in the healer's capacity to heal in order for the treatment to have any effect. This has been proved not to be the case, as on their list of successful healings, spiritual healers can include children, animals and even plants, which are presumably incapable of faith. Even the most hardened sceptic can be healed; the only thing that the patient is required to believe in is that he or she wants to be well.

Nowadays, the term 'spiritual healing' specifically refers to the type of healing practised by the National Federation of Spiritual Healers (NFSH), which has around 8,000 healers on its register. Spiritual healing is, in fact, listed as a recognized therapy within the National Health Service; GPs are permitted by the General Medical Council to refer their patients for spiritual healing, and it is possible for NFSH healers to visit hospital inpatients on request. Some enlightened doctors do actually realize that good health is more than simply an absence of illness, and that a state of spiritual imbalance can be as debilitating as a physical disorder.

Spiritual healers address themselves to the non physical aspect of being, working on the level of the spirit or soul rather than that of the body. They direct healing energy to the inner essence of an individual, and if this vital spark responds, the body's healing mechanisms can be activated.

The other definitively 'spiritual' element of spiritual healing is the source of its healing power. Where the faith healer invokes the will of God to heal, the spiritual healer calls upon the power of nature, or the all-pervasive life force that unites us.

It should be pointed out at this stage that spiritual healing is not to be confused with spiritualist healing. Spiritualism entails a fervent belief in the afterlife as its basis and effects its healing through communication with dead spirits. This form of healing is discussed later in Healing and the Occult.

There are two basic types of spiritual healing—contact and absent.

Contact healing is the more common form employed by healers, usually identified by the term 'the laying on of hands'. This phrase has distinctly mystical, and even biblical, connotations, but in fact it is a very simple procedure, performed in order to implement healing. It is perhaps the oldest, and certainly the simplest, type of healing in existence. Everyone knows the therapeutic value of the intimacy of touch. When a fellow human being is in distress we instinctively reach out a hand to place on his or her arm or shoulder, and this gesture is immediately recognized to be both comforting and reassuring.

Obviously, the laying on of hands by professional healers goes beyond simply making someone 'feel better'. It is their way of transferring vital energy to the patient, thus stimulating the body's natural restorative mechanisms and enabling the healing process to be set into motion.

The 'laying on of hands' denotes exactly that—the healer lays his or her hands either directly on, or just above, the patient's body. The hands are usually placed on the head or shoulders, or on a specifically affected part of the body. Sometimes a healer likes to move his or her hands down the spine, an important part of the human body that can reveal ailments in other regions. Many healers are able to diagnose with their hands, as well as heal, although this is not advisable in place of a proper medical examination and diagnosis. This method does, however, help to guide the healer to the areas of the body where energy levels have become depleted because of illness or injury. The healer will sense an imbalance and be able to restore lost energy by passing life force through the hands. The patient will usually experience a sensation of heat in the area where the problem is located. This is the thermal energy, visible using Kirlian photography, that is transmitted through the touch of the healer's hands and penetrates the body in much the same way as scientifically proven deep heat treatment. The process of replacing lost energy usually feels wonderful for the recipient, inducing a feeling of calmness, contentment and deep relaxation.

This transfer of energy may sound like a form of magic, but no genuine spiritual healer would ever claim to possess special, mystical powers. All honest healers acknowledge that they themselves neither create nor possess healing power or energy but merely act as channels for a higher power. Their talent is not the gift of healing but the gift of being able to tap into universal healing energy.

Most spiritual healers who practise contact healing also practise absent or distant healing. As the name suggests, the healing is performed in the patient's absence, sometimes even without their knowledge. The principles of harnessing the healing forces and channelling them to the patient remain the same, however. In this case the positive energy is transmitted in the form of a healing message. The healer sends out healing vibrations while clearly visualizing the recipient in perfect health, perhaps bathed in ethereal light. Sometimes the name of the sufferer is spoken out loud, creating a telepathic link along which the energy can travel. The nature of the illness to be cured, however, should not be uttered or even thought about, because this will add potency to the illness in the mind and make it grow stronger.

Absent healing is obviously particularly suitable for patients living far away, but also for children, animals, the mentally deranged, the chronically ill and those who are unconscious in a coma. Absent healing can be highly beneficial for anyone who is incapable of taking an active part in his or her own healing. It does not matter that the recipient may not be actively receptive to the healing vibrations—as long as he or she is not sending out negative counter-healing messages there will still be benefit.

Radionics is a slightly more dubious form of distant healing, involving specially designed instruments. A 'black box' is employed that can pick up the electromagnetic radiations emitted by all living things. The instrument can be used as a diagnostic tool by tuning into 'diseased' wavelengths and translating them into electrical frequencies, determining an individual's mental, physical and emotional state. By transmitting vibrationally suitable wavelengths, the unsatisfactory condition can be cured. This all sounds very technical, drawing from the laws of physics, but in fact the practice of radionics is highly unscientific and relies largely on the intuition and sensitivity of the practitioner. There is, in fact, no scientific evidence of the effectiveness of radionics nor any logical reason why it should work.

Now that you know a little about the basic ways in which spiritual healers operate, and the techniques they employ, we should focus on how to find a suitable healer.

Finding the name and address of a spiritual healer in your area is relatively easy, as the NFSH provides lists, but finding a healer who works for you, and with whom you feel comfortable, may be a different matter. Basically it is a question of using your intuition and listening to your instincts. Healing is a two-way process, and it is important that a mutual bond is established between healer and patient, allowing the free passage of healing energy from one to the other. The patient must therefore feel fully at ease with the chosen healer and be able to relax and express himself or herself freely in the healer's presence.

Spend a bit of time chatting to the healer before you commit yourself to undergoing a session of treatment. If you feel at all uncomfortable with him or her, do not be afraid to suggest that perhaps he or she is not the right practitioner for you and leave. Do not accept treatment from a healer who appears tired or weak; he or she obviously does not know how to harness the healing life force properly and may even drain you of whatever vital energy you have. Also, be on the lookout for anything that seems vaguely self-serving in the healer's character, behaviour or manner, such as traces of ego or lust. The role of the healer as lover is discussed in Roles of the healer, but in this situation, dishonourable intentions on either side could become a serious obstacle to effective healing. Genuine healers offer their services out of a sincere wish to use what powers they have to help people in suffering, not for the rewards, either emotional or material, that this may bring.

While on this subject, the question of whether spiritual healers should charge for their services remains a contentious issue. There are those who believe that it is wrong to make money out of desperate, suffering people, but anyone wishing to concentrate on exercising their healing abilities on a full-time basis obviously requires some kind of income. Most healers compromise by asking for donations, and those who charge a fee can usually be negotiated with if there is a real need.

To give you some idea of the different kinds of healing experience that are possible, here are four people's personal stories of spiritual healing. Each illustrates something different that can be achieved through healing while expressing something universal about the nature of the human condition and the healing phenomenon.

Case study 1

Mick Allstrap, a thirty-two-year-old journalist working in Amsterdam, visited a spiritual healer for the first time during a recent return visit to the UK. A card-carrying sceptic, Mick decided to undergo this experience, partly out of journalistic curiosity and partly out of sheer desperation after a string of doctors had been unable to help him.

Mick has suffered from recurrent back problems ever since his teens, when he was the victim of an unprovoked street attack by a gang of youths. The muscle tissues surrounding the vertebrae were damaged, resulting in frequent bouts of intense pain and slightly restricted movement.

The back and spine are complex and vulnerable areas of the body, notoriously difficult to treat effectively. There are a limited number of medical treatments available for a doctor to administer, the most commonly prescribed being painkillers and anti-inflammatory agents, which merely alleviate the discomfort temporarily.

Dissatisfied with the little that orthodox medicine had to offer, Mick decided to bite the bullet and look elsewhere. Through a friend he found the name and address of a Romanian spiritual healer living just outside Glasgow and arranged a session.

Arriving for his appointment full of trepidation, Mick was pleasantly surprised to be ushered into a brightly lit flat by an elegant middle-aged woman who did not conform to his mental image of a kaftan-wearing New Age casualty.

The woman carried out an immediate psychic appraisal, correctly identifying Mick's back as the 'sick' part of his body, as well as several minor ailments of which he had not been aware. Mick told the healer about the way in which he had sustained the original back injuries, and she nodded sagely.

After taking off his shoes, Mick was asked to lie on his stomach on the treatment bench and to relax and breath deeply. The woman then clasped his feet, one in each hand. Mick could actually feel a flow of energy running from her left hand into his left foot, up his left side and back down his right side, through his right foot into the woman's right hand. He felt the energy forming a complete circuit around his body, which felt wonderful, relaxing and revitalizing.

Then the woman focused her energy upon Mick's back, laying her hands on the affected area. It felt as if all the energy that had been circulating his body was suddenly drawn to an epicentre, creating a tremendous amount of heat where the healer's hands were placed. As well as heat, Mick began to experience a substantial amount of pain, even though the woman was not applying any pressure with her hands. She explained that, because of the traumatic way in which his back had come to be in its present state, he had been withholding the pain of the original assault. In order to heal, Mick had to confront the pain, re-experience it and release it.

Before the pain escalated to an unbearable level, the healer ran her hands swiftly down from his back to his feet. This action was accompanied by what Mick could only describe as a 'whooshing' sensation, as the heat and pain travelled down his body and out through the soles of his feet.

On standing up, Mick was delighted to find that the pains in his back had indeed gone, along with a headache he had had that morning. In fact, he felt like a new man. The healer advised him to take life slowly over the following few days as he would probably feel slightly sick and groggy because of the stale energy that had been displaced during the healing gradually eliminating itself from his system.

Several weeks on, and still feeling the benefits, Mick had to admit that the treatment had worked for him and that something remarkable and inexplicable had taken place. He still, however, remains sceptical as to the source of his healing.

Case study 2

This next story concerns a young man in his mid-twenties, whom we shall call Declan. Born and brought up in the Stockport area, the only son of an elderly Catholic couple, Declan began to develop obsessive-compulsive disorder, or OCD, at the age of eighteen.

For anyone unfamiliar with this condition, it is a severely debilitating form of mental illness that can have devastating effects on the sufferer's daily life. The disorder usually begins as a phobia, an irrational fear that escalates into an all-consuming obsession. Sufferers often believe that some terrible fate will befall them if they do not carry out particular actions. These actions are often ritualized and performed in a specific pattern, making even the simplest of tasks tortuous.

In Declan's case, his obsessive-compulsive behaviour first manifested itself in a morbid fear of coming into contact with bacteria and germs. This began in church when, during mass, he would be expected to shake hands with the people next to him. The thought of this, and the exchange of bacteria involved, repulsed him in the extreme until he could eventually no longer participate. He also began to dread handling money and having to touch the hands of shop assistants as they handed him change. He could not prevent his mind from dwelling on the idea that some coins could have been in circulation for as long as twenty years, accumulating bacteria that he could not avoid touching.

The next stage was compulsive hand-washing, a common behavioural pattern in OCD sufferers. Declan would perform numerous hand-washing rituals, both before and after completing any given task. Especially before eating or preparing food, he would wash his hands for at least half an hour, scrubbing them with a nail brush.

Declan's parents began to notice that his hands were often red raw until eventually his father confronted him and persuaded him to see a doctor. The doctor referred Declan to a psychiatrist in the hope of uncovering some psychological trigger for this obsessive-compulsive behaviour. The psychiatrist proffered several theories for Declan's condition, centring on some possibly forgotten trauma in infancy combined with Catholic guilt and repression. This diagnosis left Declan more confused and anxious than ever, his head spinning with psycho-babble.

His mother then suggested that he talk to an acquaintance of hers who carried out spiritual healings. This woman, who combined her healing with a full-time teaching job, immediately put Declan at his ease, encouraging him to express the feelings of fear and revulsion that fuelled his behaviour. Then she stood behind him and held her hands just above his shoulders, not touching so as not to activate his OCD. She told him that she was passing vital energy into him, and encouraged him to shut his eyes and imagine the energy flowing into him as a stream of liquid light. Declan could indeed feel a warm tingling sensation entering him and moving around his body. Then the healer urged him to visualize this energy, which now pervaded his body, as extending beyond his body to form a kind of aura completely surrounding him.

He was to imagine this energy force-field as a protective shell that would allow other people to pass through to make physical contact but would dissolve germs and bacteria on contact before they could reach his body.

After several healing sessions and regular self-help visualization exercises, Declan has managed to keep his obsessive-compulsive behaviour under control to an extent. As any OCD sufferer will tell you, it is not a problem that ever really goes away—you just have to learn to control and resist the compulsions that threaten you. Declan believes that he now has the strength to fight his phobias and that it was spiritual healing that helped him to achieve this.

Case study 3

Christine Booth, a fifty-seven-year-old divorcee, was diagnosed as suffering from breast cancer in 1992. After distressing chemotherapy treatment, it became evident that she would have to undergo surgery in order to remove the cancerous growth.

After much soul-searching Christine decided that surgery was indeed her only hope and went into hospital for a mastectomy. Unfortunately, she had taken the step too late, and the operation proved unsuccessful in removing every trace of cancerous tissue. The cancer continued to spread, and Christine's condition was acknowledged to be terminal.

At this point, having accepted that the doctors could do nothing for her now, Christine embarked on a spiritual journey, hoping to find something to help her come to terms with her situation. A life-long atheist, she now realized how scared she was of death and how much she desperately needed the consolation of a spiritual belief.

A chance encounter with a spiritual healer provided her with what she was seeking and marked the way towards a healing of sorts. Christine met Trevor Foster at a supermarket, where they struck up a conversation and immediately established a special rapport. Trevor, a registered healer, had recently lost his wife to cancer, having supported and treated her through several painful years of illness. Trevor extended his help and support to Christine in her hour of need and she accepted his offer of treatment and spiritual guidance.

Over the course of many weeks Trevor channelled positive spiritual energy into Christine. He also taught her meditation and visualization techniques, and counselled her through emotional low points. Through these actions, Christine's levels of self-awareness and life-awareness soared, and she began to recognize and express the feelings of anger, pain and resentment that she had bottled up all her life, particularly surrounding the breakdown of her marriage. Consequently, she felt a sense of liberation and a reconcilement with life, which in turn instilled in her a sense of calm and completion. She had reached a state of acceptance, free from inner conflict, and was ready to die, knowing that her spirit would be immortal as part of the universal life force that encompasses humankind.

It was at this point that the cancerous cells in her body ceased to multiply and the tumours started to reduce in size. Christine is in no doubt that this was a direct result of Trevor's care and treatment. She believes that when her body was eased of tension, her immune system was given an enormous boost, and her illness began to go into spontaneous regression.

She is still by no means free of the cancer, but she has already significantly stretched the life expectancy allotted to her by her doctors. She continues to battle against the disease with the power of positive belief as her weapon and Trevor as her standard-bearer.

Case study 4

Most people will be aware of the therapeutic value of animal companionship, as experiments have shown that petting a dog or a cat can significantly reduce stress levels and lower blood pressure. It is certain, however, that not everyone will have heard of a moose possessed of healing powers.

A Canadian moose hit the headlines in the early 1980s when it played the central role in a remarkable story involving a small diabetic boy. The nine-year-old, who had developed diabetes at the age of five, required twice-daily injections of insulin and a strictly controlled diet in order to regulate his blood sugar level.

The boy's parents encouraged him, however, to lead a normal, active life, as diabetes need not be a constraining condition. On this premise, they decided to take their son and his elder brother on a short camping trip. During a game the boy became separated from his family and became lost in the densely forested woodland.

As darkness fell, hampering search rescue attempts, hopes for the boy's safety faded. Having gone without insulin or food for so many hours it was unlikely that he would survive without slipping into a diabetic coma caused by dangerously low blood sugar.

When daylight returned and searches continued afresh, the boy was discovered safe and well in the company of an adult moose. The moose was unwilling to leave the boy's side, adopting an aggressive stance, and eventually had to be frightened away by gunshots being fired into the air. Paramedics who immediately examined the boy on the scene found him to be in perfect health, and a test of his blood showed his sugar level to be constant.

It transpired that the boy, realizing he was lost, had panicked and run deeper into the forest, trying to find a way out. Starting to feel faint and unsteady, the first symptoms of low blood sugar, he had stopped and huddled in a small clearing. Shortly afterwards, a large dark creature emerged from between the trees and approached the boy. Frozen with terror, as the moose is a fearsome looking beast, especially to a young child, the boy stayed completely still as the animal lay down beside him, pressing its flank against his body. Something about the creature's benign brown eyes reassured the boy, and he thinks he fell asleep, exhausted with running and distress.

He awoke the next morning, no longer feeling faint, to find the moose still at his side. Soon afterwards, the search party arrived and he was reunited with his family.

To this day doctors are baffled as to how the boy survived without insulin, and how his blood sugar level appeared normal. After the incident, the boy continued to require treatment for his diabetes and still receives daily insulin injections.

Later the moose was identified as a female who had recently lost her calf. The theory was put forward that the boy must have suckled from the still lactating moose, but even this would not have been sufficient to raise his blood sugar level to beyond danger point.

The boy, now a young man, strongly believes that the moose exercised some kind of protective healing power over him. While in its presence, he felt a feeling of warm, deep peace and a lifting of physical and mental discomfort.

It would be easy to dismiss this idea out of hand, simply because it is ridiculous. Mooses healing? Whatever next—pine cones playing ping pong?

When considered without empirical hysteria, however, it becomes apparent that this parable could be illustrative of the power of love and therapeutic touch. The moose, suffused with maternal instincts following the death of her calf, extended her protective love to what she recognized to be a young animal in danger and distress, for which the boy and his family will be eternally grateful.

Sadly, the moose, affectionately christened 'Harriet' by the Canadian public and dubbed 'The Moosiah' by the Canadian press, died shortly afterwards, perhaps in order to escape the stream of prying tourists and misguided pilgrims.

Many people may find these stories hard to believe, but they are representative of the kind of healings that occur week in, week out. They sound incredible because spiritual healing is incredible. It is true that no scientific basis has been identified for the claims made for healing, but this seems trivial and irrelevant in the light of the hundreds of successfully treated people who stand as testimony to their own healing experiences.

Detractors of spiritual healing will say that these cases can all be explained rationally and attributed to the power of suggestion or auto-suggestion, or to the charismatic influence of the healer. These explanations, however, are no more 'rational' than the idea of spiritual healing, as they too work on the unconscious level of the psyche and are intangible to scientific experimentation.

If, as stated previously, the healer simply acts as a channel for the greater forces of life, in theory anyone can develop healing skills. Meditation and contemplative, self searching thought, combined with a genuine love and compassion for humankind and peppered with a touch of intuitive sensitivity, could be the recipe for a healing disposition. The basic requirement is an ability to learn to be receptive to the messages that the mind sends the body and, in time, acquire the ability to control these messages. Self-healing can be the most fulfilling spiritual healing of all, opening up the self to others and becoming one with the universal healing life force.

Healing-related therapies

It will have already become apparent that most alternative healing processes involve the harnessing and channelling of energy from the healer to the patient. This energy is often perceived in different ways, whether it is believed to be life force, prana, ch'i, divine force, psychic or electromagnetic energy. Some say they can actually see this energy, while most sense it in a more abstract, intangible way.

There are many ways in which we can develop and expand the five senses to which we are limited in order to become sensitive to the energy vibrations that surround us somewhere where physics and mysticism meet. By tuning in to the rhythms of the universe we can learn to co-operate with nature's innate healing capacity

Here are several interconnected therapies, all of which respond to the vibrations of the life-energy around us. They also all are complementary to, and indeed contain elements of, spiritual and faith healing. Some of the same methods are employed in each of them, but they all harness and channel energy differently.

Aura therapy

Many healers believe that as well as a physical body, we all possess a psychic 'body' that extends beyond our corporal form. This is believed to be a force field of spiritual energy that surrounds all living things and connects individuals through a universal source.

The aura, as this force field is called, is thought to comprise all the radiations from the actions and interactions of cells and chemicals in the body, and therefore reflects the state of health of the individual. If the body is suffering from illness, the radiations from the affected organ will be weak, and subsequently dull patches in the aura are perceived.

The aura can stretch up to several metres from the body, or merely several centimetres, and consists of bands of different coloured light, all the colours of the spectrum as well as black, white and grey. Each person's aura is different in shape, colour and definition, and those who can perceive auras say that they can tell a lot about an individual's character and mood as well as the state of his or her physical, emotional and spiritual health.

Practitioners of aura healing are so sensitive to tuning into auras that the colours and shapes of a patient's aura are actually visible to them, not just sensed. Then they can interpret the order and the intensity of these colours, as each colour signifies different emotions, characteristics and disposition to illness. In a proper interpretation of someone's aura, the positioning of the colours in relation to each other is very important, but here is a basic outline of what each colour may signify:

- *Red*—red is the colour of vitality, passion and energy, and someone with a lot of red in his or her aura will be outgoing, physically vigorous and generous of spirit, although an excess indicates selfishness and materialism. Dark red in the aura may be indicative of anger or malice, whereas light red shows anxiety and tension.
- *Orange*—bright orange denotes a strong, ambitious personality and is also associated with good health and energy. A slightly lighter shade of orange signifies a compassionate, considerate and well-adjusted nature, but too much orange in the aura indicates overambition to the detriment of others
- *Yellow*—yellow in the aura shows mental agility and is apparent when someone is concentrating. As well as intellect, yellow also highlights optimism, and gold-yellow shows spirituality and perception. A murky yellow in the aura may indicate weakness, indecisiveness, frustration or suspicion.
- *Green*—green is a healing colour as it is the colour of nature and rebirth. In the aura it shows a vibrant sociable personality and may mean that the individual has the healing gift. A preponderance of green, on the other hand, signifies a lack of empathy with others.
- *Blue*—blue is a very positive colour, associated with idealism, inspiration and integrity. Dark blue indicates specifically religious inspiration and a deeply spiritual nature while pale blue shows a predisposition to scholarship. A dingy blue, however, means negativity.
- *Indigo*—indigo is also a spiritual colour, denoting strong moral values and the search for a higher truth. A lot of indigo in an aura signifies inner calm, serenity and good-naturedness. If it shows up blotchy or weak, this could indicate moodiness and irritability.
- *Violet*—violet is a devotional colour signifying love and spiritual enlightenment. Not everyone possesses a noticeable amount of violet in his or her aura, but those who do have profound insight and spiritual awareness.
- *White*—white represents perfection, the attainment of the highest possible spiritual enlightenment. It signifies truth and purity.

- *Black*—black in the aura shows an emotionally damaged individual. Black represents negative thoughts, destruction and despair.
- *Grey*—grey in the aura usually signifies illness or depression. In rare cases it can denote an individual devoid of personality.

As stated previously, these colours are present in different combinations in every individual and can appear mixed, layered or patchy, depending upon the ailment. Aura healing is not only a diagnostic but a curative therapy. Once the therapist has defined and interpreted the state of a patient's aura, and feels that he or she fully understands the problem, there are a number of ways in which the patient can be treated.

As with other forms of spiritual healing, the therapist acts as a channel through which universal spiritual energy can flow. Rather than use energy from their own auras, practitioners harness this greater energy and 'feed' it into the patient's aura. This could involve increasing the amount of colour that has become depleted in a particular area of the aura, or introducing a complementary colour that will even out any imbalances in the intensity of another colour.

The role of the patient in his or her own healing is heavily emphasized in this form of therapy. Patients are encouraged to take an active part in the healing process through self-awareness and positive thinking. Meditation and visualization exercises can be used to tune into and strengthen the aura.

Some auric practitioners believe that everyone has the ability to sense auras, if not actually see them. We subconsciously pick up the vibrations that another person's aura sends out, and this is the basis on which we place our impressions of him or her and gauge his or her personality and mood. If an individual makes you feel uneasy it could be because the aura is vibrating in conflict with your own, creating disharmony.

There are ways in which you can develop your ability to sense, or even see, auras. This means adopting a completely open mind and attitude, and setting aside any scepticism about the existence of auras. Watch people closely and listen very carefully to what they say, with as much empathy as possible. Notice their movements and mannerisms, and observe how they relate to their environment. It is a question of learning to notice and understand the subliminal messages that people continually send out about themselves and their situation.

Of course, there is no scientific evidence to support the existence of auras, although Kirlian photography shows that the body does emit some kind of electromagnetic energy. It could be said that the way in which auric therapists sense moods, emotions and disorders is through a form of observant intuition, itself as intangible as the idea of the aura.

Colour therapy

Colour therapy is closely linked to aura healing, and the two are often practised in conjunction. The idea of colour therapy goes back to ancient civilizations, as the Greeks and Egyptians are believed to have chosen the colours of their temple adornments for their beneficial effects on the mind, body and spirit. Colour therapy is also still practised in Tibet and India, where Buddhist monks wear orange robes because of the colour's spiritual properties. It has been proven that people are affected both psychologically and physically by different coloured light. What colour healers do is work with the various principles of certain colours to bring about effective healing.

Recent investigation has shown that there is a close correlation between certan colours and states of mind. Colour can affect people's mood, perception of time and temperature, and their ability to concentrate and function effectively. Some colours can induce anxiety and unease while others create a tranquil, restful state of mind. For example, greens and blues are commonly used in the decoration of hospitals and prisons because they have been found to have a relaxing effect, counteracting aggression and anxiety. Even fast-food restaurants know the significance of colour psychology and use the colour red to encourage people to eat quickly and move on. The strength of the colour induces a feeling of urgency and discourages the desire to linger.

Colour therapists go beyond psychology and believe that specific maladies can be treated and cured by adjusting the colour input to the body. As with aura therapy, it is believed that the body absorbs the electromagnetic energy of light and gives out its own aura of energy, which vibrates in a specific pattern. An unhealthy body creates an imbalance in this pattern, and the colour therapist strives to restore the balance through the stimulation of bodily reactions by colour. Colour healing is said to be based on the principle of attraction—the vibrations of the colour attract similar vibrations in the human body and extract the vibrations that are causing imbalance and illness.

The main colours used in colour therapy are red, orange, yellow, green, turquoise, blue, violet and magenta. Each colour is considered to be effective in the treatment of specific ailments.

- *Red*—red can be helpful in the treatment of circulatory problems, low blood pressure and anaemia.
- *Orange*—orange is effective on complaints involving the chest and the digestive system.
- *Yellow*—yellow can be used to help sufferers of skin complaints and nervous conditions.
- *Green*—green can treat stress, headaches and emotional disturbances.
- *Blue*—blue also calms the mind and can be used to help ease fevers and complaints of the nervous system.
- *Violet*—violet is helpful in the treatment of rheumatism, epilepsy and nervous disorders.

When making a diagnosis, a colour therapist will ask about your colour preferences as well as for details of your medical history and lifestyle. Most therapists will also employ an element of intuition or extrasensory perception to assess any imbalances in your aura.

Then the therapist will concentrate on your spine, stroking the length of it while focusing on your condition. Each vertebra relates to a part of the body as well as to one of the main eight colours listed earlier, which are repeated in sequence down the twenty-four vertebrae of the spinal column. In this way, any vibrations from an individual vertebra are picked up and interpreted to reveal where the colour balance is upset.

Once the balance or imbalance has been established, the practitioner will know which colours are required for effective treatment. Treatment involves the beaming of different coloured lights onto the patient by a special colour therapy instrument. Sometimes the whole body is bathed in the healing light, and at other times the colour will be focused only on a specific part of the body, depending on the patient's condition. The main colour used in the healing will usually be interspersed with a complementary colour, apparently increasing the efficacy of the former.

A session of this treatment will usually last around twenty minutes, and the patient should undergo at least seven or eight sessions over several weeks in order to receive the full beneficial effects. In addition to this formulaic treatment, the practitioner will advise the patient on what colours to wear and use around the home in the form of furnishings or lighting. Self-help techniques will also be taught and encouraged, to reinforce psychologically the benefits of the colour treatment. The therapist will guide the patient by visualization exercises, which he or she may then practise at home. These exercises may include visualizing a particular colour penetrating the body and suffusing it with coloured light, or the visualization could be based on a narrative and involve the patient imagining himself or herself enacting a journey through fields of specifically coloured flowers.

There is no doubt that colour can indeed affect mood and perhaps alter behaviour patterns, but the curative powers of colour therapy are yet to be scientifically proven. Even colour therapists recognize that this form of treatment should not replace orthodox medical diagnosis and treatment, but should be complementary.

Healing with crystals

Crystals and gemstones can be used to aid healing when used in conjunction with other alternative therapies, particularly colour therapy because of the obvious links of colour and refracted light. Some people believe that crystals are actually the tools of healing and can be used in isolation, although practices of meditation and visualization are usually also employed. As with the previous two therapies, crystals act on energy vibrations and are believed to emit their own vibrations, which amplify and focus the natural energies of the recipient's mind and body.

Crystals are believed to alleviate blockages in the flow of energy around the body, which may be causing physical or spiritual distress. It achieves this by working on the chakra points.

The chakra is a concept of Indian origin, literally meaning wheel, and its system is used in many different types of healing. The chakras are subtle points of focused energy in the human being and are believed to be the source of physical, mental, emotional and spiritual energy. They are sometimes described in physical terms as whirling vortices that can easily become blocked, but, of course, this is merely a symbolic representation of an abstract concept.

There are seven major chakras, each relating to different functions of the mind and body. Each chakra also relates to specific colours and different gemstones. Here are the seven chakras, beginning at the bottom of the body and working up:

Root or base chakra
This chakra is located at the base of the spine, near the reproductive organs. It relates to sexual activity and feelings, and links us to our basic instincts. The root chakra is associated with the elimination of waste from the system and the regeneration of cells and tissues in the body. Its colour is red, and its stones are rubies, garnets and bloodstones.

Abdominal or sacral chakra
This chakra relates to the digestive system and the reproductive system, as well as controlling the body's production of adrenaline. This chakra also signifies happiness and openness towards others. Its colour is orange, and its gemstones are coral, carnelian and amber.

Solar plexus chakra
Situated at the level of the naval, this chakra relates to the internal organs, such as the liver, spleen, pancreas and intestines. It is also to do with the intellect and communication. Its colour is yellow, and its stones include citron, topaz and yellow amber.

Heart chakra
This chakra is connected to the heart, circulation and immune system. It is also the centre of love and emotions. The colour of the heart chakra is green, and its corresponding stones are emeralds, jade and green tourmaline.

Throat chakra
Located just below the vocal chords, this chakra is connected to sound and the larynx. It is also associated with the thyroid gland and the lymphatic system. The throat chakra's colour is blue, and its stones include turquoise, sapphires and aquamarine.

Brow chakra
Situated between the eyebrows, this chakra relates to psychic or spiritual matters, and governs the pituitary gland and certain parts of the brain. The brow chakra coordinates all the other chakras, and its colour is indigo, its stones being amethyst, dark sapphires and lapis lazuli.

Crown chakra
This last chakra is located at the top of the head and is associated with the functions of the brain and spiritual aspirations. Its colours are violet and white-gold, and its stones include amethyst, rose quartz, clear crystal quartz and diamonds.

In order to unblock a chakra, a charged crystal is held above or placed directly on the area where the affected chakra is located. *(See also* Reiki, page 76, and Shiatsu, page 90.)

There are different ways in which a crystal can be charged with energy. One method is to sit quietly holding it in your palm, concentrating on positive thoughts and visualizing spiritual energy entering into it. Some people like to sleep with a crystal under their pillow, so that they can absorb their own special psychic power during dream sleep.

Another popular method of charging is to leave the crystal in direct sunlight (or moonlight) for at least six hours, or, even better, leave it outside during an electric thunderstorm.

Once a crystal has been used for healing it will have absorbed a lot of negative energy and must be cleansed before being recharged. An easy way of cleansing a crystal is to leave it to soak overnight in a bowl of spring water and sea salt, or, if there is a handy stream nearby, just give it a good dip.

When it comes to choosing a crystal, as well as bearing in mind what function you wish the stone to fulfil, you must use your intuition to guide you to what you are looking for. If you feel towards a particular stone, pick it up and handle it to see if you can sense its energy. Always inspect every crystal carefully for chips or cracks, as any imperfection may result in a dramatic loss of energy and healing sensitivity.

Here is a small selection of some of the most widely available stones and their uses:

Quartz crystal
Quartz crystal is the most easily recognizable type of healing crystal. It is the rough-cut clear stone that you will find in most New Age boutiques. Quartz is highly suitable for healing as it is believed to unblock the energy centres, allowing the body to respond and heal itself. It is a good all-round crystal to use for meditative and healing purposes as it promotes mental and spiritual well-being.

Rose quartz
Rose quartz is a beautifully coloured version of clear quartz, with its soft pink glow. This is another very important stone of healing as it deals with love and emotions. It is also a comforting stone and can ease distress in someone who has suffered trauma, as well as relieving everyday stresses and tensions.

Amethyst
Amethyst is thought to be a highly spiritual stone, associated with heightened perception and psychic insight. It is believed to have protective properties and

is therefore a good stone to carry about with you. Amethyst is also said to relieve insomnia and provoke inspired dreams if placed under the pillow.

Carnelian
Of a warm red colour, this stone is believed to help with circulatory problems. Carnelian can also help to ease feelings of anger and frustration, and induce contentment and fulfilment.

Sodalite
Sodalite is a blue stone often speckled with white. It is believed to help those suffering from neuroses and irrational thoughts by balancing the mind and lowering the blood pressure.

Tiger's-eye
This also belongs to the quartz family and is golden brown in colour. Tiger's-eye is thought to increase confidence and reduce nervousness. On a physical level it can aid the digestive system.

There is no harm in experimenting with crystal in order to find out what feels right for you. Meditation with crystals is a good way to introduce yourself to the types of energy emitted, before trying to achieve healing effects. It must also be stressed that using crystals can neither diagnose illness nor provide miracle cures. If in doubt, see a doctor.

Reiki

Reiki is a Japanese form of healing that is becoming increasingly popular in this country. This healing system contains elements of just about every other alternative healing practice under the sun—spiritual healing, auras, crystals, chakra balancing, meditation, aromatherapy, naturopathy, and homeopathy.

The word *reiki* translates as 'universal life energy', and like the preceding trio of therapies, it deals with forces that are not immediately intelligible to the human senses. The essence of reiki energy is love, 'an all-embracing divine vibration'.

Reiki energy has several basic effects: it brings about deep relaxation; destroys energy blockages; detoxifies the system; provides new vitality in the form of healing universal life energy; and increases the vibrational frequency of the body.

The laying on of hands is used in reiki therapy, as in spiritual healing when a healer, or a person strong with life energy, places his or her hands just above a particular part of the recipient's body in order to release energy into it. The difference between reiki and spiritual healing is that, rather than the healing sending out energy, the recipient draws it in. In this way the individual takes responsibility for his or her own healing, identifying specific needs and catering to them.

The implementation of reiki therapy is a fairly ritualized affair. Before beginning treatment and after removing jewellery and washing the hands, the healer will perform an invocation in prayer form as a gesture of respect towards the person to whom the reiki energy will be channelled. The reiki therapist focuses on and centres his or her own life force energy before moving on to the next ritual.

The next ritual is the smoothing out of the aura, which the therapist does with the right hand while placing the left hand on his or her abdomen. The healer strokes down the middle of the body in a fluid motion, with the hand held around twenty centimetres from the recipient's body. This can be repeated several times. This ritual establishes contact between the two people's energy fields and prepares the client for healing.

There are specific hand positions involved in reiki treatment, all of which have a particular significance to different parts of the body and different energy centres. It is not necessary to employ the exact positioning, as reiki energy can be drawn into any part of the body.

The first basic position is with the hands on the front of the head, covering forehead and eyes. This positioning relieves chronic diseases of every type, as well as combating stress, fatigue, allergies, weakness of will and discontentment.

When the hands are placed on the back of the head, the client can obtain relief from colds, headaches, eye problems, asthma and nausea.

The positioning of the hands on the body are numerous and can relieve all manner of ailments, from diabetes and indigestion to depression and fear of heights.

There are also several special positions that are used in the treatment of specific illnesses, such as arthritis, multiple sclerosis and heart disease.

Reiki can also be used in conjunction with the chakras (*see* Crystal healing). In this case the hands are held above a chakra that requires unblocking, and energy is absorbed into the invisible vortex, dissolving the blockage. How's that for psychic plumbing!

Meditation forms an important part of reiki, as it encourages the individual to cease resisting and allow life and energy to flow along their chosen course. A simple meditation exercise to help you to focus on the energy within the body and the true self is to sit on the floor with your legs drawn up, soles of the feet pressed together, and hands held, palms together, at the level of the heart. It is believed that in this position the circuit of energy around the body is complete, and the chakras are aligned and open. Concentrating on this energy flow will help you to reach a state of heightened awareness.

Reiki's healing of physical disorders is only a small part of its spiritual possibilities. Accepting reiki energy enables people to live more consciously and to develop their capacity for life and love. (*See* page 76 for a fuller discussion of Reiki)

Eastern healing philosophies

Many people today, disillusioned with the perceived spiritual and moral bankruptcy of contemporary western society, are turning to more ancient cultures for inspiration and enlightenment.

Eastern religions and philosophies, such as Buddhism, seem to embody the New Age tenets of personal development and psychic attunement, while offering a more appealingly mystical alternative to traditional western forms of organized religion.

These philosophies encourage new ways of viewing oneself and others, creating a deeper level of insight and self-understanding in daily life. Their emphasis on relating to others more positively through increased self-awareness provides a welcome antidote to our increasingly competitive and self-centred society in which people are fuelled by personal ambition and materialism.

Most eastern cultures embrace the concept of karma, a system of belief whereby everything that an individual does and says has a 'karmic value' that will be repaid to that person in the future. Good actions will therefore be rewarded by good fortune, and wrong actions will eventually have bad consequences on the original perpetrator.

This belief is similar to the Christian doctrine of 'love your neighbour as you love yourself', and is illustrated in the true, if slightly twee, adage 'The smile you send out will come back to you'.

The influence of the East on western culture is already perceptible and will continue to gain ground for as long as people continue to question the existing value system and to welcome positive change.

For those in search of healing, incorporating elements of eastern philosophy into daily life can be highly beneficial. The new perspective on life and the teaching of awareness and acceptance can help to ease inner tension and induce wellbeing. This, combined with the effects of stress-reducing techniques such as meditation, can provide effective treatment for many problems, such as depression, anxiety and phobias.

Such a state of mental, physical and spiritual attunement can also be beneficial in the treatment of more organic illnesses, as it eliminates conflict within the system, creating a state of harmony and receptivity. This, in turn, can boost the immune system, increase tolerance to pain and improve responsiveness to medication, all of which will help the healing process.

It is important, however, to emphasize that embracing these philosophies should not mean rejecting orthodox medicine. As with other alternative healing therapies, the watchword is 'complementary', and any treatment should be combined with medical consultations.

It is also important to stress that these kinds of philosophies, which focus on self-enlightenment, are not forms of psychotherapy and cannot provide easy relief from mental or emotional turmoil. In fact, the level of self-confrontation involved would make these techniques unsuitable for anyone with real psychological problems.

Buddhism

Buddhism is an ancient philosophy founded by Gautama Siddhartha Buddha in the sixth century BC in India, from where it was taken to China in 520 AD by a monk named Bodhidharma. It still flourishes as a practised religion in Asia, particularly in the Far East, and has elicited much interest in recent years amongst westerners searching for self-knowledge and inner tranquillity.

It could be said that of all the recognized religions practised today, Buddhism is the one that most embodies the healing ethic, as the ideal of 'wholeness' as we have come to understand it. The central teachings of Buddhism are concerned with exactly the ideas that are the mainstay of spiritual healing, in that it seeks to give its followers a new understanding of life through peace of mind.

Buddhism aims to eliminate the general feelings of dissatisfaction that pervade many people's lives, causing distress and, perhaps, illness.

Its teachings hinge on the 'noble truth' that life is unsatisfactory and engenders inescapable suffering. This inherent unsatisfactoriness is called *dukkha*, a word that suggests restlessness and suffering. Dukkha manifests itself in the individual as a kind of thirst for selfish desire, which is linked with ignorance, greed and hatred.

This belief in the inevitability of strife and suffering may sound negative and extremely pessimistic, but it is also believed that the individual is capable of achieving a state in which no selfish desire arises. As it is the unfulfilment of selfish desires that make one's life unsatisfactory, an absence of these desires leads to an acceptance of the world as it is.

In order to achieve this state of 'no dukkha', one must follow certain moral and spiritual disciplines, which are laid down in the Noble Eightfold Path.

The Noble Eightfold Path

1 Right understanding—here one acknowledges life as it is, in all its impermanence and unsatisfactoriness.

2 Right thought—this involves realizing the power of one's mind, which should be filled with positive thoughts of loving kindness and compassion.

3 Right speech—this includes not telling lies or saying anything that could be harmful to another, such as gossip.

4 Right action—such action as not taking life, stealing or engaging in sexual misconduct.

5 Right livelihood — one must be careful to have a job that does not involve one in destroying life or hurting others.

6 Right effort — this is needed in order to think about what one does and says.

7 Right awareness — one must be entirely alert or awake in life.

8 Right concentration — this is required to achieve a deeper level of attentiveness, characterized by peace and calm.

As you can see, each of the eight stages must be 'right', which means appropriate or effective. Through this 'rightness', the practising of an ethical lifestyle and meditation, the Buddhist hopes to find insight into the nature of existence and to transcend suffering.

As stressed before, this state of acceptance is not a resigned or indifferent one but a joyful one. Similarly, being without dukkha is not simply a passive, but a positive, dynamic state of contentment and compassion.

Indeed, compassion is fundamental to a Buddhist way of life. Alongside the emphasis on personal development, concern for other people and for life is paramount. A Buddhist develops 'mindfulness', starting with greater consciousness of oneself, one's body, mind and emotions, and radiating out to other people and the surrounding environment.

Meditation plays a vital role in developing mindfulness and is an important part of a Buddhist's daily routine. Meditation can take many forms and is a key factor in many healing therapies, as it encourages relaxation as well as self-awareness. (*See* the following passage on Zen for more details of Buddhist meditation techniques.)

Buddhism is a non-doctrinal religion that does not require its teachings to be forced upon its followers — its main concern is in the quest to help people achieve a full and aware life. So, in a sense, it is a philosophy that allows you to pick and choose the attitudes and practices that you wish to incorporate into your own life. Followers claim that through the teachings of the Buddha they find a special, personal path that will eventually lead them to realize their own enlightenment.

This kind of understanding transcends the intellectual and reaches deep into the self, a profound experience that leads to complete freedom.

Zen

Zen is a branch of Buddhism introduced into Japan in the 12th century, where it has thrived ever since. Zen is a system of sustained discipline and meditation aimed at transforming the everyday experience of its followers through the traditional Buddhist teachings of insight and self-awareness. Where Zen differs from Buddhism is in its anti-rational approach, with more of an emphasis on *zazen* (meditation) and direct experience without conscious reasoning.

Zen meditation is geared towards gaining direct insight into oneself at a level too deep to be expressed in words. This kind of transcendental meditation leads to enlightenment. As in other forms of Buddhism, Zen also teaches that accepting the world as it is and abandonng selfish desires are essential steps in the quest for enlightenment.

This acquiescence to the 'unsatisfactoriness', instability and impermanence of life, as described in the earlier section on Buddhism, reaches out into every aspect of life, including self-identity. A sense of a fixed personal identity is seen to be illusory, as everything on earth is impermanent and mutable, including the 'self'. Zen teaching therefore concentrates on encouraging the individual to discard any established self-image or notion of ego, thereby acknowledging and embracing the transience of existence. With each moment of insight, the influence exertd by the personal 'I' on the individual's way of thinking lessens and a new, more profound understanding develops.

This kind of understanding is cultivated through the use of three main techniques: daily life practice, meditation, and anecdotal wisdom.

Daily life practice

The aim is to live your life according to the Buddhist principle of 'mindfulness', which means being continually aware of all your own actions and responses. Again, this entails adhering to the Noble Eightfold Path and releasing yourself from preconceptions and driving desires, thus quashing the wilful, self-serving side of the personality. In this state, happiness and suffering are equally gratefully received as part of the ever-changing pattern of life.

Meditation

The Zen form of meditation, known as zazen, is really a way of perfecting daily-life practice. It encourages 'stillness' and 'mindfulness', eventually enabling the meditator to carry thought beyond the limits of the intellect by allowing thoughts to come and go freely, without making judgements on them. Ultimately, the person reaches a state of heightened awareness, without the intrusion of a personal 'I' who is aware.

The practising of zazen is slightly ritualized—the meditator always sits cross-legged on a cushion, with the back absolutely straight, head upright, and the centre of gravity completely aligned so that weight is evenly distributed around the body.

Many meditative exercises centre on concentrating on one's own breathing, and the simplest Zen meditation focuses on this principle. The meditator silently counts each exhalation of breath. The idea is to count from one up to ten without any other thoughts crossing the mind. When a thought does arise, the sitter must expel it and restart the count from one.

Trying this at home will show you just how hard it is to free the mind from rational interjecture, but if you persevere you will also begin to discover the profound states of calm that can be experienced.

Zen practitioners meditate daily, either privately or in groups, and the duration of a meditative session can be infinitely variable.

Anecdotal wisdom

One of the more notorious elements of Zen philosophy is its subscription to the use of symbolic stories, riddles and paradoxes. There are usually no firm conclusions to be drawn from these stories through contemplation, rather the wisdom comes from accepting that there is no right answer. These puzzles confront the intellect with a wall that no amount of logical reasoning can surmount. The hope is that intuitive insight will take over and instinctively offer a response 'born of the immediate moment'—a smile, an exclamation, the sight of an otter shaking itself, the sound of the wind in the trees—moments of experience that intrinsically define existence. The answer is, in a sense, to 'unask' the question and to realize that the problem rests in calling it a problem. Probably the best-known example of a Zen puzzle is: 'What is the sound of one hand clapping?'

If you wish to expand your mind and heighten your awareness through this particular philosophy, you must find a good teacher, as Zen is taught as a form of apprenticeship. Most major cities in Britain now have some form of Buddhist Society, where you will be able to receive information about finding a teacher in your area.

Hinduism—the Ayurvedic system

In Indian society there are many practitioners of Ayurvedic medicine, an ancient Hindu system of healing based on both natural and homoeopathic remedies. It uses mental techniques actually to alter bodily responses to disease processes—a form of 'mind over matter'. This system also involves concentration on primordial sounds, such as meaningless syllabic sounds, or mantras. The patient repeats these sounds unceasingly for long periods of time in order to concentrate the mind and focus attention away from pain. These techniques are often used in conjunction with transcendental meditation for general improvement of wellbeing.

Ayurveda is a complete system of healing that deals with every aspect of an individual's physical, mental and spiritual health. In the language of Ayurveda, these three aspects are known as the physical, the subtle and the causal, and 'health' is defined as a harmonious functioning of all three together.

The name 'Ayurveda' comprises two Sanskrit words, *ayur*, meaning 'life' or 'daily living', and *veda*, meaning 'knowledge'. Ayurveda, therefore, is the knowledge of daily living, meaning that it is a medical system that emphasizes an understanding of Nature and the individual's place within society and the universe. This emphasis on the *individual* is key to the Ayurvedic system, which is more a whole lifestyle than simply a set of treatments. An Ayurvedic practitioner will keep in close contact with his or her patient, monitoring and assessing the patient's entire way of life—diet, exercise, habits, sleep patterns, religious beliefs, occupation and conditions at work, state of personal relationships, and so on. By finding out all he or she can about the patient's personal and professional life, eating habits and medical history, the therapist can advise changes as necessary in order to prevent the onset of illness.

One of the most important teachings in the Ayurvedic diagnosis of a patient is the Tridosha theory. According to Ayurvedic law, everyone and everything in the universe is comprised of three basic elements or 'doshas'. These three doshas are called *vata*, *pitta* and *kapha* and are said to control all mental and physical processes. The nature of each dosha can be likened to the forces of the wind, the sun and the moon.

Vata
This is compared to the wind and is the moving force behind the other two doshas, which are believed to be immobile without it. Because of this, vata is considered to be the most influential of the Tridosha. It is responsible for all the body's actions and sensations, controlling the central nervous system and the respiratory and circulatory systems. It also regulates thought processes, promoting mental balance and comprehension.

Pitta
This is comparable to the sun and is a source of heat and energy. The word 'pitta' literally means 'that which digests things', and this dosha governs the digestive system, the metabolism, and all biochemical processes in the body. It is also responsible for the 'digestion' of ideas and perceptions, stimulating the intellect and the capacity for curiosity and enthusiasm.

Kapha
This is likened to the moon, with its tidal influence. Kapha controls the balance of fluids in the body and governs cell growth and structure. In fact, it provides support and structure for the whole body, giving strength and stability, both physical and psychological. Kapha also stimulates the capacity for positive emotions such as love, peace, patience and courage.

Every individual consists of a combination of these three basic forces in differing proportions. Their relative proportions in a person are thought to be determined at conception and continued throughout childhood and adult life. Good health results when all three doshas are working in harmony, with none exerting any more considerable force than the others. In his or her diagnosis, therefore, the Ayurvedic physician must first try to identify and understand the patient's inborn disposition. This he or she does through examination of the patient's eyes, skin, hair, nails, tongue, spittle, urine and stools. The practitioner will also listen carefully to the voice and take note of physical mannerisms and general physique. By all these means he or she can establish a person's basic constitution and identify which dosha 'rules' the individual's body.

Characteristics of the vata individual

Vata people have thin, bony bodies and dry, rough skin. The hair is also thin and dry, and often curly. Their eyes are small and dull, often dark in colour, and their teeth tend to be large and prone to decay. The voice is weak, hoarse and uncertain. Psychologically, these people are creative, active and intellectually sharp.

Characteristics of the pitta individual

Pitta people are of medium height and build, with reddish complexions and oily skin. Their hair is soft, fine and fair, light brown or red. The eyes are sharp and penetrating, often green or grey in colour, and teeth are medium sized and yellowish. The voice tends to be sharp and high-pitched. These people are highly intelligent, with strong leadership qualities.

Characteristics of the kapha individual

Kapha people have large, strong physiques, with a tendency to be overweight. The skin is pale and smooth, and the hair is thick, dark and wavy. They have large, attractive eyes, often blue, and large white teeth. The voice is clear, deep and well-pitched. These people learn slowly but have long memories, and their thoughts are generally logical and well-considered.

Obviously, these are purist manifestations of different dosha types, and one would not be likely to encounter an individual with all the characteristics of a particular dosha, as everyone is a combination of all three types, and where one type is dominant the other two doshas will serve to modify it.

Once the practitioner has assessed the dosha type, he or she will be able to pinpoint any imbalance that may cause distress or disease and will treat the patient accordingly. As Ayurveda has a strong doctrine of prevention, people are often treated before showing any signs of illness. If, however, illness does occur, a wide variety of treatments is available—from conventional surgery to plant-derived drugs.

Basic treatments fall into three main categories: medicinal, practical and dietary.

Medicinal remedies

There are some 8,000 different medicines designed to heal patients, made from natural substances such as herbs, vegetables and minerals. Each drug is custom-blended to create the right balance of ingredients for the individual patient. In addition, various orthodox medicines and treatments may be prescribed by the Ayurvedic physician.

Practical remedies

These include complementary therapies such as massage, yoga, oil treatments, breathing exercises and meditation. These practices are prescribed in order to promote general wellbeing as well as to treat physical and psychological disorders.

Dietary discipline

Foods are broken down into six types: sweet, sour, salty, pungent, bitter and astringent. A patient is prescribed different types of food according to his or her individual needs. Food is also prepared and consumed in accordance with external factors, such as time of year, time of day and weather conditions. It is also important that food is fully savoured, well chewed and swallowed in a relaxed, contented state of mind.

Most Ayurvedic practitioners qualify first in orthodox medicine and then attend courses in Ayurveda, so professional integrity is ensured. There are some 60 to 70 orthodox doctors practising Ayurvedic medicine in Britain.

Many Western doctors agree that Ayurveda is a highly effective health-care system, with its emphasis on preventative measures and physical, mental and spiritual wellbeing.

Sufism

Sufism is an Islamic mystical movement originating in Persia in the seventh century AD as a reaction against what the Sufis perceived as the increasing worldliness and rigidity of orthodox Islam. The orthodox rejected them at first, but today Sufi orders are fully accepted among the majority Islamic groups.

It is difficult to define clearly the distinction between Sufism and Islam, as both are contained within each other. In a way Sufism is at the heart of Islam. The Sufis aim to remain true and pure in the following of the teachings of Islam but to concentrate particularly on the idea of inner awakening, and to explore consciousness through the understanding of the relationship between the inner and outer life. Shaykh Fadhlella Haeri describes the key to Sufism as 'that of inner awakening, freedom and joy through recognition of outer restriction by choice and discrimination'. The practices of genuine Sufis result in outer discipline and inner openings and delights.

In common with most mystical traditions, the aim of the Sufi is direct experience of, and ultimately union with, God or Allah. This is achieved through ascetic practices and, more importantly, through love, both of God and of other people. Sufism has been called 'the religion of the heart', as it centres on purity of heart and feeling, relying on a largely devotional approach with the emphasis on intuition and emotion. There is no religious dogma in Sufism, nor any rigidly structured philosophical system that defines its beliefs.

Sufism stresses the ideal of equilibrium and wholeness, both in the self and in the universe. The Sufis see that the human being is potentially a microcosm of the balanced unity of the universe. The idea is not to retreat from the world by looking inwards, but to bring one's own vision and insight into the world. By gaining knowledge of God, the devotee becomes in turn a channel through which God's knowledge can act in the world.

The Sufis have always used many different methods and techniques to develop consciousness. Their practices include contemplative meditation, breathing exercises, music, visualization and controlled movement. Meditation techniques can include repetitive mantras, such as 'La ilaha illa'llah', meaning 'There is no god but Allah'. The Sufi repeats this phrase until his or her mind is free from thought.

Sufism draws several analogies from the practising of medicine. Indeed, Sufi prophets and spiritual masters are considered to be the physicians of the soul. In fact, many Sufi masters do themselves practise medicine in order to be able to treat themselves and their immediate followers. The physical body must be in a state of calm and equilibrium in order to experience inner stillness.

Sufis are constantly striving towards harmony and right action, facilitating healing of the heart through purity and calm. The main purpose of life is seen to be awake fully, to learn the disciplines of abandonment and submission, and to discover the common uniting force behind everything.

The Sufi aims to reach the peak of his or her self, overcoming the obstacles of mind and the intellect, to become spontaneously aware of 'beingness'. Each Sufi order develops its own techniques in reaching the heights of the self. Like Buddhism, Sufism enables each individual to go on a personal journey in order to arrive at his or her own particular understanding of reality.

Obviously, becoming a follower of Sufism means fully embracing the teachings of Islam and the Koran, but there are many interesting lessons that the western spiritual traveller can learn from the study of this religion.

Healing and the occult

'The Occult' is a phrase that often provokes a negative reaction amongst those for whom it has sinister connotations. For many people, the occult conjures up associations with satanic cults and the forces of evil; subjects that, understandably, inspire fear and condemnation. Those who are interested in the practices of the occult are considered to be devil-worshipping sociopaths, intent on inflicting harm on others and summoning up evil spirits.

It is true that in any section of society there are those who are going to abuse their position and act unlawfully or immorally, and the occultist community is no different. These cases, however, create a false image of the mystical arts, which have as great a capacity for good as for evil.

It is human nature to be afraid of what is unknown, and that is exactly what the occult is, its literal translation being 'that which is kept hidden'. The term covers many different disciplines, including spiritualism, paganism, white and black witchcraft, shamanism, voodoo, and more widely recognized practices such as tarot and other forms of fortune-telling.

Some people believe that it is wrong to 'dabble' in the unknown and tamper with things that are beyond our common understanding. Surely, however, it is better to strive to understand rather than remain ignorant and fearful?

It is perhaps not surprising that the world of the supernatural is particularly fascinating to those people who are interested in alternative and esoteric therapies, as both require an attitude of open-mindedness and a thirst for cosmic communion. Most importantly, they require an acceptance that there are realms of experience that cannot be explained by rational thought or scientific investigation.

The world is defined by our perceptions of it, and five has always seemed an inadequately small number of senses with which to understand such an infinite environment. It almost seems like a rational approach to acknowledge that there must be things beyond our ken, imperceptible or merely intangible. Faith healing is such a phenomenon, confounding intellect and defying explanation, and healing and occultism can be married to remarkable effect. The forces of the supernatural can be harnessed with beneficial consequence to help the sick and the troubled, if we are to believe the common reports of such cases.

One of the most significant areas of human experience that can be helped by occultist healing methods is the commonly fearful attitude towards death. The disciplines of the occult may help people to come to terms with death, their own or that of loved ones, and accept it as an inevitable part of the universe and its life cycle. For many people it is comforting to believe that there are worlds beyond our own and that death is not the end.

As with any topic of study concerning people's fundamental beliefs, investigation into the occult and its practices should not be taken on lightly, and anyone of an exceptionally superstitious or anxious nature should probably not delve too deeply into the world of the preternatural.

The witch doctors, keepers of the flame

A reason for the detachment with which doctors view the healer is the association of healing in the popular mind with occultist practices, such as seances and the activities of the witch doctor. Doctors themselves are not exempt from these popular prejudices. Yet if we take the time to examine the work of the witch doctor, we find that the Western doctor has much to learn from him. In the meeting between witch doctor and sufferer, the humanity of the patient is never disregarded. He or she does not receive the blow to one's selfdom, which is the standard in Western culture, where the patient often feels he or she has been dehumanized and reduced to the level of a simple number or case. The witch doctor would never be so crass or ignorant. This kind of therapeutic problem is alien to tribal medicine, where the soul is considered to necessitate healing along with the body.

Our distant ancestors did not see themselves as distinct from the environment. The stars, the spirits and the gods that controlled the cosmos also controlled the people. Human beings were intimately involved with nature. Shamans and medicine men use prayers, chants, talismans, herbs and potions to influence a world that humans in primitive society could not understand or influence. Faith healing of a simple kind is present still in so-called 'backward' parts of the world where medical science has made few inroads. The therapeutic powers of the local witch doctor are boosted by the implicit belief in the potency of his magic in the community. From centuries of observation and experiment, he has developed a pharmacopoeia for everyday needs, such as inducing vomiting in the case of poison; purgatives for ridding children of worms; sedatives for quieting hysterics; and potions for chest colds, headaches, whooping cough, dysentery, snakebite, swellings, and stings. If his remedies were all totally ineffective, the medicine man would soon lose his standing in the community, just as a doctor would in ours. The witch doctor's remit is to deal with a multiplicity of illnesses—sudden fevers, barrenness in women—and to help the community cope with the sudden death of a chief. The pharmaceutical knowledge of witch doctors has often preceded that of scientific medicine. Malaria was successfully treated by South American tribes prior to Old World doctors, and African Somalis diagnosed the transmission of the disease by the mosquito at least two centuries before Europeans. The modern witch doctor compares favourably with the western doctor. The comparison is especially favourable regarding illnesses of a hysterical or psychiatric nature, illnesses such as impotence and loss of speech.

A great deal of the witch doctor's treatment is psychological in essence and is in the realm of faith healing. The witch doctor flourishes in primitive societies because of the belief that good and evil govern both the spirit world and the human world. The witch doctor is on the side of the good, and his chief function is to protect the community from evil spirits. In the light of modern discoveries of the relationship between mind and body in illness, the ancient craft of the witch doctor appears surprisingly modern.

Primitive societies all over the world have their medicine men, or witch doctors. They nearly all wear colourful ceremonial costumes and use mysterious rituals to impress their suggestible patients. Native medicine is also closely bound up with the local religious cult, and involves the use of totem figures and charms to ward off sickness, which is usually attributed to evil spirits. The witch doctor is both physician, psychiatrist, chaplain and private detective. Death is rarely regarded as a natural and unavoidable event but is usually ascribed to be the work of a supernatural agency. Here the witch doctor will be required to act as a priest to decide what spirit has been affronted or abused. His capacity as private detective will be utilized, as the witch doctor must then investigate possible conspirators responsible for the illness. He is also a therapist, as part of his job is to administer herbal remedies, massage or heat treatment. He will also make ritual incantations, which will lull the patient into a state of placidity.

Many of the multicoloured ceremonial rituals, the masks and extravagant grass costumes put on by native doctors have a design. They are a visual assistance to psychiatric doctoring. Native medicine on the tribal level is almost invariably combined with psychiatry, an approach which 'civilized' practice has only newly adopted.

The visual aids, symbolic incantations and persuasive assertion used by native doctors may be regarded either as sympathetic magic or as a mild hypnotic suggestion. The doctor might say while bathing his patient: 'Your trouble is departing as this river is flowing out to sea.'

The religious mien of native psychiatry is provided by the local cult. This may entail a belief in the intercession of one of the ancestors, often recently dead, whose power as an elder is remembered. A suffering person may feel that his or her illness is accountable to the spirit of a dead uncle who beat him badly during his childhood. He will be advised to desist from the bad behaviour that has brought about this visitation from the spirit.

In parts of Ghana, there is a tradition of the use of deep hypnosis by witch doctors, who may induce a trance in a roomful of patients at a time. Authorized observers claim that the Ghanaian native doctors are able to cure serious skin disorders by this spiritual method.

The shaman

A shaman is said to use healing energies either to heal or to harm. These powers are used to maintain the order of the community. 'Voodoo' or 'hexing' has long been associated in many cultures with healing. The term 'shaman' is derived from the Tunguso-Manchurian term *saman*, which means 'he who knows'. In taking their professional vows, healers vow to harm as well as heal in their society in order to maintain order. Shamans of Siberian, Eskimo and American Indian tribes were initiated into their tribes not by their mastery of an arcane body of knowledge but by personally imposed ordeals. These ordeals would involve fasting and experiencing visions induced by trances. After this initiation the shaman would be credited with many abilities, such as healing and access to divine revelation.

The Indian shaman is said to be able to cure snakebites by methods akin to those employed by the Africans. Many Indian snakebites are not poisonous, but the shock of the bite can be so severe that it can be lethal to a suggestible person ignorant of this. Nobody really knows whether the shaman cures only the state of shock, or rather increases the bodily resistance to the poison.

In Patagonian tribes the shaman, or witch doctor, held an important position. The usual treatment of the patient involved creating as much hullabaloo and clatter as possible to drive away the aggressive demon. The shaman would also suck a part of the sufferer's body and then brandish a stone, a stick or an insect that the shaman would claim had been drawn from the body of the afflicted person. Often the patient would be strapped to the back of a horse and sent out into the day amid a great tumult and uproar. As well as disquiet, cold was thought to be a great curative next to noise. If needs be, a mare would be sacrificed in the house of the sufferer. The shaman would deliver the fatal stab to the heart. The animal would writhe in convulsions as its heart was extracted. The assembled company would then feed on the horse. What was left of the unfortunate animal would be taken to a local hill top and erected on a pole. If this failed to bring about a cure, the case was considered beyond help.

White witches: 'We died of ourselves'

The nearest cousin to the witch doctor in Europe is the art of the white witch. Practice of the 'cunning arts' was common in Britain as recently as two centuries ago. White witchery was regarded as liable to cure as it was to curse. It was only about a hundred years ago that the majority of the population lived away from the towns, away from any qualified medical aid. Anyone suffering from pneumonia stood approximately the same chance of recovery three thousand years ago as they did in the mid-1930s.

In Hanoverian England, for instance, traditional medicine had not really moved decisively beyond the language and lore of the ancient world. Even the products of the Royal College of Physicians emerged from their training with scarcely more formidable diagnostic tools than their quack counterparts. Most physicians could offer little more than laudanum and sympathy.

Prior to the beginning of medical services to rural areas in 1911, folk medicine held sway among country people. The average labourer in rural England was too poor to employ the services of a doctor. The faith healers of these communities were white witches. The most renowned of the areas where white witchcraft held sway was the North of England. Here a white witch could quite openly ply her trade of magic medicines and love charms up until the middle of the 1830s. Most famous were the Wise Man of Brompton and his female counterpart the Wise Woman of Cloughton.

A number of folk remedies used in the past are now manufactured as pharmaceutical preparations prescribed by physicians. For example, rauwolfia is an extract of the snakeroot plant, which was used in the Far East for its calming effect. It is now prescribed by physicians to lower blood pressure.

Foxglove was first brewed by Indians to treat dropsy, fluid in the legs caused by heart problems. This practice was extant centuries before it was discovered that foxglove contributed the active ingredient now known as digitalis, a treatment now employed to stimulate weakened hearts.

Folk medicine is still popular among large groups of Mexican-Americans in New Mexico, Colorado, Arizona, California, and especially in west Texas. Their healing system is based on pre-Columbian indigenous lore, and its popularity reflects the isolation of Mexican-Americans from mainstream American culture and the unwillingness of Mexican-Americans to assimilate to Anglo-Saxon culture. Prominent among Mexican-American faith healers is the *curandero*, a type of shaman who uses white magic and herbs to effect cures. In the cosmic struggle between good and evil, the curandero, using God-given powers, wards off harmful spells and hexes. As in other faith healing practices, the essence of the success of the curandero lies in the patient's faith in his abilities.

Spiritualism

The spiritualist movement began in 1848 in a house in Hydesville, New York State, where lived the Fox sisters, Leah, Margeretta and Kate. At first the whole family were disturbed by 'paranormal' happenings such as phantoms and bizarre unexplained knockings. The parents decided that an unquiet spirit was to blame, and two of the sisters, Margeretta and Kate, began a communication with the spirit. They were on the way to fame and becoming celebrated figures. The only drawback is that in 1888 the two sisters who had been principal in the occurrences, Margeretta and Kate, admitted that they had faked these altercations with the afterlife. But by then it was too late. The spiritualist church that they founded continued unabashed. Spirit healing is a branch of this minority religion, a branch that now overshadows the original movement as a church.

Generally thought of as being interested purely in communication with the spirit world, the spiritualist church has developed a growing interest in healing, confirmed when, in 1963, the National Federation of Spiritual Healing in Britain boasted of having over two thousand practitioners.

Spiritualists believe that in their work they are merely facilitating the Christian belief in the divine power of healing. Spiritual healing is distinct from faith healing in one important aspect. In faith healing, what is paramount is the patient's personal belief. In the case of spiritual healing, however, faith itself is irrelevant, and the source of the power is said to emanate from the spirits of the dead in attendance. These spirits are brought forth by means of a spiritualist medium. Needless to say, mediumistic or spiritist diagnosis made through spirit guides and clairvoyance are expressly forbidden in scripture (Deuteronomy 18:9–13).

No less a person than James Joyce satirized the pseudo-scientific language of spiritualism in that seminal work of modernist literature, *Ulysses*. In the Cyclops chapter, which opens in Barney Kiernan's bar, an unnamed bibulous Dubliner recounts how the 'apparition of the etheric double' during a seance is particularly lifelike 'owing to the discharge of jivic rays from the crown of the head'. Yet there was a more serious side to this. Spiritualism's most celebrated critic was the renowned escapologist, Harry Houdini. He was an unwilling participant in this personal crusade, in that nobody more than he would have liked to have believed in the afterlife. What dismayed him was the deceit and exploitation of human anguish that were employed in these sessions of communications with the dead. 'It ought to be stopped, it must be stopped,' he wrote. Distinguished figures from the world of science investigated the claims, and, in the case of Sir William Crookes, the eminent physicist, found in favour of the spiritualists.

Houdini bewailed the fact that it was only scientists who were sent to investigate the claims because the fact that these men were scientists did not ensure that they would not be immune to the extremely clever and sophisticated trickery that a spiritualist may employ. Indeed, even he, the 'Great Houdini', claimed that he himself could be deceived by the trickery of the spiritualists. If he could be fooled, a man who had devoted his life to the creation of illusion, who then was immune?

Harry Edwards

One of the most renowned faith healers in England in the 1950s was Harry Edwards. More than any other, he popularized healing to the public. On one occasion he managed to fill the Royal Albert Hall. As an amateur magician, Edwards went along to spiritualist meetings eager to expose the chicanery he felt was involved. Instead, the converse occurred and he became an initiate and disciple of the church.

He believed that his success was because of the fact that he was in communication with spirits when engaged in the healing process. These spirits, he believed, wished to help the living. His belief in these spirits meant that he was attended by a guide, or medium, during his healing sessions. Edwards was himself a convert to spiritualism and claimed he was in contact with the spirits of Louis Pasteur and Lord Lister.

It is a matter of documented fact that Edwards treated individuals who then made dramatic recoveries. Possibly this is merely because of the fact that he treated a very large number of sick people, and in the light of this it seems only a matter of statistics that some of the people that he treated would make dramatic recoveries, just as there will always be dramatic recoveries amongst a percentage of a number of the sick.

Edward's success and notoriety were felt to have sufficient weight and theological import for the Archbishop of Canterbury to set up a special commission in 1958 to investigate the evidence for spiritual healing. It concluded, predictably, that there was no evidence of any supernatural healing power at work with spiritualist mediums. Whatever one's views on the subject, one could hardly expect such a deeply conservative organization as the Church of England to find in favour of the spiritualists, whatever evidence was proffered. Edwards continued healing until his death.

Roles of the healer

Who are they?

Over the centuries the qualifications for being a faith healer have been as bizarre and as arbitrary as they can be. It was once believed that husbands and wives with the same surname before marriage had healing powers. Another prime candidate for healing power was a baby born with a membrane over its head. Just as the Catholic church will limit the practice of formal exorcism to well-chosen and judicious priests with the express permission of a bishop, the ability to heal in particularly gifted individuals will grudgingly be accepted by the church. The gift of healing is like many other gifts — some people will have a natural aptitude for it that marks them out.

Having been the recipient of healing, you may want to investigate the possibility of being a healer yourself. There are a few useful addresses at the back of the book. The distribution of the healing ability does not seem to favour one class over another. As with anything, practice will enhance ability, but ultimately how successful one is will be dependent on one's natural ability. Mystics, faith healers and gurus, like great painters and musicians, have to go through a long and disciplined developmental stage, as a sense of the spiritual is not enough to sustain them.

A large number of healers begin as one-time patients of healers, and to their astonishment they are told that they themselves have the healing ability. St Paul makes it clear that only some are given the ability to heal (1 Corinthians 12:9). Yet in the Gospel of Mark, Jesus says: 'Everything is possible for anyone who has faith' (Mark 9:32b).

Any would-be healer has to resolve the moral dilemma that he or she may be hurting people by giving them false hopes. This probably explains why healers have to enter the field with strong personal convictions and the tentative first steps of Arigo and the Stroker. One can have an innate capacity to 'feel' illness and diagnose it through one's hands. What is reassuring is that if someone does have the gift of healing it will not be long before it is recognized. Sometimes it may be intuitively felt by others that you have the healing gift.

If one only stops to consider it, everyone has met individuals whose physical presence was commanding in some inexpressible manner, either by sheer physicality or force of intellect. Some may even have felt a corresponding feeling that they would, if asked, bend to the will of that person, whatever they were to ask. Yet if asked to articulate precisely why this was the case, most people would be unable to do so. Everyone can recognise the 'aura' another person, perhaps even a stranger, is giving off without a word of communication between them. Some people can leave you feeling weary while others can leave you feeling inspired and revivified. It is a short leap from this to imagine the presence and ambience of the healer.

Even the most imperceptive can recognize a baleful or beautiful aura on a wordless, pre-verbal level. It is interesting that when we attempt to discuss this phenomenon, we are drawn inevitably into using a vocabulary that centres on the idea of energy and energy fields, words such as 'electric' and 'vibrations' being the most obvious examples. Perhaps this is a clue to what passes between the healer and recipient during a session, the healer projecting some positive high-intensity energy into the recipient.

The universality of healing suggests its deep resonance and significance to us. As we have seen, faith healing's resonance is multicultural and transcontinental. It has been present in some form in the Graeco-Roman world, the Indic culture of the East, on the African continent, in the Americas, and in the former Soviet Union. In advanced late capitalist post-modern urbane western society, particularly in America, where fundamentalist religion is very popular, huge crowds attend faith healing meetings.

When we study the archetypal faith healers (figures who follow the career pattern, well established in healing, of the tentative beginning followed by rise to notoriety followed by establishment clampdown) what is perplexing and ultimately uplifting about them is their endearing guilelessness. The really successful healers tend to be unassuming souls and not even markedly religious people.

At the outset we have to distinguish here between the avaricious televangelist breed of healer and the more dignified figures of healing. This is a thorny distinction, but one we have to confront. The reason it is so thorny is that both types of healer can use the same methodology to achieve their ends. What may be, and what we will examine here, is that the methodology in question has a potency that the healers are unaware of themselves. Its power exists, and one can use it to good or acquisitive ends.

If we examine the classic figures of healing—the Stroker, Quimby and Arigo, for example—instead of the cynical manipulator or the charlatan, we meet the idiot savant. A prime example of this would be Valentine Greatrakes, timorously beginning his healing in fear of looking a fool to the populace and most of all his own wife.

His powers had so much of 'the extraordinariness' about them, he wrote, that 'I thought fit to conceal [them] for some time'. Jose de Freitas (Arigo) is another example of the idiot savant, displaying amazing abilities yet comically falling into a dead faint after witnessing them played back to him on film.

These men were not imbeciles, rather their beginnings were often clownish and instinctual rather than rationally considered. It should be said that most healers enter the practice through strong personal conviction. These people are far from being fools, and, indeed, a person would have to be a fool to hold a mass healing in the way that Mesmer or Jacob did without some special healing gift. Often the end of the career of the healer has a resemblance to that other clownish figure, the King for a Day, as many healers also find—usually after a sustained attack on their confidence by the medical establishment—that their powers wane or completely disappear. Mesmer and Greatrakes are prime examples of this. Yet it goes without saying that if their abilities disappear, we must accept that there must have been something there in the first place.

Unexceptional in all other regards, these men confound any charge of charlatanism that may be brought against them in their very simplicity. Of course, the cynic could say that this is feigned simplicity. If one does subscribe to this view, then one has to ask to what end would a healer conduct such a masquerade? Healers run huge risks. Nine white witches were executed at Husband's Bosworth in the Midlands for failing to effect a cure against epilepsy. Today, if they become big enough to rock the boat of orthodox medicine they can still be imprisoned. In 1981, a German healer called Joseph Müller was imprisoned for two years in West Germany. He was found guilty of 'contravention of the laws governing medical practice'.

Neither can we see healing as the gulling of one class by another. Faith healers and the people that heal come from any and every class. We have aristocratic faith healers, such as the Earl of Sandwich and Prince Alexander von Hohenlohe. Then there are the peasant healers, such as the Cheshire woman Bridget Bostock and Arigo. Nobody is compelled to believe in the faith healer, yet millions of people use their services. The German philosopher

Schopenhauer writes that 'Belief is like love; and as any attempt to compel love produces hate, so it is the attempt to compel belief that first produces real unbelief.' (*Essays and Aphorisms*). In the face of this we must ask why faith healing persists and continues to fascinate a cynical public. The intellectual accessibility of the ideas, which would attempt to explain healing to the man on the street, is another factor that could account for the popularity of healing, and this contrasts sharply with the Latinate and obscure language of the doctor. The notion that good health can be seen as the balancing of energies within the body is eminently plausible to the layman, who probably knows that his pancreas and liver perform actions akin to this in their regulatory function. The complexities of biochemical changes within the body and physiology may be off-putting, but the healer's art is graspable. Aiding this is the healer's primary wish to communicate with the patient in a meaningful manner, a revolutionary sentiment yet to storm the medical profession.

Perhaps there are socio-biological reasons for the magnetism of the healer. There is a deep-seated need in human beings to want to submit themselves to a dominant member of the group in which they live, inherited from our monkey and ape ancestors. This must in some part explain the attraction of the healer and the witch doctor. The healer provides answers and confidence in an uncertain world. The witch doctor is a particularly salient example as he is often second only to the tribal chief in his society.

Yet more than this, the figure of the healer will occupy a number of deeply resonant roles that play to our inner psyche. We cannot view the healer as merely a kind of glorified doctor with some added mysticism thrown in for good luck. It would also be inappropriate to associate the role of a doctor with the role of the healer, as the healer's role embraces much more than the doctor's. Whereas in the West the roles of doctor and counsellor are divorced, the healer acts as both these figures and more.

Healer as lover

The psychoanalyst Carl Jung (1875–1961) wrote: 'Christ the healer is one of the eternal images or archetypes.' The healer is a tremendously potent figure in our imaginations. We have said that the witch doctor is both physician, psychiatrist, chaplain and private detective. The faith healer, his western cousin, can also boast a variety of functions. He or she is the lover, employing touch in a therapeutic way that it is difficult to imagine any doctor or counsellor ever contemplating. One cannot underestimate the potency and the primacy of touch. Embryos react to touch at just six weeks. The first contact with the external world the baby will experience will be through the medium of touch. By extension, spending 50 minutes a week with someone who is touching you and making eye contact with you, and is fully involved with you and your illness is a tremendously positive and invigorating experience. It would be a lucky patient indeed who received 50 minutes (or even 5 minutes!) of a doctor's time today. Moreover, a patient in the care of a doctor will no doubt meet different doctors from the one he or she originally saw on follow-up visits. Yet with healers there is a sense of continuity built up, which strengthens the confidence of the patient.

This demonstrates that sometimes the success of a healer can lie in quite prosaic answers. If you were an old lady living alone in a high-rise block, the very act of being physically touched and spoken to sensitively and softly with a healer's undivided attention would be therapeutic.

It has been found that one of the most compelling figures to the female psyche is that of the mysterious stranger, a figure that Emily Brontë used as a key motif in drawing the character of Heathcliff, perhaps the greatest romantic hero in all English literature. Like Heathcliff and the Byronic hero, the healer is handsome, magnetic and melancholy. We are also slightly ambivalent about him. Consciously or unconsciously, the healer taps into the resonance of this figure.

To put it less discreetly, we should not ignore the factor of sex as an element in the appeal of the healer. Mutual attraction was undoubtedly there between Baker Eddy and Phineas Quimby. No doubt it explains the appeal of a figure like Rasputin, who obviously possessed strong sexual magnetism, and clearly it was an element in the attraction of the female genteel society that surrendered their dignity to Mesmer. Striking good looks and personal magnetism also play a part in the appeal of Djuna Davitashvili.

Modern healers tend to have a disproportionately high number of female patients. A wander around any complementary health fair shows a preponderance of women over men. Two-thirds of pilgrims to Lourdes are women. A possible explanation for this is that women tend to have far less control over their lives than men and are therefore more inclined to believe in an external force over which they have no control, be it healing, horoscopes or magic crystals.

Mystery and mastery

This also ties in with another important element in the psychology of faith healing, which is the weighty factor of mystery. Every general practitioner has a catalogue of twenty or so drugs that can be administered and are well known to both practitioner and patient. This tends to kill off any sense of awe or romance in the healing process. When one is attended by a healer one feels that one is taking part in an ancient mystical rite that taps into a past of folklore, of witchery bequeathed to us from remote generations past or (and perhaps more importantly) our imagined romanticized perceptions of it gleaned from television and books. This element of mystery also manages to coexist cheerfully with the intellectual accessibility of the ideas that lie behind healing.

Not only is there the mystery of the healer to consider, but the very mystery of the rituals they perform. The allure of the church is based on the glamour of mystical rituals that, to be successful, require a kind of blind acquiescence from the follower. Once this is questioned, the entire edifice must collapse. This is analogous to the work of the faith healer, who also relies on a speechless complicity in his or her strange practices. If this is not there, the healer's work is all the more harder.

He or she is also the counsellor—the witch doctor. Healers offer sustenance where there has only been a counsel of despair from a doctor. This may not sound too grandiose a claim for healing, but one can easily imagine the effect of having someone tell you that your cancer is at least treatable, if not curable, when a few sleepless days before a synthetically sympathetic doctor has regaled you with the cheery news that there is no hope for you and you may as well submit placidly like a drugged factory animal to your unlovely fate. Hope itself has a curative power that cannot be overlooked, as it lessens one's symptoms and enlarges the pain threshold. Healers can be both Jesus himself and the slightly frightening figure that links us to the pagan past. Just as symbolism can work only if it bypasses the conscious mind and goes to the unconscious, the power of faith healing is all the stronger if the recipient is only dimly aware of what the healer represents.

Theatre

An element of theatre also augments the attraction of the faith healer. This is especially pronounced in American evangelists, who perhaps use the sense of the dramatic to a level where it becomes crass and tawdry, yet executed properly by a healer this can be utilized to add to his or her potency. Christ himself had a pronounced sense of theatre, exhibited in his organization of the triumphal entry into Jerusalem and the Last Supper and, indeed, the dramatic nature of his many healings.

It is easily conceivable that for someone who has been bedridden for ten years, the very prospect of a trip to visit a faith healer could discharge recuperative agents into the metabolism, just as Mary Baker began to feel better before her meeting with Phineas Quimby. And once in the presence of the faith healer, it is hard to maintain your critical faculties when you are surrounded by devout, friendly and well-meaning believers—to keep your head, as Kipling put it, when all about you are losing theirs. Perhaps the very practice of healing inherently plays to our sense of the dramatic. The knowledge that faith healers pose an ideological challenge and danger to a profession that has become so arrogant as to be totalitarian sets up a sense of dramatic conflict, but more than this, the dramatic defeat of illness by a healer is a Manichean battle between dark and light, and intensely appealing.

It is ironic that the very herd instinct that doctors are wont to follow in pursuit of their profession and that so disables and detracts from that very profession is the same herd instinct that contributes so much to the success of the healing process in the complementary sphere. A large contributory factor to the patient's first considering the possibility of visiting a healer will be the proximity of friends and relations who have visited a healer in the past and found it beneficial, and who will advocate it as a possible avenue.

It is interesting to note that a large part of the attraction of complementary health therapies to the general public resides in the glamour it is given by the interest that the British royal family has shown in complementary health treatments. For several generations they have had a homoeopathic doctor, and, during his term as President of the BMA, Prince Charles extolled the benefits of holistic medicine, most notably in the speech he made to the BMA in 1983. The Princess of Wales also made clear her interest in complementary therapies.

Orthodox medicine and healing

> Your long Latin words are unable to cure
> This sickening sadness I have to endure
> So from my sorrow one thing is sure;
> Doctors, your learning is simply absurd.
>
> (Molière)

It was in the middle of the 19th century that science began stumblingly and slowly to approach an explanation for the occurrence of disease, and to effectively begin to thwart it. Medical treatment became constantly more effective. During the last twenty years breathtaking strides have taken place. The infant mortality rate has dropped, antibiotics cure once lethal diseases with exciting adroitness. Surgery has advanced to a startling degree. People are living longer and welcome a more easeful old age.

Our maturing comprehension of the workings of the human body, and of the troubles that harry it, give optimism that one by one the ailments that hurt it will cede to scientific medicine. Yet despite all this, gigantic areas remain where our medical knowledge remains skeletal. Patients still yield to strange contagions, to tumours and to premature failure of vital organs, when neither drugs nor surgery are effectual.

It is at times like these that people, confronted with the diagnosis of an inoperable tumour or a debilitating disease of the nervous system, such as disseminated sclerosis, decide to turn elsewhere for an answer. They may turn to faith healing, to quack remedies or pilgrimages to religious shrines. As far as one can tell from the available evidence, these actions are essayed as a last resort, and usually achieve no more than a fleeting and short-lived lift of the spirits, or the consolation of religious faith in the face of the unfair.

Yet occasionally cures do occur that correspond with the sufferer's call to a shrine or a faith healer. There is much written evidence to this effect, which suggests that these sudden and dramatic cures are not quackery but evidence of some healing power as yet unexplained by medical science. Some of these cures are even backed up by medical evidence from qualified doctors.

For both the church and the medical profession, healing is the mad woman in the attic, the close relative that they would prefer not to talk about. But so-called 'orthodox' medicine (note the connotations of this term) is a fleeting parvenu when compared to the longevity of healing. Faith healing held sway for a full 18 centuries, from the time before Christ when the oracle at Delphi accepted the healing powers of Asclepius up to the Renaissance and beyond to the present. It is highly likely that healing is as old as mankind itself.

Beyond the Graeco-Roman world, belief in healing cures was even more common. The Persians considered the spell the most valid and trustworthy form of treatment. We should also consider the Indic culture of the East in our study. At the time from 100 to 1000 BC, the time of the Buddha and the Krishna, we find claims for magical cures alongside the use of herbal remedies. In this philosophy the *prana*, or 'life force', of yoga is equated with the healing force. Indian texts tell how this energy can be transferred by touch and through the mind for therapeutic purposes. Reports are also given of the chakras, the circular energy fields by which energy flows from the etheric to the physical body.

The sphere of orthodox medicine has at its foundation figures such as Empodocles, Hippocrates, Paracelsus, Galen (who took the cure at Pergamum, the temple erected in honour of a healing cult) and Robert Boyle (the father of modern chemistry). These were figures who were willing to attach credence to the so-called 'forgotten art'. Were all these people duped? Or were they open to something we are wilfully blind to? The symbol of medicine itself, the snake, is a symbol that arose from a story connected to Asclepius, the Greek god of healing.

The career of the faith healer follows an archetypal pattern. After a halting and tentative beginning, the healer will begin to build up a following. His or her popularity spreads and then reaches its critical mass, where he or she becomes important enough to be seen as a potential threat, as a rival power bloc, to the monopoly of the church or the medical establishment. Often the healer will have a powerful patron, but this is not enough to prevent either the physical or psychological destruction meted out to them. It is often forgotten that faith healers themselves are as much in need of positive reinforcement as their patients. A prosaic explanation will be produced by the orthodoxy in an attempt to besmirch and undermine the healer. The healer retires into seclusion, if he or she is lucky. If unlucky, he or she may end up in prison.

Sounds familiar? It should, because this is the story of virtually all faith healers, from Greatrakes to Jacob, from Rasputin to Arigo. This is a story that will be repeated until medicine begins to accept the sphere of faith healing as a legitimate branch of medicine.

In the pantheon of faith healing since the 13th century this pattern is endlessly repeated. Older (and wiser?) traditions extolled the healer as a functionary worthy of respect. In the case of Asclepius, the healer was a god. Yet now in America non-medical treatment is illegal in every state. How did such a falling-off occur? We have seen how the church itself contributed to the marginalization of faith healing, now it is time to call orthodox medicine to the dock.

It has become a commonplace in literature on healing to berate the indifference of orthodox medicine to healing and to turn members of the medical profession into bogeymen. In some cases this attitude is understandable, but the way forward must surely lie in dispensing with this mutual antagonism and bringing these two branches of medicine together. Bridging this chasm would be no mean feat, as it has been reinforced by centuries of mutual suspicion.

It is not doctors we should castigate but the system that allows them to emerge from medical schools with a mechanistic view of human illness. Medicine sees injury in a mechanistic way, studying the biochemical changes that are triggered in the immune system, and how the body naturally dams the flow of blood that is produced. While these processes are magical and amazing enough in themselves, the important question is the one that addresses the interaction and influence of the mind upon these physical processes.

The system perpetuates itself by means of a subtle (and therefore incredibly powerful) form of indoctrination. Young idealistic doctors are trained with methods stressing efficiency. They learn to treat patients no doubt as they themselves were treated and as their superiors, whom they try to imitate, treat patients. When dealing with a sick individual, the notion that one should be intuitive should never be lost sight of; otherwise we are simply 'block-booking' and forgetting that we are dealing with an individual. It is all too often the case with conventional medicine that the doctor will attempt to diminish the significance of the personal quirks of the patient to the illness in question. In contrast, the complementary practitioner sees these peculiarities as keys to the illness and the root of the cure for it. Medical students are as yet untrained in counselling skills or even rudimentary social skills.

The resentment of the spokespeople for conventional medicine is aggravated by the fact that they feel they are being undermined by people with no training in medicine. This in turn leads to resentment from the side-lined practitioners of complementary medicine, who are then driven into a more extreme position brought about by their own defensiveness. The schism between orthodox medicine and unorthodox is a corrosive one and one that is ultimately pointless. The term 'complementary medicine' is favoured over over 'alternative medicine' in this section of the book as orthodox medicine and spiritual healing are not mutually exclusive, although one could be forgiven for thinking they were.

Healers are caught in a Catch-22 situation. People with healing gifts are alienated from the church and thus tend to work in fringe religious groups, which is the precise reason they are regarded with suspicion by many Christians.

The cures that were discovered by folk medicine have now been adopted and assimilated into standard everyday medical practice. Yet the wisdom that faith healing has to offer has not made the transition into orthodoxy as yet and, apart from a few pockets of enlightenment, stands in a medicinal no-man's-land. The reasons for this are cultural and religious.

The influence of René Descartes (1596–1650), the great philosopher and mathematician who is credited with beginning modern philosophy, led to a firm dichotomizing of mind and body. Descartes believed that all animal behaviour and internal processes could be explained mechanically. On the relationship between mind and body, Descartes was a dualist, believing the two to be separate. The type of dualism he advocated was interactionism—he believed in a separate but interacting mind and body. After Descartes, some philosophers elaborated the mechanical side of his philosophy by proposing that humans were nothing but machines and the concept of mind was unnecessary.

While the influence of Cartesian ideas led us out of the Dark Ages in the physical sciences, making medicine search out physical causes for illness, these ideas were corrosive in that they denied the mind as a causal influence on the body. They led science to denigrate everything that was not explainable by theory. As well as the Cartesian outlook, the influence of the Industrial Revolution, contemporary with the prominence of Descartes, led to a growing confidence in humankind as regards the ability to master the environment. This instilled a materialistic outlook on the world, which manifested itself in an increasing emphasis on the purely physical aspects of illness. It spawned the identification of parasites, bacteria, viruses, vitamins, hormones and genetic anomalies, as well as the benefit of using chemicals to treat disease. Alexander Fleming discovered penicillin; digitalis was discovered from an old folk remedy; the physician became confident that the eradication of disease was on the horizon. Lister made innovations with the antiseptic treatment of wounds. While, of course, this is all laudable, it encouraged the practitioners of medicine to downgrade the importance of the patient's mental attitude to illness in favour of a purely physical account. It was into this gap that sects such as Christian Science leapt, filling the vacuum left when medicine became materialistic. The very word 'disease' demonstrates an awareness of the root of many illnesses—a state of absence of ease, of psychological tranquillity, yet this was a reasoning that passed by many in the medical profession. The term 'shell-shock' from the First World War was a manifestation of the unwillingness of conventional medicine to accept that war left psychological damage as well as physical. The disjunction of physical and psychological approaches to healing has prevailed from antiquity. Egyptian papyri delineate two wings of therapy—one involving charms and incantations, the other scientific approaches employing medicine.

Orthodox humanistic medicine traditionally advocated healing through regimen and diet, contrary to the claim of the complementary health fraternity that they were the authors of the holistic approach to therapy. The problem lies in the medical fraternity's apparent unwillingness to act on this knowledge. Doctors have known for years that what goes on in a patient's mind is as important as the biochemical processes within the body. At the beginning of the 19th century, Johann Heinroth, a German clergyman, invented the word 'psychosomatic', which unites two words meaning 'mind' and 'body' and emphasizes that a sick person can be cured only when his or her psychological make-up is considered as well as the disturbed organs. There are specific kinds of illness in which the state of the patient's mental attitude to the malady is of primary importance to the success or failure of its management. It is perhaps more than pure coincidence that these are the illnesses in which faith healing has much of its success.

The first and most obvious of these are afflictions that can be of a psychosomatic character, such as headaches, vomiting and rashes. Another branch includes illnesses that are short lasting and which the body's normal mechanisms will combat in due time. These include muscular aches and pains, and even warts. With these illnesses a positive mental attitude is as important as the physical cure. A further category is terminal illnesses, where there will be great fluctuations in progress as the disease moves towards its inevitable conclusion.

This knowledge, however, was ignored for a great interval of time as the discovery of the germs that caused diseases such as tuberculosis, cholera and syphilis persuaded doctors that every illness was the result of a specific germ. If they could isolate the germ, they could confidently cure the disease with drugs or by other physical means. They ignored the effects of mental experiences on the progress of disease and treated the body as a machine.

The term 'psychosomatic' is still used in a pejorative sense by doctors, with the faintly patronizing and dismissive implication that the patient is being soft and weak-willed. It has been estimated that illnesses involving a psychosomatic factor apply to some 80 per cent of diseases. As regards faith healing, one can either view this fact negatively or positively. One can say that this proves the validity and appropriateness of faith healing to deal with the kinds of illness that consume and plague the mind. Conversely, one could say that this fact demonstrates that faith healing's success can be placed in the realm of primitive psychiatry and its triumphs can be put down to suggestion rather than a divinity shaping our ends.

The limits of orthodox medicine

In fairness to conventional medicine, it is clear that we often overestimate the abilities of the medical profession. People still surrender to inexplicable viral infections, to tumours, and to premature failure of vital organs, when drugs or surgery are less than useless. Orthodox medicine has failed to provide cures for a whole array of conditions, including Aids, arthritis, cancer and heart disease. The physician or surgeon does not cure disease; he or she only assists the natural processes of cure, which are performed by the intrinsic healing and renewing ability of the human body. The English physician Thomas Sydenham wrote: 'I often think more could be left to nature than we are in the habit of leaving to her; to imagine that she always wants the help of art is an error, and an unlearned error too.'

We should remember that many mechanistic medical treatments, such as chemotherapy and radiation therapy for cancer, are toxic and deleterious and may even be of unproven value. Until recently electroconvulsive therapy was employed by the medical profession, albeit as a last resort.

Robert Buckmann reports that only fifteen per cent of medical practice can be said to be based on 'sound science'. As for the rest, the doctor will employ the very things that a healer will—that is, an amalgam of folklore, individual predilection and observation.

Many New Age commentators are often to be found bewailing the exclusivity of the orthodox medical establishment and the willingness they (whoever 'they' are) display to dismiss complementary medicine. Yet often what seems to lie behind this is a desire amongst the New-Agers to paint themselves as romantic outsiders excluded by the orthodoxy. The truth of the matter is that in some areas of medicine there is a great receptivity to complementary medicine. Oncologists (those who study tumours) have always displayed a holistic approach to medicine. Furthermore, meditation and dietary manipulation may be considered complementary to orthodox, proved therapies. What is needed is a synthesis between the wisdom of faith healing and conventional medicine. At this point holistic medicine as a mainstream idea is in its childhood. Several of the leading exponents in this new area of medicine acknowledge healing as a holistic regimen.

A Devon GP, Michael Dixon, has been referring many of his patients to the faith healer Gill White for over three years. Initially, his fellow doctors in practice were sceptical but eventually they became receptive to the idea once the results became evident.

Dr Dixon used the first fifty of his patients who had seen the healer to conduct an enquiry into the success of the referral. These results were published in *Connection*, the membership journal of the Royal College of General Practitioners. Seventy-five per cent said that their symptoms were 'much better' and 30 per cent said they were 'very much better'. The success of the healer was so impressive that Dr Dixon is now funded by the Family Health Services Authority in researching the effects of healing, and a second healer has been taken on. Interestingly, the ailments that seem to respond to treatment more readily are arthritis, eczema, back pain, stress and depression.

What this illustrates is that we cannot generalize about the receptivity of orthodox medicine to what healing has to offer. As long as there are men with the open-mindedness and vision of Michael Dixon, it is unfair to defame the medical profession for its narrow-mindedness towards complementary medicine. Particular branches, such as oncology, will be more receptive than others to what healing has to offer.

Perhaps the increasing receptivity of the medical profession towards complementary medicine is born not of a healthy intellectual openness but of desperation in the face of its own failure to combat a growing number of illnesses that conventional medicine is impotent against.

One should always be mindful of the propensity for advances in medical knowledge to come from the most unlikely quarters. The old wives' cure for a wound entailed binding it in cobwebs. Cobwebs, we now know, are rich in penicillin. Who are we to say that the practice of faith healing does not contain some hidden truth as yet unreachable by the current grasp of medicine?

The limits of our understanding

We rely on direct demonstration of the curative value of a treatment to believe in the efficacy of a particular therapy. This relies on the availability of a viable method by which we can test the claim. In some cases, however, this simply does not exist. For example, the Ancient Romans knew that disease within the arteries caused angina. Yet verification of this knowledge was only really available in the 1930s, when Werner Forsmann put a catheter into his own heart finally to prove the truth of this assertion.

It is quite possible that a relevant test of what precisely happens during the healing process is not yet available to us, and as yet it is simply inappropriate to dismiss it as a form of therapy. It may be premature to perform experiments on healing without first knowing the essence of the processes that take place. Not knowing the very nature of these processes may bias what is found.

It is conceivable that there might be an aptitude in humankind to cure, which is reliant on some dimly understood emanation that is now an enigma to humanity. It may be that, in terms of getting near to a fuller understanding of precisely what is happening when a healer cures, we are like a caveman trying to comprehend chaos theory. An element of suggestion is assuredly a factor in these healings, but this falls woefully short of explaining the cures. Whatever the interaction that occurs between healer and patient—presupposing that there is one—no one has as yet offered any definitive explanation of what it might be composed.

We should remind ourselves that what is today regarded as pseudo-science may in the future become part of medical practice, and one can never be entirely certain that one is right to dismiss new claims. It is quite possible that there might be an ability in humans to heal, which is not the doing of a deity or a devil but accountable to some mysterious force, as yet unexplained or unexplainable with the current vocabulary of medical science. An article in *New Scientist* magazine in 1995 bewailed the fact that we are not prepared to discuss the extent of what we simply do not know. Instead we swagger and preen and talk complacently of what we do understand.

It is important to consider the idea that the beneficial aspects of having visited a healer do not easily lend themselves to being quantified in a scientific way. After you have seen a healer or a healing doctor, you may behave slightly differently, and people may perceive you differently, leading to a chain of positive effects that bolsters your sense of wellbeing, reducing your symptoms and increasing your pain threshold. These are all very subtle changes, and changes that we ourselves may not even be consciously aware of.

This means examining the psychological, cultural and social aspects of illness and health, and the importance of understanding not only the means by which a patient's physical system comes to work properly but also the way in which the patient comes to feel well again and is re-integrated into his or her society as a full participant.

There is a detectable shift in some medical quarters at least from placing the emphasis on relieving symptoms and curing disease to the broader question of how healing itself occurs. What we need is a synthesis between the wisdom of faith healing and conventional medicine. Just as the nature-nurture debate can be resolved only by the bringing together of sociology and socio-biology, so too can medicine proceed only when it comes to some meaningful rapprochement with healing and the rest of complementary medicine. We should denigrate neither conventional medicine nor healing but begin the peace process between the two in the spirit of human enterprise.

The healing goes on . . .

The debate about the validity of faith healing will continue, as will the battle between scientific empiricism and age-old mysticism. It may be fatuous to argue the case for a subject that is dimly understood and of which, moreover, there can be no one authoritative definition.

It does, however, seem churlish to question the validity of anything that eases suffering, even if that relief is branded as imaginary. Are we really so confused and deluded that we do not know how we feel, and, if so, is it really so bad to make someone believe that they feel better?

At a recent alternative health exhibition in Glasgow, a woman had a stall covering the subject of 'spiritual healing'. This was no crank, but an ordinary human being with an open mind and a curiosity into the faith healing phenomenon. What was especially heartening was her willingness to express her doubts and worries about the subject; some of the religious groups that she had had attachments with had been too doctrinal, too intent upon making every one of their followers think the same. She confessed that she did not truly understand what powers were at work when her healer colleagues used their skills, but that the results spoke for themselves.

And there it is; however mired in quackery we may believe it to be, and however contrary to our beliefs, we have to accept faith healing if it can relieve just one ounce of pain in one individual.

Indeed, the one thing that we can be emphatic about is the imperative of healing. Perhaps the question should not be 'Does faith healing exist?' but 'Why do we need faith healing?' It does not take long to figure out. We live in an instant culture that is fragmented and self-absorbed. Saturated with cynicism, we have declared ideology dead.

We get our reality second-hand from a flickering box, waste our faith on Saturday night lottery draws, and pay strangers to listen to our fears. Gone are the days when you went to your minister or priest for spiritual guidance. People have lost faith in the church and never had faith in the government, which is why they are turning inwards to find faith in themselves.

If, as many religions espouse, God is indeed inside every one of us, churchmen all over the world must be laughing into their cassocks. It would appear that what we thought we had rejected, we have simply re-invented and accepted in a different form.

It seems ironic that from such cultural rubble, such a bright hope has emerged. Perhaps our high-rise existence has brought us closer to God. Or perhaps the higher power that we long for, and sometimes feel we can sense, is in fact the sum total of our projected individual faiths. Perhaps this is the force that heals, and *all* healing is faith healing. Still, that's a lot of maybes.

One thing that is certain is that we are a sick society, and it is not hard to see that our world is itself wracked with disease and in desperate need of healing. War, poverty and pollution are the earth's equivalent of anger, despair and anxiety, and are ravaging the planet in the same devastating ways in which these emotions affect our bodies. Indeed, perhaps these global 'illnesses' are manifestations of our own sickness as we project our accumulated rage and fear out into the wider environment.

Each individual is a microcosm of the universe, and the way towards a healthy planet lies in healing ourselves and each other. Through healing ourselves we heal the world, and vice-versa, and the first step towards self-healing is self-love.

So as we limp into the next millennium, a message has to be sent around the world—a message of positivity and love. Love that has the power to heal.

The Natural Way to Combat Stress

The body's internal reaction to external pressure

Stress is the 'wear and tear' our minds and bodies experience as we attempt to cope with our continually changing environment. People often think of stress as pressure at work, a sick child or rush-hour traffic. These events may be triggers, but stress is actually the body's internal reaction to such factors. Stress is the automatic 'fight-or-flight' response in the body, activated by adrenaline and other stress hormones, which stimulate a variety of physiological changes, such as increased heart rate and blood pressure, faster breathing, muscle tension, dilated pupils, dry mouth and increased blood sugar. In simple biological terms, stress is the state of increased arousal necessary for an organism to defend itself when faced with danger.

Whenever we feel anxious, tense, tired, frightened, elated or depressed, we are undergoing stress. Few aspects of life are free from the events and pressures that generate such feelings, and stress has become an acceptable and unavoidable part of normal everyday existence. In fact, contrary to popular assumptions, stressed lifestyles are not an exclusively modern phenomenon—stress has *always* been intrinsic to human existence, and life without stress would be unbearable. For example, certain types of stress, such as physical and mental exercise, sex, and intense creativity, are actually very desirable. It is only when real or perceived change overwhelms the body's ability to cope, that stress becomes harmful (distress), leaving us prone to unwanted physical, mental or emotional reactions and illnesses.

Types of stress

The causes of stress ('stressors') are multiple and varied, but they can be divided into two general categories—external and internal:

External stressors

- *physical environment*—noise, bright lights, heat, confined spaces
- *social interaction*—rudeness, bossiness or aggressiveness by others
- *organizational*—rules, regulations, 'red tape', deadlines
- *major life events*—death of a relative, lost job, promotion, new baby
- *daily hassles*—commuting, misplacing keys, mechanical breakdowns

Internal stressors

- *lifestyle choices*—caffeine, not enough sleep, overloaded schedule
- *negative self-talk*—pessimistic thinking, self-criticism, over-analysing
- *mind traps*—unrealistic expectations, taking things personally, all-or-nothing thinking, exaggerating, rigid thinking
- *stressful personality traits*—type A, perfectionist, workaholic

These factors generate various symptoms of emotional and mental stress, the most common including: anger, anxiety, worry, fear, and depression.

Negative stress

Excessive, prolonged and unrelieved stress can have a harmful effect on mental, physical and spiritual health. If left unresolved, the feelings of anger, frustration, fear and depression generated by stress can trigger a variety of illnesses. It is estimated that stress is the most common cause of ill health in modern society, probably underlying as many as 80 per cent of all visits to family doctors. Stress is a contributory factor in relatively minor conditions, such as headaches, digestive problems, skin complaints, insomnia and ulcers, but also plays an important role in the leading causes of death in the western world—cancer, cardiovascular disease, respiratory disorders, accidental injuries, cirrhosis of the liver and suicide.

Positive stress

Stress can also have a positive effect. It is essential in spurring motivation and awareness, providing the stimulation needed to cope with challenging situations. Tension and arousal are necessary for the enjoyment of many aspects of life, and without them existence would be pretty dull. Stress also provides the sense of urgency and alertness needed for survival when confronting threatening situations, such as crossing a busy road or driving in poor weather conditions. An overly relaxed approach in such situations could be fatal.

Stress and the individual

There is no single level of stress that is optimal for all people. Everyone is different, with unique perceptions of, and reactions to, events: what is distressing to one person may be a joy to another. A person who loves to work alone would be stressed in a job that involved high levels of social interaction, whereas the person who thrives as part of a team would very likely be stressed in a job that involved working from home.

Even when we agree that a particular event is distressing, we are likely to differ in our physiological and psychological responses to it. Some individuals are more sensitive to stress than others, owing to experiences in childhood and the influence of teachers, parents, religion, etc. It is also important to note that most of the stress that we experience is actually *self-generated*. How we perceive life—whether an event makes us feel threatened or stimulated, encouraged or discouraged, happy or sad—depends to a large extent on how we perceive ourselves.

Self-generated stress is something of a paradox, because so many people think of external causes when they are upset. Recognizing that we create most of our own upsets is an important first step towards coping with them.

The stress response

It is tempting to think that mental and physical stress is an ailment only of modern civilization; that our fast-paced urban lifestyles, straining under the relentless pressure of greater competitiveness and automation, has created a culture that lives on its nerves and feeds off crisis. This is a misconception; stress has been part of the human condition since the beginning of time. Like the air we breath, stress is an integral factor in human survival. Think about any challenge or stimuli, and stress has been a factor in our response. It is an active force that helps us rise to meet whatever everyday life throws at us and we thrive on taking up challenges, meeting that deadline and adapting to difficult situations.

How our bodies respond to stress was first described in the 1930s by two American doctors, Walter B. Cannon and Hans Selye. They found that the first reaction to severe stress is what is known as the 'fight-or-flight' response, which activates the body's protective mechanism either to fight (confront the stressor) or flee (act to avoid the stressor or threat of it). Initially, the fight-or-flight response alerts us to danger and is, in fact, beneficial—providing the strength, speed and stamina necessary for survival.

The stress response is controlled by the endocrine system, which regulates various bodily functions, including the reproductive system, the immune system, growth, metabolism, allergic response and stress tolerance. Any unusual demand on the body's physical and mental resources stimulates the endocrine glands—mainly the adrenal, pituitary and hypothalamus—to secrete chemical messengers, called hormones, into the blood stream. These stress hormones include powerful stimulants, such as adrenaline, noradrenaline, cortisol, testosterone and thyroxin, which produce a variety of physical responses. The most common include:

- increased pupil dilation
- perspiration
- increased heart rate and blood pressure (to get more blood to the muscles, brain and heart)
- rapid breathing (to take in more oxygen)
- muscle tenseness (in preparation for action)
- increased blood flow to the brain, heart and muscles (the organs that are most important in dealing with danger)
- less blood flow to the skin, digestive tract, kidneys and liver (where it is least needed in times of crisis)
- increased mental alertness and sensitivity (to assess the situation and act quickly)
- increased blood sugar, fats and cholesterol (for extra energy)
- a rise in platelets and blood-clotting factors (to prevent haemorrhage in case of injury)

Unfortunately, although this natural physical response would have been invaluable at an earlier stage in human evolution, fighting and running away are rarely appropriate responses to stressful situations in the modern world. Under long term, unrelieved stress our bodies remain in a constant state of arousal, which can result in the gradual onset of various health problems.

Primitive human beings frequently faced life and death situations, when alertness, strength, speed and performance were vital and the primary, instinctive response was to survive. The type of challenges we all meet with today, however, are rather different and, as they rarely require a physical response, the body's reaction to the situation is often inappropriate.

The stresses of modern life are more complex and last over longer periods of time. In the past, challenges were instantaneous and had to be resolved instinctively; today, we are subjected to long-term emotional, occupational and environmental anxieties, which demand that we maintain a certain level of mental and physical health. We also have to prepare ourselves for times of crisis and events that test us to our fullest, such as divorce, redundancy, bereavement or illness. This means that we have to be poised to 'fight or flight' at another level and in a completely different way from our forebears.

The rapid way in which our society now changes and constantly throws up fresh challenges places an unhealthy strain on a system that may be struggling to keep up. The extra mental exertion we all expend just to keep 'on top of things' can create a bottleneck of energy as pressure builds up with nowhere to go. If nothing is done to relieve the situation the mechanisms we have for dealing with stress will eventually fail us, causing illness and exhaustion. It is vital, therefore, that we make a priority of finding ways of easing our bodies and minds out of 'fight or flight' mode and put ourselves on a better footing to be able to deal with the ever-changing pressures of the modern world.

In order to do this we need a greater understanding and awareness of how our bodies work. Our automatic physical response to danger or stress involves an intricate chain reaction of bodily and biochemical effects, involving the brain, the nervous system and hormones. As soon as we perceive a threat, our body explodes with energy and strength, and thousands of messenger hormones flood into the bloodstream to call the alarm. Our minds and bodies instantly become clear, alert and poised—ready for action. In this alarm reaction the main players are the lungs, brain, nervous system, muscle systems and hormones. Arousal is initially registered by the hypothalamus—a tiny crowd of cells at the base of the brain—which controls all automatic bodily functions and reactions. It releases chemicals called endorphins, which act as natural painkillers. They dull the perception of pain and mental turmoil and help us to deal with the situation by blocking out factors that may otherwise prevent us from giving less than our peak performance.

Adrenaline, also helps us rise to the situation. It causes a quickening of the heart rate, a raising of blood pressure and a release of vital nutrients. It also creates muscle tension and affects breathing patterns, making them faster and shallower. But it is only one of the arousal hormones released by the adrenal gland near the kidneys. Noradrenaline, associated with positive ecstatic arousal, is also released into the bloodstream. The hormone cortisol is the agent involved in converting glycogen, stored in the liver, into blood sugar, creating instant energy and alerting the brain. The required surge of strength and effort comes from the male hormone testosterone. The thyroid gland also plays a part in our body's arousal response. It releases thyroxin, a hormone that stimulates the metabolic system, increasing its work rate and regulating oxygen consumption. This is vital, as the body anticipates that it will need increased resources of energy. Our digestive system also slows down during this process, as blood is diverted from the skin and stomach. We instinctively shut down the unnecessary systems in order to concentrate on mobilizing those vital for survival. As the digestive system is not deemed essential in a life or death situation it slows down and is effectively put on hold.

The body has undoubtedly evolved an efficient and prompt survival response but, as already mentioned, the goalposts have moved slightly. The things that cause stress today are more complex and require more sophisticated solutions over a longer period of time. Our hormonal system suffers if it stays in 'fight' mode, as lengthy periods with our bodies on red-alert are not healthy for our mental or physical wellbeing. What begins as a positive range of responses, therefore, can eventually have a negative effect on our health.

Research shows that we put our bodies on challenge alert without realizing it. Emotions such as anger, anxiety and impatience produce the same chemical reactions in the body as standing in front of a speeding car—our nervous systems and hormones will still be poised for 'fight-or-flight'. But the same physiology that leaves us feeling poised and alert can create havoc over a long period of time. A build-up of energy can lead us to become stress addicts, who become hooked on the adrenaline rush that stressful situations create. Or we can become so used to living on such a psychological and physical 'tilt' that we don't realize the harm it is causing.

Overdoses of adrenaline can cause irritability and agitation, while too much noradrenaline can leave us feeling disconnected and high. If arousal continues, the adrenal glands create anti-flammatory chemicals to speed tissue repair, but cortisol will also suppress the immune system, leaving it vulnerable to illness and disease. Extra sodium is retained, endangering the performance of the cardiovascular system by causing fluid retention, raising the heart rate, increasing blood pressure and possibly inducing blood clots. Stomach ulcers are a classic symptom of stress, as the stomach cannot deal with the extra secretion of acid that occurs during times of turbulence. Acute and cumulative stress over a period of time can even cause death.

General Adaptation Syndrome

How the body adapts to prolonged stress is described by Dr Hans Selye in terms of the General Adaptation Syndrome. Selye divides the stress response into three phases: the Alarm Response, Adaptation, and Exhaustion. The Alarm Response is the fight-or-flight response that prepares the body for immediate action. If the source of stress persists, then the body prepares for long-term protection through the secretion of further hormones that increase blood sugar levels to sustain energy and raise blood pressure. This Adaptation phase, resulting from exposure to prolonged periods of stress, is common, and not necessarily harmful, but without periods of relaxation and rest to counterbalance the stress response, sufferers become prone to fatigue, concentration lapses, irritability and lethargy as the effort to sustain arousal slides into negative stress. Under persistent chronic stress, sufferers enter the Exhaustion phase: mental, physical and emotional resources suffer heavily, and the body experiences 'adrenal exhaustion', where blood sugar levels decrease as the adrenals become depleted, leading to decreased stress tolerance, progressive mental and physical exhaustion, illness and collapse.

Symptoms of stress

Exposure to excessive stress results in hormonal imbalances, which can produce a variety of symptoms:

Physical symptoms
- changes in sleep patterns
- fatigue
- changes in digestion—nausea, vomiting, diarrhoea
- loss of sexual drive
- headaches
- aches and pains in different areas of the body
- infections
- indigestion
- dizziness, faintness, sweating and trembling
- tingling of hands and feet
- breathlessness
- palpitations
- missed heartbeats

Emotional symptoms
- deterioration in personal hygiene and appearance
- bouts of depression
- impatience and irritability
- fits of rage
- tearfulness

Mental symptoms
- lack of concentration
- memory lapses
- difficulty in making decisions
- confusion
- disorientation
- panic attacks

Behavioural symptoms
- appetite changes—eating too much or too little
- eating disorders—anorexia, bulimia
- increased intake of alcohol and other drugs
- increased smoking
- hypochondria
- restlessness
- fidgeting
- nail-biting

Stress-related illness

Cardiovascular disease

The term 'cardiovascular' refers to the heart and to the body's system of blood vessels. Cardiovascular disease is probably the most serious health problem that can be linked to stress—it is the most common cause of death in Britain and the USA. The primary causes of heart disease include smoking and high-fat diets, but stress is a significant contributory factor.

Adrenal hormones act to increase blood pressure; temporary rises in blood pressure present no threat to health, but a frequent or perpetual state of high blood pressure can have a serious effect on health in the long term. High blood pressure is linked with the development of arteriosclerosis, or hardening of the arteries. Arteriosclerosis is the result of the development of blood plaque in the arteries, which progressively narrows the pathway through which the blood flows. Eventually an artery can become blocked, leading to angina, stroke and heart failure.

The immune system

The immune system protects the body from infection. It fights foreign invaders (such as viruses and harmful bacteria) and cancer. Excessive stress can damage the immune system by affecting the thymus gland. This manufactures white blood cells, called T-cells, for regulating immunity and also produces various immune-related hormones. The stress reaction diverts resources to the main parts of the body that need to deal with stress, mainly the brain, heart and muscles. Other systems are deprived of resources, including the immune system. Hormones produced by the adrenal glands can cause the thymus gland to shrink and also degrade the activity of white blood cells, causing damage to the body's ability to fight infection. As a result high stress can result in reduced resistance to common infections, such as colds, influenza and herpes (cold sores). Because certain types of white blood cells produced by the thymus are active in preventing the development of cancer cells in the body, any damage to the thymus may effect the body's ability to resist cancer.

Asthma

Asthma is a respiratory disorder marked by the temporary constriction of the bronchi, the airways branching from the trachea to the lungs. Attacks usually are brought on by allergic reaction to antigens, such as grass and tree pollens, mould spores, fungi, animal dander, and certain foods, but may also be caused by chemical irritants in the atmosphere or by infections of the respiratory tract. Susceptibility to an asthma attack is based on hyperactivity of the bronchial muscles, which constrict on exposure to one or other of these agents. Chronic stress reduces the efficiency of the adrenal glands, reducing the output of anti-inflammatory and anti-allergic adrenal hormones, which may make an asthma attack more likely.

Diabetes

Diabetes is caused by the inability of the body to metabolize sugar correctly, leading to excessively high levels of sugar in the blood. Sugar metabolism is the responsibility of the hormone insulin, which is secreted by the pancreas. Most diabetics can produce insulin, but various factors limit the hormone's efficiency, known as 'insulin sensitivity'.

As we know from the physiology of the stress response, the release of adrenal hormones under stress can have significant impact on blood-sugar levels. Adrenaline causes sugar in the liver to be dumped into the blood stream, and cortisol acts to reduce metabolism of glucose by cells. Large amounts of corti-

sol act to decrease insulin sensitivity. High blood-sugar levels are not dangerous in normally healthy individuals, but chronic stress, combined with other
factors such as obesity, act to increase the likelihood of developing diabetes.

Ulcers

Ulcers are frequently associated with stress, although no conclusive link has
yet been demonstrated. Normally the lining of the stomach is covered with a
layer of mucus to protect it from the digestive acids and enzymes used in the
breaking down of food. Over time, chronic stress can stimulate the overproduction of gastric juices, which break down the protective mucus and act upon the
walls of the digestive tract, resulting in ulceration. Ulcers usually occur singly
as round or oval lesions; the erosions are usually shallow but can penetrate the
entire wall, leading to haemorrhage and possibly death.

Digestive disorders

Many problems with the digestive tract, such as constipation, diarrhoea and irritable bowel syndrome, are linked to stress. The nerves in the digestive tract
receive messages from the brain in the form of hormones, which tell the intestinal muscles to expand or contract. Hormonal imbalances can cause alterations
in intestinal function, such as spasms, constipation and diarrhoea. Chronic
stress tends to shut down the digestive system altogether, exacerbating intestinal problems.

Skin complaints

Stress increases levels of toxicity in the body and contributes to hormonal imbalances, both of which have an effect on the skin. The visible effects of stress
on the skin include:
- acne
- spots
- eczema
- psoriasis
- excessive pallor
- skin diseases

Headaches and migraines

Headaches are one of our most common afflictions. Millions of people seek
medical help for this problem every year, and millions of pounds are spent on
headache remedies annually.

Most headaches are caused not by disease but by fatigue, emotional disorders, or allergies. Intermittent tension headaches are caused by worry, anxiety,
overwork, or inadequate ventilation. The most common type—a chronic tension headache—is often caused by depression. Brain tissue itself is insensitive
to pain, as is the bony covering of the brain (the cranium). Headache pain results from the stimulation of such pain-sensitive structures as the membranous
linings of the brain (the meninges) and the nerves of the cranium and upper
neck. This stimulation can be produced by inflammation, by the dilation of
blood vessels of the head, or by muscle spasms in the neck and head. Headaches brought on by muscle spasms are classified as tension headaches; those
caused by the dilation of blood vessels are called vascular headaches.

Almost 90 per cent of all people seeking medical help for headaches suffer
from tension headaches. These are characterized by a diffuse ache that either
spreads over the entire head or feels like a tight headband. Tension headaches
are often associated with poor sleep and persistent tension in the muscles of
the neck, shoulders and forehead. These muscles must relax before the pain
eases.

Migraine is the most common form of vascular headache. About 60 per cent of all migraine sufferers are women, and most sufferers first develop symptoms between the ages of 10 and 30. In approximately 30 per cent of all cases, migraine attacks are preceded by warning signs such as blind spots, zigzag flashing lights, numbness in parts of the body, and distorted visual images. Migraine pain almost always occurs on only one side and is usually accompanied by nausea. Many things seem capable of triggering migraine attacks, including stress, fatigue, changes in the weather, fasting, menstruation, drugs, such as birth control pills, that contain oestrogen, and foods, such as cheese, alcohol, and chocolate, that contain substances that affect the blood vessels. Many migraine patients have family histories of the problem.

Many of the relaxation techniques and alternative therapies outlined later in this book will help to alleviate headaches. However, chronic headaches may be physical symptoms of depression or other kinds of severe emotional problems. If you suffer from persistent headaches, then be sure to consult your doctor for professional treatment.

Premenstrual Syndrome (PMS)

Stress has a debilitating effect on the nerves in general, and certain premenstrual symptoms may be aggravated by stress. Many sufferers of PMS have abnormal levels of the adrenal hormone aldosterone, which may account for some of the problems of excessive fluid retention and weight gain, breast tenderness and abdominal bloating. Further release of aldosterone caused by stress will exacerbate these problems.

Depression

Chronic stress can produce severe depression, because of its debilitating psychological effects. The physiological changes produced by stress can also contribute to depression. Adrenaline and noradrenaline are not only adrenal hormones but also chemical messengers in the brain. Deficiencies of noradrenaline have been linked to depression in certain individuals, and so adrenal exhaustion through chronic long-term stress may be a contributory factor in depressive illness.

The causes of stress

Environmental stress

Urban decay and deprivation are a major source of distress for large sections of the population. Inadequate housing, noise, pollution, overcrowding, violence and poverty create some of the most cumulative and pervasive forms of stress. These factors affect how we live, work and play. Their impact depends on the infrastructure of the location, transport requirements, and availability of opportunities to spend time away from the environment.

We all have different reactions to stress, and experience helps us to develop our own methods of dealing with it. While some of us may lead *less* stressful lives, it is impossible to lead a completely stress-free life, as things happen to all of us unexpectedly and 'out of the blue'. The trick comes in weeding out as much of the trivial stress as possible and learning how to control our response to unavoidable, accumulative stress. If we can do this then we can be better prepared for the surprises life springs on us and learn to enjoy rising to the challenges they present.

All of us will have times in our lives that cause us great distress and leave us feeling unable to go on. Bereavement, family break-up and redundancy are devastating events, but even moving house or changing jobs, usually seen as happy occasions, can produce high levels of stress. This is because stress doesn't just occur when we feel angry or are in grief. Welcomed events can be just as stressful if they create self-doubt or anxiety. Any sort of change, with relationships, homes or occupations, can induce stress, as human beings are essentially creatures of habit. The fight for homeostasis—internal and physiological equilibrium—is a relentless process and is made more difficult when drastic changes in the way we organize and live our lives are forced on us. The amount of stress we experience, therefore, is largely dependent on how we adapt to circumstances.

One of the most prevalent causes of stress is our immediate environment. Urban living, in particular, with its associated problems of inadequate housing, noise, pollution, crowding, violence and poverty creates some of the most cumulative and pervasive forms of stress. These factors affect how we live, work and play, and much may depend on the infrastructure of the location, transport provision, and our ability to spend time away from our environment. If we feel unable to escape stressful surroundings, even for a brief time, then feelings of helplessness can grow to the point where they become very damaging to our self-image and the way we interact with other people.

There are ways of improving how we live and deal with stress that most of us recognize only subconsciously. For example, our home to most of us is more than a place to eat and sleep. In an increasingly hostile society we use our home as an oasis of calm. In our own homes we can shut the door on the outside world and surround ourselves with our personal possessions, family and friends. The 'feathering the nest' syndrome is well documented—it is an instinctive need to create a comfortable environment, one where we can relax and be ourselves.

In creating comfort, space is one of the most important factors. We all have invisible boundaries which outline our personal space. But these are difficult to maintain when our personal space is constantly being invaded. We should all be able to retreat inside ourselves and find peace, but many of us experience a physical lack of space that has an affect on our mental wellbeing as overcrowding and lack of privacy make personal calm all the more difficult to achieve. Also, advances in technology have led to increasing numbers of people working from home, and in many instances this has put a further strain on space allocation, as work space is carved out of resources already stretched between family members and various activities.

Our individual space requirements depend heavily on what we are used to. In Hong Kong, for example, where overcrowding has reached epidemic proportions, what most of us are used to in Britain would look positively luxurious. Building and space cost money, however, and in all societies those with lower incomes are usually restricted in their choice of accommodation or, increasingly, deprived of it altogether. Without privacy and space, quality of life undoubtedly suffers, as certain activities such as meditation, relaxation or making love need uninterrupted peace and quiet.

Light

Light is another important factor in determining the quality of our everyday lives. In the depths of winter most of us look forward to the long summer days ahead. This is because natural light is almost as vital for healthy living as the air we breath. It regulates levels of the hormone melanonin, which influences sleep, mood and the reproductive cycle. Our instinctive love of light and the sun explains our annual migration to hotter climates. A lack of daylight can influence the natural production of melanonin, creating lethargy and depression. SAD—seasonal affective disorder—is increasingly seen in the winter months. Sufferers feel antisocial, tired and depressed. In order to counter such feelings it is advisable to work beside windows and let as much daylight into the workplace or home as possible. Fluorescent lighting, the most unnatural from of light, should be avoided wherever possible. As artificial light is a necessary evil, it is best to use full spectrum lights, as they simulate daylight.

Natural light is as vital for healthy living as the air we breath. It regulates levels of the hormone melatonin, which influences sleep, mood and the reproductive cycle. Our instinctive love of light and the sun explains our annual migration to hotter climates.

Colour

Colour affects many aspects of our lives and can have a significant effect on our moods and perceptions. We are all colour biased—we may chose colour as a response to their innate properties or we may just have a distinctive preference for it. Colours have physical as well as psychological effects. Research has shown that physiological responses such as blood pressure and brain-wave patterns vary according to which colour we are being exposed to. For example, exposure to red, the most stimulating colour, can lead to an increase of blood pressure while exposure to blue light has the opposite effect.

Colour can have a huge effect on our moods and ability to relax. Effective and intelligent use of colour is one of the easiest and cheapest ways to improve our surroundings. This is increasingly being recognized by health and education authorities, and more thought now goes into selecting the decor for classrooms, hospital wards and waiting rooms. Scientific research has also shown that colours can have physical as well as psychological effects. It has been found, for example, that exposure to red light can often raise blood pressure, while exposure to blue light can actually lower it.

Life events and the pace of change

In the following table of stressful events, compiled by two American doctors, T. H. Holmes and R. H. Rahe (*Journal of Psychosomatic Research No. 11, 1967*), specific events are weighted on a scale from 0 to 100.

The chart suggests that it is *change itself* that is stressful—moving house, getting married, redundancy, etc—regardless of whether the change is regarded as favourable or unfavourable. Scores of about 300 supposedly indicate a major life crisis, scores of 200 to 299 a moderate life crisis, and 100 to 199 a mild life crisis.

Event	Life Change Units	Event	Life Change Units
Death of a spouse	100	Large mortgage or loan	31
Divorce	73	Foreclosure of mortgage or loan	31
Marital separation	65	Change in job responsibilities	29
Imprisonment	63	Son or daughter leaving home	29
Death of a close relation	63	Outstanding personal achievement	28
Personal injury or illness	53	Beginning or end of school or college	26
Marriage/engagement/ cohabitation	50	Change in living conditions	25
		Change in personal habits (more or less exercise)	24
Loss of job	47		
Marital reconciliation	45	Trouble with the boss	23
Retirement	45	Change in working or conditions	20
Illness in the family	44	Moving house	20
Pregnancy	44	Change of school or college	20
Sexual problems	39	Change in recreation	19
Birth of a child	39	Change in social activities	18
Business readjustment	39	Change in sleeping habits	16

Event	Life Change Units	Event	Life Change Units
Change in financial state	38	Holiday	13
Death of a close friend	37	Christmas	12
Change to a different job	36	Minor violations of the law	11

Personal relationships

The quality of personal relationships is traditionally regarded as one of the main sources of stress. The relationship between partners is the key factor, followed by the parent–child relationship. Factors that contribute to successful and relatively stress-free relationships include:

- communication
- honesty with yourself and partner
- listening
- respect for yourself and partner
- realistic expectations
- quality time together
- quality time apart

Home and family

Many sources of stress, such as bereavement, financial worries and relationship breakdowns, which feature prominently in the Holmes and Rahe scale, orginate within the family.

Increases in stress over the last 30 years can be partly explained by changing social factors. Within the context of a large extended family, and a close working and social environment, an individual benefits from contact and communication with others, receives feedback to establish realistic life goals and meaning, as well as useful information and practical help to overcome problems. The dissolution of these close social support networks makes the individual more vulnerable to various stress-related chronic illnesses.

In the same period it has also become clear that, as well as being a source of support, affection and love, the home can also be the place where individuals, especially women and children, are most likely to suffer varying degrees of physical and emotional abuse.

Parenthood

Parenthood imposes heavy physical, emotional and financial burdens, which can crush the less resilient. Combining childcare and full-time employment is the most stressful of all, especially for the working mother, who is more likely to be responsible for a bigger share of the housework and childcare than the father. In this situation, arguments, disagreements, misunderstandings, resentments and depression are more likely to surface. The following advice can help to reduce parental stress levels:

- care for yourself as well as the children
- keep a sense of self, apart from the role of parent
- plan, prepare and prioritize to exploit free time
- use free time in a creative and stimulating way
- partners should acknowledge and define shared responsibilities
- preserve healthy communication
- avoid self recrimination—no one is perfect
- be prepared to use family, friends and agencies for support

Occupational stress

Work provides an income and also fulfils a variety of other human needs—mental and physical exercise, social contact, a feeling of self-worth and competence. Work, however, is also a major source of stress, arising from the nature of the relations between management and employees, and that between colleagues in the workplace in general.

The modern world thrives on the work ethic, and we are taught at a very early age to equate personal adequacy with material success and professional status. Few of us are immune to the pressures placed on us by society to desire things—bigger televisions, faster cars, exotic holidays—that are symbols of status. Advertising and marketing strategies tap into this competitive urge we all have and create in us a need to go one better than people around us, in other words succumb to the 'keeping up with the Joneses' syndrome. This starts at an early age—basically in tandem with the learning process. The fear of failure and the challenge of peer pressure motivates us to work to achieve. In moderation, this can be healthy, as achievement goes hand in hand with self-esteem, but it also creates a cumulative stress that follows us from school to higher education, through to our working lives.

For many of us, however, it is a struggle to keep up, and we often work unnaturally long hours in unfortunate working conditions just to keep our heads above water. It has become a truism nowadays to say that no job is for life. Temporary employment contracts and the threat of unemployment are now features of more and more peoples' working lives, and many feel lucky to have a job at all. Society, therefore, is forcing us to change our expectations of how we work, and this is taking its toll on our physical and emotional security.

In coping with the structural changes of our working lives, it is vital to try to embrace the positives among the negatives. Flexitime, job sharing and increased communication through technology and the 'information superhighway', offer new ways of working, which, if we are able to adapt to them, can offer us greater freedoms. More emphasis on leisure time and recreation should also mean more time to relax and relate to family and friends. We are starting to see worth in activities not necessarily related to the working environment. This control can be used to create a healthy, more relaxed style of living. Stress is a plague of current working practices, and even if we can't change our overall working situation, there are certain steps we can take to de-stress our days.

There is a lot of truth in the saying that a messy desk portrays a messy mind. Being chronically disorganized can be debilitating at work, where lack of planning is one of the most common causes of stress. Stressful environments are minimized when we impose a form of structure that can offer security against problems appearing 'out of the blue'. Too inflexible a pattern would be impractical, but keeping a diary, writing lists and prioritizing duties all help to stem stressful situations. Writing down objectives, duties and activities helps to make them seem more tangible and surmountable. Don't try to overload your mind with too much information—if you are already stressed there is more chance of you forgetting vital references and data—but if you take steps to keep control of things then you will work more efficiently.

People have different tolerances for routine and variety. Some personalities thrive under the security of a routine working day. In many ways it can be quite liberating, as adhering to a pattern means that you can fully concentrate on one task at a time and not get in a muddle attempting things that there may not be adequate time for. On the other hand, too much routine can be boring and demoralizing and eat away at your enthusiasm for the job. Variety at work holds interest and enthusiasm, but too little structure leads to overloading, confusion and stress.

Most of us need to strike a balance between routine and variety in order to enjoy work and maintain levels of efficiency. Monotony can be broken by looking ahead and planning when to switch from one job to another. Perhaps there is a way to inject some variety into your tasks—can you open up your job description? Those suffering under too great a workload should learn to say 'no', and not be afraid of the consequences. Pacing yourself is one of the most vital practices in achieving a relaxed lifestyle. Learn when to stop and stand back from your activity, the odd moment of calm will increase efficiency when you do return to your task.

Most people suffer from time deprivation, as it is perhaps one of life's most precious commodities. We have to juggle everything—work, family, friends, leisure, eating and sleeping—in only 24 hours. Every day most of us have to strip demands on our time down to the essentials, and usually it is the time spent working and commuting that dictates how much we can give to other activities.

Time deprivation leaves us feeling harassed, hurried and guilty. It may also damage relationships, as it can mean breaking arrangements because we 'just don't have the time'. Some people make the situation worse—as the saying goes, 'less haste, more speed'. They will procrastinate and waste time worrying about commitments in their social life and deadlines at work. Often they take on too much and end up fulfilling few or none of their aims. Work will pile up and relationships suffer as commitments are neglected, and the individual is left feeling panicked and chaotic.

It can be very difficult to change habits formed over a lifetime. Often the best way is to recognize weak points in time management and learn to deal with them. Prioritize and look at the steps mentioned earlier for dealing with organization. Also, don't punish yourself for not having the time to do everything or be everywhere—it is not humanly possible or desirable.

The drive for success

Western society is driven by the work ethic. We are taught at a very early age to equate personal adequacy with professional success, making us crave status and abhor failure. Our culture demands a monetary success together with professional identity, and it takes a strong personality to step off the ladder.

Changing work patterns

In our post-industrial society's climate of unemployment and greater leisure time, many people feel lucky to have a job at all. Unemployment, redundancy, a shorter working week and the impact of new technology are affecting our physical and emotional security. Careers for life are no longer guaranteed, and more employers offer short-term contracts that preclude them from offering sickness or holiday pay. Financial and emotional burnout is therefore increasingly common among all levels of the workforce.

Working conditions

There can be little doubt that an individual's physical and mental health is adversely affected by unpleasant working conditions—such as high noise levels, too much or too little lighting, extremes of temperature, and unsocial or excessive hours.

Overwork

An individual may experience stress through an inability to cope with the technical or intellectual demands of a particular task. On the other hand, no matter how competent you are at your job, circumstances, such as long hours, unrealistic deadlines, and frequent interruptions, will all produce stress.

Underwork

An employee may experience boredom because there is not enough to do, or because a particular job is dull and repetitive.

Uncertainty

Uncertainty about an individual's work role—work objectives, responsibilities, colleagues' expectations and a lack of communication and feedback can result in confusion, frustration, helplessness, and stress.

Conflict

Stress may arise from work that an individual does not want to do or that conflicts with their personal, social and family values.

Responsibility

The greater the level of responsibility, the greater the level of stress.

Relationships at work

Good relationships at work with superiors, subordinates and colleagues are crucial. Within an organization, open discussion of problems is essential to encourage positive relationships.

Change at work

Changes that alter psychological, physiological and behavioural routines, such as promotion, retirement and redundancy, are extremely stressful.

Working conditions survey

Causes of stress
3 points each

- ❏ company has been taken over recently
- ❏ staff reductions/lay-offs in the past year
- ❏ department/company had major reorganization
- ❏ staff expect company to be sold or relocated
- ❏ employee benefits significantly cut recently
- ❏ mandatory overtime frequently required
- ❏ employees have little control over their work
- ❏ consequences of making mistakes are severe
- ❏ workloads vary greatly
- ❏ most work is machine-paced or fast-paced
- ❏ staff must react quickly and accurately to change

2 points each

- ❏ few chances of opportunities for advancement
- ❏ red tape hinders getting things done
- ❏ inadequate staffing, money or technology
- ❏ pay is below the going rate
- ❏ sick and holiday benefits are below the norm
- ❏ employees are rotated between shifts
- ❏ new machines/work methods have been introduced
- ❏ noise/vibration levels are high or temperature keeps changing
- ❏ employees normally isolated from one another
- ❏ performance of work units normally below average

Remedies
3 points each

- ❏ staff recognized and rewarded for their contributions
- ❏ management takes firm action to reduce stress
- ❏ mental health benefits are provided
- ❏ company has formal employee communications programme
- ❏ staff given information on coping with stress
- ❏ staff given clear job descriptions
- ❏ management and staff talk openly with one another
- ❏ employees are free to talk with one another

2 points each

- ❏ work rules are published and are the same for everyone
- ❏ child care programmes are available
- ❏ employees can work flexible hours
- ❏ perks are granted fairly
- ❏ employees have access to necessary technology
- ❏ staff and management are trained in resolving conflicts
- ❏ staff receive training when assigned new tasks
- ❏ company encourages work and personal support groups
- ❏ staff have space and time for relaxation

1 point each

- ❏ staff assistance programme is available
- ❏ each employee's work space is not crowded
- ❏ staff can have personal items in their work areas
- ❏ management appreciates humour in the workplace
- ❏ programmes for care of the elderly are available

Subtract the total points for stress reducers from the total for stress producers. Results will range from minus 50 for excellent working conditions, to plus 60 points for a very stressful working environment.

Personality traits

Type-A and Type-B personalities

Two American cardiologists, Friedmann and Rosenman, noticed that many of their patients with heart disease shared similar personality characteristics and tended to find it difficult to adjust their lifestyle in a way that would aid recuperation. After detailed research they discovered a significant relationship between certain habitual behavioural patterns and stress-related illness. They reported that males with Type-A behaviour were six times as likely to suffer heart disease as men who exhibited Type-B behaviour. Type-A behaviour features four main patterns:

- *intense sense of time urgency*—always rushed, trying to achieve more in less time
- *inappropriate hostility and aggression*—excessively competitive, finds it difficult to relax and have fun; slight provocation may trigger hostility
- *multiple behaviour*—engages in two or more things simultaneously at improper times
- *lack of proper planning*—lack of planning to achieve required goals

Many studies of people who exhibit Type-A personalities in a wide range of contexts show that common characteristics include:

- work longer hours
- spend more time in classes (students)
- travel more for business
- get less sleep
- more involved in voluntary work, clubs, etc
- spend less time resting or relaxing
- work more around the home
- communicate less with their partners
- less marital sex
- derive little pleasure from socializing

Type-A behaviour places more stress on the cardiovascular system, stimulating high blood pressure, high heart rate and increased risk of heart attacks.

Type-B behaviour is the opposite: more relaxed, less hurried, less competitive. The main character traits include:

- *able to take the long view*—they don't try to meet unrealistic targets or to take on more than they can cope with; better at delegating
- *speed is not that important*—don't worry if not every task can be completed to deadline
- *sense of personal identity*—don't feel they have to earn respect and love; secure in who they are and what they do
- *sense of proportion*—no sense of constant struggle; always maintain a sense of balance at events in their lives

Classifying individuals as either Type-A or Type-B personalities helps to explain why some people are more prone to stress-related disease. It should be emphasized, however, that the distinction between these two personality types is not absolute; most people will fall between the two extreme types described.

Personality type questionnaire

In the list of attributes, circle the number that most closely represents your own behaviour.

At one end of the scale is Type-A behaviour, the other is Type-B behaviour. High Type-A scores are obtained on the right side of the scale for questions 2, 5, 7, 11, 13, 14; high Type-A scores are obtained on the left side of the scale for questions 1, 3, 4, 6, 8, 9, 10, 12. Give yourself 10 points if you score at the end of the scale towards Type-A, working down to 0 points at the other end of the scale, which represents Type-B.

1 Never Late 5 4 3 2 1 0 1 2 3 4 5 Casual about appointments

2 Not competitive 5 4 3 2 1 0 1 2 3 4 5 Very competitive

3 Anticipates what others 5 4 3 2 1 0 1 2 3 4 5 Good listener
are going to say (nods,
interrupts, finishes for them)

4 Always rushed 5 4 3 2 1 0 1 2 3 4 5 Never feels rushed

5 Can wait patiently 5 4 3 2 1 0 1 2 3 4 5 Impatient while waiting

6 Goes all out 5 4 3 2 1 0 1 2 3 4 5 Casual

7 Takes things one at a time 5 4 3 2 1 0 1 2 3 4 5 Tries to do too much

8 Emphatic in speech 5 4 3 2 1 0 1 2 3 4 5 Slow deliberate talker

9 Wants good job 5 4 3 2 1 0 1 2 3 4 5 Seeks self-satisfaction
recognised by others regardless of others

10 Fast (eating, walking, etc.)5 4 3 2 1 0 1 2 3 4 5 Slow doing things

11 Easy going 5 4 3 2 1 0 1 2 3 4 5 Hard-driving

12 Hides feelings 5 4 3 2 1 0 1 2 3 4 5 Expresses feelings

13 Many outside interests 5 4 3 2 1 0 1 2 3 4 5 Few outside interests

14 Satisfied with job 5 4 3 2 1 0 1 2 3 4 5 Ambitious

Childhood influences and upbringing

A traumatic childhood is likely to lead to greater levels of stress as an adult. A difficult childhood is also more likely to lead to low self-esteem, low self-assertiveness, difficulty expressing personal beliefs, attitudes and feelings, and a tendency to depend on others to provide a sense of emotional wellbeing and self-worth. Over-dependence upon others is likely to lead to frustration as expectations are inevitably dashed—leading to feelings of frustration, anger, depression and hopelessness in adulthood.

Unrealistic expectations

Unrealistic expectations are a common source of stress. People often become upset about something, not because it is innately stressful but because it does not concur with what they expected. Take, for example, the experience of driving in slow-moving traffic. If it happens at rush hour, you may not like it but it should not surprise or upset you. However, if it occurs on a Sunday afternoon, especially if it makes you late for something, you are more likely to be stressed by it.

When expectations are realistic, life feels more predictable and therefore more manageable. There is an increased feeling of control because you can plan and prepare yourself (physically and psychologically). For example, if you know in advance when you have to work overtime or stay late, you will take it more in your stride than when it is dropped on you at the last minute.

Attitudes and beliefs

A lot of stress results from our beliefs. We have literally thousands of premises and assumptions about all kinds of things that we hold to be the truth—everything from, 'You can't beat the system' and 'The customer is always right', to 'Men shouldn't show their emotions' and 'Children should tidy their rooms'. We have beliefs about how things are, how people should behave and about ourselves ('I can never remember people's names'). Most of our beliefs are held unconsciously so we are unaware of them. This gives them more power over us and allows them to run our lives.

Beliefs cause stress in two ways. The first is the behaviour that results from them. For example, if you believe that work should come before pleasure, you are likely to work harder and have less leisure time than you would otherwise. If you believe that people should meet the needs of others before they meet their own, you are likely to neglect yourself to some extent. These beliefs are expressions of a personal philosophy or value system, which results in increased effort and decreased relaxation—a formula for stress. There is no objective truth to begin with. These are really just opinions but they lead to stressful behaviour. Uncovering the unconscious assumptions behind actions can be helpful in changing one's lifestyle.

The second way in which beliefs cause stress is when they are in conflict with those of other people. However, it should always be remembered that personal assumptions are not the truth but rather opinions and, therefore, they can be challenged. In situations of conflict it is always helpful if the protagonists attempt to revise their beliefs, or at least admit that the beliefs held by the other person may be just as valid as their own. This mind-opening exercise usually helps to diminish stressful antagonism.

Relaxation response

Just as the body has an automatic process to prepare it for a 'fight or flight' situation, it can also go into what is called the 'relaxation response'. This stage of low arousal is less well known than the body's red-alert status, and it initially takes a concentrated effort in order to experience it. The symptoms of the 'fight or flight' response—increased metabolic rate, quickened heart rate and faster breathing—are the direct opposite of those experienced by the body while in a state of deep relaxation.

We need to be truly relaxed for the process to begin and for the body to feel the full benefits. Two branches of the automatic nervous system are responsible for most of the changes that take place. What is known as the 'sympathetic branch' slows down, allowing the 'parasympathetic branch' to assume a greater role, calming the body and mind and decreasing metabolism until it reaches a hypometabolic state—it was in a hypermetabolic state during the 'fight or flight' process.

During relaxation our bodies require very low maintenance, and the decrease in metabolism is similar only to that found in deep sleep. Our breathing becomes more regular and the heart rate decreases. In a sustained period of relaxation oxygen consumption actually falls below that measured during deep sleep. There is also a significant fall in blood lactate, a substance that enters the blood through the metabolism of skeletal muscles. This occurs three times faster during meditation than while sitting at rest.

Blood pressure is also lowered, but only to normal pre-stress levels. All these things allow the body to recover from the strains placed on it by everyday life.

The relaxation response also elicits a marked alteration in brain activity. The brain emits four types of waves, each with its own rhythm. Beta waves signify everyday conscious rhythms; delta waves are present during sleep; theta waves appear while in a dreamlike state; and alpha waves are more prominent when the mind is active, yet relaxed. Effective meditation manufactures a predominance of alpha and theta waves—signifying a state of restfulness and deep relaxation, where the mind is alert but not strained or confused. These waves appear almost as soon as the body starts to relax, increasing in frequency as the process intensifies, allowing clearer and more constructive thinking.

A prolonged period of relaxation will also increase the body's secretion of particular mood-altering chemicals, known as neurotransmitters. One of these, serotonin, is a powerful hormone that is associated with feelings of happiness and contentment. Recent medical research suggests that a deficiency in this hormone is a contributory factor in cases of clinical depression.

Achieve relaxation and combat stress through self help

It would not be possible, or desirable, to eliminate all the effects of stress in our lives. The aim of stress management should be to harness and control the effects of stress to help to enrich our physical, mental and emotional well-being. Positive stress management involves recognizing the existence and type of stress and then taking remedial action. By getting to the root causes of your stress, you can not only relieve current problems and symptoms, but you can also prevent recurrences.

Remedial action falls into three main categories:
• change your thinking   • change your behaviour   • change your lifestyle

Change your thinking

Reframing

Reframing is one of the most powerful and creative stress reducers. It is a technique used to change the way you look at things in order to feel better about them. We all do this inadvertently at times. The key to reframing is to recognize that there are many ways to interpret the same situation. It is like the age-old question: Is the glass half empty or half full? The answer of course is that it is both or either, depending on your point of view. However, if you see the glass as half full, it will feel different than seeing it as half empty because the way we feel almost always results from the way we think. The message of reframing is this: there are many ways of seeing the same thing — so you might as well pick the one you like. Reframing does not change the external reality, but simply helps you to view things differently — and less stressfully.

Positive thinking

When faced with stressful situations try to avoid becoming preoccupied with debilitating negative thoughts of powerlessness, dejection, failure and despair. Chronic stress can leave us vulnerable to negative suggestion, so try to focus on positives:
• focus on your strengths
• learn from the stress you are under
• look for opportunities in the stressful situation
• seek out the positive — make a change

Change your behaviour

Be assertive

Being assertive means taking control and advancing your own needs and aspirations whilst remaining aware of the wishes of others. Assertiveness helps to manage stressful situations, and will in time help to reduce their frequency. Lack of assertiveness is often a function of low self-esteem and low self-confidence, factors that aggravate stress levels and can turn even relatively benign situations and events into potential crises.

The key to assertiveness is verbal and non-verbal communication. People who cannot adequately communicate their needs or wishes will create various problems for themselves. For example, the person who cannot say 'no' to others' requests is likely to be overwhelmed by external demands; the person who finds it difficult to express personal feelings and thoughts will lack self-fulfilment and not be comfortable with his or her own identity; an overly aggressive style of communication will prevent an individual from forming close personal relationships.

We all display different degrees of passive, aggressive or assertive behaviour, at different times and in different situations. Problems arise when a particular response is unhelpful for a particular situation, and we find it difficult to change to a more appropriate style of response. Improving assertiveness is about learning how to extend the range of our communication style to allow a greater flexibility of responses in different situations.

It is important to acknowledge that we are all equal and have the same basic rights (*see* Assert your rights below). Being too passive means denying one's rights by failing to express honest feelings, thoughts and beliefs, and allowing others to violate oneself. A passive person may express thoughts and feelings in such an apologetic, self-effacing manner that others can easily disregard them. Being non-assertive means allowing people to walk all over you, denying the validity of your own needs, and surrendering control over a situation to others. This leads to stressful feelings of anxiety, powerlessness, frustration and anger.

Being assertive involves standing up for your personal rights and expressing your thoughts, feelings and beliefs directly, honestly and spontaneously in ways that don't infringe the rights of others. Assertive people respect themselves and others, and take responsibility for their actions and choices. They recognize their needs and ask openly and directly for what they want. If they fail in these efforts, for whatever reason, they may feel disappointed, but their self-confidence remains intact. They are not reliant on the approval of others.

Useful verbal and non-verbal assertive skills include the ability to:
- Establish good eye contact, but do not stare.
- Stand or sit comfortably without fidgeting.
- Talk in a firm steady voice instead of rambling or shouting.
- Use gesture to emphasize points (hands, facial expressions, body posture).
- Use statements such as 'I think', 'I feel'.
- Use empathetic statements of interest such as 'What do you think', 'How do you feel?'
- Be concise and to the point. State clearly the message you want the other person to hear.

The more you stand up for yourself the higher your self-esteem. Your chances of getting what you want out of life improve greatly when you let others know what you want and you stand up for your own rights and needs. Expressing negative feelings at the appropriate time avoids the build-up of resentment. Being less self-conscious and anxious, and less driven by the need for self-protection and control, you will be able to manage stress more successfully, and to love and appreciate yourself and others more easily.

Assert your rights:

1 I have the right to express my feelings.
2 I have the right to express my opinions and beliefs.
3 I have the right to say 'yes' and 'no' for myself.
4 I have the right to change my mind.
5 I have the right to say 'I don't understand'.
6 I have the right simply to be myself, and not act for the benefit of others.
7 I have the right to decline responsibility for other people's problems.
8 I have the right to make reasonable requests of others.
9 I have the right to set my own priorities.
10 I have the right to be listened to, and taken seriously.

Any of the above can be personalized: if your boss asks you to work late at short notice, then by rights 3 and 7, your decision may be: 'I have the right to refuse this unreasonable request, I should have been given more warning

Get organized

Being chronically disorganized, either at work or in the home, is one of the most common causes of stress. Stressful environments are minimized when you impose a form of structure: this offers security against problems appearing 'out-of-the-blue'. Too inflexible a pattern would be impractical, but keeping a diary, writing lists and prioritizing duties all help to stem stressful situations. Writing down objectives, duties and activities helps to make them seem more tangible and surmountable. Don't try to overload your mind with too much information—if you are already stressed there is more chance of you forgetting vital references and data. If you keep control over what you are doing there is less chance of spiralling into professional and personal chaos.

Ventilation

There is an old saying that 'a problem shared is a problem halved'. People who keep things to themselves carry a considerable and unnecessary burden. Talking through a problem with others can be the first step to eliminating it. It is worth developing a support system—a few trusted relatives, colleagues or friends to talk to when you are upset or worried. Often it's not events themselves that are stressful but how we perceive them. Another form of communication that may be helpful is writing, for example in a private journal at home, or even letters to oneself, which should then be destroyed. The value is in expressing the feelings and getting them out. Rereading the letter just reinforces the upset and reawakens the anger.

Humour

Humour is a wonderful stress-reducer and antidote to upsets, both at home and at work; we often laugh hardest when we have been feeling most tense. Laughter relieves muscular tension, improves breathing, regulates the heart beat and pumps endorphins—the body's natural painkillers—into the bloodstream.

Diversion and distraction

Take time out (anything from a short walk to a holiday) to get away from the things that are bothering you. This will not resolve the problem, but it gives you a break and a chance for your stress levels to decrease. Then, you can return to deal with issues feeling more rested and in a better frame of mind.

Change your lifestyle through nutrition and exercise

Relaxation is virtually impossible if your body isn't maintained properly. Nutrition and exercise are the cornerstones of a healthy lifestyle, and so it is vital to achieve an equilibrium between the two.

Food is the fuel we put into our bodies in order to survive, and exercise creates the process that turns it into energy. In times past, the equation was relatively easy to achieve—the balance between energy input and output occurred naturally. We burnt up a lot of energy just keeping warm and doing a lot of physical work. Today's society, with its increased automation and sedentary jobs, makes it more difficult to maintain any equilibrium. Western society offers us abundant food and warmth with minimum physical outlay, so it has become all the more important consciously to monitor the balance of our diets.

Being overweight or underweight can create serious health problems. Obesity can cause diabetes, high blood pressure and heart problems. Being underweight is no more desirable in terms of health. An underweight body can lack the energy and strength to carry out effectively its functions, leaving the individual tired and listless. Add bad habits such as smoking or excessive alcohol consumption to either of these conditions and it often becomes very difficult for the body to cope.

Food management is important not just when it comes to checking weight, it can also improve your ability to relax and cope with stress. Food affects every organ of our bodies, including the heart, lungs and brain. The correct diet will encourage fitness and energy, nourish nerves, feed muscles, improve circulation and breathing, and support the immune system. It will promote a general feeling of positiveness and calm.

The eating process itself can create a feeling of wellbeing. What, and how, we eat says a lot about our emotional state—think of how a baby is calmed by the act of feeding, even if it is not hungry. We instinctively link eating to nurturing, comfort and security. At one extreme, anorexia nervosa and bulimia nervosa are examples of how emotional distress can affect our relationship with food. Yet all of us skip meals or overeat when we are feeling under pressure. As the digestive system shuts down during periods of stress, this is particularly dangerous and can lead to stomach problems and 'executive' ulcers.

To guard against ill-health it is vital to be aware of your body's needs. Often this means re-educating your body in terms of nutrition and taste—it can take a while for a 'junked-out' palate to become accustomed to unprocessed foods.

But information has never been more accessible. Nutritional education is now seen as a step in preventive medicine, and the general principles are easy to follow.

Every food has its own nutritional make-up and has a unique effect on the mechanics of your body. What each food does for you depends on its core attributes and composition, and it can either enhance or aggravate your sense of wellbeing.

Most experts agree that a well-balanced diet is crucial in preserving health and helping to reduce stress. Certain foods and drinks act as quite powerful stimulants to the body and so are a direct cause of stress. This stimulation may be pleasurable in the short term, but more harmful with prolonged consumption.

Caffeine

In small doses caffeine can be a good thing. Its initial effects are increased alertness and activity in the muscles, nervous system and heart. Unfortunately, people often use caffeine to fuel an already overloaded system, thinking that it will improve their performance. Too much caffeine has the same effects on the system as prolonged stress—anxiety, over-stimulation, headache, migraine, emotional instability, palpitations—and should be avoided wherever possible.

Caffeine is a drug commonly found in food and drinks such as coffee, tea, chocolate and Coca-Cola. It is a strong stimulant that actually generates a stress reaction in the body by causing a rise in the relase of adrenaline. In small doses caffeine can have a positive effect on our health. People often use caffeine to fuel an already overloaded system. Some studies have also indicated a possible link between caffeine intake and high blood pressure and high cholesterol levels.

The best way to observe the effect of caffeine is to get it out of the system long enough to see if there is a difference in how you feel. After about three weeks many people notice a benefit. You feel more relaxed, less jittery or nervous, sleep better, have more energy (a paradox, since you are removing a stimulant), less heartburn and fewer muscle aches. To avoid withdrawal symptoms it is best to decrease intake by one drink per day until they you are down to zero, then abstain for three weeks.

Fats

There are some foods that, quite simply, are not good for you. It is important to cut back or drop these foods from your diet. Most people know that fat intake should be carefully monitored. Fats generally fall into two groups: saturated and unsaturated. Saturated fats are found in dairy produce, vegetable fats, palm oil, hard margarines, sauces and biscuits, and are the most dangerous. Polyunsaturated fats are a sub-group of unsaturated fats and are present in sunflower, corn and soya oil, nuts and soft margarines. Eating too much fat can lead to obesity, heart disease, strokes and cardiac arrest. Polyunsaturated fats do not raise cholesterol levels in the same way as saturated fats, and they can also help to restore everyday wear and tear.

It is important to limit the amount of fat in our diet. Too much fat causes obesity and puts unnecessary strain on the heart. There is also evidence that high-fat diets contribute to the growing incidence of breast, colon and prostate cancers in Western society.
- saturated fats—in milk, cheese, butter, animal fats, vegetable fats, biscuits, cakes and sweets
- unsaturated fats—which include polyunsaturated fats are found in sunflower oil, corn oil, soya oil, nuts, trout, mackerel and herring.
Nutritionists advise that we should substitute polyunsaturated fats for satu-

rated fats wherever possible. This will help to avoid the tendency towards obesity and raised cholesterol levels in the blood, which can lead to cardiovascular disease and premature death.

Salt

Most of us eat much more salt than is healthy. Part of the reason our intake is so high is that salt is present in most foods as a preservative, making it difficult to avoid.

Salt should be minimized in your diet. Foods high in salt, such as refined convenience foods, bacon, ham, sausages and pickled items, should be avoided. The dangers of high salt intake are similar to our responses to stress. It can induce high blood pressure, irritate the menstrual cycle and have a stimulating and weakening effect on the adrenal glands, muscles and nervous system. Instead of salt use a salt substitute that is rich in potassium rather than in sodium.

Preservatives

Preservatives, antioxidants, colourings, raising agents, flavour enhancers and sweeteners, emulsifiers and stabilizers are all included in the 3,500 different additives frequently used by food manufacturers. Some are natural and some are completely synthetic, and most are silently injected into our diet. It is difficult to check the label on everything we buy in the supermarket, but it is well worth the effort to make ourselves aware of what we are taking home. Some of these additives have been found to have negative effects on our health and emotional wellbeing, and the only way to guard against them is through conscious awareness and nutritional education.

Sugar

Sugar is one of the most common food additives, and, unfortunately, it is also one of the most 'empty' of all foodstuffs. It induces a short-term boost of energy, but when we eat too much of it our adrenal glands are overloaded and become sluggish. This reduces our ability to relax and causes irritability and a lack of concentration. An overly high sugar intake will also strain our insulin-producing glands, perhaps inducing diabetes. More obvious problems include obesity, tooth decay and mood swings. These are particularly difficult problems for children to deal with, and parents must be aware of the dangers of placating a disruptive child with a bar of chocolate or a bag of sweets.

Sugar consumption can be reduced by eating fresh fruit for dessert instead of sugary puddings; drinking unsweetened fruit juices and sugar-free squashes and carbonated drinks; leaving out sugar in coffee and tea; looking for sugar-free labels on products in supermarkets; and avoiding junk foods.

Alcohol

The amount of alcohol we consume can also create health problems and contribute to stress levels. A limited intake can actually be very beneficial—red wine in particular contains things that are very good for us—but taken in excess, alcohol will destroy organs as well our emotional wellbeing. Dependency on alcohol is a disease in itself, which can create great distress not only for the alcoholic but for his or her family and friends as well.

Like caffeine, alcohol stimulates the secretion of adrenaline, producing the same problems of nervous tension, irritability and insomnia. Alcohol in excess will increase fat deposits in the heart and decrease immune function. Alcohol is also a toxin to the bone marrow, and has a severe impact on the liver, inhibiting that organ's ability to detoxify the body. These toxins include hormones released during stress, which will continue to circulate in the body if liver function is impaired.

Balance and nutrition

It should be clear by now that it is important to avoid too much salt, sugar and dairy products in our diet. These foods tend to promote adrenaline release, which decreases stress tolerance, and they also have a negative effect on cardiovascular health. As part of a balanced diet, the following foods will encourage fitness and energy, nourish nerves, feed muscles, improve circulation and breathing, support the immune system and promote a general feeling of positivity and calm:

- *whole grains* — wheat, rice, oats, barley, rye, corn — are a source of complex carbohydrates and essential vitamins and minerals and other nutrients that are of great value in improving stress tolerance
- *beans* — soybeans, kidney beans, broad beans, lentils, chick peas — are an excellent source of anti-stress B-vitamins
- *fresh fruit and vegetables* — are an excellent source of essential vitamins and dietary fibre.

Nutrients

If you seek a more relaxed lifestyle, you should start by caring for yourself from the inside, and feed your body with only 'good' fuel. The general maxims of a healthy diet are to increase our intake of fruit, vegetables, carbohydrates and low fat proteins, such as fresh fish or lean meat. Fibre became a buzz word of the 1980's and it is still valued — but fortunately a healthy diet should preclude the need for endless bowls of bran. Fat is essential but, as discussed, only in restricted quantities.

Of course there are many foods that aid the mental and physical balance of our bodies. When we are under a lot of pressure and feel worn down by life, the body will benefit from supplements of substances that are devoured by a system under stress. Unfortunately, vitamins and nutrients can have a short shelf-life. Food has to be very fresh, as some vitamins are easily eroded by heat, light and storage. Overcooking can destroy the nutritional value of many foods, and it is always best to eat food raw or lightly cooked whenever possible. Buying organic food is another way of ensuring that our bodies get the nutrients they need.

Although nutrients are best taken in their most natural form, modern diets do not always allow this, and we often need to supplement our intake. It is now possible to obtain vitamins and minerals that are specifically targeted to help with stress. A deficiency of vitamin C is a common problem, as stress hampers our ability to create and absorb it. Such a deficiency can also damage our absorption of iron. Supplements of vitamin B6 are recommended when under stress, pregnant or during times of anxiety and worry. A lack of B6 can lead to physical and mental exhaustion. Zinc deficiency is a common sign of stress and can induce stomach problems, a breakdown of the immune system, poor healing, low appetite and fatigue. Iodine, linked to the thyroid gland, has a direct effect on the metabolic rate of the body, so a deficiency can cause exhaustion while supplements have a stimulant effect. For more information make time to visit your local health food shop or chemist — staff there will be glad to advise.

It is important to keep your diet and dietary behaviour as balanced as possible. The demands of modern-day life sometimes make it difficult to adhere to a well-balanced diet. There will always be times when the processed, over-cooked oven meal is just too convenient, or when you really don't have time to sit down for a bite. Given this inevitability, it is all the more important to monitor what you eat and try to make up for the days when you do not have the time or inclination to prepare something more wholesome. This is the only way to let your body cope and to lessen any anxiety you may have about not eating properly.

Vitamins and minerals

Vitamins are a group of chemically unrelated, organic nutrients that are essential in small quantities for normal metabolism, growth, and physical wellbeing. These nutrients must be obtained through diet, since they are not synthesized in the body. In general, all the vitamins required by the average person can be obtained from a natural, well-balanced diet. However, stress increases cellular activity, which leads to increased nutrient usage, and under chronic stress certain vitamin deficiencies may occur.

The following vitamins and supplements are available from most chemists and health shops. For more information contact your doctor, local health shop, pharmacist or alternative health practitioner.

Vitamin C

Vitamin C deficiency is a common problem caused by stress, which hampers the body's ability to create and absorb the vitamin. Vitamin C deficiency has been linked to a range of illnesses and disorders, including scurvy, lethargy and fatigue, a weakened immune system and degenerative diseases such as arthritis and arteriosclerosis. Alcohol and cigarettes are also thought to inhibit the action of vitamin C. Foods rich in vitamin C include fresh fruit and vegetables.

Vitamin B_6

Vitamin B_6 is essential to the health of the nervous system. It is important in maintaining a healthy immune system, and there is evidence that B_6 plays a role in limiting the growth of certain tumours and skin cancers. B_6 relieves a wide variety of PMS symptoms, such as breast tenderness, weight gain (water retention) and irritability. This very important vitamin has also been shown to be helpful in reducing or eliminating symptoms of nervous tremors and epileptic seizures. A lack of B_6 can lead to physical and mental exhaustion, and has been linked to anaemia.

Supplements of vitamin B_6 are recommended when under stress, for morning sickness during pregnancy, and for anxiety. Foods rich in vitamin B_6 are fish, fresh vegetables, pulses and whole grain cereals.

Vitamin B_{12}

Vitamin B_{12} is vital for blood formation and a healthy nervous system. Living with persistent and unmanaged stress can and will eventually result in symptoms of physical deterioration and mental and emotional breakdown. B_{12} helps you to fight disease, recover more quickly from viral infections and helps to restore a sluggish appetite. Foods rich in B_{12} are red meats, fish and dairy products.

Vitamin B_5 (pantothenic acid)

Pantothenic acid is essential for the proper functioning of the adrenal glands, the health of which is so important to the management of stress. Most experts agree that pantothenic acid supplements are recommended to help to alleviate the symptoms of chronic stress.

Selenium

This trace element is essential for normal growth and development. It acts as an anti-oxidant, an anti-polluting agent and helps to strengthen the immune system. Research indicates a possible a link between heart disease and selenium deficiency. Nutritionists advise that selenium supplements are best taken together with vitamin E.

Iron

Iron deficiency leads to tiredness and exhaustion, anaemia and moods of depression. A deficiency in iron can result from vitamin C deficiency, which limits the absorption of iron in the body. Symptoms of iron deficiency include brittle nails, paleness and mouth ulcers. Foods rich in iron include pulses, grains, fish, poultry, meat, spinach, potatoes and peas.

Zinc
Zinc deficiency is a common sign of stress, and can cause stomach problems, a breakdown of the immune system, poor healing, low appetite and fatigue. Foods rich in zinc include seafood, dairy products, meat, ginger root and soya beans.

Iodine
The body's supply of iodine is dependent on a healthy thyroid gland, which determines the metabolic rate of the body—so a deficiency can cause exhaustion, whilst iodine supplements have a stimulant effect. Foods rich in iodine include seafoods, spinach and green peppers.

Calcium
Calcium is essential for healthy bones, joints, teeth, nerves, muscles and for efficient blood clotting. Foods rich in calcium include dairy products, pulses, apples and cabbage. Some foods, such as bread and milk, have added calcium and are advertised as calcium-fortified.

Super health foods
There are certain foods that are super foods—packed full of nutritional value in such beautifully balanced forms that they are easy to assimilate. Much richer in specific nutrients than ordinary or processed food, if you incorporate these super foods into your diet, you will boost your energy levels and achieve a personal equilibrium that is one of the most basic—and long-lasting—aspects of relaxation in the truest sense of the word.

Almonds
Almonds are an important source of the minerals zinc, magnesium, potassium and iron, so that a small handful of the nuts can transform a light salad into a well-balanced meal. You should eat vitamin C-rich foods at the same time, because almonds also contain oxalic and phytic acid, which can prevent your absorption of this vitamin.

Apricots
The brighter the fruit, the more beta-carotene it contains, and apricots are very high in vitamin A. Dried apricots are a wonderful source of beta-carotene during the winter months.

Avocado pears
Avocados are an almost complete food—so much so that in some parts of the world babies are weaned using mashed avocado. They are rich in potassium and vitamin A.

Barley
This grain has a very high mineral content. It has lots of calcium, potassium and B-complex vitamins, making it especially useful for anyone suffering from stress or fatigue. Add a handful of barley to home-made chicken soup ('Jewish penicillin') for a soothing and nourishing meal. It also lowers the level of cholesterol in the body.

Beetroot
For hundreds of years, beetroot has been used as a folk remedy for anaemia and liver problems. It helps the digestive system—especially when grated raw, perhaps served with grated apple and carrot and dressed with lemon juice and olive oil. It is much better eaten in this way rather than drowned in vinegar.

Broccoli
Like other members of the crucifer family—cabbage, cauliflower, Brussels

sprouts, etc—broccoli has a protective effect against disease. It is rich in vitamin C, iron, beta-carotene and folic acid. Like all green vegetables, it should be lightly cooked (steaming is ideal) to preserve most of its nutrients.

Carrots
A single carrot will supply all your vitamin A needs for a whole day. Nibbling carrot sticks is a much healthier pastime than grazing on salted peanuts and crisps. Research has shown that carrots have a protective effect against ultra-violet rays, so they can help you to look younger for longer as well.

Celery
According to Hippocrates, celery calms the nerves—perhaps because of its high calcium content. It helps eliminate waste via the urine, due to the effect it has on the kidneys.

Cider vinegar
Made by fermenting the juice of whole, fresh apples, cider vinegar's beneficial effects come from the high mineral content of apples. It is unusually high in potassium, calcium, phosphorus, sodium and trace elements. It increases blood oxygenation, improves metabolism, strengthens digestion and increases blood clotting ability. Two teaspoonfuls of cider vinegar in a glass of water on an empty stomach first thing in the morning is helpful to people with weight problems.

Garlic
Like sprouts, garlic has been used as a cure-all for millennia. Inscriptions on the Great Pyramid at Gizeh in Egypt mention garlic as one of the foods eaten by its builders.

Some naturopaths believe that common infectious diseases, like flu and bronchitis, are caused by an accumulation of toxins in the body that gradually undermines the functions of internal organs. Garlic has been shown to be an excellent antiseptic. It was used with amazing success in treating soldiers with infected wounds during both World Wars. In the Second World War, the wounds of British soldiers were treated with garlic. Some of the wounds were already gangrenous, but garlic checked the spread of the gangrene and resulted in the shedding of gangrenous tissue. As recently as 1965 the Russians flew 500 tons of garlic to Moscow to fight a flu epidemic, and some people still call garlic 'Russian penicillin'.

Garlic also helps clear fat accumulations from the blood vessels, lower cholesterol, and protect against bacterial and viral infections.

Grapes
Grapes are very cleansing and regenerating. Grape fasts—eating nothing but grapes and drinking water for a day or two—are a well-known method of detoxifying the body. They are an ideal food, not only for convalescents, but for anyone suffering from fatigue or depression,

Kelp
Kelp—or seaweed—is a wonderful source of iodine, which helps protect the body against the radioactivity in the atmosphere that contributes to early ageing. It is rich in B-complex vitamins, vitamins D, E and K, magnesium and calcium. It is particularly good for hair and nails.

Kelp tablets are not concentrated; they are simply dehydrated seaweed, so six or eight of them should be taken after each meal for good results.

Lecithin
Lecithin is important in maintaining a healthy nervous system and is vital in helping the body resist stress. Daily lecithin consumption means that body fats are converted into energy more quickly, and existing fat deposits will slowly

disperse. It breaks up cholesterol so that it can pass through artery walls, and has been shown to increase immunity to virus infections and help prevent gall-stones. It also helps to cleanse the liver and purify the kidneys and, because of its choline and unsaturated fatty acid content, it is very good indeed for the condition of the skin.

Lecithin can be bought in granule form from health food shops.

Mixed three seeds

Pumpkin, sunflower and sesame seeds, ground in a blender or coffee grinder in equal proportions, make a wonderful complete protein to sprinkle on salads or fruits. They are extremely rich in vitamins, and are excellent for hair and skin as well as general health. Pumpkin seeds are rich in B vitamins, phosphorus, iron and zinc. Sesame seeds are rich in magnesium and potassium and have been used for generations to treat fatigue, insomnia and sexual dysfunctions. They also contain more calcium than milk, cheese or nuts and are a good source of vitamin E. Sunflower seeds are rich in iron, the B-complex vitamins, magnesium and zinc.

Molasses

A tablespoonful of black-strap molasses supplies as much calcium as a glass of milk, as much iron as nine eggs, more potassium than any other food, and the B-complex vitamins in good balance. It is also rich in magnesium, vitamin E and copper, and is a very valuable food for women who tend to be anaemic. It is an alkali-forming food, beneficial for maintaining a proper acid-alkaline balance in the body. A tablespoon of molasses and the juice of half a lemon in a mug of hot water is a good way to start the day. It is also very good for the condition of your skin and hair.

Warning: Diabetics must not use molasses.

Oats

Oats are a uniquely soothing food for the nerves. They are amazingly high in calcium, potassium and magnesium, together with lots of B-complex vitamins, which are all vital to a healthy nervous system. They also help lower cholesterol levels. A bowl of porridge, perhaps with a spoonful of honey or molasses, makes a uniquely calming breakfast for a child on the morning of an exam.

Potatoes

Potatoes have a well-known soporific effect: they contain a substance very like chloroform. Research suggests that certain foods cause contentment and lifting of depression by altering brain chemistry in a similar way to drug therapy. To prevent downward mood swings, a chemical called serotonin must be present in the brain in proper amounts. The body makes serotonin from the amino acid tryptophan. Under ordinary circumstances, tryptophan has to compete with other amino acids to get into the brain. But when more carbohydrate than protein is eaten, tryptophan has much less trouble getting in. A potato is not only an ideal carbohydrate: a medium potato contains only about 90 fat-free calories, as well as vitamins A, C, B_1, B_6, niacin, iron, potassium and fibre. What could be more comforting or soothing than a creamy mass of freshly whipped up potato with a swirl of olive oil or a knob of fresh, cold butter melting on top?

Rabbit

Much lower in fat than beef or lamb, rabbit—especially wild rabbit, if you can get it—makes delicious slow-cooked dishes to warm and soothe on a cold winter's evening. Rabbit with prunes and Guinness is bursting with nutrients. Serve with barley instead of rice or potatoes for the ultimate nourishing and relaxing treat.

Sprouted grains

Sprouted grains and seeds have been used in diets for thousands of years, especially by the Chinese. They are amazing powerhouses of live food nourishment. They are rich in vitamins A, C, D, E, K and B complex, in calcium, phosphorus, potassium, magnesium, iron, high quality protein and enzymes. Sprouts are rich in vitality factors because, unlike most vegetables, they are eaten at the peak of their freshness — when they are still growing.

Sprouts contain an amazing quantity of enzymes. As we age, our bodies become less efficient at producing enzymes from food, which often leads to indigestion or flatulence. Sprouts, by giving us lots of enzymes, produce more efficient digestion and improved metabolism of food into energy. As well as being highly nutritious, sprouts are extremely low in calories.

How to grow sprouts:

Seeds to sprout include alfalfa (considered to be the richest in minerals), wheat, mung beans, buckwheat, lentils, sesame seeds, soya beans and chickpeas.

Put a heaped tablespoonful of seeds or grains into a jar, cover it with lukewarm water and leave it overnight. In the morning, covering the jar with a piece of muslin or cheesecloth held in place with a rubber band, pour off the water and rinse the seeds in fresh lukewarm water (not hot — or you will kill them). Pour off the excess water through the cloth and put the jar on the windowsill. In the evening, rinse again and pour off excess. Repeat the rinsing twice a day, and, in three to six days — depending on the kind of seeds used — you will have sprouts to sprinkle on your salads or steam lightly and enjoy with a sprinkling of olive oil and lemon juice. Patent plastic sprouters are now available that make sprouting even easier.

Spirulina

Spirulina is a blue-green, single-celled alga, microscopic in size and spiral in shape — hence its name. It thrives in warm alkaline lakes such as Lake Texcoco in Mexico. It was so highly valued by the Aztecs that it was used as currency.

The B_{12}, folic acid and chlorophyll content of spirulina makes it useful in the treatment of anaemia and liver disorders.

Spirulina is helpful in weight control. Its protein contains a high proportion of the amino acid phenylalanine, which is transformed into brain neurotransmitter substances that control appetite, energy level and mood. The appetite is curbed and a state of wellbeing is maintained. The usual dose is three tablets taken half an hour before each meal.

Wheat germ

Wheat germ is the richest known source of vitamin E. It is also rich in magnesium, copper, manganese, calcium and phosphorus. Sprinkled on yoghurt or cereal, it a superb source of protein. But it is rich in fat — a tablespoonful a day is enough.

Hypoglycaemia

If you are suffering from hypoglycaemia — often called 'the great imitator' because it mimics so many mental and emotional disorders — you will find it almost impossible to relax completely. A large proportion of patients receiving psychotherapy — more than half, it is thought — are in fact hypoglycaemic. Symptoms include: irritability, exhaustion, nervousness, depression, faintness and dizziness, cold sweats, headaches, confusion, heart palpitations, lack of sex drive, lack of concentration, blurred vision, phobias and allergies.

Hypoglycaemia, or low sugar levels in the blood, was discovered in 1924 by Dr Seale Harris. At that time it was called hyperinsulinism because it was thought to be caused by excessive insulin secretion due to an overactive pancreas. The excess insulin causes rapid uptake of glucose by the cells and tissues of the body, leaving the blood depleted of glucose. When glucose is in short supply, cell function is impaired, leading to physical and mental problems.

Low blood sugar may impair mental health even more than physical health because it deprives the brain and nervous system of oxygen.

During digestion, all ingested carbohydrates (sugars and starches) are converted to glucose, which is the only carbohydrate the body can use. After a meal, particularly one with a high sugar content, surges of glucose enter the blood, causing the pancreas to secrete insulin. Insulin causes rapid uptake of glucose by almost all of the tissues of the body and also promotes the conversion of excess glucose to glycogen, a more compact form of glucose that can be stored in the liver for future use. The pancreas, however, is only part of the mechanism that controls blood sugar. The whole process originates in glucoreceptor (glucose-sensitive) nerve cells in the brain from which impulses travel to the pituitary gland, adrenal glands, liver and finally the pancreas. In this sophisticated sugar-control chain, there are also hormones that convert glycogen back to glucose to raise the blood glucose level. The hormones that do this are glucagon, also secreted by the pancreas, and adrenaline, secreted by the adrenal glands. In this way, opposing forces are constantly at work, balancing each other, so that blood sugar levels are kept within fairly narrow limits. But they do not always succeed and, if the blood sugar level gets too low, hypoglycaemia occurs.

Some people inherit or develop an overactive pancreas, which secretes excessive amounts of insulin even when only small amounts of sugar enter the blood. Sometimes, the pancreas may react slowly and insulin does not enter the blood until the sugar level has already fallen—this is retarded hypoglycaemia. On the other hand, secretion of glucagon and adrenaline, the hormones that balance the action of insulin, may be too low. Hypoglycaemia can also be caused by allergies or an imbalance in the autonomic nervous system. Other causes are excessive consumption of alcohol, tobacco, coffee, overeating and emotional stress. Whatever the reason, hypoglycaemia develops when the delicate balance of the systems and substances that control blood sugar is upset.

Theoretically, sugar would appear to be the ideal food to raise blood sugar levels. But sugar is the one food that hypoglycaemics should avoid. In fact, sugar will eventually contribute to lower blood sugar levels.

When we eat sugar, it is readily absorbed into the blood, where it raises blood sugar levels, triggering the pancreas to secrete insulin, which will cause glucose to be absorbed into the tissues. Insulin, because it breaks down much more slowly than sugar, remains circulating in the blood for several hours, lowering blood sugar level even lower than the original level. It triggers the hypoglycaemic symptoms again, creating a craving for more sugar. So the hypoglycaemic eats more sugar, which deepens the vicious circle. The high consumption of refined sugar is thought to be the main cause for the higher rates of hypoglycaemia.

When we start consuming huge amounts of white sugar, our pancreas becomes highly stressed. The occasional binge can be dealt with, but when large intakes of refined carbohydrates are the norm, the strain on the sugar-regulating mechanism becomes intolerable and it breaks down. The pancreas may develop an over-sensitivity to sugar and produce more insulin than is really needed to keep a normal sugar level. This results in a consistently low blood sugar level, which deprives the brain and the nervous system of vital oxygen and produces all the symptoms of hypoglycaemia.

Coffee (especially when taken with sugar) and soft drinks that are high in caffeine contribute to hypoglycaemia by acting on the adrenal glands, brain and liver while sugar is flooding the blood stream. Too much salt in the diet depletes potassium and stress and allergies overtax the adrenal glands. Vitamin deficiencies—particularly zinc, chromium, B vitamins, magnesium, potassium and vitamin E—also contribute to hypoglycaemia. So it is easy to see that the condition, which has such a devastating effect on so many people's equilibrium, is mainly a nutritional disorder.

The influence of sugar in the body goes far beyond carbohydrate metabolism. Fatty acid synthesis and oxidation, cholesterol synthesis and the accumulation of ketone bodies, are all in part controlled by the rate at which glucose is broken down within cells.

Refined sugar causes more build-up of fat than any other carbohydrate except alcohol. This, in turn, means a greater susceptibility to heart attacks and high blood pressure.

Changes in Western eating habits over the last couple of generations have been in the direction of fewer complex carbohydrates (cereals, potatoes etc) and more simple sugars.

Life stresses are also an important factor. Under conditions of stress, more adrenaline is secreted, releasing more sugar from the liver. Repeated stress can impair the function of the adrenal glands, reducing the body's ability to cope with stress. When this happens we get depressed easily, and also develop hypoglycaemic symptoms. Persistent stress is a major cause of depression.

Like diabetes, hypoglycaemia is diagnosed by means of a glucose tolerance test, which can be arranged through your doctor.

A healthy diet, which means only rarely consuming simple sugars or junk food, can keep hypoglycaemia at bay. Plenty of complex carbohydrates and vegetables, together with a good multivitamin and multimineral supplement will go a long way towards this.

There are some simple rules that will improve your diet. These are not to be followed slavishly of course, the occasional sweet treat will do little harm if the mainstay of your diet is good, fresh food.

1 Eat good quality food
If we are what we eat, we do not want to put substandard materials into our bodies. Stick to good, natural foods that have nourished people for generations: fresh vegetables and fruit; fresh fish; poultry, game, beef and lamb—reared organically, if possible; wholegrains; nuts; seeds; pulses, free-range eggs; cold-pressed oils; cheeses, butter and milk.

2 Eat regularly
It is better to eat four or five small meals spread throughout the day, rather than starving all day and bingeing on a large dinner at night. This is also very important for keeping your blood sugar level constant.

3 Eat fresh foods in season
It is sensible to eat a really fresh, locally grown carrot, rather than some green beans that have been flown from Kenya and will have lost some nutrients in transit. It is also cheaper. Local produce is also more likely to have been harvested at its peak. Exotic fruits and vegetables are often chemically treated to ripen them artificially in transit.

4 Avoid over-processed and refined foods
Use wholemeal rather than white flour and eat brown rice rather than white. Try not to eat mass-produced cakes and pastries and sugary cereals. It is easy to munch your way through a packet of high-fat, high-salt crisps merely out of habit, without enjoying them. If you change your diet for a healthier one, after a while the artificial cream gateau will lose its appeal.

5 Eat in moderation
Exercise a little self control. It is not necessary to weigh every wedge of cheese

or count out the strands of spaghetti. Listen to your body. A glass of wine occasionally is fine—but not if you go on to down the entire bottle.

6 Eat slowly and calmly

Take time to sit down and enjoy your meal. Grabbing some food and bolting it, when short of time, will play havoc with your digestion.

7 Don't mix foods that fight

All foods belong in one of three groups: protein, starch and neutral. Many people believe that a particularly harmonious way of eating is one in which protein and starch foods are not eaten at the same meal. People who follow this regime (sometimes called the Hay system after Dr Hay who developed it) eat neutral foods with any of the protein foods or any of the starch foods. They aim to eat one starch meal, one protein meal and one made up mainly of fruit, vegetables and salads every day. Four hours should be allowed between starch and protein meals.

If you would like to try this eating plan, the chart below shows which foods can be combined.

The Three Food Groups

Protein	Neutral	Starch
meat	all vegetables except potatoes, yams and sweetcorn	potatoes
poultry		yams
game	all nuts except peanuts	sweetcorn
fish	butter	bread
shellfish	cream	flour
eggs	cream cheese	oats
all fruit except those in the starch group	yoghurt and milk (these are protein foods, but their protein content is low and they can be used in very small amounts only with starch foods)	wheat
all dried fruit except raisins, which are neutral		barley
		rice
		millet
tomatoes (but when cooked their acidity is increased, making them unsuitable for eating with starch foods)		rye
		buckwheat
	cold-pressed sesame sunflower and olive oils	very sweet fruits such as ripe pears, bananas, papaya, mango and sweet grapes
peanuts	all salad stuffs	beer
soya beans	lentils	
tofu	dried split peas	
milk	dried or tinned beans, chickpeas etc	
yoghurt	seeds and sprouted seeds	
all cheeses except cream cheese	herbs and spices	
wine	raisins	
cider	honey	
	maple syrup	

It is a good idea to begin meals with a salad; this will encourage your digestion to work efficiently, as well as curbing your appetite. Base your meals as much as possible around fresh fruit and vegetables. At first it may seem strange giving up classic combinations like fish and chips or shepherd's pie. But it is possible to eat very enjoyably—from a delicious mushroom and barley casserole, to a corn-fed chicken, cooked with olive oil and tarragon, and served with a wide range of appetizing vegetables and a glass of good wine.

Following this regime, many people are pleasantly surprised to find that they lose weight without really trying.

Exercise

But getting the diet right is only part of the picture. It is impossible to overestimate the significance of exercise in a healthy and relaxed lifestyle. If a body is never pushed beyond its regular pace, relaxation periods will invariably have less benefit. Exercise doesn't just promote an increase in physical fitness; people who exercise regularly can enjoy a range of secondary benefits.

Regular exercise improves sleep, reduces headaches, improves concentration and increases stamina. Endorphins are released into the brain during exercise and these chemicals promote a sense of positiveness and happiness that will last for some time after the actual activity. This is an effective tool in the fight against depression and a vital move in the preparation for a relaxed life.

People are often accused of putting too much time into their careers or families, and strenuous physical activity is a great antidote to that. In today's society there is a general emphasis on sedentary lifestyles, and it is trend that shows little sign of slowing down. This makes it difficult to find an appropriate outlet for mental negativity and accumulated physical frustration. Physical exertion is great for releasing the toxic emotions that threaten a relaxed sense of wellbeing. You can thrash out tension, anger, frustration and aggression, exercising your mental muscles along with your physical ones.

Exercise, like relaxation, is a personal thing. Just as you will prefer one relaxation method over another, you probably won't like all forms of activity. Your preferences will be affected by your individual personality, physical capabilities and the time you have available. Realistically tailoring your activity to your lifestyle is the best way to ensure that the exercise is kept up.

Skilled sports such as skiing or golf are obviously more appealing if you have the time to invest in learning the game and developing your ability to a certain level. Highly competitive sports such as squash should be viewed with caution if you already have an exceptionally stressful lifestyle. Most experts would advise some form of noncompetitive exercise, like swimming, weight-training or walking, for those with limited time and resources. Even as little as twenty minutes a day put aside for such activities will be of great benefit.

Aerobic exercises

Aerobic activities include swimming, long-distance running, cycling, rowing, cross-country skiing and even walking—if it is brisk enough. These differ from the other sorts of exercise because they demand your body's efficient use of oxygen throughout the whole time you are doing them.

Oxygen is the ignition factor in the burning of energy from the foods you eat. A good supply is always necessary for your body's metabolic processes to take place efficiently. When your cells—particularly your brain cells—have a good supply, you have stamina, feel well and don't tire easily. If you often feel tired, become depressed easily and have trouble concentrating, it is likely that your body is not getting enough exercise. Taking aerobic exercise will change all that. Any movement of sustained rhythm that puts a constant demand on your heart—raising your pulse rate to between 120 and 160 beats a minute—will bring about several important changes in your body.

It will tone your muscles and improve your circulation. It will increase the number and the size of the blood vessels that carry blood from your heart all over your body so you will have better transport of oxygen. It will increase your body's capacity to take in oxygen by strengthening the chest wall and making you breathe more easily. This oxygen will generate energy. It will make your bones, joints and ligaments stronger so they are more resistant to injury. It will increase the level of energy-rich compounds and enzymes in your body, making it easier for you to use the nutrients in your food. As the efficiency of your heart increases, pumping more blood with each beat, your basic pulse rate will decline.

Walking

Walking is often overlooked as an aerobic activity. A brisk, purposeful walk will improve your muscle condition, your circulation and your posture.

All you need is a good pair of strong shoes and a lightweight, waterproof jacket. Start off by walking for thirty minutes a day. Walk fast enough to make yourself a little out of breath and vary your route so you are not walking on flat ground all the time.

After a week or two, you can increase the time you walk to about forty-five minutes. By now you should be seeing the benefits: you will probably be sleeping better, your concentration will be sharper and you will feel better balanced emotionally.

Walking is an ideal aerobic exercise because you can do it wherever you are—in the country or the city. You need no equipment to measure your progress—you do not need to stop and take your pulse. Get into the habit of walking briskly every day and you will be rewarded with a fit body, glowing skin and a new sense of wellbeing.

Running

Running is the most satisfying form of aerobic exercise for many people. No special training is needed and it can be done anywhere—at home or on holiday. All you need is a good pair of running shoes and the self-discipline to get started. You may be surprised to find that before long you too are hooked and can't imagine life without this liberating activity.

Before you start on a programme of running, it is important to check your fitness. If you are over thirty-five, suffer from high blood pressure, have a family history of heart disease or have recently been ill, it is a good idea to have a check-up with your doctor to make sure that running is safe for you.

There is a simple way to check your own fitness level. Simply walk two miles in thirty minutes at a brisk pace and ask yourself how you feel afterwards. If you feel no nausea or dizziness you are fit enough to start a graded programme of running. If, however, you find the two-mile walk difficult, persevere until you can do it comfortably in half an hour. You may be surprised how quickly this happens—walking for half an hour each day can have a marked effect on your condition. Here is a programme that you can follow:

First week:
Take a brisk walk of one mile, breaking into a jog of roughly 50–100 metres whenever you feel like it. In between these jogs, walk at a steady pace but do not force yourself. Pushing yourself too hard in the beginning is counter-productive and you could end up with strains or injuries that set you back. You should feel relaxed enough that you are able to appreciate your surroundings.

Second week:
Walk/jog for a mile, alternating about 100 strides of each at a stretch.

Third week:
Walk/jog for one and a half miles, increasing your jogging intervals to 150 strides with 100 strides of walking in between.

Fourth week:
Jog for a while at the speed that you find most comfortable. Don't worry if you have to stop from time to time to walk, although by now you should be finding that minor discomforts are fleeting and that you can run through them.

Fifth week:
Run a mile in less than nine minutes.

Sixth week:
Jog/run for one and a half miles or more. By now you should have passed through the initial barrier and be beginning to reap all the rewards of your perseverance. You will be more aware of your body and able to listen to what it is telling you. Your stamina will be increased and you can vary your running by pushing yourself more on the days when you feel in top condition and ready for a challenge.

By the end of six months, you should be able to run easily and steadily for between half an hour and an hour, covering a distance between three and nine miles. This programme leads on to a flexible regime of running. Enjoy running and don't get fixated with rigid training schedules. To reap the true benefits of running, aim to run for thirty minutes at least three times a week. This is more effective at building fitness than one running session of one and a half hours. If you want to run every day, it is a good idea to take one day off each week to give your muscles a chance to restore themselves and build up their store of glucose again. This day of rest will only improve the quality of your running.

Running has knock-on effects for health and relaxation. The more you run, the more you will feel in touch with your body. You will find yourself naturally drawn towards healthier foods, your skin will be clearer, and health problems like constipation and insomnia will disappear. As you look better and feel better, you may feel that running is addictive in the best sense of the word.

What to wear
Clothes made from fabrics that breathe, like cotton, are much better than those made from man-made fibres. In summer a pair of shorts and a T-shirt are ideal: running in bare legs increases the sense of freedom. In winter a cotton tracksuit with a fleecy lining is fine, perhaps with a lightweight waterproof jacket when it's raining. If it is very cold outside a wool cap will protect your ears.

Proper running shoes are not cheap, but they are an excellent investment. They should be not too flexible, without studs and with a high-density sole. Some excellent soles are made of microcellular rubber. Some soles on running shoes extend up the toe and heel to take account of the rocking movement from heel to toe that comes with running. The padded instep helps to absorb shock from running on hard ground. These special design features make you far less likely to risk the sort of injury to tendons or muscles that can come if you run in an old pair of tennis shoes. There should be plenty of room inside for your toes to move about and the heel should be slightly raised to help prevent injury to your Achilles tendon that comes with overstretching. It should have at least five set of holes for laces, so the shoe hugs your foot: in fact, the shoes should feel, when you are out and running, as if they are part of your feet. Plastic shoes are not a good idea because they make your feet sweat: light leather or nylon is a much better bet.

Cotton socks help absorb shock and, because you can change them every time you run, they keep your shoes fresh.

Warm up
It is not a good idea to jump straight out of bed and go running. You need to warm up your muscles and get your metabolic rate up first. If you run when your muscles are stiff or cold after a long period of inactivity, you are much more likely to pull a muscle or injure a joint. Simply moving about the house briskly for ten minutes will ease your body into action but, if you have time, it is a good idea to do some warm-up exercises. These will also limber the back of your legs, tighten your tummy muscles and strengthen your ankles—cover-

ing the muscle areas that running leaves out. Here are six stretching and firm-
ing exercises that many regular runners rely on:

1 For your calf muscles and Achilles tendons: stand a little under a metre from
a tree or wall. With your feet flat on the ground, lean into it until the backs of
your legs hurt a little. Hold the position for ten seconds and then relax. Repeat six times.

2 For tight hamstrings at the back of your legs: keeping your legs straight, put
one heel up on a table at waist level (lower, if you cannot reach that high).
Now lower your head down to your knee until you feel the strain. Hold the
position for ten seconds, holding on to your leg or foot to steady yourself if
you need to. Repeat (with each leg) six times.

3 For lower back and hamstrings: lie on your back, arms at your sides. Keeping
your legs straight, bring them up over your head. Now lower them as far as
possible above your head—touching the floor if you can. Hold for ten seconds and relax. Repeat six times.

4 For your shin muscles: sit on the edge of a table and hold a weight of about
two kilograms on the front part of your foot just behind the toes (a small
bucket or old paint tin filled with stones is ideal). Keep them there for a few
seconds and then lower. Repeat a few times with each foot.

5 For your quadriceps: sit on the table and hang the weight over the toes of one
foot so the bucket or tin is resting on the floor and you are not stretching the
knee ligaments. Now straighten your knee, raising the weight. Hold for a few
seconds and then lower. Repeat six times with each leg.

6 For tummy muscles: do twenty sit-ups with your knees bent and your feet
tucked under a heavy piece of furniture if this helps you keep your balance.
Clasp your hands behind your head and keep your chin in, curling your body
up from the floor.

If you don't have time to go through this routine before you run, start running
very slowly and keep to a slow, steady jog for the first five minutes or so until
your muscles start to warm up. This is very important if you want to protect
yourself from injury.

Never run after a meal, a hot bath, or when you are feeling really cold.

Cool down

It is just as important to cool off properly after a run, and your muscles should
cool off gradually. A good way of achieving this is by walking for five or ten
minutes after every run. This keeps extra blood flowing through the muscles
and helps your body to eliminate the waste products of exercise such as lactic
acid, which can otherwise make you stiff or sore.

If you like, do some stretching exercises, such as bending over from the hips.
You should find that any muscular aches and pains vanish quickly as your body
responds to your new regime and works itself into condition.

Problems

Don't worry if you get a stitch while you are running. Stop and walk or jog
slowly through it until it passes. As you become fitter, stitches will become
fewer. If you find areas of skin becoming irritated where they rub together—
between the thighs, for example—apply a little petroleum jelly to the spot.

If you experience a sharp pain in a muscle, you should stop running. You may
have torn some fibres and the muscle may harden and swell, which is a sign
that it is bleeding inside. Place a cold compress—like a bag of frozen peas—on
the area and, if the pain doesn't go away in a couple of days, it is a good idea to
see your doctor. Of course, if you experience a sharp pain in your chest, you
must stop running at once and seek medical advice.

Progress

When you first start running you will find yourself breathing deeper and faster as your body seeks more oxygen to meet the new demands being made on it. You may feel some stiffness in your chest as your muscles expand to help you to breathe more fully. After some minutes of running, you will probably experience the 'oxygen debt', when your body demands more oxygen than it is able to process efficiently at that moment. It is quite common at this point to feel that you want to stop. Walk slowly for a while, breathing deeply.

You may also find that your joints feel stiff, with your legs as heavy as lead. They are merely letting you know that they are being used in a way that is unusual for them. This is perfectly normal and will pass.

You will find, however, that when you are able to run for between six and ten minutes without having to stop and walk, you will come into your second wind. Suddenly your running is easier and you find yourself breathing more freely, coursing forward in a fresh and unrestricted way. If you are new to running, it will take time to reach this phase but, as you persevere, eventually it will come every time you run.

After several weeks running, when you can run for half an hour or so without stopping, you may experience your 'third wind'. You run until your legs are beginning to feel heavy and you are breathing hard. You are just thinking that you should stop, when your running suddenly changes gear, becoming almost automatic. Your body feels lighter and you feel as if you could run on and on. This kind of euphoria is known as 'runner's high' and is one of the reasons that running is such a good tool for anyone seeking relaxation in the deepest sense of the word. Perceptions are heightened and, as your mind clears, problems are seen in their proper perspective. It doesn't happen during every run, but it is an experience well worth working towards.

If you make running part of your routine, you will find that you gain energy in every area of your life—mental and physical.

It is important not to push yourself too hard in the beginning, especially if you are not used to regular exercise. It is always a good idea to seek advice on which form of sport to take up and to consult your doctor before you begin. Ease yourself into an exercise programme, as doing too much too soon could lead to physical exhaustion or injury. Also remember that the body benefits more from short periods of regular exercise than from infrequent bursts.

It is impossible to overestimate the importance of exercise in managing stress. The stress reaction encourages a state of high energy but there is usually no place for that energy to go; therefore, our bodies can stay in a state of arousal for hours at a time. Exercise is the most logical way to dissipate this excess energy. It is what our bodies are trying to do when we pace around or tap our legs and fingers. It is much better to channel it into a more complete form of exercise like a brisk walk, a run, a bike ride or a game of squash. During times of high stress, we could benefit from an immediate physical outlet—but this often is not possible. However, regular exercise can drain off ongoing stress and keep things under control: it improves sleep, reduces headaches, creates a feeling of wellbeing, helps concentration and increases stamina. Chemicals called endorphins are released into the brain during exercise. Morphine-like in their effect, these substances promote a sense of positivity and happiness, which will last for some time after exercising.

At the very least, it is important to exercise three times per week for a minimum of 30 minutes each time. Aerobic activities like walking, jogging, swimming, cycling, squash, skiing, aerobics classes and dancing are suitable. Choose things you like to do or they will feel like a chore and you will begin to avoid them. It is important not to push yourself too hard in the beginning, and to seek medical advice on which form of sport to take up. The body benefits more from short periods of regular exercise rather than infrequent bursts. Ease yourself into an exercise programme, as doing too much too soon could lead to physical exhaustion or injury.

Sleep

As mundane as it sounds, sleep is an important way of reducing stress. Fatigue is a common component of chronic stress (in some cases resulting from stress-induced insomnia), and when tired it is more difficult to cope with stressful situations. These dynamics can create a vicious cycle. When distressed individuals get more sleep, they feel better and are more resilient and adaptable in dealing with day-to-day events.

Most people know what their usual sleep requirement is (the range is five to ten hours per night; the average being seven to eight), but a surprisingly large percentage of the population is chronically sleep-deprived. If you do feel constantly tired, go to bed 30 to 60 minutes earlier and monitor the results after a few days or a week. If you are still tired, go to bed 30 minutes earlier than this. Eventually, there will be a pattern which does help to reduce stress. The three criteria of success are:
• waking refreshed
• plenty of daytime energy
• waking naturally before the alarm goes off

Sleeping-in is fine, but if you sleep too long, it throws off your body rhythms during the following day. It is better to go to bed earlier.

Daytime naps are an interesting phenomenon. They can be valuable if they are short and timed properly (i.e. not in the evening). The catnap is a short sleep (five to 20 minutes) that can be rejuvenating. A nap lasting more than 30 minutes can make you feel groggy. If you suffer with insomnia daytime naps are not a good idea. Beyond these cautionary notes, getting more sleep can be important in reducing stress and helping you to cope and function better.

Leisure

No one would expect a tennis player to complete an entire match without taking breaks. Surprisingly though, many otherwise rational people think nothing of working from dawn to dusk without taking a break and then wonder why they become distressed.

Stop smoking

Many people use cigarettes as a coping mechanism in times of stress, and it seems that smoking can help to reduce stress in the short term. The long-term hazards of smoking, however, far outweigh its palliative properties. Smoking is one of the major causes of illness and death worldwide. Cigarettes unquestionably cause a variety of cancers, especially of the lung and bladder, and also contribute to the development of hypertension, respiratory illness and heart disease.

Pacing

It is important to learn to monitor stress and energy levels, and then pace ourselves accordingly. Pacing is about awareness and vigilance—knowing when to extend ourselves and when to ease up. It is also about acting on the information supplied by our bodies. The graph below illustrates the relationship between stress and performance, and leads to the following important conclusions:
• Increased stress produces increased performance, initially.
• Once you pass a certain point (the hump), any more stress results in decreased

performance. Trying harder at this point is unproductive or even counterproductive. The only sensible option is to take a break.

- We need a certain amount of stress to function well. However, stress becomes harmful when there is too much, when it lasts too long, or when it occurs too often.
- One of the first symptoms of distress is fatigue, which we tend to ignore. It is a good idea to take steps to reduce stress levels at this point, before fatigue becomes exhaustion.

The other key to pacing is taking periodic rest. Too many people go far too long without breaks. Just as we all have cycles of deep sleep and dream sleep throughout the night (at roughly 90- to 120-minute intervals), we also have cycles through the day (peaks of energy and concentration interspersed with troughs of low energy and inefficiency). These cycles are called ultradian rhythms because they happen many times per day (as opposed to the 25-hour circadian rhythm). We need to watch for these troughs and take 20-minute breaks when they occur, as opposed to working through them and building up stress.

It is not always convenient for us to take breaks when nature tells us to, but we can all become better at this. A mid-morning break, lunch, a mid-afternoon break and supper divide the day into roughly two hour segments. These time-outs can include catnaps, meditation, daydreaming, a social interlude, a short walk, a refreshment break, a change to low-concentration tasks, or listening to music. Like the catnap, it is simply a good investment of time that pays itself back quickly in increased productivity and reduced stress.

Work/leisure balance

Optimizing the balance between work and leisure is an important means to eliminating unwanted stress in our lives. Despite all our labour-saving devices, leisure is still an elusive commodity for most people. Statistics show that we are working an extra three hours per week compared with 20 years ago. That translates into an extra month of work each year. Add to that the phenomenon of the two career family (which makes family and leisure time even more scarce) and you start to get a picture of society on an accelerating treadmill.

Leisure time and levels of distress are inversely proportional—the less leisure, the more stress. It may be useful to divide your life (excluding sleep time) into four compartments (work, family, community and self) and then to assess what percentage of your time and energy in an average week goes into each part. There is no normal range, but when work is over 60 per cent and/or when self is less than 10 per cent this indicates there may be a problem with stress. We all require time to meet our own needs (self-care, self-nurturing, etc) and when that is neglected, trouble usually follows. Self-directed activities can include exercise or recreation, relaxation, socializing, entertainment and hobbies.

The word leisure is derived from the Latin word *licere,* which means 'permission'. The main reason so many people do not have enough leisure is that they are not giving themselves permission to make the time to enjoy it. Leisure is one of the most pleasant stress relievers ever invented, and it is strange that people resist it so much.

Conventional treatment for stress

It may not always be possible to alleviate all the causes and symptoms of stress without professional help. In addition to the family doctor, there is a great variety of various alternative therapies and medicines available, many of which provide excellent stress relief.

Tranquillizers

There are a variety of tranquillizing drugs that act to suppress the central nervous system, thereby reducing anxiety and other stress-related symptoms. Benzodiazepines, such as Valium, Librium or Ativan, are the most commonly prescribed minor tranquillizers. Because these products have few side effects and are relatively safe in overdose, they have come to replace barbiturates as prescribed sedatives and sleeping pills.

Benzodiazepines depress mental activity and alertness, but do not generally make you drowsy or clumsy as do barbiturates, but they do affect driving and similar skills. Alone, benzodiazepines cannot produce the 'high' that alcohol or barbiturates produce, and after up to two weeks' continuous use, they may become ineffective as sleeping pills, and after four months may become ineffective against anxiety. Long-term dependence is more likely to be psychological; the pills become a means of coping with stressful events, and there may be severe anxiety if the drug is unavailable. Withdrawal symptoms appear in many users if they suddenly stop taking such drugs after about eight years' treatment with normal doses. Symptoms include insomnia, anxiety, tremor, irritability, nausea and vomiting. Such symptoms are more noticeable with shorter-acting benzodiazepines such as lorazepam and temazepam.

In the 1950s and 1960s doctors would prescribe minor tranquillizers almost indiscriminately and for indefinite periods. Nowadays the medical profession is more aware that the short-term benefits of these drugs can be outweighed by long-term problems of dependency and withdrawal. In Britain in 1988, the Committee on Safety of Medicines recommended that minor tranquillizers should be prescribed for a period of no longer than two to four weeks.

Counselling and psychotherapy

There are various support organizations and counselling services available to help with stress management. These range from expensive specialist stress-management experts to free stress clinics run by local doctors. Counselling is especially good for short-term problems: trained experts help you to examine the causes of problems and devise strategies to avoid negative behaviour patterns and restore a sense of physical and emotional wellbeing.

Psychotherapy is used for resolving deeper, long-term emotional and psychological problems. Psychotherapy is usually offered by psychiatrists, clinical psychologists, and psychiatric social workers. Psychiatric social workers are trained in treatment methods and often work as part of a treatment team in hospitals or clinics. Today psychotherapy is being practised more and more by paraprofessionals, who have less training but may be supervised by a professional or may be trained to work with specific problems using specific methods.

Psychotherapy is conducted in several formats. Individual therapy refers to a therapist's work with one person on his or her unique problem; the relationship between client and therapist may be particularly important in producing change. In group therapy, a therapist meets with a group of patients, and the interactions between patients become an important part of the therapy process.

Many different theories or schools of psychotherapy exist. Two of the more common are psychodynamic therapy and behavioural therapy.

Psychodynamic therapy

Psychodynamic therapy makes the fundamental assumption that emotional disorders are merely symptoms of internal, unobservable and unconscious conflicts between personality components. These conflicts result from unresolved family conflicts, experienced in early stages of childhood, that become reactivated in problem situations in adulthood. The aim of psychodynamic therapies is to revive the early conflict and to transfer it to the relationship with the therapist. The symptoms are removed when the therapist helps the patient to resolve the conflict in the transference relationship. The therapist interprets the transference to the patient and helps him or her overcome resistances to accepting the interpretation. Additional methods, such as dream interpretation or word-association techniques, are used to aid in uncovering unconscious material. Sigmund Freud's psychoanalysis is the primary example of a psychodynamic therapy.

Behavioural therapy

Behavioural approaches assume that all behaviour is learned. Emotional disorders are considered to be conditioned responses or habits that can be modified by the same principles of learning that govern all behaviour. From this perspective psychotherapy means providing corrective learning or conditioning experiences. Different therapy techniques are employed for remedying specific disordered behaviours. In social-skills training, for instance, patients practise handling difficult interpersonal situations via role playing.

Natural methods of therapy—relaxation techniques

An effective way to reduce stress in the body is through certain disciplines that fall under the heading of relaxation techniques.

Just as we are all capable of mounting and sustaining a stress reaction, we have also inherited the ability to put our bodies into a state of deep relaxation, called the 'relaxation response'. In this state, all the physiological events in the stress reaction are reversed: the pulse slows down, blood pressure falls, breathing becomes slower, and the muscles relax. But whereas the stress reaction is automatic, the relaxation response has to be deliberately induced. Fortunately, there are many ways of doing this. Sitting quietly in a park or beside the fireplace, gently petting the family cat, reclining on the sofa and other restful activities can generate this state. There also are specific skills that can be learned that are efficient and beneficial.

A state of deep relaxation achieved through meditation or self-hypnosis is actually more physiologically restful than sleep. These techniques are best learned through formal training courses, which are taught in a variety of places. Books and relaxation tapes can be used when courses are not available or are beyond your budget. On days when exercise is not possible, relaxation techniques are an excellent way to bring down the body's stress level. Whereas exercise dissipates stress energy, relaxation techniques neutralize it, producing a calming effect. As little as 20 minutes once or twice per day confers significant benefit.

Planning ahead

Making time in a busy schedule is probably the hardest of all the relaxation criteria to satisfy. You may need to obtain the cooperation of your friends, family or colleagues. If people close to you see you disappearing behind a locked door for twenty minutes or so, they may start wondering... so explain to them what you are doing. You may have to endure a bit of leg-pulling until other people come to appreciate the importance of it to you. If you fail to get support, then you will have to change your itinerary (or your friends).

Choose a time when you are least likely to be disturbed: early morning or late at night, if necessary. You should prepare yourself for relaxation by exercising moderately for five to ten minutes beforehand. You should also exercise moderately for up to three minutes afterwards to help you reorientate. Twenty minutes is the minimum time to spend on this three-part routine.

Get comfortable

It is up to you to ensure that you relax in a completely disturbance-free atmosphere. There must be no radio, no TV, no background music, no incense. Turn on the telephone answering machine and turn down the ringer if it is in the same room. It is best to avoid meals just before relaxation.

Find a comfortable chair in which to sit. Your back and neck should be straight, your shoulders not hunched forward. Your hands should rest comfortably in your lap half open. Your feet should be on the floor and your legs should not be crossed, just sit naturally. Next make sure there is nothing in the room to distract you, such as insects, draughts, direct sunlight. If you're relaxing in a group do so with experienced people—there's nothing less conducive to relaxation than an outburst of giggles from your flatmate or the person who shares your office.

Loosen off tight clothing like belts, ties and shoe laces. If you must lie down to get comfortable, rest your hands about an inch away from your body either side and don't cross your legs. Physical discomfort of any sort will provoke the secretion of adrenaline to spur you into remedial action, creating a sense of restlessness. Listen to what your body is trying to tell you about avoidable discomfort in your posture and remove the source before you go on.

Correct breathing

Breathing for relaxation should be moderate, slow and rhythmic. Don't hold your breath, and conversely, don't take short gasping breaths. Your whole chest should be involved in breathing—not just the top half—so use both chest and diaphragm muscles. Don't fully inhale or exhale and above all, don't force your breathing, make it natural. Sigh or take deep breaths if you need to—but do try to make it moderate, slow and rhythmic.

'Don't hold your breath' is an often heard expression, and one that suggests that we are always in full control of our breathing. Usually, of course, we are, but that is not always the case. During a normal day we take between 16,000 and 21,000 breaths. This automatic action is one of the first things to go when we become stressed. Our breathing gets shallower and accelerates erratically. Erratic breathing patterns lead to disorientation and emotional wavering, which can create even more stress—thus a vicious cycle begins. Investigating the breathing pattern and learning to control it is an important step in learning to control stress.

The brain controls our breathing by checking the ratio between oxygen and carbon dioxide in the blood. We exhale when the carbon dioxide makes the blood too acidic. Hyperventilation (fast, deep breathing) makes us expend too much carbon dioxide, leaving the blood in an alkaline state. This induces dizziness and disorientation, as the brain is starved of carbon dioxide.

Habitual hyperventilation causes fainting, numbness, palpitations, sweating and chest aches—all symptoms of carbon dioxide deficiency. These create a cause and effect cycle—erratic breathing induces other unpleasant symptoms, which in turn make our breathing worse.

Obviously, these symptoms occur when we are very stressed. But there are more subtle signs that breathing patterns could be better—gulping, holding the breath, moving the upper chest when talking and breathing, and frequent yawning.

Try a simple test to find out if you are breathing correctly. Lay a hand on the upper section of your chest and the other hand on the lower part of your rib-cage. If only your chest moves when you breathe, then you are breathing ineffectively. If the lower edge of the rib cage expands and the stomach rises at the start of each breath, then you are breathing correctly.

When stress hits, regular breathing is the first thing to go. To enable you to maintain easy breathing under stress, it is important to practise breathing exercises. It can sometimes seem difficult to slow down and become conscious about such an automatic act, but regular controlled breathing exercises are a very good way of getting your whole body to relax and to work out stress. Just a few minutes each day given over to fully concentrating on these exercises will bring great relief from stress.

Bad posture can effect the flow of air in and out of the body. Try lying down on your back to give the lungs and diaphragm freedom to move and leave the body relaxed and flexible. By removing the upright strain on your body and lungs there is more chance of developing an easy breathing pattern.

While breathing, focus on raising the abdomen, and filling lower, mid and upper sections with air. Be aware of the expansion of your ribs as you hold your breath—concentrate on that feeling. To exhale, pull in your diaphragm towards the back of your spine, slowly and smoothly. Try to ensure that you fully empty your lungs before inhaling again. This is commonly overlooked when breathing, which means that the lungs are never used to their full potential.

Correct attitude

The human mind is a highly complex, mostly automatic processing machine. If you have expectations that are not met, your mind will unconsciously generate a stress response as the first stage in remedying the situation. That stress response will initiate a host of subliminal physiological reactions that make you feel like doing something—the heart rate increases, muscles tense, and a lowering of the body's surface temperature makes you feel uncomfortable. Your attitude, your expectations and your intent are the foundation of your thoughts and your actions. If this foundation is not in keeping with your reality your relaxation will not be complete. Therefore, set your intent on relaxing without expectations and when you get it right it will be a very peaceful, restful and invigorating twenty minutes.

Thought control

Thinking is a form of internalized action, a visualization of consequences. Through thought we are distinguished from animals who act on instinct alone. However, the mind is an imperfect mirror, and every thought carries with it a kind of charge capable of setting off a stress response before rational decision making can take its turn. For relaxation this is a problem because that thought charge is just as potent as any external stimulus, as anxiety sufferers know only too well.

In order to relax effectively, that is, to reduce the stress response to a minimum for a meaningful period of time, thought has got to be put on hold—you have to stop the internal dialogue.

In the mind there are preconscious entities that float around, dragging you into self-dialogue. Recognizing these entities and avoiding their lure is a skill arrived at only with practice, and you must practise this skill every time you relax.

Perseverance

It may look easy to start with, but the benefits of this exercise are mainly long term. Other than noticing an improvement in your ability to sleep at night (or catnap during the day) you may spend many sessions doubting that benefit until you have grown stronger mentally and physically. It is important to persevere—20 minutes minimum—every day.

Meditation

Meditation is central to the Hindu way of life, and is also an integral part of the other great oriental religions, Buddhism and its close cousin, Zen. It also has its place in Sufism, Christianity and Judaism. (That said, meditation does not require adherence to any of the faiths and religions that advocate it.)

Many people view meditation as peaceful but ineffectual self-centredness. They are wrong: the benefits to be gained from meditation in any of its various forms are many. Those who meditate regularly believe that it leads to a significant lowering of mental tension and negative emotions, while at the same time increasing efficiency at work and deepening the sense of inner calm. This feeling of wellbeing brings physical benefits: regular meditation eliminates or reduces stress; can ease migraine and tension headaches; reduces blood pressure; benefits the heart; and reduces the pain of menstrual cramps.

In its simplest form, meditation is nothing more than allowing the mind to be lulled by a simple repetitive sensation—waves lapping on the beach, the tinkling of a fountain, repeating a word or sound over and over again, even something as mundane as the sound of machinery, any of these, and countless others, can be used as something on to which the mind focuses so strongly that problems and anxieties are crowded out. In its more refined, mystical guise, it is a means to total self-fulfilment, being completely at one with the universe.

Meditation is neither a time-consuming process—20 minutes a day are all that is needed—nor is it, as many suspect, a form of self-hypnosis. Practised properly, it is a life-enhancing voyage during which preconceived opinions and ideas fade, the senses and the intellect are refined and the ability to concentrate is increased.

A simple meditation technique

Sit in a comfortable chair, with your feet flat on the floor, your legs and arms uncrossed. (This can also be done lying down, but you might fall asleep). Rest your hands on your upper legs, with your palms down. Close your eyes, so your mind won't be distracted by what is going on around you.

Direct your focus of awareness to a place six inches (about 20 centimetres) directly above the centre of the top of your head. Here is a location in consciousness which is always calm and radiant, no matter what is going on elsewhere in your mind or body, or around you. It is called the 'upper room'. Think of a point of pure, crystal-white light here. Don't 'try' to visualize it. If you see it, fine, but if you don't, it doesn't matter. As you think of the point of white light, it grows brighter, expanding into a little star, three inches (about 10 centimetres) in diameter.

Think and let the star burn away the veils that have kept it hidden all these years. Direct the star to open, releasing a downpour of cleansing and purifying life energy. This energy is crystal-clear, like fresh spring water.

Let the energy flow through your hair, scalp, into the bones of your head and face, into your brain, eyes, ears, nose, mouth, down the neck, through your shoulders, arms and hands. Experience it flowing through your chest and back, abdomen, hips, pelvic area, upper legs, knees, lower legs, ankles and feet. Think and let the soles of your feet open, releasing the energy into the earth beneath your feet. Now it is flowing through your whole body.

Think of the bottoms of your feet closing, so the energy begins to reflow up through the areas you have cleared out. Experience it in your legs, hips, torso, shoulders, arms, hands, neck and head. Let it overflow out of the top of your head, surrounding your body with an aura of crystal-clear white light.

Bring your hands together, almost but not quite touching, palms facing each other, out in front of your body. Experience the energy flowing through your hands. You could use this energy to heal others, by laying your lighted hands on the person's head, heart, or wherever they have discomfort. Whatever you touch with your hands lighted this way will be filled with inner light-fire-energy.

If you experience discomfort anywhere in your body as you are working with the inner light, think of the 'consuming fire' aspect of the energy. Hold the focus of it in the area of discomfort to burn through the obstructions to the flow of your pure life energy. Afterwards, take a few minutes to assimilate the radiant essence of the light into any area that you have cleared out with the consuming fire aspect.

In addition to your focusing of the energy during meditation, as described above, you can work with the downpour anytime and anywhere, day or night, with your eyes open or closed, as appropriate to the situation. You can use it as an inner shower while you take your outer shower in the morning. Every time you think of the star and the white light downpouring, it continues for about 30 minutes. So you can literally fill your day with inner light. It's also a great way to go to sleep at night. For stress-reduction it is best to practice the technique for at least a few minutes every day.

See page 130 for more on Meditation.

Autogenic training

Autogenic training is a form of therapy that seeks to teach the patient to relax, thereby relieving stress. This is achieved by the patient learning a series of six basic exercises that can be undertaken either lying flat on the back, sitting in an armchair or sitting towards the edge of a chair with the head bent forwards and the chin on the chest. The six exercises concentrate on (a) breathing and respiration (b) heartbeat (c) the forehead to induce a feeling of coolness (d) the lower abdomen and stomach to induce a feeling of warmth (e) the arms and legs to induce a feeling of warmth (f) the neck, shoulders, arms and legs to induce a feeling of heaviness.

It is now well established that a number of illnesses and disorders are related to, or made worse by, stress. By learning the techniques and exercises of autogenic training, the person is able to achieve a state of relaxation and tranquillity, sleeps better and generally has more energy and a greater feeling of wellbeing. Autogenic training is taught at group sessions involving a small number of people (about six is usual).

Patients with a variety of disorders may benefit from autogenic training, which can also help people who feel under stress without particular physical symptoms. Illnesses that may be helped include irritable bowel syndrome, digestive disorders, muscular aches and cramps, ulcers, headaches and high blood pressure. Also, anxieties, fears and phobias, insomnia and some other psychological illnesses. This form of therapy can benefit people of all age groups, although it is considered that children under the age of six may not be able to understand the training. Therapists in autogenic training usually hold medical or nursing qualifications and expect to obtain a full picture of the patient's state of health before treatment begins. Therapy is both available privately and through the National Health Service in some areas of Great Britain.

Massage

Inactive lifestyles and sedentary occupations have created a society of people with cramped, stooped, and neglected postures. By realigning our bodies, massage can help to repair damaged postures. Not only does massage help to coax the spine and corresponding physiology back into position, it also makes us more aware of our bodies. Relieved of muscle tension, the body feels lighter and can therefore be borne more naturally and with more poise. Used in conjunction with postural therapies such as the Alexander technique (*see* page 15), massage is a valuable contribution towards a relaxed yet controlled posture.

Many of the benefits of massage come through the healer–patient contact. Our hands are one of the most sensitive parts of our body—we experience much of our sense of touch through our hands. Hand healers are believed to help people through their hands, often without even touching the body. There is a certain element of this in massage techniques. The masseur is communicating feelings of harmony and relaxation through their hands, allowing a benign force to flow into the client. Many practitioners therefore believe that it is important for the masseur to be in a positive state of mind.

During a massage the patient is coaxed from emotional and occupational stresses and brought into the intense arena of the here and now. Such one-on-one non-verbal communication is a valuable element in our overstressed lifestyles.

For more on the benefits and techniques of massage *see* page 29.

Yoga

Yoga is a technique of self-awareness that has been practised in the East as a physical, psychological and philosophical discipline for over 5,000 years. The word 'yoga' derives from the Sanskrit *yuk,* meaning 'to bind together', and the aim of yoga is to integrate the mind and the body and commune with the universal process of being.

Yoga is not a religion and does not require adherence to any particular dogma; it is basically a technique for personal development, enabling people to explore and fulfil their physical and spiritual needs. Over the last twenty-five years yoga has become increasingly popular in the West, and its effectiveness in relieving stress is widely acknowledged within the medical profession. Practised regularly, yoga creates mental clarity, emotional stability, deep relaxation and body awareness.

See page 48 for a fuller explanation of the benefits and positions of Yoga.

Traditional Chinese medicine

About 2,500 years ago, deep in the mountains of Northern China, Taoist priests practiced Ki Gong—meditative movement revealing and cultivating the vital life force. They believed this force, ki (pronounced 'chi' in China, 'ki' in Japan), was inseparable from life itself. They discovered that ki animated not only body and earth, but was the energetic force of the entire universe. Traditional Chinese medicine is a philosophy of preserving health, and is based first and foremost on an understanding of the ultimate power of ki. In contrast to much of Western medicine, traditional Chinese medicine is a preventative practice, strengthening the immune system to ward off disease.

In traditional Chinese medicine, ki is manifested both as *yin* (cold, dark, and 'interior'), and *yang* (warm, light, and 'exterior'). In fact, ki is present in all the opposites we experience, such as night and day, hot and cold, growth and decay. And although yin and yang may be perceived as opposites, they are actually inseparable. The recognition of one is essential to the recognition of the other. The balance between them is like the motion of night and day; at the instant darkness reaches its zenith at midnight, the cycle has begun to flow steadily towards dawn. At noon, the zenith of light, the day begins slowly to turn towards the darkness of night. All the internal organs of the body are subject to this nocturnal–diurnal swing of the universe.

This world view further holds that ki, manifesting as yin/yang, makes up the universe in the form of five elements: wood, fire, earth, metal, and water. These five elements also represent our bodily constitution as human beings, making us one with the universe. Ki flows into our bodies, up from the earth in its yin form and down from the heavens in its yang form. The energy channels in our bodies through which it moves are called 'meridians'.

These meridians do not directly correspond to any anatomical component recognized by Western medicine. The best way to understand the flow of ki through the meridians is to compare it to the flow of blood in our veins and arteries. If our blood does not reach our toes, they become dead. If our blood does not flow freely, we have high or low blood pressure. If our blood clots, we have an embolism or a stroke. Similarly, unbalanced or stagnant ki can cause many diseases and ailments. In fact, traditional Chinese medicine is based on the principle that every illness, ailment, and discomfort in the body can be explained in terms of an imbalance of ki.

Each meridian is related to one of the five elements. For example, the heart meridian is related to the element fire, the kidney and bladder to water. Along the meridians are pressure points, or 'gateways', special places where ki can become blocked. With the help of a trained practitioner, its flow can be freed and balance restored.

Out of the belief system of traditional Chinese medicine arose many healing methods, all directed to the balancing of ki. These include acupuncture, shiatsu, Tai Chi Ch'uan and herbalism.

Acupuncture

This is a form of traditional Chinese medicine that uses the gentle insertion of hair-fine needles into specific points on the body to stimulate the flow of one's ki, or natural healing energy. As we have already seen, according to ancient Chinese medicine Ki flows through the body in channels, called meridians, and illness is the result of an imbalance of ki.

Most people are surprised to learn that acupuncture needles are very thin (from ten to fifteen acupuncture needles can fit into one conventional hypodermic needle). Acupuncturists can attain a high level of skill in gently placing these tiny needles into the skin with a minimum of discomfort.

Acupuncture excels in those areas in which conventional medicine offers limited relief—chronic disease, pain control, and stress-related disorders. Acupuncture treatments are drug-free; you avoid side effects or dependency. However, you should always inform any practitioner about all pre-existing conditions, the names of all medicines you are taking, whether you are, or could be, pregnant, and if you have a cardiac pacemaker or cosmetic implants. Your acupuncturist will be able to evaluate your specific situation with this information to ensure the best form of treatment.

See also Acupuncture page 11.

Shiatsu

Shiatsu is a Japanese healing art combining the principles of traditional Chinese medicine with practices similar to those of acupuncture but performed without needles. Shiatsu is a balance—a dance—between practitioner and receiver, in which the healing power of both build upon each other to clear and balance the vital life force known as ki.

Shiatsu is a Japanese word: *shi* meaning 'finger', and *atsu* meaning 'pressure'. But shiatsu is more than acupressure. It is a combination of many different techniques, including pressing, hooking, sweeping, shaking, rotating, grasping, vibrating, patting, plucking, lifting, pinching, rolling, brushing, and, in one variation—barefoot shiatsu—it includes walking on the person's back, legs, and feet.

But these are merely the physical techniques. With an awareness of psychological and spiritual implications, shiatsu has become, indeed, a kind of dance between giver and receiver. A unique rapport develops between the practitioner and client, because shiatsu relies on the simple but powerful experience of touch to awaken the client's own self-healing powers. This 'touch communication' between practitioner and client is fundamental to all healing methods.

See page 90 for more on Shiatsu.

Aromatherapy

In the past the human sense of smell was crucial to our survival—we could smell intruders, sense which plants were poisonous and track game through their odour. Obviously, the need for this ability has lessened, and we are now more likely to appreciate the smell of the latest perfumery sensation, or suffer under the stench of cigarettes or cigars. However, we are still extremely susceptible to smell—both personal and environmental. We all have our own unique smell (pherones), apart from body odour, and while our recognition may be subconscious, it has more effect on our responses and behaviour than we may realize. Our emotions and physical harmony can be affected through our sense of smell. The effect of pleasant or unpleasant smells on the harmony of our bodies is well documented, and utilized through the art of aromatherapy.

Aromatherapy uses essential oils, which are extracted from aromatic plants and trees. A holistic medicine, it shares the same principles as acupuncture, reflexology and herbal medicine, to name a few. These arts are complementary and work on the principle of promoting mental serenity and bodily health— treating the person as one entity.

The therapy works from the principle that life itself is utterly intangible, that its core or essence cannot be seen, felt or analysed. When we talk about life, we talk about our souls and emotions, as well as our physical and physiological presence. The Chinese call it ki, and it represents the energy that propels us through each day of our lives and creates the world around us. This force is present in every plant and tree, and aromatherapy deals with extracting this organic 'essence' and using it to enhance, cure and protect. Essential oils can affect mood, alleviate fatigue, reduce anxiety and promote relaxation. When inhaled they work on the nervous system and brain through stimulation of the olfactory nerves. When absorbed through the skin, stronger components are released into the bloodstream.

See page 295 on Aromatherapy.

Biofeedback

This refers to the use of monitoring equipment to measure and control levels of relaxation. Training can be given after the scientific data is examined.

Although great feats of body and mind control have been reported in Eastern medicine for centuries, it has only been in the past two decades that Western medicine has accepted the fact that humans can, indeed, regulate their own heart rate, circulation, temperature, muscle tension, and other body functions that were mostly thought to operate only automatically. That acceptance came largely through the development of the biofeedback machine, which teaches people to become aware of various body functions and to control them with conscious intent, using relaxation and mental imagery techniques.

Today biofeedback is widely used for the treatment of chronic pain and stress-related disorders. Even astronauts have used biofeedback to control the nausea of space sickness.

If you go for biofeedback therapy, you will be asked to sit in a comfortable chair in front of a machine that looks like a TV set. Electrode sensors (wires) from the biofeedback machine will be taped to your body, usually on your forehead, neck, back, or forefinger. With the help of relaxing music or a taped voice that suggests relaxation techniques, you will be asked to reduce the muscle tension throughout your body. Later you way also be asked to slow your heart rate, even warm your hands by increasing their blood flow. While you're trying to accomplish these feats, the machine measures your muscle tension, heart rate and blood flow, and 'feeds back' how well you are doing. This feedback can be in the form of audible beeps, pictures, or graphic lines.

After learning what the correct response feels like by working with the machine and practising at home, you should eventually be able to achieve the same response without the machine.

Hydrotherapy

Floatation

A form of sensory deprivation, floatation involves lying face up in an enclosed, dark tank of warm, heavily salted water. There is no sound, except perhaps some natural music to bring the client into a dream-like state. It is exceptionally refreshing and induces a deep, relaxing sleep.

Neutral bath

Before the development of tranquillizers, the most dependable and effective method of calming an agitated patient was the use of a neutral bath. The patient was placed in a tub of water, the temperature of which was maintained at between 33.5°C and 35.6°C (92°F to 96°F), often for over three hours, and sometimes for as long as twenty-four hours. Obviously, this is not a practical proposition for the average tense person.

As a self-help measure, the neutral bath does, however, offer a means of sedating the nervous system if used for relatively short periods. It is important to maintain the water temperature at the above level, and for this a bath thermometer should be used. The bathroom itself should be kept warm to prevent any chill in the air.

Half an hour of immersion in a bath like this will have a sedative, or even soporific, effect. It places no strain on the heart, circulation or nervous system, and achieves muscular relaxation as well as a relaxation and expansion of the blood vessels: all of these effects promote relaxation. This bath can be used in conjunction with other methods of relaxation, such as breathing techniques and meditation, to make it an even more efficient way of wiping out stress. It can be used daily if necessary.

Hot bath

Most people know the relaxing benefits of a hot bath. A bath with the temperature between 36.5°C and 40°C (98°F and 104°F) is very useful as a means of muscle relaxation. To begin with, five minutes immersion in a bath of this temperature is enough. This can be stepped up to ten minutes a day, as long as no feelings of weakness or dizziness arise. It is important to realize that a brief hot bath has quite a different effect from a long one.

For other methods of hydrotherapy see page 22.

Herbalism

The use of medicinal herbs to alleviate illness is based on ancient techniques. When used properly, traditional herbs are non-addictive, have no side effects and can have impressive results. Herbs are particularly useful in treating nervous tension, depression, insomnia, PMS, nervous headaches and migraines. Herbal remedies are also extremely important in helping to reduce stress by their effects on the immune, circulatory and neuromuscular systems.

See page 311 for Herbal Remedies.

Homoeopathy

Put most simply, homoeopathy is based on the belief that substances which are poisonous in large doses can be beneficial in small doses. Various substances can be taken in the form of pills, capsules, sachets of powder, sachets of granules or liquids. These homoeopathic remedies can be bought in chemists and health shops, or obtained from a practitioner. *See* page 402 for Homoeopathy.

Hypnotherapy

Because it can be used to treat conditions where psychological aspects are important, hypnotherapy is a valuable means of treating stress-related illnesses; although it is not clear how hypnosis works, and the links between hypnosis and entertainment have contributed to prejudice against its use as a therapeutic tool.

See page 126 for Hypnotherapy.

Pet therapy

The evidence is clear that owning and caring for a family pet can help to reduce stress levels. Pets provide their owners with unconditional love and loyalty. In return, the experience of caring for the animal imparts a sense of belonging and opportunities for play and amusement. Relationships with animals are largely free of the threats and responsibilities inherent in human intercourse. The rewards may not be so great, but for many animal lovers there can be no substitute for the emotional rewards of owning a pet.

Physiological tests have shown that stroking and petting animals can improve general health, lower blood pressure, reduce anxiety and produce a reduction in stress levels.

Certain institutions, such as hospitals, old people's homes, and even prisons, have noticed an improvement in their inmates' mental, physical and emotional health and behaviour when given access to animals.

Reflexology

Reflexology is a method for activating the natural healing resources of the body. Forms of reflexology have been in use for at least 3000 years (paintings depicting the art have been discovered in an Egyptian doctor's tomb dating back to 2330 BC). The science of reflexology as it is practised today was developed fairly recently, and its use as a complementary therapy has been on the increase ever since.

Reflexology works on the principle that the body is divided into ten zones that run lengthwise from head to toe, where the reflex areas for all the organs, glands and body parts are found. Energy runs through these zones. Reflexologists believe that if this constant flow of energy is impeded by a blockage or congestion, illness sets in. A reflexologist, by using constant, rhythmic pressure on the reflexes of the patient's feet, breaks down the blockage, allowing the return of free-flowing energy and deep relaxation to occur, thus enabling the body's own healing mechanisms to take effect.

See also page 55 for more on reflexology.

Tai Chi Ch'uan

The aim of Tai Chi (the ch'uan is usually dropped) is to combine motion, unity and dance so that those who practise its art surrender to the natural flow of the universe and become one with it—exactly the aim of more passive meditation.

Tai Chi is a means of exploring the processes of mind and body through creative movement and reflects the I Ching belief that nature is always in motion. It is said to have originated with the meditation of a Taoist monk, Chang Sanfeng, who one day saw a magpie trying to attack a snake. The reptile teased the bird by writhing and curling in a spiral motion, always remaining just out of the bird's reach. Similar movements are now an integral part of Tai Chi.

In Tai Chi, the image of water symbolizes the flow of energy and the way it yields to the form of its container. Earth is seen as a link between person and planet. The use of circular forms of expression shows unity and containment.

It is not possible to learn Tai Chi from the pages of a book. Traditionally, the practise was handed down from master to pupil. Today most large towns offer Tai Chi classes, and anyone wishing to learn its ways and mysteries should join a group.

The classes always begin with a period of meditative stillness, and then the pupils step forward on the right foot—an energy step with fire being visualised shooting from the palms of the hands. The energy is pulled back into the body and the weight transferred to the left foot, everyone now visualizing water cascading over them. With the body turning to the left, the palms are rotated and curved back to the right. The body continues to turn to the right with both feet firmly fixed to the floor, then the left foot is brought round, returning the body to the centre.

Tai Chi is a processs of self-discovery and, like yoga, demonstrates the link between body movement and posture and contemplative states of being. In the words of one expert, Al Huang, who wrote the classic *Embrace Tiger, Return to Mountain*, 'Tai Chi is to help you get aquainted with your own sense of personal growth, the creative process of just being you.'

3

MEDICINAL PLANTS AND NATURAL REMEDIES

This section covers the topics of aromatherapy, herbalism and homoeopathy, three therapies that make use of plant and herb extracts. The substances used in aromatherapy and herbal medicine can be very potent—sometimes potentially poisonous—and no course of treatment should be undertaken without a consultation with a qualified herbalist or aromatherapist.

Homoeopathy is a very complex medicine and it is wise to seek an expert opinion as to what treatment is ideal for you although the actual treatment itself is very safe and non-addictive.

Aromatherapy

Healing through aromatherapy

Aromatherapy is a method of healing using very concentrated essential oils that are often highly aromatic and are extracted from plants. Constituents of the oils confer the characteristic perfume or odour given off by a particular plant. Essential oils help the plant in some way to complete its cycle of growth and reproduction. For example, some oils may attract insects for the purpose of pollination; others may render it distasteful as a source of food. Any part of a plant—the stems, leaves, flowers, fruits, seeds, roots or bark—may produce essential oils or essences but often only in minute amounts. Different parts of the same plant may produce their own form of oil. An example of this is the orange, which produces oils with different properties in the flowers, fruits and leaves.

Art and writings from the ancient civilizations of Egypt, China and Persia show that plant essences were used and valued by priests, physicians and healers. Plant essences have been used throughout the ages for healing—in incense for religious rituals, in perfumes and embalming ointments and for culinary purposes. There are many Biblical references that give an insight into the uses of plant oils and the high value that was attached to them. Throughout the course of human history the healing properties of plants and their essential oils has been recognized and most people probably had some knowledge about their use. It was only in more recent times, with the great developments in science and orthodox medicine, particularly the manufacture of antibiotics and synthetic drugs, that knowledge and interest in the older methods of healing declined. However, in the last few years there has been a great rekindling of interest in the practice of aromatherapy with many people turning to this form of treatment.

Extraction of essential oils
Steam distillation, solvent extraction, maceration, defleurage, enfleurage

Since any part of a plant may produce essential oils, the method of extraction depends upon the site and accessibility of the essence in each particular case. The oils are produced by special minute cells or glands and are released naturally by the plant in small amounts over a prolonged period of time when needed. In order to harvest the oils in appreciable amounts, it is usually necessary to collect a large quantity of the part of the plant needed and to subject the material to a process that causes the oil glands to burst. One of the most common methods is *steam distillation*. The plant material is placed tightly into a press or still and steamed at a high temperature. This causes the oil glands to burst and the essential oil vaporises into the steam. This is then cooled to separate the oil from the water. Sometimes water is used for distillation rather than steam. Another method involves dissolving the plant material in a solvent or alcohol and is called *solvent extraction*. This involves placing the material in a centrifuge, which rotates at high speed, and then extracting the essential oils by means of a low temperature distillation process. Substances obtained in this way may be called *resins* or *absolutes*. A further method is called *maceration* in which the plant is soaked in hot oil. The plant cells collapse and release their essential oils, and the whole mixture is then separated and purified by a process called *defleurage*. If fat is used instead of oil, the process is called *enfleurage*. These methods produce a purer oil that is usually more expensive than one obtained by distillation. The essential oils used in aromatherapy can be costly as vast quantities of plant material are required to produce them and the methods used are complex and costly.

Storage and use of essential oils

Essential oils are highly concentrated, volatile and aromatic. They readily evaporate and change and deteriorate if exposed to light, heat and air. Hence pure oils need to be stored carefully in brown glass bottles at a moderate temperature away from direct light. They can be stored for one or two years in this way. For most purposes in aromatherapy, essential oils are used in a dilute form, being added either to water or to another oil, called the *base* or *carrier*. The base is often a vegetable oil such as olive or safflower, which both have nutrient and beneficial properties. An essential/carrier oil mixture has a short useful life of two or three months and so they are usually mixed at the time of use and in small amounts.

Techniques used in aromatherapy

Massage

Massage is the most familiar method of treatment associated with aromatherapy. Essential oils are able to penetrate through the skin and are taken into the body, exerting healing and beneficial influences on internal tissues and organs. The oils used for massage are first diluted by being mixed with a base and should never be applied directly to the skin in their pure form in case of an adverse allergic reaction.

An aromatherapist will 'design' an individual whole body massage based on an accurate history taken from the patient and much experience in the use of essential oils. The oils will be chosen specifically to match the temperament of the patient and also to deal with any particular medical or emotional problems which may be troubling him or her.

Although there is no substitute for a long soothing aromatherapy massage given by an expert, the techniques are not difficult to learn and can be carried out satisfactorily at home.

Bathing

Most people have experienced the benefits of relaxing in a hot bath to which a proprietary perfumed preparation has been added. Most of these preparations contain essential oils used in aromatherapy. The addition of a number of drops of an essential oil to the bath water is soothing and relaxing, easing aches and pains, and can also have a stimulating effect, banishing tiredness and restoring energy. In addition, there is the added benefit of inhaling the vapours of the oil as they evaporate from the hot water.

Inhalation

Inhalation is thought to be the most direct and rapid means of treatment. This is because the molecules of the volatile essential oil act directly on the olfactory organs and are immediately perceived by the brain. A popular method is the time-honoured one of *steam inhalation*, in which a few drops of essential oil are added to hot water in a bowl. The person sits with his or her face above the mixture and covers the head, face and bowl with a towel so that the vapours do not escape. This can be repeated up to three times a day but should not be undertaken by people suffering from asthma. Some essential oils can be applied directly to a handkerchief or onto a pillow and the vapours inhaled in this way.

Steam inhalation with essential oils constitutes a wonderful, time-honoured way of alleviating the symptoms of colds and flu, and can also be beneficial to greasy skins. Steam inhalations should, however, be avoided by asthmatics unless under direction from a medical practitioner, as the steam can occasionally irritate the lungs.

Compresses

Compresses are effective in the treatment of a variety of muscular and rheumatic aches and pains as well as bruises and headaches. To prepare a compress, add 5 drops of oil to a small bowl of water. Soak a piece of flannel or other absorbent material in the solution. Squeeze out excess moisture (although the compress should remain fairly wet) and secure in position with a bandage or cling film. For acute pain, the compress should be renewed when it has reached blood temperature, otherwise it should be left in position for a minimum of two hours and preferably overnight. Cold water should be used wherever fever or acute pain or hot swelling require treatment, whereas the water should be hot if the pain is chronic. If fever is present, the compress should be changed frequently.

Hair treatments/scalp tonics

Many hair conditions such as dryness, excessive grease, or dandruff will respond to aromatherapy using specific recipes of essential oils diluted in a nourishing base oil. For instance, 60 drops of an essential oil diluted in 100 mls of base oil (such as olive or sweet almond) will make a wonderful conditioning treatment. Simply rub the oils thoroughly into the scalp, then wrap the hair in warm towels and allow the oil to penetrate the hair and the scalp for an hour or two. The choice of oil depends of course upon the desired effect: chamomile and rosemary, for instance, will condition and promote healthy hair growth, bergamot and tea tree are helpful in dandruff control whilst lavender has repellent qualities which will deter lice and fleas.

Face creams, oils and lotions

For the face, essential oils should be mixed with base oils in much the same way as for massage, the main difference being that more nourishing oils such as apricot kernel and avocado should be used in preference to ordinary vegetable oils. (It should be noted that avocado is a fairly heavy oil and its use is best reserved for dry skin.) Essential oils can also be added to a non-perfumed cold cream or lotion and used for problem complexions.

Most essential oils have antiseptic properties and can be used to treat infective skin conditions. Certain oils (such as rose and neroli) are anti-inflammatory and have a soothing effect, whereas sandalwood is useful in the treatment of superficial broken veins. Rose and neroli are also excellent for care of mature skins. For dry cracked skin, the addition of wheatgerm and avocado oil (with their high vitamin E content) to preparations will relieve the condition. In general, aromatherapy can improve the skin by encouraging toxin removal, stimulating cell growth and renewal and improving circulation. A gentle circular massage with the tips of the fingers should be used on the face, and special care must be taken not to stretch or drag the delicate skin around the eye area.

Flower waters

Flower waters constitute a refreshing and soothing aid in the treatment and prevention of skin conditions such as eczema and acne, and can be easily prepared at home. Simply add around 20 drops of essential oil to an amber glass bottle containing 100 mls of spring water, then leave it to stand in a dark place for a few days. Filter the water through some coffee or similar filter paper, then apply to the skin as required using a cotton wool pad.

Bathing and showering

Add a few drops (5–10) of essential oil to the bath water after the water has been drawn, then close the door to retain the aromatic vapours. The choice of oils is entirely up to the individual, depending on the desired effect, although those with sensitive skins are advised to have the oils ready diluted in a base oil prior to bathing.

Bathing in essential oils can stimulate and revive or relax and sedate depending on the oils selected: rosemary and pine can have a soothing effect on tired or aching limbs, chamomile and lavender are popular for relieving insomnia and anxiety, etc. A similar effect (although obviously not quite as relaxing) can be achieved whilst showering by soaking a wet sponge in essential oil mix, then rubbing it over the body under the warm spray.

Sitz bath

A sitz, or shallow, bath in the appropriate essential oil can bring enormous relief in conditions such as haemorrhoids, thrush and cystitis.

Foot bath

Tired, swollen feet can be refreshed by bathing in a basin of hot water containing 4–5 drops of lavender, peppermint, rosemary or thyme.

Hands

Dry, chapped hands may be soothed by soaking in a bowl of warm water containing a few drops of essential oil such as patchouli or rose.

Mouthwash and gargles

Used strictly in the correct dilutions, essential oils provide a natural, gentle way to help clear up mouth ulcers, oral thrush and infected gums, but it cannot be stressed too much that essential oils should never be swallowed.

Neat application and internal use

Generally, the application of undiluted essential oils directly to the skin should be avoided as many are highly irritant. However, there are one or two exceptions which have been safely applied to the skin undiluted for centuries. These include lemon oil, which can be applied neat to warts (Vaseline can be applied around the wart to protect the surrounding skin); lavender, which can be safely applied directly to burns, cuts, bites and stings; and tea tree, which may be dabbed on spots. Any other oils must be used in dilution unless under careful direction from a trained aromatherapist.

Many essential oils are highly toxic when taken orally and there are **no circumstances** in which they may safely be taken at home in this way.

Mode of action of essential oils

Although the subject of a great deal of research, there is a lack of knowledge about how essential oils work in the body to produce their therapeutic effects. It is known that individual essential oils possess antiseptic, antibiotic, sedative, tonic and stimulating properties, and it is believed that they act in harmony with the natural defences of the body such as the immune system. Some oils, such as eucalyptus and rosemary, act as natural decongestants whereas others, such as sage, have a beneficial effect upon the circulation.

Conditions that may benefit from aromatherapy

A wide range of conditions and disorders may benefit from aromatherapy and it is considered to be a gentle treatment suitable for all age groups. It is especially beneficial for long-term chronic conditions, and the use of essential oils is believed by therapists to prevent the development of some illnesses. Conditions that may be relieved by aromatherapy include painful limbs, muscles and joints due to arthritic or rheumatic disorders, respiratory complaints, digestive disorders, skin conditions, throat and mouth infections, urinary tract infections and problems affecting the hair and scalp. Also, period pains, burns, insect bites and stings, headaches, high blood pressure, feverishness, menopausal symptoms, poor circulation and gout can benefit from aromatherapy. Aromatherapy is of great benefit in relieving stress and stress-related symptoms such as anxiety, insomnia and depression.

Many of the essential oils can be safely used at home and the basic techniques of use can soon be mastered. However, some should only be used by a trained aromatherapist and others must be avoided in certain conditions such as pregnancy. In some circumstances, massage is not considered to be advisable. It is wise to seek medical advice in the event of doubt or if the ailment is more than a minor one.

Consulting a professional aromatherapist

Aromatherapy is a holistic approach to healing hence the practitioner endeavours to build up a complete picture of the patient and his or her lifestyle, nature and family circumstances, as well as noting the symptoms which need to be to be treated. Depending upon the picture that is obtained, the aromatherapist decides upon the essential oil or oils that are most suitable and likely to prove most helpful in the circumstances that prevail. The aromatherapist has a wide ranging knowledge and experience upon which to draw. Many oils can be blended together for an enhanced effect and this is called a 'synergistic blend'. Many aromatherapists offer a massage and/or instruction on the use of the selected oils at home.

Base oils

Because essential oils are extremely concentrated and also because of their tendency to evaporate rapidly, they need to be diluted with carrier or base oils. Generally it is not advised that essential oils should be applied undiluted to the skin, although there are one or two specific exceptions. It is very important to use a high quality base oil, as oils such as baby or mineral oil have very poor penetrating qualities which will hamper the passage of the essential oil through the skin. Indeed, it would be better to use a good quality vegetable or nut oil for babies in preference to proprietary baby oils as the vegetable oil is more easily absorbed and contains more nutrients.

Although the choice of base oil is largely a matter of personal preference, it is useful to note that many vegetable oils possess therapeutic properties of their own. Any of sweet almond, soya bean, sunflower, jojoba, olive, grapeseed, hazelnut, avocado, corn or safflower will provide a suitable base for essential oils, although these should preferably be of the cold-pressed variety that has higher nutrient levels.

Pure essential oils should retain their potency for one to two years, but once diluted in a base oil will only last for three months or so before spoiling. They should also be stored at a fairly constant room temperature in corked dark glass bottles or flip-top containers as they will deteriorate quickly when subjected to extremes of light and temperature. Adding some vitamin E or wheatgerm oil to the mixture can help prolong its usefulness. For massage oils, it is best to make up a very small quantity of essential oil in base oil for each application because of its poor keeping qualities.

Below is a very rough guide to the dilution of essential oils. However, you will find many variations and differing opinions on this depending on the preference of individual therapists, and their recipes will differ accordingly.

Base Oil	Essential Oil
100 ml	20–60 drops
25 ml	7–25 drops
1 teaspoon (5 ml)	3–5 drops

Blending essential oils

Essences can be blended to treat specific ailments, and some aromatherapy books contain precise recipes for blends. When two or more essential oils are working together in harmony, this is known as a synergistic blend. Obviously, it takes many years of experience to know which combinations of plant essences will work most effectively together, but as a rough guide, oils extracted from plants of the same botanical family will usually blend and work well together, although it is by no means necessary to stick rigidly to this rule as other combinations may be just as successful. Really, a number of factors need to be taken into account when preparing a blend of oils for a patient, such as the nature of his/her complaint, his personality or frame of mind. For home use, it is not usually beneficial to blend more than three oils for any one preparation.

Around the home

There are a variety of ways in which your home can be enhanced by the use of essential oils. Fragrances, pomanders, ring burners and diffusers can all be used in conjunction with essential oils to impart a wonderful scent to a room. (Essential oils should be put into water and vapourized and not burned as they are inflammable. Follow the instructions on ring burners carefully and never put essential oils directly onto a hot light bulb.) Most essential oils also have antimicrobial properties which make them extremely useful when the occupants of the room are suffering from colds and flu. Oils such as myrtle and eucalyptus also seem to have a soothing effect on coughs and can be used in the bedroom where they will release their aroma throughout the night.

Fragrancers, pomanders, and ring burners can all be purchased quite cheaply from shops and indeed make very welcome gifts, but it is not neccessary to use any extra equipment to benefit from essential oils in the home. By adding a few drops of essential oil to a bowl of water or soaking a cotton ball in the oil and placing it in a warm place the same effect can be achieved. You can also sprinkle logs and twigs before placing them on the fire or barbecue to create a soothing aroma.

In case of colds or flu, a bowl of water is actually preferable as it has a humidifying effect on the air. Three or four drops of an appropriate essential oil such as eucalyptus or cypress sprinkled on a handkerchief can also be inhaled periodically to alleviate the worst symptoms of sinusitis, colds and headaches. Similarly, 2–3 drops of a relaxing essential oil on the pillow at night can help to alleviate insomnia.

How essential oils work

Inhalation, application and bathing are the three main methods used to encourage the entry of essential oils into the body. When inhaled, the extremely volatile oils may enter via the olfactory system, and permeation of the skin occurs when they are diluted and applied externally. By bathing in essential oils, we can inhale and absorb the oils through the skin simultaneously.

Little is known about how essential oils actually affect the mind and the body, although research is currently ongoing in the USA and the UK. However, the effectiveness of aromatherapy has been supported by recent research in central Europe, the USA, the UK and Australia. It appears that most essential oils are antiseptic and bactericidal to some degree, whilst some even seem to be effective in fighting viral infections.

On inhalation, essential oil molecules are received by receptor cells in the lining of the nose, which will transmit signals to the brain. Electrochemical messages received by the olfactory centre in the brain then stimulate the release of powerful neurochemicals into the blood which will then be transported around the body. Molecules inhaled into the lungs may pass into the bloodstream and be disseminated in the same way.

When rubbed or massaged into the skin, essential oils will permeate the pores and hair follicles. From here, they can readily pass into the tiny blood vessels (known as capillaries) by virtue of their molecular structure, and then travel around the body.

Once absorbed, the action of the oil depends upon its chemical constituents. Most essential oils are high in alcohols and esters, although a few contain a high concentration of phenols, aldehydes and ketones. The latter are powerful chemicals and their use should be avoided by all save the skilled professional.

Special care

You may find that your professional aromatherapist will use some of the following oils, but these are generally unsafe for use by the lay person.

Generally

Aniseed, cinnamon bark, cinamon leaf, clove bud, clove leaf, clove stem, fennel (bitter), pine, parsley, nutmeg.

During pregnancy

Basil, cedarwood, clary sage, fennel, juniper, marjoram, myrrh, rosemary, sage, thyme, parsley, nutmeg.

Prior to exposure to sun

Bergamot, lemon, mandarin, orange, fennel.

Hypertension

Sage, thyme, cypress.

Aromatherapy massage at home

Before beginning an aromatherapy massage, there are a number of steps that should be taken in order for the subject of the massage to derive full benefit from the treatment.

1 It is important to take a brief history from the patient in order to be able to select the correct oils. This will involve an assessment of his/her emotional state as well as any physical complaints.

2 At least an hour should have elapsed since the last meal prior to receiving or giving a massage.

3 Make sure your clothing is loose and will not obstruct your movements.

4 Ensure that hands are clean and nails short.

5 Have some tissues ready, and make sure your oil is easily accessible.

6 Make sure your hands are warm before touching your subject.

The room should be warm so that your subject will be comfortable even though only partly dressed. Lighting should be subdued, and the telephone should be disconnected to avoid interruption. Perhaps music could be played softly in the background, but this is a matter of preference and convenience. It is a good idea to have a compatible essence evaporating in the room prior to commencement. The massage surface needs to be firm, therefore a normal sprung bed is unsuitable—instead, pad the floor or use a futon or similar firm mattress.

First of all the subject may have a warm bath or shower in order that the pores are open and receptive to the essential oil. This, however, is a matter of personal preference on the part of the therapist. The subject should be positioned comfortably and should be covered with towels, exposing only the area that is to be massaged at any one time in order to avoid embarrassment and cold. Hair should be tied out of the way.

Basic techniques

The following constitutes only a very basic guide to massage movements and is no substitute for a comprehensive aromamassage course. However, massage can be used to great benefit at home using the following simple movements and suggestions:

Effleurage

This is the most often used therapy movement, and constitutes a simple, gentle stroking movement. Note that deep pressure should *never* be used by an untrained person. The strokes may be long or short, gentle or firm, but the whole hand should be used, always pushing the blood towards the heart, thus promoting venous return. This stroke promotes muscle relaxation and soothes the nerve endings.

Petrissage

In petrissage, the flesh is gently rolled between the thumbs and fingers in a movement not unlike kneading dough. This technique is best used on the back and on fatty areas. The idea is to stimulate the circulation and lymphatic flow and thereby increase the rate of toxin expulsion.

Head massage

Put a little of the essential massage oil on the fingertips and massage in circular movements over the scalp and temples.

Massage for tension headaches and migraine

Work from the base of the neck and scalp for a few moments, using effleurage strokes firmly, again with the chosen oil(s) on the fingertips

Neck massage

Neck massage should be carried out with the patient sitting on a chair with some support in front. Working around the base of the neck and scalp, use small upward and outward circular movements. Move slowly up, down and around the sides of the neck, alternating firm and gentle movements.

Shoulder massage

Using gentle anticlockwise effleurage movements, stroke firmly from the shoulders to the neck.

Arm massage

Use effleurage and petrissage movements upwards in the direction of the armpit, concentrating on muscular and fatty areas. Avoid bony areas.

Back massage

Avoiding the vertebrae, use gentle or firm petrissage or effleurage movements.

Stroke all the way from the lumbar to the shoulders, move the hands outwards across the shoulders and return slowly down the outer area of the back. Repeat this movement to induce deep relaxation.

Abdominal massage

Use a clockwise effleurage stroke, taking care not to apply too much pressure.

Leg massage

Always massage the legs in an upward direction. Avoid bony area, and *never* massage varicose veins.

Massage for menstrual or gynaecological problems

Always use gentle effleurage movements and do not exert any pressure on the lower abdomen. Begin at the lower back and slide forwards and downwards across the hips. Repeat several times.

Feet massage

Work in the direction of toe to heel, using the fingers uppermost and the thumb under the foot.

Common ailments

Stress-related disorders

Anxiety	basil, bergamot, geranium, lavender, marjoram (sweet), melissa, neroli, sandalwood, vetiver.
Mild shock	basil, chamomile, melissa, peppermint, rosemary.
Depression	bergamot, chamomile, geranium, jasmine, lavender, neroli, patchouli, rose, rosemary, sage*.
Fatigue	clary sage, eucalyptus, juniper berry, peppermint, rosemary.

Skin complaints/disorders

Dry skin	bergamot, hcamomile, geranium, jasmine, lavendar, melissa, neroli, patchouli, sandalwood, ylang ylang.
Oily skin	cypress, lemon, tea tree.
Acne	bergamot, chamomile, cedarwood, cypress, eucalyptus, fennel, geranium, juniper berry, lavender, lemon, myrrh, parsley*, patchouli, petitgrain, rose, rosemary, sandalwood, tea tree.
Eczema	chamomile, geranium, juniper berry, lavender, melissa.
Psoriasis	bergamot, chamomile, eucalyptus, lavender, peppermint.

Feminine/gynaeological disorders

Amenorrhoea	chamomile, clary sage, fennel, geranium, sage*.
Dysmenorrhoea	cypress, geranium, rose.
Hot flushes	chamomile, clary sage, jasmine, lavender, neroli, petitgrain, sandalwood, ylang ylang.
Mastitis	chamomile, clary sage, geranium, lavender, rose.
Period pain	clary sage, lavender, marjoram
PMT	geranium, lavender, neroli, petitgrain, rose.

* oils marked with an asterisk can have adverse effects and are normally recommended to be used under the guidance of a professional aromatherapist

A – Z of Essential Oils

The following section is by no means an exhaustive one, but aims to include the most popular oils readily available today. Similarly, whilst therapeutic uses have been suggested, therapists will differ in the choice of oils for particular complaints, just as a general practitioner may prescribe one remedy for a specific complaint, whereas his partner in the same practice may favour another treatment for the same complaint.

Aniseed
Pimpinella anisum

Aniseed seems to have a carminative (flatulence-expelling) effect on the alimentary canal and is therefore useful in the treatment of flatulence and indigestion. It has a strong antiseptic effect, and its antispasmodic properties can be effective against period pains. It also seems to stimulate lactation post-natally and is used in lozenges and cough sweets for its decongestant effect. Its anti-parasitic effect makes it useful in the treatment of lice and scabies.

CAUTION: Can be irritant to sensitive skins and narcotic in large doses. It is not suitable for home use and should only be used by a qualified aromatherapist.

Basil
Ociymum basilicum

Basil is now grown in many countries of the world although it originates from Africa. The herb has a long history of medicinal and culinary use, and was familiar to the Ancient Egyptian and Greek civilizations. Basil is sacred in the Hindu religion and has many medicinal uses in India and other Eastern countries. The whole plant is subjected to a process of steam distillation to obtain the essential oil used in aromatherapy. Basil is valued for its soothing and uplifting effects — its sweet, liquorice-like fragrance alleviates fatigue and depression and has a general tonic effect. Basil has a refreshing, invigorating effect and also has antiseptic properties. It can be effective in treating respiratory infections such as colds, bronchitis, asthma and sinusitis. It can also alleviate the symptoms of fever, gout and indigestion. It seems to be equally effective in relieving tired and over-worked muscles and is widely used in baths, inhalation and massage. Its strongly antiseptic effect soothes skin abrasions and as-

sists the healing process. It also has insect repellent qualities. As a digestive aid, basil's antispasmodic effect has made it a favoured herb in cookery throughout the ages.

CAUTION: Basil should be avoided during pregnancy. It can also have a depressant effect, so it should be used in moderation. It is relatively non-toxic, but should be well diluted to avoid possible skin irritation.

Bay
Laurus nobilis

Both *Laurus nobilis* and its West Indian cousin *Pimenta racemosa* are valuable in the treatment of colds, flu and bronchitis. As discovered by the ancients, it also promotes digestion, and combats dyspepsia and flatulence. The West Indian oil is favoured in the treatment of rheumatic pain because of its anti-inflammatory properties and is widely used as a general tonic. Both can be used in inhalation, baths and massage.

CAUTION: Avoid application to sensitive skins.

Benzoin
Styrax benzoin

For skin complaints, benzoin is indicated in the treatment of chapped, inflamed or irritated skin. Its antiseptic properties make it a popular choice for urinary, respiratory and throat infections. Benzoin also has uplifting qualities which can relieve stress and nervous tension when used in a massage oil. As an expectorant, many therapists recommend a few drops of benzoin in a pint of hot water as an inhalation.

CAUTION: Compound tincture of benzoin (which contains other substances including aloe, tolu balsam and storax) occasionally causes sensitivity, but benzoin itself is generally non-toxic and non-irritant.

Bergamot
Citrus bergamia

Oil of bergamot is obtained from a plant that

is a native species of some Asian and Eastern countries. The oil was first used and traded in Italy and derives its name from the northern city of Bergamo. In Italian medicine, it was popular as a remedy for feverish illnesses and to expel intestinal worms. It has also been used in cosmetics and perfumes, as the flavouring of Earl Grey tea, and in other foods. Recent research carried out in Italy indicates a wide variety of therapeutic applications for bergamot, including urinary tract and respiratory infections.

Its strong antiseptic effect makes it a good choice for the treatment of skin, throat and mouth infections.

In particular, scalp and skin conditions such as psoriasis, acne and ulcers will often respond to treatment with bergamot, especially where stress and depression may have played a part in lowering resistance to infection. When combined with eucalyptus, its soothing effect will afford relief to sufferers of cold sores and shingles. Insomnia, anxiety and depression can be alleviated by the uplifting and refreshing nature of this oil. It also has a natural deodorizing effect and can be used both as a breath freshener and as a personal deodorant.

CAUTION: Bergamot can irritate the skin if used in concentrations in excess of one per cent. It is phototoxic and should not be used in homemade suntan oil.

Cajeput
Melaleuca cajeputi

Therapists have found cajeput helpful for relief of a wide variety of complaints. Used in baths, diffusers, inhalation and massage, cajeput can bring relief from asthma, bronchitis, sinusitis and throat infections. Occasionally it has been used to treat diarrhoea and indigestion.

CAUTION: It may be irritant to the skin if used in high concentrations.

Cedarwood
Juniperus virginiana

Cedarwood seems to be beneficial in skin and scalp conditions such as alopecia, acne, dandruff and eczema. It also helps the body to fight respiratory infections and problems and has a mild diuretic effect which can be useful in the treatment of urinary tract infections. Cedarwood has been credited with aphrodisiac qualities.

CAUTION: High concentrations may irritate the skin, and on **no account** must cedarwood be

used during pregnancy as it is a powerful abortifacient.

Chamomile (Roman)
Chamaemelum nobile

There are several varieties, but Roman chamomile is the essential oil of choice for home use. It is used by therapists to treat many skin complaints and promotes the healing of burns, cuts, bites and inflammations. It is also effective in allergic conditions and can have a beneficial effect on menstrual problems when used regularly in the bath. It seems to be effective in reducing stress and anxiety and problems such as headache, migraine and insomnia. As an analgesic, it is used in the treatment of earache, toothache, neuralgia and abscesses, and is popular for treating childhood illnesses.

CAUTION: Camomile is generally non-toxic and non-irritant, but may cause dermatitis in very sensitive individuals.

Cinnamon
Cinnamomum zeylanicum

This oil possesses a warm, spicy aroma and has been favoured in the treatment of nausea, dyspepsia, flatulence and other digestive disturbances. Its warm, soothing qualities can be beneficial to rheumatism when used in massage oil on the affected parts.

These soothing, relaxing qualities also impart a strong stress-relieving effect.

CAUTION: Cinnamon can be irritant to the mucous membranes in large doses. Oil distilled from the bark is especially irritant to skin and mucous membranes and should never be directly applied. It is unsafe for home use and must only be used by a trained aromatherapist.

Clary Sage
Salvia sclarea

Clary sage is possessed of antispasmodic, antidepressant, balsamic, carminative, tonic, aperitive, astringent, anti-inflammatory, bactericidal and antiseptic qualities. It is valuable in stress-related conditions and has an anti-hypertensive effect. A thick mucilage can be made from the seeds, which was traditionally used for removing particles of dust from the eyes. Clary sage is also indicated in the treatment of colds and throat infections. It is also good for regulating menstrual problems and for soothing problem skin, particularly if dry or sensitive.

CAUTION: It should be avoided during pregnancy and also in conjunction with alcohol consumption. However, in general, clary sage has very low toxicity levels and is therefore preferable to garden sage for use in aromatherapy.

Clove
Eugenia aromatica

Clove is a useful antiemetic and should also be used for dyspepsia. It has a powerful antiseptic and a mild analgesic action which make it popular in the relief of gum infections and aching teeth. Its expectorant effect is valuable in the treatment of bronchitis and catarrh. It is widely used as an antihistamine and an antirheumatic and to treat skin conditions such as scabies and athlete's foot. It is also good for treating infections, especially colds and flu, and is often an ingredient of commercially available digestive tonics and mouthwashes.

CAUTION: It can cause mucous membrane irritation and is therefore best used in small doses. It can be dangerous and is best used only by a trained aromatherapist.

Cypress
Cupressus sempervirens

Cypress is thought to be beneficial to the urinary system and seems to help in conditions involving a loss of fluid. These include excessive perspiration, diarrhoea and menorrhagia. Used in the bath, cypress brings great relief to tired aching legs and feet. On the skin, or in a massage oil, its antiseptic and astringent actions can have a balancing effect on oily skin and provide an aid to healing. Cypress is often used by therapists to reduce swellings and nasal congestion, and it is useful in the treatment of colds and flu.

CAUTION: Not to be used by those suffering from hypertension, otherwise non-irritant and non-toxic.

Eucalyptus
Eucalyptus globulus

Eucalyptus is a native species of Australia and Tasmania but is now grown in many countries throughout the world. The plant has a characteristic pungent odour, and the oil obtained from it has disinfectant and antiseptic properties, clears the nasal passages and acts as a painkiller. The leaves and twigs are subjected to a process of steam distillation in order to obtain the essential oil used in aromatherapy. The diluted oil is used for muscular and rheumatic aches and pains, skin disorders such as ringworm, insect bites, headaches and neuralgia, shingles, respiratory and bronchitic infections and fevers. Eucalyptus is used in many household products and in remedies for coughs

and colds. Its analgesic properties are often used to ease the discomfort of shingles, chicken pox and herpes as well as to soothe muscular aches and sprains.

CAUTION: When diluted, eucalyptus is safe to use externally, but can be fatal if taken internally.

Fennel (Sweet)
Foeniculum vulgare

Fennel has properties similar to those of aniseed, so that it is frequently used to treat colic and flatulence. It is also a mild natural laxative. It is credited with an action similar to oestrogen and is thought to stimulate milk production in nursing mothers. This action also indicates fennel in the treatment of menopausal symptoms. As a mild diuretic, it slows the build-up of toxic waste, which is a causative factor in gout and liver problems. Fennel is also suitable for children's complaints.

CAUTION: Avoid use on sensitive skin or prior to exposure to sun. It should not be used by epileptics or pregnant women. Bitter fennel oil can be dangerous and is best used only by a trained aromatherapist.

Frankincense
Boswellia carteri

The inhalation of frankincense is used to relieve the symptoms of bronchitis and laryngitis, and its soothing effect is useful in the treatment of asthma, attacks of which may be brought on by anxiety or emotional stress. It is also indicated in urinary tract problems such as cystitis and is sometimes used as a uterine tonic. Its healing properties have long been valued in the treatment of wounds, and it is often used in skin preparations for mature skins. It has an extremely relaxing aroma and is ideal in the bath for soothing away the day's stress.

Geranium
Pelargonium graveolens

Geranium is an excellent 'all-round' oil, with a wide range of uses, particularly for menopausal problems and pre-menstrual tension. Its diuretic quality makes it a wise choice for fluid retention, and cellulitis and mastitis often respond well to it. For skin conditions and emotional disorders, it is a popular choice in the bath and in massage oil. Serious skin conditions often respond to its antiseptic and antifungal qualities.

CAUTION: Generally non-toxic and non-irritant, it may cause contact dermatitis in hypersensitive individuals.

Jasmine
Jasminum officinalis

Because jasmine is so costly, it is not much used in home aromatherapy, but like all essential oils it does have therapeutic uses. Its heady, uplifting scent makes it useful in the treatment of stress-related illnesses. It also has a smoothing effect on skin and is a valuable component in skin care preparations. It also seems to have a regulating effect on the menstrual cycle, and has been successfully used for throat problems, coughs and catarrh. However, as there are many less expensive oils that will perform these functions, jasmine's main use is as a fragrance ingredient in perfumes.

CAUTION: Although non-toxic and non-irritant, it has, on occasion, caused an allergic reaction

Juniper Berry
Juniperus communis

Juniper is a native species of many northern countries and has a long history of medicinal use. It has stimulant, tonic and antiseptic properties. It is beneficial in the treatment of stress and sleeplessness. In cases of debility, it helps by acting as a tonic for the digestion and boosting the appetite.

Juniper seems to be beneficial to the digestive system, the female reproductive system and the menstrual cycle. It also helps regulate problem skin and is favoured by therapists in the treatment of acne, eczema, dermatitis and haemorrhoids. It helps disperse uric acid build-up and is therefore useful in the treatment of gout and other joint problems. It is a good stress-reliever, especially when used in the bath, and has a mild diuretic action which indicates its use in cystitis. Juniper also acts as an appetite stimulant, and is often used to get rid of intestinal parasites. It can be used in massage and baths.

CAUTION: Juniper stimulates uterine contractions and therefore should not be used in pregnancy. It should also be avoided by those with kidney disease. Generally non-toxic, but it may be slightly irritant.

Lavender
Lavendula vera

The highly perfumed lavender is a native species of the Mediterranean but has long been popular as a garden plant in Britain and many other countries. It has antiseptic, tonic and relaxing properties, and the essential oil used in aromatherapy is obtained by subjecting the flowers to a process of steam distillation. It is considered to be one of the safest preparations and is used in the treatment of a wide range of disorders.

Lavender is an appetite stimulant, a tonic and an antispasmodic. It is particularly effective in the treatment of minor burns and scalds, wounds, sores and varicose ulcers, and is generally one of the most versatile and widely used oils for healing. It also has a strong antiseptic effect and is employed in many cosmetic preparations and as an insect repellent. It is also used in the treatment of muscular aches and pains, respiratory problems, influenza, digestive problems, and genito-urinary problems such as cystitis and dysmenorrhoea. Its soothing effect is recommended for headaches and pre-menstrual tension. Lavender is a very safe oil and can even be applied undiluted to the skin.

Lemon
Citrus limonium

As a massage oil lemon can have a very stimulating effect on the circulation, and seems to have the ability to stimulate the body's own immune system. Therefore, it is frequently used to treat circulatory problems and respiratory ailments such as asthma, bronchitis and catarrh. As a digestive aid, lemon can have a calming effect on dyspepsia. As a natural cosmetic, lemon has an astringent and toning effect.

CAUTION: It is generally safe but should not be used prior to exposure to sunlight.

Lemongrass
Cymbopogon citratus

Combined with neroli in a massage oil, lemongrass brings relief to muscular aches and pains. It also has a sedative effect on the central nervous system, inducing a deep sense of relaxation when used in the bath. Lemongrass has an extremely strong bactericidal and fungicidal effect, which indicates its use in a variety of infections such as athlete's foot and thrush. It is also helpful in digestive disturbances such as colitis and indigestion, especially where stress or anxiety is a factor.

CAUTION: It is generally non-toxic, but occasionally dermatitis has been reported in sensitive individuals. Use under the guidance of a trained therapist.

Mandarin
Citrus nobilis

Mandarin is still a popular oil in the treatment of digestive weaknesses and liver disturbances and is especially preferred for children and the elderly because of its gentle nature. For stress, anxiety, insomnia and nervousness, its use is recommended in conjunction with other citrus oils. Like neroli, it is also a wonderful skin tonic, particularly for acne and oily skins. It is also indicated in the treatment of fluid retention.

CAUTION: Generally very safe, although its use on the skin is not recommended prior to exposure to sunlight.

Marjoram (Sweet)
Origanum marjorana

Marjoram can be extremely effective in reducing the pain and swelling of muscular damage, bruises and sprains, and arthritis. It has an extremely hypnotic effect, which is useful in inducing sleep and calming emotions, especially when used in the bath. It can also be effective in menstrual problems. Marjoram is also a popular treatment for colds and coughs, bronchitis and asthma, and has a carminative and antispasmodic action on colic, constipation and flatulence.

CAUTION: It should be avoided by pregnant women as it has a strong emmenagogic effect.

Melissa True
Melissa officinalis

Melissa is used in the treatment of respiratory disorders, nausea, indigestion and skin disorders. It is said to regulate menstruation and fertility, and is helpful in the treatment of anxiety and depression because of its revitalising properties. It also relieves wasp and bee stings and aids their healing. *The British Herbal Pharmacopoeia* recommends it for flatulent dyspepsia, neurasthenia and depressive illness.

CAUTION: It has caused occasional sensitization and dermal irritations and is therefore best used in low concentrations. Rarely stocked commercially, most melissa oils are blends and should be labelled so.

Myrrh
Commiphora myrrha

Myrrh has a stimulant effect on the mucous membranes and is therefore a useful expectorant. It is still used in Chinese medicine to treat menstrual disturbances and complaints, haemorrhoids and sores. It is also indicated for dental problems and is an effective antiseptic gargle for throat infections. It has long been known as an appetite stimulant and is a valuable ingredient in beauty treatments for mature skin.

CAUTION: Myrrh has an emmenagogic action

and therefore should not be used by pregnant women.

Neroli
Citrus aurantium

Neroli is an extremely expensive oil to produce because of the volume of flowers required, but it is very much in demand because of its wonderful aroma. This is frequently harnessed in massage oil because of its power to uplift, calm and relax. It is also believed to have qualities that are beneficial to the skin, and is widely used to prevent stretch marks and scarring, to reduce thread veins and as an aid for dry, sensitive skin. Neroli's stress-relieving qualities indicate its use in a wide variety of complaints, ranging from colitis and diarrhoea to palpitations, insomnia and premenstrual tension.

Niaouli
Melaleuca viridiflora

Niaouli has a sweet, fresh fragrance and is strongly antiseptic and non-irritant, making it popular in the treatment of acne, boils and other skin irritations. It also makes a very stimulating chest rub and is good when vaporized.

Nutmeg
Myristica fragrans

Nutmeg is recommended in *The British Herbal Pharmacopoeia* for a variety of digestive complaints such as dysentery, nausea, dyspepsia, flatulence and diarrhoea. It has powerful stimulant properties that lend it to the treatment of poor circulation, poor appetite and menstrual irregularities. It can also be applied locally in massage to soothe aches and pains and to relieve rheumatism. Its warming effects are particularly welcome in the winter, and it has strong stimulant properties that lend it to the treatment of poor circulation.

CAUTION: It must not be used in high doses or for extended periods of time, as essential oil of nutmeg can induce hallucinations and hypnosis. Avoid its use during pregnancy. Nutmeg should always be well diluted, even for bathing purposes, as it can cause skin irritation. It can be dangerous and should be used only under the supervision of a trained aromatherapist.

Orange (Sweet)
Citrus sinensis

Sweet orange essential oil is very useful in the treatment of respiratory infections such as colds, bronchitis and influenza, and is thought to increase bronchial secretions. It can also help oily and dull complexions when used as part of a skin care routine. Having similar stress-relieving qualities to neroli, it is also helpful in the alleviation of stress-related complaints. As a gentle aid to digestion, it is often used to ease dyspepsia and constipation.

CAUTION: It is generally safe but should not be applied to the skin prior to exposure to sunlight.

Parsley
Petroselinum Crispum

Parsley has a diuretic and emmenagogic effect, which makes it useful for menstrual problems. It also has the power to reduce fever and has a soothing effect on colic, flatulence and indigestion. It is used for treating bladder and kidney problems, and is also indicated in the treatment of arthritis, rheumatism and sciatica, cystitis and urinary tract infections.

CAUTION: Oil of parsley is moderately toxic, therefore it is wise to use it in moderation and to avoid it completely in pregnancy. It should be used only under the supervision of a trained aromatherapist.

Patchouli
Pogostemon patchouli

Patchouli possesses a soothing, calming earthy scent. It is a good antiseptic with anti-inflammatory properties, which makes it a sensible choice in the treatment of minor burns. Patchouli has also been credited with aphrodisiac powers, and is excellent for relieving a variety of skin disorders including acne, athlete's foot, eczema and dry and cracked skin. It is also used for treating poisonous snakebites in Japan and Malaysia.

Peppermint
Mentha piperita

Peppermint is a native plant of Europe with a long history of medicinal use dating back to the ancient civilizations of Egypt, Greece and Rome. Oil of peppermint is obtained by subjecting the flowering parts of the plant to a process of steam distillation. The essential oil of peppermint has a calming effect on the digestive tract and is excellent for the relief of indigestion, colic-type pains, nausea, travel and morning sickness. It is also an extremely gentle inhalation for asthma. It is cooling and refreshing, and useful in the treatment of colds, respiratory symptoms and headaches.

Peppermint is widely used in remedies for

colds and indigestion, as a food flavouring, especially in confectionery, and in toothpaste.
CAUTION: Possibly irritant to sensitive skin— use in moderation always.

Petitgrain
Citrus bigordia

Petitgrain can be used as a mild antidepressant substitute for neroli, and is effective in the alleviation of anxiety and insomnia. It is also valuable in skin care, having a balancing and toning effect on greasy skin conditions. In the digestive system, it reduces the symptoms of dyspepsia and flatulence.

Pine
Pinus sylvestris

Pine has a strong antiseptic quality, valued for its effectiveness in treating respiratory conditions and relieving asthma, blocked sinuses and catarrh when used as an inhalation. Its stimulating effect also makes it a good choice as a warming massage oil for muscular pains and strains. It has a multitude of other applications for cuts and sores, arthritis and rheumatism, cystitis and urinary tract infections, fatigue, stress, anxiety and neuralgia.

CAUTION: Those with a tendency towards sensitive skin should avoid bathing in pine oil. Pine oil should only be used under the direction of a trained aromatherapist and is unsafe for home use.

Rose
Rosa centifola

Rose has a supremely feminine and deeply sensual aroma, which is the traditional mainstay of the perfume industry. Rose oil has a wonderful antidepressant effect that may be harnessed in body and face massages, baths or vaporizers to treat anxiety, stress and depression. It also has a gentle balancing effect on gynaecological disorders and is said to have aphrodisiac properties.

Rosemary
Rosemarinus officinalis

Rosemary has a wide application and is effective in the treatment of numerous complaints. Possessing a powerful aroma, rosemary is favoured as a decongestant in inhalation and an invigorating muscle-strengthening massage oil. Skin and hair problems can respond well to rosemary, and gargling with it will freshen the breath. Above all, rosemary seems to possess remarkable memory and concentration-enhancing properties. Other therapeutic uses are in digestive disorders, headaches and stress.

CAUTION: It should be avoided during pregnancy and should not be used by epileptics.

Sage
Salvia officinalis

Sage is a native plant of the northern coastal regions of the Mediterranean and has a long history of medicinal and culinary use dating back to the ancient civilizations of Greece and Rome. The essential oil used in aromatherapy is obtained by subjecting the dried leaves to a process of steam distillation. Sage has an expectorant effect when used in inhalations, and its astringent and cooling properties make it a popular choice as a tonic, an appetite stimulant and as a fever reducer. Its antiseptic effects are beneficial to sore throats and mouth problems if used in a gargle or mouthwash. It is also used to improve poor circulation, sore throats, colds and viral infections, bronchitic and catarrhal complaints, rheumatism, arthritic pains, joint sprains and strains, mouth infections and headaches. Sage is widely used as a flavouring in foods and in some household preparations and toiletries.

CAUTION: It should be avoided during pregnancy and if epileptic. Sage is toxic if ingested and is best substituted with clary sage for home use.

Sandalwood
Santalum album

Its preservative powers are often employed to lengthen the life of creams and potions. Sandalwood is a wonderful facial oil, with a soothing emollient effect on dry or sensitive skin. This oil also has a powerful relaxing effect and can alleviate upset stomachs, especially where nervous tension or stress has been a causative factor. Sandalwood also seems to have a powerful antiseptic effect that is particularly useful in the treatment of cystitis and urinary tract infections. It is also favoured for menstrual problems, as a sedative and for catarrh.

Tea Tree
Melaleuca alternifolia

Tea tree contains four substances that do not occur anywhere else in nature and, next to thyme, is the most antiseptic of all oils. It is also strongly disinfectant, antibacterial, antifungal, and antiviral—all qualities that make tea tree an invaluable weapon in the treatment of a multitude of infections. Similarly, it also seems to offer a boost to the body's own immune system whenever threat of infection occurs. Tea tree should be considered when treating any of the following problems: colds, influenza, bronchitis and asthma, warts and verrucas, burns and inflammation, thrush and similar fungal infections, mild shock and hysteria. It can be used undiluted on facial spots and, in a cream, on sunburn.

CAUTION: It is generally very safe, but may cause sensitization in some people.

Thyme (Sweet)
Thymus vulgaris

Thyme is a strong antiseptic, perhaps the strongest of any oil, and is also a powerful stimulant to the appetite, the immune system, and the central nervous system. Respiratory infections, coughs and asthma all seem to respond well to thyme oil, especially if used in inhalations and gargles. Note, however, that gargles must not be swallowed and care must be taken to use the thyme in low dilutions. Its use is indicated in a wide variety of fungal, bacterial and viral infections, in the treatment of wounds and sores and as an aid to the immune system.

CAUTION: It should not be applied undiluted to the skin or used during pregnancy, or on children's skin. Always dilute prior to use in the bath. In fact, generally it is best used in low concentrations. There are several types of thyme, some of which can be dangerous. Only sweet thyme is safe for home use.

Ylang ylang
Cananga odorata

Ylang ylang is a native species of the Far Eastern islands of Indonesia, the Philippines, Java and Madagascar. To obtain the essential oil used in aromatherapy, the flowers are subjected to a process of steam distillation. Like most essential oils ylang ylang has a strong antiseptic effect, but it is best known for its euphoric and aphrodisiac properties. The nervous system can also benefit greatly from its relaxing powers, and its antidepressant powers can also be harnessed to treat mild shock, anger and stress. It has a calming effect on the heart-beat rate and can be used to relieve palpitations, tachycardia, hypertension (raised blood pressure), depression and shock.

It is used widely as an ingredient in skin care, having a wonderful tonic effect and gentle action.

CAUTION: It is generally very safe, although sensitization has been reported in a small number of cases. Used excessively, it can cause nausea or headache.

Herbal Remedies

History of the use of herbal remedies

Herbalism is sometimes maligned as a collection of home-made remedies to be applied in a placebo fashion to one symptom or another, provided the ailment is not too serious and provided there is a powerful chemical wonder-drug at the ready to suppress any 'real' symptoms. We often forget, however, that botanical medicine provides a complete system of healing and disease prevention. It is the oldest and most natural form of medicine. Its record of efficacy and safety spans centuries and covers every country worldwide. Because herbal medicine is holistic medicine, it is, in fact, able to look beyond the symptoms to the underlying systemic imbalance; when skillfully applied by a trained practitioner, herbal medicine offers very real and permanent solutions to concrete problems, many of them seemingly intractable to pharmaceutical intervention.

Early civilizations

The medicinal use of herbs is said to be as old as mankind itself. In early civilizations, food and medicine were linked and many plants were eaten for their health-giving properties. In ancient Egypt, the slave workers were given a daily ration of garlic to help fight off the many fevers and infections that were common at that time. The first written records of herbs and their beneficial properties were compiled by the ancient Egyptians. Most of our knowledge and use of herbs can be traced back to the Egyptian priests who also practised herbal medicine. Records dating back to 1500 BC listed medicinal herbs, including caraway and cinnamon.

The ancient Greeks and Romans also carried out herbal medicine, and as they invaded new lands their doctors encountered new herbs and introduced herbs such as rosemary or lavender into new areas. Other cultures with a history of herbal medicine are the Chinese and the Indians. In Britain, the use of herbs developed along with the establishment of monasteries around the country, each of which had its own herb garden for use in treating both the monks and the local people. In some areas, particularly Wales and Scotland, Druids and other Celtic healers are thought to have had an oral tradition of herbalism, where medicine was mixed with religion and ritual.

The first publications

Over time, these healers and their knowledge led to the writing of the first 'herbals', which rapidly rose in importance and distribution upon the advent of the printing press in the 15th century. John Parkinson of London wrote a herbal around 1630, listing useful plants. Many herbalists set up their own apothecary shops, including the famous Nicholas Culpepper (1616–1654) whose most famous work is *The Complete Herbal and English Physician, Enlarged,* published in 1649. Then in 1812, Henry Potter started a business supplying herbs and dealing in leeches. By this time a huge amount of traditional knowledge and folklore on medicinal herbs was available from Britain, Europe, the Middle East, Asia and the Americas. This promoted Potter to write *Potter's Encyclopaedia of Botanical Drugs and Preparations*, which is still published today.

The decline of herbal medicine

It was in this period that scientifically inspired conventional medicine rose in popularity, sending herbal medicine into a decline. In rural areas, herbal medicine continued to thrive in local folklore, traditions and practices. In 1864 the National Association (later Institute) of Medical Herbalists was established, to organize training of herbal medicine practitioners and to maintain standards of practice. From 1864 until the early part of this century, the Institute fought attempts to ban herbal medicine and over time public interest in herbal medicine has increased, particularly over the last 20 years. This move away from synthetic drugs is partly due to possible side effects, bad publicity, and, in some instances, a mistrust of the medical and pharmacological industries. The more natural appearance of herbal remedies has led to its growing support and popularity. Herbs from America have been incorporated with common remedies and scientific research into herbs and their active ingredients has confirmed their healing power and enlarged the range of medicinal herbs used today.

Its rise and relevance today

Herbal medicine can be viewed as the precursor of modern pharmacology, but today it continues as an effective and more natural method of treating and preventing illness. Globally, herbal medicine is three to four times more commonly practised than conventional medicine.

Nowhere is the efficacy of herbalism more evident than in problems related to the nervous system. Stress, anxiety, tension and depression are intimately connected with most illness. Few health practitioners would argue with the influence of nervous anxiety in pathology. Nervous tension is generally acknowledged by doctors to contribute to duodenal and gastric ulceration, ulcerative colitis, irritable bowel syndrome and many other gut-related pathologies.

We know also, from physiology, that when a person is depressed, the secretion of hydrochloric acid—one of the main digestive juices—is also reduced so that digestion and absorption are rendered less efficient. Anxiety, on the other hand, can lead to the release of adrenaline and stimulate the over-production of hydrochloric acid and result in a state of acidity that may exacerbate the pain of an inflamed ulcer. In fact, whenever the voluntary nervous system (our conscious anxiety) interferes with the autonomic processes (the automatic nervous regulation that in health is never made conscious), illness is the result.

Herbalists rely on their knowledge of botanical remedies to rectify this type of human malfunction. The medical herbalist will treat a stubborn dermatological problem using 'alternatives' specific to the skin problem, and then apply circulatory stimulants to aid in the removal of toxins from the area, with remedies to reinforce other organs of elimination, such as the liver and kidneys. Under such natural treatment, free of any discomforting side effects, the patient can feel confident and relaxed–perhaps for the first time in many months.

Curiously, this is an approach that has never been taken up by orthodox medicine. There, the usual treatment of skin problems involves suppression of symptoms with steroids. However, the use of conventional antihistamines or benzodiazepines often achieves less lasting benefit to the patient because of the additional burden of side effects, such as drowsiness, increased toxicity, and long-term drug dependence.

Herbs, on the other hand, are free from toxicity and habituation. Because they are organic substances and not manmade synthetic molecules, they possess an affinity for the human organism. They are extremely efficient in balancing the nervous system. Restoring a sense of wellbeing and relaxation is necessary for optimum health and for the process of self-healing.

Naturally, the choice of a treatment should be based upon a thorough health assessment and the experience and training of a qualified herbal practitioner. The herbalist will then prepare and prescribe herbal remedies in a variety of different forms, such as infusions, loose teas, suppositories, inhalants, lotions, tinctures, tablets and pills. Many of these preparations are available for home use from chemists, health shops and mail-order suppliers.

Herbs for stress management

Camomile

This has a relaxing effect on the mind and body. It is an excellent sedative for anxiety and muscle tenseness. Many people enjoy its benefits in the form of camomile tea.

Valerian

This is the ideal tranquillizer. The rhizomes of this plant contain a volatile oil (which includes valerianic acid), volatile alkaloids (including chatinine), and iridoids (valepotriates), which have been shown to reduce anxiety and aggression. So effective is Valerian in relieving anxiety while maintaining normal mental awareness, that it enables us to continue the most complicated mental exercise without drowsiness, loss of consciousness or depression. Valerian has been usefully taken before an examination or a driving test!

Peppermint

This is effective for treating digestive discomfort: it relieves indigestion, flatulence, constipation and nausea. Peppermint is also a good mind tonic, helping to clarify ideas and focus concentration. It is also helpful in alleviating the symptoms of colds and influenza. peppermint and camomile tea is thought to be effective in reducing the pain of tension headaches and migraines.

Vervain

This is not only effective against depression but also strongly supports the detoxifying function of the liver. Its French name is still 'Herbe Sacre'; an old English name is 'Holy Wort' — it was one of the seven sacred herbs of the Druids. Today we know that the antispasmodic qualities of Verbena are largely due to the glycoside verbenalin. Recent Chinese research has linked the plant with dilation of arteries in the brain: a likely explanation of its usefulness in treating migraine, especially when this problem is accompanied by liver congestion. It is certainly of use to treat exhaustion and depression.

St John's Wort

Also called *Hypericum perforatum*, St John's wort has analgesic and anti-inflammatory properties, with important local applications to neuralgia and sciatica. Systemically, its sedative properties are based on the glycoside hypericin (a red pigment), which makes it applicable to neurosis and irritability. Many herbalists use it extensively as a background remedy.

Lemon balm

This herb is both carminative and antispasmodic, and is active specifically on that part of the vagus nerve that may interfere with the harmonious functioning of the heart and the stomach. Recent research has indicated that the action of the volatile oil begins within the limbic system of the brain and subsequently operates directly upon the vagus nerve and all the organs that are innervated by it. Accordingly, neurasthenia (complete nervous prostration), migraine, and nervous gastropathy are amenable to its healing power.

Lime flowers

These are thought to be helpful in controlling anxiety and hyperactivity. They are also effective for treating insomnia, high blood pressure and for soothing muscles and nerves.

Borage

This is an effective mind tonic, which helps to alleviate headaches, migraine and depression.

Oats

Oats is one of the great herbal restoratives of the nervous system. The plant contains a nervine alkaloid that is helpful in angina and in cardiac insufficiency. It has also been used in the treatment of addiction to morphine, narcotics, tobacco and alcohol.

Soothing herbal drinks

Warm milk and honey

Perhaps with a dash of cinnamon, this is an ideal drink to take at bedtime. It will help you relax and ward off insomnia.

Hop tea

Three hop cones, or heads, infused in a cup of boiling water whenever you begin to feel excessively tense, is a marvellous remedy for anxiety and insomnia.

A soothing herb tea to sustain a feeling of equilibrium

25g (1 oz) each dried chamomile flowers, lime flowers, hibiscus blossoms and marigold flowers
15g ($\frac{1}{2}$ oz) each dried peppermint leaves and vervain
1 teaspoon whole fenugreek seeds
100g (4 oz) Lapsang Souchong tea

Mix all the ingredients together and store in a dark airtight container. Use 1 teaspoon to 300 ml ($\frac{1}{2}$ pint) of boiling water in a tea pot and leave to infuse for five minutes before straining and serving with a slice of lemon and a teaspoon of honey if desired. This is a very calming tea that soothes feelings of anxiety. It also helps to clear your head and settle an upset tummy. One cup taken morning and night will promote a feeling of wellbeing.

Another calming tea, especially good for the nerves

1 teaspoon each grated valerian root and dried mint
$\frac{1}{2}$ teaspoon each dried chamomile and lavender flowers
600 ml (1 pint) boiling water

Infuse the dry ingredients in the water for 15 minutes then strain and take a glass three times a day for one week only.

Two tonic teas to sip when feeling depressed

Sip either 2 teaspoons of dandelion and 1 of basil infused in 600 ml (1 pint) of boiling water, or 2 teaspoons each of nettle, basil and melissa infused in 600 ml (1 pint) of boiling water.

A tonic tea to relieve stress and anxiety

1 tablespoon each fresh dandelion and nettle tops
1 teaspoon each fresh blackcurrant and borage leaves
600 ml (1 pint) boiling water

Steep the greenery in the water for five minutes. Strain and drink with lemon and honey.

Dock wine

Dock is one of the great tonic herbs because it is extremely high in iron. Here is a recipe for an old-fashioned dock wine.

175g (7 oz) dock root
15g (¹/₂ oz) liquorice wood
7g (¹/₄ oz) juniper berries
100g (4 oz) raw cane sugar
2 litres (3¹/₂ pints) organic red wine

Put all the ingredients together in a china container, cover and place either in a very slow oven or in a bain marie. Continue to heat gently until the mixture is reduced by half. Strain, bottle and seal tightly. Drink a sherry glass of the dock wine every morning for two weeks.

Rosemary in wine

Steep 6 sprigs of rosemary in a well-sealed bottle of sweet white wine for 14 days. Take 1 wineglass as a daily tonic.

Sage tonic

Take 100g (4 oz) of fresh sage leaves and put them in a bottle of organic white wine for two weeks. Sweeten to taste with honey and leave for another day. Press and strain through muslin. Bottle, and take 1 sherry glass before lunch and dinner.

You can also infuse sage leaves in boiling water, strain and sweeten with honey for an uplifting sage tea.

A-Z of Herbal Remedies

Aconite *Aconitum napellus*. COMMON NAME: Monkshood, blue rocket, friar's cap, wolfsbane.

OCCURRENCE: indigenous to mountain slopes in the Alps and Pyrenees. Introduced into England very early, before 900 AD.

PARTS USED: the leaves used fresh and the root when dried. It contains alkaloidal material—aconitine, benzaconine and aconine amongst other compounds.

MEDICINAL USES: the plant is poisonous and should not be used except under medical advice. It is an anodyne, diaphoretic, febrifuge and sedative. Used for reducing fever and inflammation in the treatment of catarrh, tonsillitis and croup. It may be used in controlling heart spasm.

ADMINISTERED AS: tincture, liniment and occasionally as injection.

Agrimony *Agrimonia eupatoria*. COMMON NAME: Church steeples, cockeburr, sticklewort.

OCCURRENCE: field borders, ditches and hedges throughout England. Found locally in Scotland.

PARTS USED: the herb. Contains a particular volatile oil, tannin and a bitter principle.

MEDICINAL USES: mild astringent, tonic, diuretic, deobstruent. It has a reputation for curing liver complaints and is very good for skin eruptions and blood diseases. Also recommended to treat the sting and bite of snakes.

ADMINISTERED AS: liquid extract.

Alder *Alnus glutinosa*. COMMON NAME: Betula alnus.

OCCURRENCE: commonly found throughout Britain, usually in moist woods or by streams.

PARTS USED: the bark, wood, shoots, catkins and leaves have all been used as dyes. The bark and leaves contain tannic acid.

MEDICINAL USES: tonic and astringent. Used as a decoction to bathe swelling and inflammation, particularly of the throat.

ADMINISTERED AS: decoction.

Allspice *Pimento officinalis*. COMMON NAME: Pimento, jamaica pepper, clove pepper.

OCCURRENCE: indigenous to the West Indies and South America; cultivated in jamaica and central America.

PARTS USED: the fruit, which contains a volatile

oil made up of eugenol, a sesquiterpene and other unknown chemicals.

MEDICINAL USES: aromatic, stimulant, carminative. Allspice acts on the gastro-intestinal tract and is usually added to drinks tonics and purgatives for flavouring. The spice may also be used for flatulent indigestion and hysteria. Allspice is frequently used as a spice and condiment in food or drinks.

ADMINISTERED AS: essential oil, distilled water, powdered fruit, fluid extract.

Aloes *Aloe perryi, Aloe vera*.

OCCURRENCE: indigenous to East and South Africa and introduced into the West Indies.

PARTS USED: the drug aloes is described as "the liquid evaporated to dryness which drains from the leaves." It contains two aloin compounds, barbaloin and isobarbaloin, as well as amorphous aloin, resin and aloe-emodin in differing proportions.

MEDICINAL USES: emmenagogue, purgative, vermifuge, anthelmintic. It is generally administered along with carminative and anodyne drugs, and acts on the lower bowel. The liquid form may be used externally to ease skin irritation.

ADMINISTERED AS: fluid extract, powdered extract, decoction, tincture.

Almond, Sweet *Amygdalus communis* var. *dulais*. **Almond, Bitter** *Amygdalus commis* var. *amara*.

OCCURRENCE: native trees of western Asia and North Africa and cultivated in most Mediterranean countries and Great Britain.

PARTS USED: the nut and the oil expressed from it.

MEDICINAL USES: sweet almonds have demulcent and nutritive properties, but since the outer skin can cause irritation of the alimentary canal, almonds are normally blanched and the skin removed before being used as food. The oil produced is emollient, demulcent, nutritive and slightly laxative, and is mainly used in cosmetics but is also taken internally as a medicine. It is of benefit in allaying acrid juices, softening and relaxing solid materials, bronchial diseases, tickling coughs, hoarseness and nephritic pains. Sweet almonds are made into emulsions with barley water or gum arabic to treat gravel, stone, kidney disorders and bladder and biliary duct problems, with more success than almond oil.

Bitter almonds yield a volatile oil upon distillation with water which is used as a flavouring agent. These almonds contain the glucoside amygdalin and the chemical emulsin that acts on the glucoside to produce glucose, prussic acid and benzaldehyde in the presence of water. Prussic acid is poisonous and use of bitter almond oil must be carefully monitored. In the Middle Ages, the oil was used for intermittent fevers, hydrophobia and as an aperient, diuretic and vermifuge drug, but it is seldom administered medicinally now. The cake left after expressing the oil has a special dietary value and is often made into flour for cakes and biscuits for diabetic patients. Almond oil is used in trade as a lubricant for watches, and in soaps and toiletries.
ADMINISTERED AS: expressed oil, bitter almond oil (with prussic acid removed).

Anemone, Pulsatilla *Anemone pulsatilla*. COMMON NAME: Pasqueflower, meadow anemone, wind flower.
OCCURRENCE: found locally in chalk downs and limestone areas of England.
PARTS USED: the whole herb. It produces oil of anemone upon distillation with water.
MEDICINAL USES: nervine, antispasmodic, alterative and diaphoretic. It is beneficial in disorders of mucous membranes and of the respiratory and digestive passages. Can be used to treat asthma, whooping cough and bronchitis.
ADMINISTERED AS: fluid extract.

Anemone, Wood *Anemone nemorosa*. COMMON NAME: crowfoot, windflower, smell fox.
OCCURRENCE: found in woods and thickets across Great Britain.
PARTS USED: the root, leaves and juice.
MEDICINAL USES: this species of plant is much less widely used than it has been previously. It used to be good for leprosy, lethargy, eye inflammation and headaches. An ointment made of the leaves is said to be effective in cleansing malignant ulcers.
ADMINISTERED AS: decoction, fresh leaves and root, ointment.

Angelica *Angelica archangelica*. COMMON NAME: Garden Angelica, *Archangelica officinalis*.
OCCURRENCE: found native to some sites in Scotland although more abundant in Lapland and is a common garden plant in England.
PARTS USED: the root, leaves and seeds. The

leaves contain volatile oil, valeric acid, angelic acid, a bitter principle and a resin called angelicin. The roots contain terebangelene and other terpenes while the seeds also yield two acid compounds.
MEDICINAL USES: Angelica has carminative, stimulant, diaphoretic, diuretic, aromatic, stomachic, tonic and expectorant properties and is good for colds, coughs, pleurisy, wind, colic and rheumatism. It is used as a stimulating expectorant and is good for digestion.
ADMINISTERED AS: powdered root, liquid extract, infusion or as a poultice.

Angostura *Galipea officinalis*. COMMON NAME: Cusparia bark, *Cusparia febrifuga*, *Bonplandia trifoliata*, *Galipea cusparia*.
OCCURRENCE: a small tree native to tropical South America.
PARTS USED: the dried bark, which has the active ingredients angosturin, the alkaloids galipine, cusparine, galipidine, cusparidine and cuspareine, as well as a volatile oil and an unidentified glucoside.
MEDICINAL USES: aromatic, bitter, tonic, stimulant, purgative. There is a long history of usage by native South Americans as a stimulant tonic. It is useful in bilious diarrhoea and dysentery, but in large doses it has a purgative and cathartic effect on the body.
ADMINISTERED AS: infusion, powdered bark, tincture, fluid extract.

Anise *Pimpinella anisum*. COMMON NAME: Aniseed.
OCCURRENCE: native to Egypt, Greece, Crete and western Asia, its cultivation spread to central Europe and North Africa.
PARTS USED: the fruit. Upon distillation, the fruit yields a fragrant volatile oil that is made up of anethol, choline, a fixed oil, sugar and mucilage.
MEDICINAL USES: carminative and pectoral. It is very useful against coughs and chest infections and is made into lozenges or smoked to clear the chest. Aniseed tea is good for infant catarrh, and aids digestion in adults. Anise seed is an ingredient of cathartic and aperient pills, to relieve flatulence and lessen the griping caused by purgative herbs. It can also be given in convulsions quite safely.
ADMINISTERED AS: essence, essential oil, tincture, powdered seeds, tea and pills.

Apple *Pyrus malus*. COMMON NAME: Wild Apple, *Malus communis*, crab-tree.
OCCURRENCE: native to Great Britain and found

throughout the temperate regions of the northern hemisphere.

PARTS USED: the fruit and bark. Apples contain water, protein material, carbonaceous matter, vitamins, organic acids, salts of potassium, sodium, carbon and magnesium.

MEDICINAL USES: diuretic, slightly astringent. The organic acids in the fruit benefit sedentary people and ease liver problems, gout and indigestion. Apple juice or cider is drunk frequently in some areas e.g. Normandy, where problems of stone or calculus are unknown because of the diuretic effects of apples. Apples can also help cure constipation, scurvy, sleeplessness or bilious complaints. They act as an excellent dentifrice (tooth cleanser) and are applied as a poultice to sore eyes when rotten. A decoction of the bark is used against intermittent and bilious fevers, while cooked apples are used in sore throats, eye problems, and in skin and tissue infected with the *Streptococcus pyogenes* bacterium. Dropsy is helped by drinking cider in which horseradish was steeped.

ADMINISTERED AS: fresh fruit, expressed juice, fermented drink, infusion, decoction, poultice.

Apricot *Prunus armeniaca.* COMMON NAME: Apricock, *Armeniaca vulgaris.*

OCCURRENCE: originally found in northern China, the Himalaya region and temperate Asia. Now cultivated across temperate regions of Europe and introduced into England in the sixteenth century.

PARTS USED: the kernels and the oil expressed from them. The oil contains olein and the glyceride of linolic acid. The cake left after oil removal produces an essential oil upon distillation that contains the glucoside amygdalin and is chemically identical to the essential oil from the almond. It is used in confectionery and as a food flavouring.

MEDICINAL USES: apricot oil is substituted for oil of almonds in cosmetics, because of its lower cost. It has a softening action on the skin.

ADMINISTERED AS: expressed oil, essential oil.

Areca Nut *Areca catechu.* COMMON NAME: Betel nut, pinang.

OCCURRENCE: a tree cultivated in the East Indies, India and Sri Lanka.

PARTS USED: the seeds contain a large amount of tannin, gallic acid, a fixed oil, lignin and a volatile oil. They also contain three alkaloids, arcoline, arecain and guracine with the second listed being the active principle.

MEDICINAL USES: aromatic, astringent, taenacide and mydriatic. The native people chew these nuts, which stain the teeth, lips and excrement red. Taken internally, the seeds expel tapeworms and cause contraction of the pupil of the eye. Areca nut is also made into a toothpaste in Britain.

ADMINISTERED AS: powdered nut, fluid extract.

Arnica *Arnica montana.* COMMON NAME: Mountain tobacco, leopard's bane.

OCCURRENCE: indigenous to central Europe but found in England and southern Scotland.

PARTS USED: the rhizome and flowers. They contain arnicin, tannin, phullin and a volatile oil.

MEDICINAL USES: stimulant, vulnerary and diuretic. It is used in external application to bruises and sprains but is rarely used internally as it irritates the stomach, and may cause severe poisoning. A tincture of arnica has been used to treat epilepsy and seasickness.

ADMINISTERED AS: tincture, poultice.

Arrach *Chenopodium olidum.* COMMON NAME: Stinking motherwort/arrach/goosefoot, dog's arrach, goat's arrach, netchweed.

OCCURRENCE: an annual herb found on waste ground or roadsides throughout Great Britain.

PARTS USED: herb. contains trimethylamine, osmazome and nitrate of potash.

MEDICINAL USES: nervine, emmenagogue, antispasmodic. This is used in female hysteria and was formerly said to cure barrenness.

ADMINISTERED AS: an infusion, fluid extract or injection.

Arrowroot *Maranta arundinacea.* COMMON NAME: *Maranta indica, M. ramosissima,* maranta starch or arrowroot, araruta, Bermuda arrowroot, Indian arrowroot.

OCCURRENCE: indigenous to the West Indies and central America. It is cultivated in Bengal, Java, the Philippines, mauritius and West Africa.

PARTS USED: the dried, powdered starch from the rhizome.

MEDICINAL USES: nutritive, demulcent, non-irritating. Well suited for infants and convalescents, particularly after bowel complaints. The jelly made of water or milk may be flavoured with sugar, lemon juice or fruit. The fresh rhizomes are mashed and applied to wounds from poisoned arrows, scorpion or spider bites and to stop gangrene. The freshly expressed juice of the rhizome, when mixed with water, is said to be a good antidote against vegetable poisons.

ADMINISTERED AS: fresh root, expressed juice, dietary item.

Asarabacca *Asarum europaeum*. COMMON NAME: Hazelwort, wild nard.

OCCURRENCE: Asarabacca is the only British species of the birthwort family and is very rare in. It is found in woodlands.

PARTS USED: the root and herb.

MEDICINAL USES: stimulant, tonic, emetic, purgative, aromatic and sternulatory. As dried powdered leaves of the herb, it is used in the preparation of snuffs, causing sneezing and giving relief to headaches and weak eyes. It has been utilized to remove mucus from the respiratory passages and may be an antidote to the bite of venomous snakes. The herb was formerly used as an emetic or purgative but its use has been replaced by safer drugs.

ADMINISTERED AS: tincture, emulsion.

Asparagus *Asparagus officinalis*. COMMON NAME: Sparrow grass.

OCCURRENCE: a rare native in Britain, but found wild on the south-west coast of England. It is cultivated as a food crop in parts of Scotland.

PARTS USED: the root.

MEDICINAL USES: this plant has diuretic, laxative, cardiac and sedative effects. It is recommended in cases of dropsy.

ADMINISTERED AS: expressed juice, decoction or made in a syrup.

Avens *Geum urbanum*. COMMON NAME: Colewort, herb bennet, city Avens, wild rue, way bennet, goldy star, clove root.

OCCURRENCE: a common hedgerow plant in Britain and Europe.

PARTS USED: the herb and root. The herb contains a volatile oil composed of eugenol and a glucoside, while the root also contains tannin.

MEDICINAL USES: an astringent, styptic, febrifuge, sudorific, stomachic, antiseptic, tonic and aromatic. It is useful in diarrhoea, sore throat, chills, fevers and headache amongst other complaints. An infusion may be used for skin problems, as a wash.

ADMINISTERED AS: an infusion, decoction or tincture.

Balm *Melissa officinalis*. COMMON NAME: Sweet balm, lemon balm, honey plant, cure-all.

OCCURRENCE: a common garden plant in Great Britain, which was naturalized into southern England at a very early period.

PARTS USED: the herb.

MEDICINAL USES: as a carminative, diaphoretic,

or febrifuge. It can be made into a cooling tea for fever patients and balm is often used in combination with other herbs to treat colds and fever.

ADMINISTERED AS: an infusion.

Balmony *Chelone glabra*. COMMON NAME: chelone, bitter herb, snake head, shellflower, turtlehead, turtle bloom, salt-rheum weed, glatte, the hummingbird tree, white chelone.

OCCURRENCE: it grows in swamps, wet woods and rivers in the eastern United States and Canada.

PARTS USED: the whole herb.

MEDICINAL USES: the fresh leaves are anti-bilious, anthelmintic, tonic and detergent in action and are used against consumption, dyspepsia, debility and jaundice. It has a peculiar action on the liver and diseases of that organ, while it is also effective in removing worms from children. When made into an ointment, balmony is recommended for inflamed tumours, ulcers, inflamed breasts and piles.

ADMINISTERED AS: a decoction, powdered herb, fluid extract, tincture.

Balsam of Peru *Myroxylon pereirae*. COMMON NAME: Peruvian balsam, *Toluifera pereira*, *Myrosperum pereira*.

OCCURRENCE: this comes from a large tree that grows in the forest of El Salvador, central America.

PARTS USED: the balsam is an oleoresinous liquid that exudes from the tree after the bark has been beaten and scorched. It is soaked from the tree and boiled in water.

MEDICINAL USES: stimulant, expectorant, parasiticide. It is used in scabies, irritant skin diseases and acute eczema. The balsam is good in all chronic mucous afflictions, catarrh, leucorrhoea, diarrhoea and dysentery. It stimulates the heart and raises blood pressure. The liquid may be applied to sore nipples and discharges from the ear to effect healing.

ADMINISTERED AS: liquid form.

Baneberry *Actaea spicata*. COMMON NAME: Herb Christopher, bugbane, toadroot.

OCCURRENCE: a rare plant in Britain, found only in limestone districts of the Lake District and Yorkshire.

PARTS USED: the root.

MEDICINAL USES: antispasmodic. The plant is acrid and poisonous. The root is used as a remedy for catarrh and some nervous disorders, but the plant must be used with great caution.

ADMINISTERED AS: infusion, dried or fresh root.

Barberry *Berberis vulgaris*. COMMON NAME: Berbery, pipperidge bush, *Berberis dumetorum*.

OCCURRENCE: a common bush that grows wild in some parts of England but is unlikely to be native to Scotland and Ireland.

PARTS USED: the root, root-bark and berries. The bark contains berberine, a bitter alkaloid, along with several other compounds.

MEDICINAL USES: as a tonic, purgative and antiseptic. It is normally used to treat jaundice and liver complaints, and is an aid to regulating digestion and stopping constipation. The berries are used to produce an acid drink that helps ease diarrhoea and fevers.

ADMINISTERED AS: powdered bark, fluid extract and solid extract.

Barley *Hordeum distichon* and *Hordeum vulgare*. COMMON NAME: Pearl barley, *Perlatum*

OCCURRENCE: throughout Britain.

PARTS USED: decorticated seeds; composed of eighty per cent starch and six per cent proteins, cellulose, etc.

MEDICINAL USES: Barley is used to prepare a nutritive and demulcent drink for ill and fevered patients. Barley water is given to sick children suffering from diarrhoea or bowel inflammation etc. malt extract is also used medicinally.

ADMINISTERED AS: an infusion and beverage.

Basil *Ocimum basilicum*. COMMON NAME: Sweet basil, garden basil.

OCCURRENCE: as a garden plant throughout Britain.

PARTS USED: the herb, which contains a volatile, camphoraceous oil.

MEDICINAL USES: aromatic with carminative and cooling properties. It is used to treat mild nervous disorders and an infusion of basil is said to be good for obstructions of the internal organs and in stopping vomiting and nausea.

ADMINISTERED AS: a flavouring in food, dried leaves or an infusion.

Bayberry *Myrica corifera*. COMMON NAME: Candleberry, waxberry, tallow shrub, wax myrtle.

OCCURRENCE: widely distributed through America, Europe and Great Britain.

PARTS USED: the bark, which contains volatile oil, starch, lignin, tannic and gallic acids along with lesser compounds.

MEDICINAL USES: a powerful stimulant, astringent and tonic. The powdered bark may be used in poultices, often together with elm. A decoc-

tion is used to treat the throat and sore gums.

ADMINISTERED AS: an infusion, decoction, powder and injection.

Bearberry *Archostaphylos uva-ursi*. COMMON NAME: *Arbutus uva-ursi, uva-ursi*.

OCCURRENCE: on heaths of the Scottish Highlands, south to Yorkshire, and in high mountains of Europe, Asia and America.

PARTS USED: the leaves, which contain arbutin as the chief constituent.

MEDICINAL USES: when made into an infusion, the leaves have a soothing, astringent and diuretic effect. This is of benefit in diseases affecting the bladder, and the kidneys, e.g. urethritis, cystitis, etc.

ADMINISTERED AS: an infusion.

Beech *Fagus Sylvatica*. COMMON NAME: Buche, boke, faggio, fagos.

OCCURRENCE: found in Europe, including Britain, although only indigenous to England.

PARTS USED: the oil of beech nuts, and beech tar.

MEDICINAL USES: beech tar is stimulating and antiseptic so is used internally as a stimulating expectorant to treat chronic bronchitis. It is used externally applied to various skin diseases.

ADMINISTERED AS: beech oil or beech tar.

Beetroot *Beta vulgaris*. COMMON NAME: Spinach beet, sea beet, garden beet, whit beet, mangelwurzel.

OCCURRENCE: *Beta vulgaris* is native to southern Europe and is derived from the sea beet, *Beta maritima* which grows wild on the coasts of Europe, England, North Africa and Asia. There are many cultivated forms and varieties of beetroot with similar properties.

PARTS USED: the leaves and root. The root contains a pure fruit sugar which is easily taken up by the body, as well as starch and gum.

MEDICINAL USES: the juice of the white beet was said to be of a "cleansing, digestive quality" to "open up obstructions of the liver and spleen" and ease headaches. Beetroot is used to produce refined sugar, as a vegetable and to make wine or ale.

ADMINISTERED AS: dietary item, decoction, expressed juice.

Belladonna *Atropa belladonna*. COMMON NAME: Deadly nightshade, devil's cherries, dwale, black cherry, devil's herb, great morel.

OCCURRENCE: native to central and southern Europe but commonly grows in England.

PARTS USED: the roots and leaves. The root contains several alkaloid compounds including hyoscyamine, atropine and belladonnine. The same alkaloids are present in the leaves but the amount of each compound varies according to plant type and methods of storing and drying leaves.

MEDICINAL USES: as a narcotic, diuretic, sedative, mydriatic, antispasmodic. The drug is used as an anodyne in febrile conditions, night-sweats and coughs. It is valuable in treating eye diseases and is used as a pain-relieving lotion to treat neuralgia, gout, rheumatism and sciatica. Belladonna is an extremely poisonous plant and should always be used under medical supervision. Cases of accidental poisoning and death are well-known. Despite this, it is a valuable drug used to treat a wide range of disease.

ADMINISTERED AS: a liquid extract which is used to produce alcoholic extracts, plasters, liniment, suppositories, tincture and ointment.

Bergamot *Monarda didyma.* COMMON NAME: Scarlet monarda, oswego tea, bee balm.

OCCURRENCE: a plant which is indigenous to North America.

PARTS USED: the oil extracted from the whole plant, and the leaves.

MEDICINAL USES: used in a similar manner to other plants containing thymol as an active chemical. Oil of bergamot has antiseptic, aromatic, carminative, tonic and antispasmodic properties. An infusion of the young leaves was a common beverage in the USA before tea became more common. The infusion is also good for coughs, sore throats, fevers and colds.

ADMINISTERED AS: essential oil, infusion, fluid extract.

Bethroot *Trillium pendulum, Trillium erectum.* COMMON NAME: Indian shamrock, birthroot, lamb's quarters, wake-robin, Indian balm, ground lily.

OCCURRENCE: a native North American plant found in the western and middle United States.

PARTS USED: the dried root and rhizome; the leaves.

MEDICINAL USES: antiseptic, astringent, tonic, expectorant, pectoral and alterative. It is useful in all cases of internal bleeding, profuse menstruation and pulmonary complaints. It is used to promote safe childbirth and delivery. The leaves may be applied to ulcers and tumours while the root makes a good antiseptic poultice to stop gangrene spreading or for skin diseases. It was used by the Native Americans as a medicine.

ADMINISTERED AS: the powdered root, fresh leaves and infusion.

Betony, Wood *Stachys bentonica, Betonica officinalis.* COMMON NAME: Bishopswort.

OCCURRENCE: found wild in woodlands, or on heath or moorland but less common in Scotland.

PARTS USED: the herb.

MEDICINAL USES: aromatic, astringent and alterative. Betony was thought to be one of the best treatments for headaches and hangover. It is normally combined with other herbs to produce a tonic for nervous affections, dyspepsia and rheumatism. The dried herb was also used to make a tea substitute and was smoked as tobacco.

ADMINISTERED AS: an infusion.

Bindweed, Greater *Convolvulus sepium.* COMMON NAME: Hedge convolvulus, old man's night cap, hooded bindweed, bearbind.

OCCURRENCE: a native of Britain which is abundant in England but rarer in Scotland.

PARTS USED: the resin produced from the roots.

MEDICINAL USES: the resin is normally made into a tincture. This preparation is then applied internally and has a purgative effect. The effects are not as pronounced as in the related plant species *Convulvus jalapa* (jalap bindweed) and *Convulvus scammonia* (Syrian bindweed).

ADMINISTERED AS: tincture.

Birch, Common *Betula alba.* COMMON NAME: White birch, bouleau, berke, bereza.

OCCURRENCE: common in Europe, from Sicily to Iceland and also found in northern Asia.

PARTS USED: the bark and leaves. The bark contains tannic acid, behilin and behils camphor while the leaves contain betulorentic acid.

MEDICINAL USES: bitter and astringent. The bark yields oil of birch tar upon destructive distillation, which is very similar to oil of WINTER-GREEN. The oil is used in skin disease ointments, e.g. treating eczema while it is also used as a component of insect repellent. Birch tea made of the leaves is recommended for gout, rheumatism and dropsy and is also said to be good for breaking up kidney stones. Sap from the tree is used to produce beer, wine, spirits and vinegar in various parts of Europe.

ADMINISTERED AS: oil, infusion.

Birthwort *Aristolochia longa.* COMMON NAME: Long-rooted birthwort.

OCCURRENCE: throughout Europe and Great Britain.

PARTS USED: the root, which contains aristolochine.

MEDICINAL USES: aromatic and stimulant. It is useful in treating gout and rheumatism and may be used to clear obstructions after childbirth.

ADMINISTERED AS: powdered root.

Bistort *Polygonum bisorta*. COMMON NAME: Snakeweed, adderwort, twice writhen, osterick, Easter marigiant, English sepentary

OCCURRENCE: a native of many parts of northern Europe, common in the north of England and southern Scotland.

PARTS USED: the root-stock which contains tannin, starch, gallic acid and gum.

MEDICINAL USES: a strong astringent and is mainly used in external and internal bleeding and haemorrhages from the lungs or stomach. Can be used to treat diarrhoea, dysentery, cholera and bowel complaints. Bistort is important in alleviating diabetes and as a mouth wash or gargle to "fasten loose teeth" and heal gum problems.

ADMINISTERED AS: a powder, fluid extract, decoction or injection.

Bitter root *Apocynum androsaemifolium*. COMMON NAME: milkweed, dogsbane, fly-trap, wild cotton.

OCCURRENCE: found in mountainous regions of Europe and North America.

PARTS USED: the dried rhizome and roots. The active chemicals in the plant are a bitter principle called cymarin, and to a lesser extent the glucoside apocynamarin.

MEDICINAL USES: cardiac tonic, hydragogue, alterative. Bitter root is similar to foxglove in action and is very powerful in slowing the pulse and it also has a strong action on the vaso-motor system. It may irritate the mucous membranes, causing nausea and purging of the bowels, so that it cannot be tolerated by all people. As a powerful hydrogogue it is good against fluid accumulation in the abdomen (ascites), particularly when it is linked to liver cirrhosis. It is also highly effective in treating dropsy which is related to heart failure. The plant's alterative powers are used against syphilis, scrofula and rheumatism. Because of irregular absorption of the drug through the gastro-intestinal tract, great care must be taken with the dosage administered and the patient's condition.

ADMINISTERED AS: powdered root, liquid extract.

Bittersweet *Solanum dulcamara*. COMMON NAME: Woody nightshade, violet bloom, scarlet berry, felonwood, felonwort, dulcamara.

OCCURRENCE: a climbing plant found in hedgerows in Britain

PARTS USED: the twigs and root-bark. The twigs contain the alkaloid solamine and the glucoside dulcamarine which gives bittersweet its characteristic taste. It also contains sugar, gum, starch and resin.

MEDICINAL USES: narcotic, resolvent, diuretic and alterative. Bittersweet promotes all secretions, particularly of the skin and kidneys, and is generally used to clear up stubborn skin infections and eruptions, scrofula and ulcers and has been recommended in chronic bronchial catarrh, asthma or whooping cough. In large doses, the drug can cause paralysis of the central nervous system and lead to death.

ADMINISTERED AS: a fluid extract, decoction.

Blackberry *Rubus fructicosus*. COMMON NAME: Bramble, bumble-kite, bramble-kite, bly, brummel, brameberry, scaldhead, brambleberry.

OCCURRENCE: common throughout Britain in hedgerows and ditches.

PARTS USED: the root and leaves, which both contain tannin.

MEDICINAL USES: as astringent and tonic. It is valuable against dysentery and diarrhoea. A decoction of the root was used to treat whooping cough. A cordial or vinegar drink was made and is useful in treating looseness of the bowels, piles or a feverish cold.

ADMINISTERED AS: decoction, fluid extract or made into cordial, wine or vinegar.

Blackcurrant *Ribes nigrum*. COMMON NAME: Quinsy berries, squinancy berries.

OCCURRENCE: a common garden plant throughout Britain, but is only truly native to Yorkshire and the Lake District. It is also found in Europe.

PARTS USED: the fruit, leaves, bark and root.

MEDICINAL USES: diuretic, diaphoretic, febrifuge, refrigerant, detergent. The fruit juice is excellent in febrile diseases and can be made to an extract which is good for sore throats. The leaves when infused are cleansing while a root infusion is used in eruptive fevers and has been used to treat cattle. A decoction of the bark is effective against calculus, oedema and haemorrhoids. The fruit was commonly used to make jelly, wine and cheese.

ADMINISTERED AS: juice, infusion or decoction.

Black root *Leptandra virginica*. COMMON NAME: Culver's root, culver's physic, physic root, leptandra-wurzel, *Veronica virginica, Veronica purpurea, Paederota virginica, Eustachya purpurea, Eustachya alba.*

OCCURRENCE: found in the eastern United States.

PARTS USED: the rhizome which contains a crystalline principle and an impure resin, which together are called leptandrin and are said to be the active principles.

MEDICINAL USES: violent cathartic, emetic, tonic, antiseptic, diaphoretic. The action of the root on the body depends upon whether the root is dried or fresh. Fresh root is violently cathartic and emetic in action while the dried root has milder effects. It is used to excite the liver and promote the secretion of bile without harming the bowels and it is a good stomach tonic of benefit to diarrhoea, dysentery, cholera and torpid liver problems. The fresh root, however, may induce abortion and gives rise to bloody stools, but a decoction of the fresh root is used for intermittent fevers. The dried root has been used successfully in leprosy, dropsy, cancer, pulmonary tuberculosis and malaria.

ADMINISTERED AS: powdered root, decoction and fluid extract.

Bladderwrack *Fucus vesiculosus.* COMMON NAME: Bladder fucus, seawrack, kelp ware, black-tang, cutweed, seetang, blasentang, meeriche.

OCCURRENCE: common around the coasts of the North Atlantic Ocean including Britain.

PARTS USED: the root, stem and leaves, the thallus. The seaweed contains a volatile oil, cellulose, mucilage, mannite, soda and iodine along with the bromine compounds of sodium and potassium.

MEDICINAL USES: a deobstruent, antifat. It has been used to cause weight loss and reduce obesity by stimulation of the thyroid gland. The wine made from grapes and dried fucus has been of benefit in diseases of the hip, joints and bones in children. It may also be applied externally as a poultice to treat enlarged glands.

ADMINISTERED AS: a liquid extract, decoction, infusion, fluid extract, or charcoal derived from *Fucus vesiculosus.*

Bloodroot *Sanguinaria candensis.* COMMON NAME: Indian paint, tetterwort, red pucoon, red root, paucon, coon root, snakebite, sweet slumber.

OCCURRENCE: a spring flower found in woods from Canada to Florida and west to Arkansas and Nebraska in the United States.

PARTS USED: the rhizome. It has the alkaloids sanguinarine, chelerythrine, protropine and B. homochelidonine as its active components. Protropine is one of the most widely used opium alkaloids.

MEDICINAL USES: emetic, cathartic, expectorant, emmenagogue. The plant is of great benefit in dyspepsia, asthma, bronchitis, croup and pulmonary consumption. It can be used in heart disease, heart weakness and palpitations, nervous irritation, torpid liver, scrofula, dysentery and to lower the pulse rate. Externally, it can be applied to cure ringworm, fungal growths, ulcers, eczema and cancerous growths. Care must be taken as toxic doses of *Sanguinaria* can be deleterious to the person.

ADMINISTERED AS: fluid extract, tincture, powdered root and solid extract.

Bluebell *Scilla nutans, Hyacinthus nonscriptus.*

COMMON NAME: Calverkeys, culverkeys, auld man's bell, ring-o' bells, jacinth, wood bells, *Agraphis nutans.*

OCCURRENCE: abundant in western Europe, Great Britain and Italy.

PARTS USED: the bulb, dried and powdered.

MEDICINAL USES: diuretic, styptic. This medicine is little used today but it was considered a very powerful remedy for leucorrhoea. It may also have been used to cure snake bite. The fresh bulbs are poisonous, so the plant is always used when dried.

ADMINISTERED AS: powdered bulb.

Blue flag *Iris versicolor.* COMMON NAME: Poison flag, flag lily, liver lily, snake lily, dragon flower, dagger flower, water flag.

OCCURRENCE: indigenous to North America and was introduced into Britain and Europe and is now a common garden plant.

PARTS USED: the rhizome which contains starch, gum, tannin, isophthalic acid, salicylic acid and oleoresin of which the latter compound contains the medicinal properties.

MEDICINAL USES: alterative, diuretic, cathartic, stimulant. It is chiefly used for its alterative properties being useful as a purgative in disorders of the liver and the duodenum. Also, combined with other herbs as a blood purifier, or used alone against syphilis, scrofula, skin afflictions and dropsy.

ADMINISTERED AS: powdered root, solid extract, fluid extract or tincture.

Bogbean *Menyanthes trifoliata.* COMMON NAME: Buckbean, marsh trefoil, water trefoil, marsh clover, boonan.

OCCURRENCE: found in spongy bogs, marshes and shallow water throughout Europe and is more common in northern England and Scotland.

PARTS USED: the herb which consists of volatile oil and a glucoside called menyanthin.

MEDICINAL USES: as a tonic, cathartic, deobstruent and febrifuge. A liquid extract is used to treat rheumatism, scurvy and skin complaints. It has also been recommended as an external application to reduce glandular swelling. In the Highlands of Scotland it was used to remedy stomach pains, particularly due to ulcers, and bogbean was also brewed into beer and smoked as herb tobacco. It is thought to cure ague (malaria) where all other cures have failed.

ADMINISTERED AS: the liquid extract, infusion or as tea.

Boneset *Eupatonium perfoliatum.* COMMON NAME: thoroughwort, Indian sage, feverwort.

OCCURRENCE: found in meadows and damp ground in North America and Europe.

PARTS USED: the herb. The important constituents are volatile oil, tannic acid, gum, resin, sugar and the glucoside eupatonin.

MEDICINAL USES: a diaphoretic, tonic, febrifuge, expectorant, stimulant, and laxative. It is used successfully to treat rheumatism, colds and influenza, catarrh and skin diseases. It acts slowly on the stomach, liver, bowel and uterus but it has a persistent beneficial effect. In large doses it has an emetic and purgative effect.

ADMINISTERED AS: powdered herb, fluid extract and solid extract.

Borage *Borago officinalis.* COMMON NAME: Burrage.

OCCURRENCE: naturalized in Britain and Europe and is found in gardens, rubbish heaps and near houses.

PARTS USED: the leaves and flowers consist of potassium, calcium, mineral acids along with nitrogen salts.

MEDICINAL USES: diuretic, demulcent, emollient, refrigerant. It is effective in treating fevers and pulmonary complaints as it activates the kidneys. It is applied externally as a poultice against inflammation and swelling and has been developed into a cream which treats itch and skin complaints, e.g. eczema and psoriasis. The flowers may be eaten raw, candied or made into a conserve to strengthen people weakened by prolonged illness.

ADMINISTERED AS: an infusion, poultice or lotion.

Box *Buxus sempervirens.* COMMON NAME: Dudgeon.

OCCURRENCE: native to Europe and western Africa but was introduced into Great Britain and the USA.

PARTS USED: the wood and leaves. The bark contains chlorophyll, wax, resin and tallow along with carbonate, sulphate and phosphate compounds. The leaves contain three alkaloids—buxine, parabuxine and parabuxonidine, as well as tannin.

MEDICINAL USES: the wood is diaphoretic, narcotic and sedative in full doses. It is generally prepared as a decoction for rheumatism and syphilis. The tincture was thought to be a bitter tonic, antiperiodic and cured leprosy. A volatile oil distilled from the wood has been used in epilepsy, piles and toothache. The leaves are sudorific, alterative and cathartic when powdered. The powder is poisonous so thus it makes an excellent purgative, vermifuge and is anthelmintic.

ADMINISTERED AS: powdered leaves, tincture, distilled oil, and decoction.

Brooklime *Veronica beccabunga.* COMMON NAME: Water pimpernel, becky leaves, cow cress, horse cress, housewell grass, limewort, brooklembe, limpwort, wall-ink, water-pumpy, well-ink.

OCCURRENCE: very common in all part of Great Britain

PARTS USED: the herb. This plant contains tannin, a bitter principle, a volatile oil and sulphur.

MEDICINAL USES: alterative, diuretic. It is used as an infusion as an antiscorbutic and to treat impurities of the blood.

ADMINISTERED AS: infusion or poultice.

Broom *Cytisus scoparius.* COMMON NAME: Broom tops, Irish tops, basam, bizzom, browne, brum, bream, green broom.

OCCURRENCE: indigenous to England and commonly found on heathland throughout Britain, Europe and northern Asia.

PARTS USED: the young herbaceous tops which contain sparteine and scoparin as the active components.

MEDICINAL USES: diuretic and cathartic. The broom tops may be used as a decoction or infusion to aid dropsy while if the tops are pressed and treated broom juice is obtained. This fluid extract is generally used in combination with other diuretic compounds. An infusion of broom, AGRIMONY and DANDELION root is excellent in remedying bladder, kidney and liver trouble. *Cytisus* should be used carefully as the sparteine has a strong effect on the heart and, depending upon dose, can cause weakness of the heart similar to that caused by HEMLOCK (*Conium maculatum*). Death can occur in extreme cases if the respiratory organ's activity is impaired.

ADMINISTERED AS: fluid extract and infusion.

Bryony, Black *Tamus communis*. COMMON NAME: Blackeye root.

OCCURRENCE: native to Great Britain and is common in woods and hedges.

PARTS USED: the root.

MEDICINAL USES: as a rubefacient and diuretic. The drug is seldom used internally now due to its poisonous nature, but was formerly used to treat asthmatic complaints. Externally the fresh root is scraped, pulped and applied as a plaster to areas affected by gout, rheumatism or paralysis. A root pulp poultice was used on bruises and black eyes to remove discolouration from the skin. Chilblains were treated using a tincture made from the roots.

ADMINISTERED AS: a plaster, poultice, tincture, rarely as expressed juice.

Bryony, White *Bryonia dioica, Bryonia alba*. COMMON NAME: English mandrake, wild vine, wild hops, lady's seal, tetterbury, wild nep, tamus.

OCCURRENCE: a native of Europe, frequently found in England but rare in Scotland

PARTS USED: the root.

MEDICINAL USES: irritative, hydragogue, cathartic. It was previously used as a purgative drug but these and other uses have been discontinued on account of its highly irritant nature. It is still used in small doses for coughs, influenza, bronchitis and pneumonia. It is useful in cardiac disorders caused by gout or rheumatism and in malarial and contagious diseases. Care should be taken when used, due to its poisonous nature.

ADMINISTERED AS: liquid extract.

Buchu *Barosma betulina*. COMMON NAME: Bucco, *Diosma betulina*.

OCCURRENCE: found at the Cape of good Hope in South Africa

PARTS USED: the leaves, which contain volatile oil, mucilage and diosphenol. They are collected from wild plants and this is strictly controlled by the government.

MEDICINAL USES: diuretic, diaphoretic, stimulant. The plant has a direct effect on the urinary organs,

benefiting gravel, inflammation and catarrh of the bladder, cystitis, nephritis and urethritis. It has been classed as an official medicine in Great Britain since 1821.

ADMINISTERED AS: fluid extract, tincture and solid extract.

Bugle *Ajuga reptans*. COMMON NAME: Common bugle, carpenter's herb, middle confound, middle comfrey, sicklewort, herb carpenter, bugula.

OCCURRENCE: abundant throughout Great Britain in damp pastures and woods.

PARTS USED: the herb.

MEDICINAL USES: bitter, astringent and aromatic. As an infusion this herb is considered very good in arresting haemorrhages, easing irritation and coughs. It acts in a similar way to that of FOXGLOVE (*Digitalis purpurea*) in lowering the pulse rate and is said to be one of the mildest and best narcotics in existence. It is also considered good for the bad effects of excessive drinking.

ADMINISTERED AS: a decoction and infusion.

Burdock *Artium lappa*. COMMON NAME: Lappa, fox's clote, thorny burr, beggar's buttons, cockle buttons, love leaves, philanthropium, personata, happy major, clot-bur.

OCCURRENCE: freely found in ditches and hedgerows throughout England and Europe but rare in Scotland

PARTS USED: the root, herb and seeds (fruits). They contain the chemicals inulin, mucilage, sugar and tannic acid along with a crystalline glucoside, lappin.

MEDICINAL USES: alterative, diuretic and diaphoretic. It is an excellent blood purifier and very effective in remedying all skin diseases. The root is most powerful and has anti-scorbutic properties which make it very useful for boils, scurvy and rheumatism. Also used as a wash for ulcers, a poultice for tumours, gouty swellings and bruises. An infusion of the leaves aids the stomach and eases indigestion. The tincture obtained from the seeds is relaxant, demulcent and a tonic for the skin.

ADMINISTERED AS: a fluid extract, infusion, tincture and solid extract.

Burnet, Greater *Sanguisorba officinalis*. COMMON NAME: garden burnet, common burnet, salad burnet.

OCCURRENCE: found in moist meadows and shady areas almost all over Europe and in British gardens.

PARTS USED: the herb and root.

MEDICINAL USES: astringent and tonic. Decoc-

tion of the whole herb is useful in haemorrhages. Both the herb and root are taken internally to treat abnormal discharges such as diarrhoea, dysentery and leucorrhoea. It is also
used to make herb beer.

ADMINISTERED AS: a powder and infusion.

Burr Marigold *Bidens Impartica.* COMMON NAME:
Water agrimony.

OCCURRENCE: commonly found in wet places in
England but less frequently seen in Scotland.

PARTS USED: the whole plant.

MEDICINAL USES: astringent, diaphoretic, diuretic. This plant has been useful in dropsy, gout,
haematuria and fevers. It is very good in treating diseases of the respiratory organs where
bleeding occurs and also in uterine haemorrhage.

ADMINISTERED AS: an infusion.

Butcher's Broom *Ruscus aculeatus.* COMMON
NAME: Kneeholm, knee holy, jew's myrtle,
sweet broom, pettigree.

OCCURRENCE: a low shrubby plant found in
woods and waste ground, primarily in the south
of England.

PARTS USED: the herb and root.

MEDICINAL USES: diaphoretic, diuretic, deobstruent and aperient. It is used in jaundice,
gravel, urinary and female obstructions and is
said to be good in clearing phlegm from the
chest and relieving difficult breathing.

ADMINISTERED AS: a decoction.

Butterbur *Petasites vulgaris.* COMMON NAME:
Langwort, umbrella plant, bog rhubarb,
plapperdock, blatterdock, capdockin,
bogshorns, butterdock.

OCCURRENCE: in low wet grounds, marshy meadows and riversides in Great Britain.

PARTS USED: the rhizome or root-stock.

MEDICINAL USES: as a cardiac tonic, stimulant,
and diuretic. It is good as a remedy for fevers,
asthma, colds, urinary complaints, gravel and
plague. It is also taken as a homoeopathic remedy for severe neuralgia in the back and loins.
Recently, the use of butterbur has been recommended in easing the pain of migraine and
painful menstruation. One of the most important developments is the treatment of cancer
with *petasites* where the drug attacks tumours
and abnormal cell changes very strongly and,
in clinical tests, it has been shown to slow or
stop the cancer spreading through the body. It
has also become an effective remedy for severe asthma.

ADMINISTERED AS: a decoction and tincture.

Buttercup, Bulbous *Ranunculus bulbosus.* COM-
MON NAME: St. Antony's turnip, crowfoot,
frogsfoot, goldcup.

OCCURRENCE: found in meadows and fields
throughout Britain.

PARTS USED: the juice and herbs.

MEDICINAL USES: this plant has various uses including easing headaches and as a cure for shingles. The herb inflames and blisters the skin
upon contact and is used to aid gout, sciatica
and rheumatism. It has also been used as a
poultice on the stomach.

ADMINISTERED AS: a poultice, decoction and tincture.

Cacao *Theobroma cacao.* COMMON NAME: Cocoa,
chocolate tree.

OCCURRENCE: found in tropical America and
cultivated in most tropical countries, e.g. Sri
Lanka and Java

PARTS USED: the seed which contain about two
per cent of the chemical theobromine and forty
to sixty per cent solid fat.

MEDICINAL USES: emollient, diuretic, stimulant
and nutritive. The seeds are ground into a paste
between hot rollers, with sugar and starch being added to produce cocoa. The cocoa butter
(or oil of theobroma) produced forms a hard
solid which is used in cosmetics, suppositories and coating pills. It has very good emollient qualities and is used to soften chapped
hands and lips. The alkaloid, theobromine,
which is contained in the beans is similar to caffeine in action on the central nervous system,
but less powerful. It acts on the heart, kidneys
and muscle and is used as a diuretic and stimulant of the kidneys. This is useful after fluid has
accumulated in the body after heart failure and
it is given in conjunction with digitalis (FOX-
GLOVE). The drug is also of benefit in high blood
pressure.

ADMINISTERED AS: expressed oil, theobromine.

Calamint *Calamintha officinalis.* COMMON NAME:
Mill mountain, mountain balm, basil thyme,
mountain mint.

OCCURRENCE: a bushy plant found in hedgerows
and lanes all over Great Britain and Europe.

PARTS USED: the herb. This contains a camphoraceous, volatile, stimulating oil similar to
those found in other mint plants.

MEDICINAL USES: diaphoretic, expectorant and
aromatic. It can be infused into a tea to treat
weak stomachs, colic and flatulence. Can also
be brewed into a syrup or decoction to heal the
spleen, gall bladder and jaundice.

ADMINISTERED AS: an infusion, decoction and syrup.

Calamus *Aconus calamus*. COMMON NAME: Sweet flag, sweet sedge, sweet root, gladdon, sweet rush, sweet cane, myrtle grass, sweet myrtle, cinnamon sedge, myrtle wedge.

OCCURRENCE: grows freely in all European countries except Spain and it is common on river banks in Great Britain

PARTS USED: the rhizome, which produces a volatile oil after steam distillation, which is made up of pinene and asaryl aldehyde. It also contains alkaloidal material including choline and the glucoside acorin.

MEDICINAL USES: aromatic, carminative, stimulant, tonic and stomachic. It is used to remove the discomfort of flatulence, wind, colic, ague and dyspepsia. It can increase the appetite and aid digestion. Calamus oil is used in inhalations.

ADMINISTERED AS: a fluid extract, infusion, tincture and distilled oil.

Calotrophis *Calotrophis procera*, *Calotrophis gigantea*. COMMON NAME: mudar bark, mudar yercum, *Asclepias onocera*.

OCCURRENCE: native to India but is cultivated in the East and West Indies and Sri Lanka.

PARTS USED: the dried bark. This contains several chemicals including madaralbum, madarfluavil, caoutchouc, mudarine, two resins and calatrophin which is an active poison similar to digitalis (FOXGLOVE).

MEDICINAL USES: in India, it is used as a remedy for elephantiasis, leprosy and chronic eczema. It may be taken internally for diarrhoea and dysentery. It has also been used to induce abortion and as a means of suicide. Atropine (from BELLADONNA, *Atropa belladonna*) may be used as an antidote to poisoning with calotrophis.

ADMINISTERED AS: powdered bark, tincture.

Calumba *jateorhiza calumba*. COMMON NAME: *Cocculus palmatus*, colombo, *jateorhiza palmata*.

OCCURRENCE: indigenous to the forests of Mozambique and found throughout East Africa.

PARTS USED: the dried root. It contains three alkaloids — columbamine, jateorhizine and palmatine, which are closely related to berberine (from BARBERRY). There is also the crystalline principle, columbine, starch and mucilage in the root.

MEDICINAL USES: bitter tonic, febrifuge. Due to its lack of astringent qualities, it does not cause nausea, headache, sickness or fevers as other similar remedies do. It is very good against pulmonary consumption, weakness of the digestive organs, dysentery and for flatulence in combination with GINGER and SENNA. Calumba can stop sickness in pregnancy and gastric irritation.

ADMINISTERED AS: cold infusion, tincture, fluid extract, powdered root, solid extract.

Camphor *Cinnamonum camphora*. COMMON NAME: gum Camphor, laurel camphor, camphire, *Laurus camphora*, *Camphora officinarum*.

OCCURRENCE: found in China, Japan and parts of East Asia.

PARTS USED: the gum and distilled oil.

MEDICINAL USES: sedative, anodyne, antispasmodic, diaphoretic, anthelmintic, aromatic. It is mainly used in colds, chills, fevers, inflammatory complaints and for severe diarrhoea. It is taken internally for hysteria, nervousness, neuralgia and is used as an excitant in cases of heart failure due to infections, fevers and pneumonia. Camphor is highly valued in all irritations of the sexual organs. Large doses of camphor should be avoided as they can cause vomiting, palpitations and convulsions due to the effects it has on the human brain.

ADMINISTERED AS: tincture, distilled oil, injection, capsules.

Caraway *Carum Carvi*. COMMON NAME: Caraway seed, caraway fruit, alcaravea.

OCCURRENCE: common in Europe and Asia and naturalized in Britain.

PARTS USED: the fruit, which produces a volatile oil containing a hydrocarbon, carvene and an oxygenated oil, carvol.

MEDICINAL USES: aromatic, stimulant and carminative. It was widely used as a cordial to ease dyspepsia and hysteria. The oil is applied to treat flatulence and stomach disorders. Distilled caraway water is used to ease flatulent colic in infants and is an excellent children's medicine. The bruised fruits were used to remove pain from bad earache and was also used as a poultice to take away bruises. Caraway is widely as a flavouring for cheeses and seedcakes.

ADMINISTERED AS: a liquid extract and poultice.

Cardamom *Elettaria cardamomum*. COMMON NAME: Mysore cardamon seeds, malabar cardamom, ebil, kakelah seghar, capalaga, gujalatti elachi, ilachi, ailum, *Amomum cardamomum*, *A. repens*, *Alpina cardamom*, *matonia Cardamomum*, *Cardamomum minus*, *Cardamomi Semina*.

OCCURRENCE: native to southern India and cultivated in Sri Lanka.

PARTS USED: the dried ripe seed containing volatile and fixed oil, starch, mucilage, potassium salts, resin and lignin.

MEDICINAL USES: carminative, stimulant, aromatic. They have a warming aromatic effect which is useful in indigestion and flatulence. If chewed, they are said to be good for colic and headaches. Cardamom is used chiefly as a flavouring for cakes, liqueurs, etc. and forms part of curry powder mixtures used in cookery.

ADMINISTERED AS: powdered seeds, tincture and fluid extract.

Caroba *jacaranda procera.* COMMON NAME: Carob tree, carobinha, caaroba, *jacaranda caroba, Bignonia caroba.*

OCCURRENCE: found in South America and Africa.

PARTS USED: the leaves contain many compounds including caroba balsam, caroborelinic acid, carobic acid, steocarobic acid, caroban and carobin.

MEDICINAL USES: alterative, diaphoretic, diuretic. The active principles have proved to be of benefit in treating syphilis and other venereal diseases. The soothing qualities of the herb have also been used to help epilepsy, as it has a sedative effect upon the nervous system. Caroba is rarely used in medicine today.

ADMINISTERED AS: dried, powdered leaves.

Carrot *Daucus carota.* COMMON NAME: Philtron, bird's nest, bee's nest.

OCCURRENCE: a native wild plant common everywhere in Great Britain. The wild and cultivated parts both exist today.

PARTS USED: the whole herb, seeds and root.

MEDICINAL USES: diuretic, stimulant, deobstruent. The herb infused in water is an active remedy in treating dropsy, chronic kidney infections and bladder disorders. Carrot tea was good for gout, while a strong decoction is good against gravel and flatulence. The roots have antiseptic properties and were formerly used as a laxative, vermifuge or a poultice. The wild carrot was particularly well thought of as a poultice for cancerous sores, while the seeds act in a similar manner to CARAWAY in treating stomach and gastric complaints. Carrot seed also has properties as an emmenagogue and in clearing obstructions of the viscera and jaundice. Carrots are made into jam, wine, spirit and can be roasted to produce a coffee substitute.

ADMINISTERED AS: an infusion, tea and poultice.

Cassia *Cinnamomum cassia.* COMMON NAME:

Bastard cinnamon, Chinese cinnamon, cassia bark, canton cassia, *Cassia lignea, Cassia aromaticum.*

OCCURRENCE: indigenous to China and cultivated in Japan, Sumatra, Java, South America, Mexico and Sri Lanka.

PARTS USED: the bark. The bark of this tree is regarded as a substitute for cinnamon and it produces a volatile oil similar to oil of cinnamon. Cassia oil contains cinnamic aldehyde, cinnamylacetate, cinnamic acid, tannic acid and starch amongst other compounds.

MEDICINAL USES: stomachic, carminative, tonic, astringent and emmenagogue. The tincture is used in uterine haemorrhage, menorrhagia and to decrease the flow of breast milk. It is also used to assist and flavour other drugs and benefits diarrhoea, vomiting, nausea and flatulence. Cassia oil is a powerful germicide but is not normally used in medicine as such as it is very irritant. It may be used for gastric pain, flatulent colic and gastric debility as it is a strong local stimulant.

ADMINISTERED AS: expressed oil, powdered bark.

Castor oil plant *Ricinus communis.* COMMON NAME: palma Christi, castor oil bush.

OCCURRENCE: a native of India, but has been cultivated in many tropical, sub-tropical and temperate countries around the globe.

PARTS USED: the oil expressed from the seeds.

MEDICINAL USES: cathartic, purgative, laxative, vermifuge, galactogogue. Castor oil is regarded as one of the best laxative and purgative preparations available. It is of particular benefit for children and pregnant women due to its mild action in easing constipation, colic and diarrhoea due to slow digestion. The oil expels worms from the body, after other suitable remedies have been given. When applied externally, Castor oil eases cutaneous complaints such as ringworm, itch and leprosy, while it is used as a carrier oil for solutions of pure alkaloids, e.g. atropine or cocaine, from BELLADONNA (*Atropa belladonna*), that these drugs can be used in eye surgery. Castor oil is used for a range of industrial purposes from soap-making to varnishes.

ADMINISTERED AS: expressed oil.

Catmint *Nepeta cataria.* COMMON NAME: Catnep, nep.

OCCURRENCE: a wild English plant in hedges, field borders and waste ground. It is found on a localized basis in Scotland.

PARTS USED: the herb.

MEDICINAL USES: carminative, tonic, diaphoretic, refrigerant, mildly stimulating and slightly emmenagogue. This herb is good in treating colds, fevers, restlessness and colic. It is also used in nervousness and insanity and to calm children and soothe nightmares when taken as an infusion or conserve. Catmint can be applied to swellings and bruises as a poultice.

ADMINISTERED AS: an infusion, injection or poultice.

Cayenne *Capsicum minimum, Capsicum frutescens*. COMMON NAME: African pepper, chillies, bird pepper.

OCCURRENCE: native to Zanzibar but is now cultivated in most tropical and sub-tropical countries, e.g. Sierra Leone, Japan and Madagascar

PARTS USED: the fruit, both fresh and dried.

MEDICINAL USES: stimulant, tonic, carminative, rubefacient. It is possibly the purest and best stimulant in herbal medicine. It produces natural warmth and helps the blood circulation, and eases weakness of the stomach and intestines. Cayenne is added to tonics and is said to ward off disease and can prevent development of colds and fevers.

ADMINISTERED AS: powdered fruit, tincture, capsules, dietary item.

Cedar, Yellow *Thuja occidentalis*. COMMON NAME: Tree of life, arbor vitae, false white cedar, *Cedrus lycea*, hackmatack, thuia de Canada, Lebensbaum.

OCCURRENCE: the United States and Canada.

PARTS USED: the leaves and twigs. The plant contains the bitter principle pinipicrin, volatile oil, sugar, wax, resin and a colouring principle called thujin. The leaves and twigs yield an essential oil similar to camphor, which contains pinene, fenchone, thujone and carvone.

MEDICINAL USES: aromatic, astringent, diuretic, anthelmintic, irritant, expectorant, emmenagogue. A decoction of the twigs can help intermittent fevers, coughs, gout, amenorrhoea, dropsy and scurvy. When made into an ointment, the leaves ease rheumatism. An infusion is good at removing warts and fungal growths. A preparation of the twigs may induce abortion by reflex action on the uterus from severe gastro-intestinal irritation. This plant should be used with some care.

ADMINISTERED AS: infusion, decoction, injection, poultice, tincture, ointment.

Celandine *Chelidonium majus*. COMMON NAME: Garden celandine, common celandine, greater celandine.

OCCURRENCE: common all over Great Britain and Europe.

PARTS USED: the herb, which contains the alkaloids chelidanine, chelerythrin (of which the latter is narcotic), homochelidonine A and B. Three other major chemicals are found in the plant.

MEDICINAL USES: alterative, diuretic and purgative. It is of benefit to jaundice, eczema, scrofulous diseases and scurvy. The fresh juice was used to cure warts, ringworm and corns but should not otherwise be allowed to come into direct contact with the skin. In various forms, it has previously been effective against itching, piles, toothache and cancer.

ADMINISTERED AS: infusion, fluid extract, decoction, lotion, poultice.

Celery *Apium graveolens*. COMMON NAME: Smallage, wild celery.

OCCURRENCE: native to southern Europe and cultivated in Britain.

PARTS USED: the ripe seeds, herb and root of which the seeds contain two oils and apiol.

MEDICINAL USES: carminative, stimulant, diuretic, tonic, nervine and aphrodisiac. It is utilised as a tonic in combination with other herbs, promoting restfulness, sleep and lack of hysteria and is excellent in relieving rheumatism.

ADMINISTERED AS: fluid extract, essential oil and powdered seeds.

Chamomile *Anthemis nobilis*. COMMON NAME: Roman chamomile, double chamomile, manzanilla (Spanish), maythen (Saxon).

OCCURRENCE: a low growing plant found wild in the British Isles.

PARTS USED: the flowers and herb. The active principles therein are a volatile oil, anthemic acid, tannic acid and a glucoside.

MEDICINAL USES: tonic, stomachic, anodyne and anti-spasmodic. An infusion of chamomile tea is an extremely effective remedy for hysterical and nervous afflictions in women, as well as an emmenagogue. Chamomile has a powerful soothing and sedative effect which is harmless. A tincture is used to cure diarrhoea in children and it is used with purgatives to prevent griping, and as a tonic it helps dropsy. Externally, it can be applied alone or with other herbs as a poultice to relieve pain, swellings, inflammation and neuralgia. Its strong antiseptic properties make it invaluable for reducing swelling of the face due to abscess or injury. As a lotion, the flowers are good for resolving toothache and earache. The herb itself is an ingredient in herb beers. The use of chamomile can be dated back to ancient Egyptian times when they dedicated the plant to the sun because of its extensive healing properties.

ADMINISTERED AS: decoction, infusion, fluid extract and essential oil.

Cherry laurel *Prunus laurocerasus*

OCCURRENCE: native to Russia and now cultivated in many temperate European countries.

PARTS USED: the leaves. The main constituent is prulaurasin which resembles amygdalin and hydrocyanic acid.

MEDICINAL USES: sedative, narcotic. The leaves are used to produce a distilled water which is the main herbal preparation used of this herb. It is good against coughs, dyspepsia, indigestion, whooping cough and asthma.

ADMINISTERED AS: cherry laurel water.

Chestnut, Horse *Aesculus hippocastanum*. COMMON NAME: *Hippocastanum vulgare*.

OCCURRENCE: a tree native to northern and central Asia from which it was introduced into England and Scotland.

PARTS USED: the bark and fruit, from both of which a fluid extract is made.

MEDICINAL USES: tonic, narcotic, febrifuge and astringent. The bark is used in intermittent fevers as an infusion, while it is also used externally to treat ulcers. The fruits are employed in easing neuralgia, rheumatism as well as rectal complaints and haemorrhoids.

ADMINISTERED AS: an infusion and fluid extract.

Chestnut, Sweet *Castanea vesca*. COMMON NAME: *Fagus castanea*, sardia nut, Jupiter's nut, hushed nut, Spanish chestnut, *Castanea vulgaris*.

OCCURRENCE: very common in Britain, Europe and North America.

PARTS USED: the leaves.

MEDICINAL USES: tonic, astringent. It is used in a popular remedy to treat fever and ague. Its reputation is due to the great effectiveness in treating violent and convulsive coughs, particularly whooping cough and in other irritable respiratory organ conditions. The nut is commonly eaten as food or as a stuffing for meat.

ADMINISTERED AS: an infusion.

Chickweed *Stellania media*. COMMON NAME: Starweed, star chickweed, *Alsine media*, passerina.

OCCURRENCE: native to all temperate and North Arctic regions and is naturalized wherever Man has settled. A common weed.

PARTS USED: the whole herb, both fresh and dried.

MEDICINAL USES: demulcent, refrigerant. It is good as a poultice to reduce inflammation and heal indolent ulcers, but is most important as an ointment in treating eye problems and cutaneous diseases. It will also benefit scurvy and kidney disorders as an infusion.

ADMINISTERED AS: an infusion, poultice and ointment.

Chicory *Cichonium intybus*. COMMON NAME: Succory, wild succory, hendibeh, barbe de capucin.

OCCURRENCE: common in England and Ireland but rarer in Scotland.

PARTS USED: the root.

MEDICINAL USES: tonic, diuretic and laxative. A decoction of the root has benefit in jaundice, liver problems, gout and rheumatic complaints. The root, when dried, roasted and ground, may be added to coffee or may be drunk on its own as a beverage.

ADMINISTERED AS: a decoction, poultice, syrup or distilled water.

Chives *Allium schoenoprasum*. COMMON NAME: Cives.

OCCURRENCE: native to temperate and northern Europe and Great Britain and has been cultivated over a large area of the northern hemisphere.

PARTS USED: the herb.

MEDICINAL USES: this herb stimulates the appetite and helps digestion during convalescence. It is also said to be effective against infections and prevent anaemia. They are also widely used in food dishes and add vitamins and colour to many meals.

ADMINISTERED AS: fresh herbs.

Cicely, Sweet *Myrrhis odorata*. COMMON NAME: Smooth cicely, British myrrh, anise, great sweet chervil, smelt chervil, sweet bracken, sweet-fern, sweet humlock, sweets, The Roman plant, shepherd's needle, cow chervil.

OCCURRENCE: native to Great Britain and also found in mountain pastures across Europe.

PARTS USED: the root and herb.

MEDICINAL USES: aromatic, carminative, stomachic, expectorant. The fresh root may be eaten or used as a tonic in brandy. It eases coughs, flatulence, indigestion and stomach upsets. The herb, as an infusion, is good for anaemia and a tonic for young girls. The antiseptic roots have been used for snake or dog bites while the distilled water is diuretic and effective in treating pleurisy. Sweet Cicely essence is said to have aphrodisiac properties.

ADMINISTERED AS: a root infusion, herb infusion, decoction, essence and distilled water.

Cinnamon *Cinnamomum zeylanicum*. COMMON NAME: Lauris cinnamomum.

OCCURRENCE: native to Sri Lanka but is cultivated in other Eastern countries.

PARTS USED: the bark.

MEDICINAL USES: carminative, astringent, stimulant, antiseptic, aromatic. It is used as a local stimulant as a powder and infusion, generally combined with other herbs. Cinnamon stops vomiting and nausea, relieves flatulence and diarrhoea and can also be employed to stop haemorrhage of the womb.

ADMINISTERED AS: powder, distilled water, tincture or an essential oil.

Clematis *Clematis recta*. COMMON NAME: Upright virgin's bower, *Clammula jovis*.

OCCURRENCE: a perennial plant common to Europe.

PARTS USED: the roots and stem.

MEDICINAL USES: diuretic, diaphoretic. When bruised, the leaves and flowers irritate the eyes and throat prompting tears and coughing. If applied to the skin, it produces inflammation and blisters appear. The herb is used both as a local external application, and internally against syphilis, cancer and other ulcers. It is used by homoeopaths for eye complaints, gonorrhoea and inflammatory conditions.

ADMINISTERED AS: dried leaves, fluid extract.

Clivers *Galium aparine*. COMMON NAME: Cleavers, goosegrass, borweed, hedgesheriff, hayriffe, eriffe, grip grass, hayruff, catchweed, scratweed, mutton chops, robin-run-in-the-grass, love-man, goosebill, everlasting friendship.

OCCURRENCE: an abundant hedgerow weed in Europe, Great Britain and North America.

PARTS USED: the herb, which contains chlorophyll, starch, galitannic acid, citric acid and rubichloric acid.

MEDICINAL USES: diuretic, tonic, aperient and alterative. It is successfully administered to treat obstruction of the urinary organs, gravel, suppression of urine, etc. A wash of the herb helps sunburn and freckles, while an ointment provides benefit against cancerous growths and tumours. The expressed juice or infusion will help scurvy, scrofula, psoriasis and other skin complaints as well as stopping insomnia and inducing sleep.

ADMINISTERED AS: an infusion, decoction, ointment, expressed juice or lotion.

Clover, Red *Trifolium pratense*. COMMON NAME: Trefoil, purple clover.

OCCURRENCE: widely distributed in Britain and Europe.

PARTS USED: the flowers.

MEDICINAL USES: alterative, sedative, antispasmodic. The fluid extract or infusion are excellent in treating bronchial and whooping coughs. External applications of the herb in a poultice has been used on cancerous growths.

ADMINISTERED AS: fluid extract and infusion.

Cloves *Eugenia caryophyllata*. COMMON NAME: *Eugenia aromatica*, *Eugenia caryophyllus*, clavos.

OCCURRENCE: grows on the Molucca Islands in the southern Philippines.

PARTS USED: the underdeveloped flowers.

MEDICINAL USES: stimulating, carminative, aromatic. It is given as powder or an infusion for nausea, vomiting, flatulence, languid indigestion and dyspepsia. The volatile oil contains the medicinal properties and it is a strong germicide, antiseptic and a local irritant. It has been used as an expectorant to aid bronchial troubles. Clove oil is often used in association with other medicines.

ADMINISTERED AS: powdered cloves, infusion, essential oil, fluid extract.

Club moss *Lycopodium clavatum*. COMMON NAME: Lycopodium, lycopodium seed, vegetable sulphur, wolf's claw, muscus terrestris repens.

OCCURRENCE: occurs throughout Great Britain being most plentiful on heath or moorland in northern countries and is also found all over the world.

PARTS USED: the fresh plant and spores.

MEDICINAL USES: spores are diuretic, nervine and aperient. The fresh plant has been used as a stomachic and a diuretic herb in calculus and kidney complaints. The spores are currently applied externally to wounds and taken internally for diarrhoea, dysentery, gout and scurvy.

ADMINISTERED AS: dried spores, fresh moss.

Coca, Bolivian: *Erythroxylum coca*; **Peruvian**: *Erythroxylum truxillense*. COMMON NAME: Cuca, cocaine.

OCCURRENCE: native to Peru and Bolivia; cultivated in Java and Sri Lanka.

PARTS USED: the leaves. They contain the alkaloids cocaine, amamyl cocaine and truxilline or cocamine when grown in South America.

Eastern-grown plants contain additional chemicals and glucosides.

MEDICINAL USES: nerve stimulant, anodyne, tonic, aphrodisiac. The leaves are used as a cerebral and muscle stimulant during convalescence relieving nausea, vomiting and stomach pains. It is utilized as a general nerve tonic and in treating asthma. In South America, the locals chew the leaves to relieve hunger and fatigue, but this does cause health damage when done over a long period of time. There is a danger of developing an addictive habit to this drug and the possible medicinal benefits are less than the potential health damage. People with a cocaine habit can appear emaciated, suffer loss of memory, sleeplessness and delusions. In Great Britain, the distribution and use of this drug is controlled by the Dangerous Drugs Act.

ADMINISTERED AS: tincture, powdered leaves, fluid extract.

Coffee *Coffea arabica*. COMMON NAME: Caffea.

OCCURRENCE: native to a province of Abyssinia and cultivated throughout the tropics.

PARTS USED: the seed and leaves. When roasted, coffee contains oil, wax, caffeine, aromatic oil, tannic acid, caffetannic acid, gum, sugar and protein.

MEDICINAL USES: stimulant, diuretic, anti-narcotic, anti-emetic. Coffee is commonly used as a beverage but it can also be applied as a medicine. It is a brain stimulant, causing sleeplessness and hence is useful in cases of narcotic poisoning. For this reason it is very good against snake bite in that it helps stop people falling into a coma. Caffeine can be valuable for heart disease, fluid retention and it is used against drunkenness. As a powerful diuretic, it can help ease gout, rheumatism, gravel and dropsy.

ADMINISTERED AS: beverage, caffeine preparation.

Cohosh, Black *Cimicifuga racemosa*. COMMON NAME: Black snakeroot, bugbane, rattleroot, rattleweed, squawroot, *Actaea racemosa*, *Macrotys actaeoides*.

OCCURRENCE: a native of the United States and Canada and was introduced into England around 1860.

PARTS USED: the rhizome. The main constituents are a resinous substance known as cimicifuga (or macrotin) and racemosin which gives the drug its bitter taste.

MEDICINAL USES: astringent, emmenagogue, diuretic, alterative, expectorant. This root is said to be effective in many disorders including whooping cough and rheumatism. It is supposed to be an antidote to poison and rattlesnake bites. The drug can help ease children's diarrhoea, and in consumption acts by slowing the pulse rate, inducing perspiration and easing the cough. In overdoses, black Cohosh can cause vomiting and nausea.

ADMINISTERED AS: tincture, infusion, decoction, powdered root.

Cohosh, Blue *Caulophyllum thalictroides*. COMMON NAME: Papoose root, squawroot, blueberry root, *Leontice thalichoides*.

OCCURRENCE: found in the United States and Canada.

PARTS USED: the rhizome. It contains gum, starch, salts, soluble resin and a chemical similar to saponin.

MEDICINAL USES: diuretic, antispasmodic, vermifuge, emmenagogue, athelmintic, diaphoretic. This drug has been used in rheumatism, epilepsy, uterine inflammation, hysteria and dropsy. It is also taken to expedite childbirth and induce menstruation.

ADMINISTERED AS: decoction, infusion, tincture, solid extract.

Coltsfoot *Tussilago farfara*. COMMON NAME: Coughwort, hallfoot, horsehoof, ass's foot, foals-wort, fieldhove, bullsfoot, donnhove.

OCCURRENCE: commonly found wild on waste ground and riverbanks in Great Britain.

PARTS USED: the leaves, flowers and root.

MEDICINAL USES: demulcent, expectorant and tonic. Coltsfoot is one of the most popular cough remedies and is generally taken in conjunction with HOREHOUND, MARSHMALLOW or GROUND IVY. It has been called "nature's best herb for the lungs" and it was recommended that the leaves be smoked to relieve a cough. Today, it forms the basis of British herb tobacco along with BOGBEAN, EYEBRIGHT, WOOD BETONY, ROSEMARY, THYME, LAVENDER and CHAMOMILE which is said to relieve asthma, catarrh, bronchitis and lung troubles.

ADMINISTERED AS: syrup or smoked when dried.

Columbine *Aquilegia vulgaris*. COMMON NAME: Culverwort.

OCCURRENCE: found as both a wild and garden plant in Great Britain.

PARTS USED: the leaves, roots and seeds.

MEDICINAL USES: astringent. It must be administered in small doses where it is used as a lotion for sore mouths and throats. It was also used for stone, jaundice and liver obstructions. Large doses can cause poisoning, so care must be taken in utilizing this drug.

ADMINISTERED AS: fresh root and infusion.

Comfrey *Symphytum officinale*. COMMON NAME: Common comfrey, knitbone, knitback, bruisewort, slippery root, gum plant, consolida, ass ear, blackwort.

OCCURRENCE: a native of Europe and temperate Asia but is common throughout England by rivers and ditches.

PARTS USED: the root and leaves. The roots contain a large quantity of mucilage, choline and allantoin.

MEDICINAL USES: demulcent, mildly astringent, expectorant and vulnerary. It is frequently used in pulmonary complaints, to soothe intestinal trouble and is a gentle remedy for diarrhoea and dysentery. A strong decoction or tea is administered in cases of internal haemorrhage whether it is the lungs, stomach, bowels or haemorrhoids. Externally, the leaves have been used as a poultice to promote healing of severe cuts, ulcers and abscesses and to reduce swelling, sprains and bruises. Allantoin is known to reduce swelling round damaged or fractured bones, thus allowing healing to occur faster and more thoroughly.

ADMINISTERED AS: a decoction, poultice and liquid extract.

Coolwort *Tiarella cordifolia*. COMMON NAME: Foam flower, mitrewort.

OCCURRENCE: found in North America from Canada to Virginia.

PARTS USED: the herb.

MEDICINAL USES: diuretic, tonic. Very good in cases of gravel, suppression of urine and other bladder diseases. It is taken as a tonic in indigestion and dyspepsia where it corrects acidity and aids liver function.

ADMINISTERED AS: infusion, decoction.

Coriander *Coriandrum sativum*

OCCURRENCE: indigenous to southern Europe and found occasionally in Britain, at riversides, fields and waste ground.

PARTS USED: the fruit and leaves.

MEDICINAL USES: stimulant, aromatic and carminative. It is generally used with active purgatives as flavouring and to lessen their griping tendencies. Coriander water was formerly used for windy colic.

ADMINISTERED AS: powdered fruit, fluid extract.

Corkwood tree *Duboisia myoporoides*. COMMON NAME: Duboisia.

OCCURRENCE: found in Australia in the states of New South Wales and Queensland.

PARTS USED: the leaves which contain alkaloidal sulphates, mainly hyoscyamine and hyoscine.

MEDICINAL USES: sedative, hypnotic, mydriatic. The drug aids the activity of the respiratory system and it is sometimes used as a replacement for atropine, from BELLADONNA (*Atropa belladonna*). The tincture of the drug is used in treating eye afflictions and paralysis.

ADMINISTERED AS: tincture.

Cornflower *Centaurea cyanus*. COMMON NAME: bluebottle, bluebow, hurtsickle, blue cap, bluet.

OCCURRENCE: common in cultivated fields and roadsides in Britain.

PARTS USED: the flowers.

MEDICINAL USES: tonic, stimulant and emmenagogue properties. A water distilled from cornflower petals was said to be a remedy for eye inflammation and weak eyesight.

ADMINISTERED AS: distilled water and infusion.

Costmary *Tanacetum balsamita*. COMMON NAME: Alecost, balsam herb, costmarie, mace, balsamita.

OCCURRENCE: an old English herb, naturalized from the Orient in the sixteenth century.

PARTS USED: the leaves.

MEDICINAL USES: it was formerly used as an aperient, antiseptic and astringent herb in treating dysentery. Used as an infusion to heal stomach and head problems but also as flavouring for ale and in salads.

ADMINISTERED AS: infusion and tincture.

Cotton root *Gossypium herbaceum* (and other species)

OCCURRENCE: indigenous to India and cultivated in Greece, Turkey, Sicily and Malta.

PARTS USED: the root-bark which contains a peculiar acid resin, sugar, gum, chlorophyll, fixed oil and tannin.

MEDICINAL USES: this drug is used to induce abortion or miscarriage as it causes contraction of the uterus. It is useful in treating abnormal uterine bleeding particularly when linked to fibroids, and in cases of difficult or obstructed menstruation. A preparation is given to induce labour (at full term) to aid safe delivery. It is said to be of use in sexual lassitude.

ADMINISTERED AS: fluid extract, decoction, solid extract.

Couchgrass *Agropyrum repens*. COMMON NAME: Twitchgrass, Scotch quelch, quickgrass, dog's grass, *Triticum repens*.

OCCURRENCE: abundant in fields and waste

ground in Britain, Europe, northern Asia and North and South America

PARTS USED: the rhizome, which contains triticin (a carbohydrate).

MEDICINAL USES: diuretic, demulcent, aperient. Widely used in complaints of the urinary organs and bladder. Also recommended for gout and rheumatism.

ADMINISTERED AS: an infusion, decoction and liquid extract.

Cowslip *Primula veris.* COMMON NAME: Herb peter, paigle, peggle, key flower, key of heaven, fairy cups, petty mulleins, patsywort, plumrocks, mayflower, Our Lady's keys, arthritica.

OCCURRENCE: a common wild flower in all parts of Great Britain.

PARTS USED: the flower.

MEDICINAL USES: sedative, antispasmodic. It is very good in relieving restlessness and insomnia. Commonly brewed into a wine which was a good children's medicine in small doses.

ADMINISTERED AS: an infusion or wine.

Cramp bark *Viburnum opulus.* COMMON NAME: guelder rose, snowball tree, king's crown, high cranberry, red elder, rose elder, may rose, whitsun rose, dog rowan tree, silver bells, whitsun bosses, gaitre berries, black haw.

OCCURRENCE: indigenous to Great Britain and North America, although rare in Scotland.

PARTS USED: the bark whose chief constituents are the glucoside viburnine, tannin, resin and valerianic acid.

MEDICINAL USES: antispasmodic, nervine, sedative. This drug is of benefit in all nervous complaints, debility, cramps and spasms of all types, asthma and hysteria. It has been effective in treating convulsions, fits, lockjaw, heart disease, palpitations and rheumatism.

ADMINISTERED AS: tincture, decoction, infusion, fluid extract.

Croton *Croton tiglian.* COMMON NAME: Tiglium, *Tiglium officinale.*

OCCURRENCE: a tree found on the Malabar coast of India and on the Indian archipelago.

PARTS USED: the oil expressed from the seeds, croton oil contains glycerides of stearic, palmitic, myristic, lauric and oleic acids; the glycerin ethers of formic, acetic, isobutyric and isovaleranic acids. The active principle is probably Crotonic acid.

MEDICINAL USES: irritant, rubefacient, cathartic, purgative. A drastic purgative drug which acts quickly, often evacuating the bowels in less

than one hour. In large doses, it causes vomiting and severe griping pains which can possibly be fatal. The drug is only used in cases of obstinate constipation where other drugs have failed. It is applied externally as a counter-irritant to relieve rheumatism, gout, neuralgia and bronchitis. The use of this oil should be monitored most carefully, only administered in small doses, and never given to children or pregnant women.

ADMINISTERED AS: expressed oil.

Crowfoot, Upright meadow *Ranunculus acris.* COMMON NAME: gold cup, grenouillette.

OCCURRENCE: native in meadows, pastures and fields in all parts of northern Europe and Great Britain.

PARTS USED: the whole herb.

MEDICINAL USES: the expressed juice is used to remove warts. A poultice of the fresh herb is good at removing violent, painful headaches or in relieving gout. The fresh herb once formed part of a famous cure for cancer practised in 1794.

ADMINISTERED AS: fresh leaves, expressed juice.

Cuckoopint *Arum maculatum.* COMMON NAME: Lords and Ladies, starchwort, arum, adder's root, friar's cowl, kings and queens, parson and clerk, ramp, Quaker, wake robin.

OCCURRENCE: the sole British species of the arum, aroidae family and is also widely distributed over Europe.

PARTS USED: the root. This contains starch, albumen, sugar, lignin, saponin a an unidentified alkaloid.

MEDICINAL USES: diaphoretic, expectorant, diuretic, stimulant. The fresh root can be prepared into a tincture and given to remedy sore, feverish throats. The dried root can be stored for long periods, but is rarely employed as a medicine today. An ointment prepared of the fresh root was used to cure ringworm.

ADMINISTERED AS: tincture, expressed juice and ointment.

Cucumber *Cucumis sativa.* COMMON NAME: Cowcumber.

OCCURRENCE: a native of the East Indies, but was first cultivated in Britain around 1573.

PARTS USED: the whole fruit, peeled or unpeeled, raw and cooked.

MEDICINAL USES: the seeds are diuretic and are an excellent taeniacide and purge. The fruit is very good as a skin cosmetic as it has cooling, healing and soothing effects on irritated skin.

Cucumber juice is widely utilised in emollient ointments or creams and is good for sunburn.

ADMINISTERED AS: expressed juice, lotion or ointment.

Cudweed *Graphalium uliginosum*. COMMON NAME: Cottonweed, marsh everlasting, cotton dawes.

OCCURRENCE: found in marshy areas in all parts of Europe.

PARTS USED: the herb.

MEDICINAL USES: astringent. It is a very good remedy for quinsy when used as a gargle and can also be taken internally.

ADMINISTERED AS: an infusion.

Cumin *Cuminum cyminum*. COMMON NAME: Cummin, *Cumino aigro*.

OCCURRENCE indigenous to upper Egypt and is cultivated in Arabia, India, China and Mediterranean countries since early times.

PARTS USED: the fruit. The chief constituents are a volatile oil, a fatty oil with resin, mucilage, gum, malates and albuminous matter.

MEDICINAL USES: stimulant, carminative, antispasmodic. This herb has similar effects to FENNEL and CARAWAY but its use has declined due to its disagreeable taste. It had a considerable reputation in helping correct flatulence due to languid digestion and as a remedy for colic and dyspeptic headache. Applied externally as a plaster, it eased stitches and pains in the side and has been combined with other herbs to form a stimulating liniment.

ADMINISTERED AS: dried, powdered fruit, whole fruit.

Cup moss *Cladonia pyxidata*. COMMON NAME: Chin cups.

OCCURRENCE: indigenous to north-west America but is also a common weed through Great Britain and Europe.

PARTS USED: the whole plant.

MEDICINAL USES: expectorant—used as a decoction to treat children's coughs and whooping cough with great effectiveness.

ADMINISTERED AS: decoction.

Daffodil *Narcissus pseudo-narcissus*. COMMON NAME: Narcissus, porillion, daffy-down-dilly, fleur de coucou, Lent lily.

OCCURRENCE: found wild in most European countries including the British Isles.

PARTS USED: the bulb, leaves and flowers. The bulbs contain an alkaloid called lyconine.

MEDICINAL USES: the flowers, when powdered, have emetic properties and as an infusion are used in pulmonary catarrh. The bulbs are also

emetic and, indeed, can cause people to collapse and die due to paralysis of the central nervous system due to the action of lyconine, which acts quickly. Accidents have resulted from daffodil bulbs being mistaken for ONIONS and eaten. Since high temperatures and cooking does not break down the poisonous alkaloid, considerable care should be taken to avoid problems. The bulbs are used externally as an astringent poultice to dissolve hard swellings and aid wound healing.

ADMINISTERED AS: powder and extract.

Daisy, Ox-eye *Chrysanthemum leuconthemum*. COMMON NAME: great ox-eye, goldens, marguerite, moon daisy, horse gowan, maudlin daisy, field daisy, dun daisy, butter daisy, horse daisy, maudlinwort, white weed, gowan.

OCCURRENCE: found in fields throughout Europe and northern Asia.

PARTS USED: the whole herb, flowers and root.

MEDICINAL USES: antispasmodic, diuretic, tonic. This herb's main use has been in whooping cough, asthma and nervous excitability. When taken as a tonic, it acts in a similar way to chamomile flowers and calms night-sweats and nightmares. An infusion of ox-eye daisy flowers is good at relieving bronchial coughs and catarrh. It is also used as a lotion for wounds, bruises and ulcers.

ADMINISTERED AS: an infusion and lotion.

Damiana *Turnera aphrodisiaca* or *Turnera diffusa* var. *aphrodisiaca*.

OCCURRENCE: indigenous to Texas and Mexico; cultivated in other areas of sub-tropical America and Africa.

PARTS USED: the leaves which contain a volatile oil, resins, tannin and the bitter principle damianin.

MEDICINAL USES: mild purgative, diuretic, tonic, stimulant, aphrodisiac. This drug acts as a tonic to the nervous system and has a direct and general beneficial effect on the reproductive organs.

ADMINISTERED AS: fluid extract, solid extract.

Dandelion *Taraxacum officinale*. COMMON NAME: priest's crown, swine's snout.

OCCURRENCE: widely found across the northern temperate zone in pastures, meadows and waste ground.

PARTS USED: the root and leaves. The main constituents of the root are taraxacin, a bitter substance, and taraxacerin, an acid resin, along with the sugar inulin.

MEDICINAL USES: diuretic, tonic and slightly

aperient. It acts as a general body stimulant, but chiefly acts on the liver and kidneys. Dandelion is used as a bitter tonic in atonic dyspepsia as a mild laxative and to promote increased appetite and digestion. The herb is best used in combination with other herbs and is used in many patent medicines. Roasted dandelion root is also used as a coffee substitute and helps ease dyspepsia, gout and rheumatism.

ADMINISTERED AS: fluid and solid extract, decoction, infusion and tincture.

Dill *Peucedanum graveolus, Fructus anethi*. COMMON NAME: Dill seed, dill fruit, *Anethum graveolus, Fructus anethi*.

OCCURRENCE: indigenous to Mediterranean districts and South Russia and is cultivated in England and Europe.

PARTS USED: the dried ripe fruit. An oil obtained from the fruit is almost identical to oil of CARAWAY, both containing limonene and carvone.

MEDICINAL USES: stimulant, aromatic, carminative and stomachic. It is usually given as dillwater which is very good for children's flatulence or disordered digestion. Oil of dill is used in medicine in largely the same way, but is also used in perfuming soaps.

ADMINISTERED AS: distilled water, essential oil.

Dock, Yellow *Rumex crispus*. COMMON NAME: Curled dock.

OCCURRENCE: normally found on roadside ditches and waste ground, all over Great Britain.

PARTS USED: the root and whole herb.

MEDICINAL USES: the root has laxative, alterative and a mildly tonic action and is used in rheumatism, bilious complaints and haemorrhoids. It is very useful in treating jaundice, diseases of the blood, scurvy, chronic skin diseases and as a tonic on the digestive system. Yellow dock is said to have a positive effect on slowing the development of cancer, due to its alterative and tonic properties. It has similar effects to that of RHUBARB and has been used in treating diphtheria.

ADMINISTERED AS: dried extract, syrup, infusion, tincture, ointment, fluid extract and solid extract.

Dodder *Cuscuta europea*. COMMON NAME: Lesser dodder, dodder of thyme, beggarweed, hellweed, strangle tare, scaldweed, devil's guts.

OCCURRENCE: a parasitic plant found in most areas of the world.

PARTS USED: the herb.

MEDICINAL USES: hepatic, laxative, purgative. A decoction made with dodder, GINGER and ALLSPICE has been used against urinary complaints, kidney, spleen and liver disorders. The herb is good in treating sciatica, scorbutic problems, scrofulous tumours and it acts as a purge due to its very bitter taste.

ADMINISTERED AS: decoction, infusion.

Dog-rose *Rosa canina*. COMMON NAME: Wild briar, hip tree, cynosbatos.

OCCURRENCE: indigenous to Great Britain.

PARTS USED: the ripe fruit which contain invert fruit sugars, a range of mineral salts and a large proportion of vitamin C or ascorbic acid.

MEDICINAL USES: astringent, refrigerant and pectoral. The fruit is used in strengthening the stomach and digestion, as well as easing coughs. It is made into an uncooked preserve, a syrup which is excellent for infants and children and rose-hip tea has very beneficial effects. An infusion of dog-rose leaves has been used as a tea substitute and has a pleasant aroma.

ADMINISTERED AS: an infusion, syrup or dietary item.

Dropwort, Hemlock water *Œnanthe crocata*. COMMON NAME: Horsebane, deadtongue, five-fingered root, water lovage, yellow water dropwort.

OCCURRENCE: common in ditches and watering places in England, particularly the southern counties.

PARTS USED: the roots.

MEDICINAL USES: the beneficial uses are few because this plant is virulently poisonous. A tincture is used to treat eruptive diseases of the skin, but with very small dosages and great caution. Poultices have been used to heal whitlows or ulcers. This wild plant is the most poisonous of our indigenous plants and many deaths have resulted from adults and children eating the leaves or roots mistakenly.

ADMINISTERED AS: tincture, poultice.

Dropwort, Water *Œnanthe phellandrium*. COMMON NAME: fine-leaved water dropwort, water fennel, fine-leaved oenanthe, *Phellandrium aquaticum*.

OCCURRENCE: a common plant in ditches and water courses across Europe and Great Britain.

PARTS USED: the fruit, which yields an ethereal oil called water fennel oil. The main chemical in the oil is the terpene, phellandrene.

MEDICINAL USES: expectorant, alterative, diuretic. The fruits are used to ease chronic pectoral conditions like bronchitis, consumption and asthma and also works well against dyspepsia, intermittent fevers and ulcers. Applied externally, the root has been utilized as a remedy for haemorrhoids. When taken in too large amounts, causing an overdose, the fruit prompts vertigo, intoxication and other narcotic effects. If the root is eaten by mistake, it can prove fatal in the same manner as with HEMLOCK WATER DROPWORT (*Oenanthe crocata*) where stomach irritation, circulation failure, giddiness, convulsions and coma can occur.

ADMINISTERED AS: powdered fruit, tincture, essence.

Dwarf elder *Sanbucus ebulus*. COMMON NAME: Danewort, wallwort, ground elder, walewort, blood hilder.

OCCURRENCE: found in ruins and waste ground throughout Europe and the British Isles.

PARTS USED: the leaves, roots and berries.

MEDICINAL USES: expectorant, diuretic, diaphoretic, purgative. The leaves are used internally to ease inflammation of the kidney and liver, and have a healing effect when used as a poultice on swellings and contusions. Dwarf elder tea was prepared from the dried root, when ground, and is one of the finest remedies for dropsy. The fresh root, when used as a decoction, is a drastic purgative. Overall, the dwarf elder is much more drastic in action than the common ELDER (*Sambucus nigra*).

ADMINISTERED AS: fresh root, decoction, poultice, infusion.

Echinacea *Echinacea angustifolia*. COMMON NAME: Black sampson, coneflower, rudbeckia, *Brauneria pallida*.

OCCURRENCE: a native plant of the prairie regions of the United states, west of Ohio. Also cultivated in Britain.

PARTS USED: the dried root and the rhizome. The wood and the bark contain oil, resin and large quantities of inulin, inuloid, sucrose, betaine, two phytosterols and oleic, cerotic, linolic and palmatic fatty acids.

MEDICINAL USES: alterative, antiseptic. This herb is considered sacred by many North American Indian tribes including the Sioux Indians. The herb boosts the immune system and increases bodily resistance to infection. It is used for boils, septicaemia, cancer, syphilis and gangrene. Echinacea is of particular value in treating diphtheria, typhoid and other infectious fevers. The herb can be used to improve appetite and digestion and can ease haemorrhoids when administered via injection.

ADMINISTERED AS: poultice, infusion, injection, fresh herb.

Elder *Sambucus nigra*. COMMON NAME: Black elder, common elder, european elder, pipe tree, bore tree, bour tree.

OCCURRENCE: frequently seen in Europe and Great Britain.

PARTS USED: the bark, leaves, flowers and berries.

MEDICINAL USES: the bark is a strong purgative and in large doses is emetic. It has been used successfully in epilepsy, and a tincture of the young bark relieves asthmatic symptoms and croup in children. A tea made from elder roots was highly effective against dropsy. The leaves are used both fresh and dried and contain the alkaloid sambucine, a glucoside called sambunigrin, as well as hydrogenic acid, cane sugar and potassium nitrate amongst other compounds. The leaves are used in preparation of green elder ointment which is used domestically for bruises, haemorrhoids, sprains, chilblains and applied to wounds. Elder leaves have the same purgative effects as the bark (but produce more nausea) and have expectorant, diaphoretic and diuretic actions.

The elder flowers are either distilled into elderflower water or dried. The water is used in eye and skin lotions as it is mildly astringent and a gentle stimulant. When infused, the dried flowers make elderflower tea which is gently laxative, aperient and diaphoretic. It is an old-fashioned remedy for colds and influenza when taken hot, before bed. The tea is also recommended to be drunk before breakfast as a blood purifier. Elder flowers would also be made into a lotion or poultice for use on inflamed areas and into an ointment which was good on wounds, scalds and burns. The ointment was used on the battlefields in World War I and at home for chapped hands and chilblains.

ADMINISTERED AS: an infusion, tincture, ointment, syrup, lotion, distilled water, poultice and dried powder.

Elecampane *Inula helenium*. COMMON NAME: Scabwort, elf dock, wild sunflower, horseheal, velvet dock.

OCCURRENCE: a true native of southern England, temperate Europe and Asia, but cultivated for medicinal purposes in northern England and Scotland.

PARTS USED: the root. This plant is a rich source of the drug inulin.

MEDICINAL USES: diuretic, tonic, diaphoretic, expectorant, antiseptic, astringent, and gently stimulant. It is used principally in coughs, consumption and pulmonary complaints, e.g. bronchitis. It is also used in acute catarrhal afflictions, dyspepsia ans asthma. Internally, it is normally combined with other herbs, as a decoction. Applied externally, it is rubefacient, and used in treating sciatica and facial neuralgia. The active bitter principle in the herb, helenin, is a very powerful antiseptic and bacterial chemical. This has meant elecampane has been used against the Tubercle bacteria and in surgical dressings.

ADMINISTERED AS: powdered root, fluid extract, tincture, poultice, infusion.

Elm, Common *Ulmus campestris.* COMMON NAME: Field elm, ulmi cortex, broad-leaved elm.

OCCURRENCE: common in Britain, Europe, Asia and North Africa.

PARTS USED: the dried inner bark.

MEDICINAL USES: tonic, demulcent, astringent and diuretic. It was formerly employed as an antiscorbutic decoction recommended in skin diseases such as ringworm. Also used as a poultice to relieve pain from gout or rheumatism.

ADMINISTERED AS: tincture, fluid extract or tea.

Ephedra *Ephedra vulgaris.* COMMON NAME: Ephedrine, epitonin, mattuang.

OCCURRENCE: grows in west central China, southern Siberia and Japan.

PARTS USED: the stems, of which ephedrine is the active alkaloidal chemical.

MEDICINAL USES: nerve stimulant, antispasmodic. The herb resembles adrenaline in effect and it relieves swellings of the mucous membranes quickly. It has been used to treat asthma, hay fever and rheumatism as well as being a prophylactic drug to help low blood pressure in influenza or pneumonia.

ADMINISTERED AS: tablets, injection.

Ergot *Claviceps purpurea.* COMMON NAME: Ergot of rye, smut of rye, spurred rye, *Serale cornutum.*

OCCURRENCE: this herbal remedy is the fungal mycelium which grows parasitically on rye, wheat and other grasses.

PARTS USED: ergot contains two alkaloids— ergotoxine and ergotamine as the active chemicals.

MEDICINAL USES: emmenagogue, haemostatic, uterine, stimulant, and sedative. It is normally used as a muscle stimulant in menstrual disorders such as leucorrhoea and painful or lacking menstruation and can be used to stop internal haemorrhage with best results against uterine haemorrhage. It is used as a sedative in cases of delirium, asthma or hysteria and also acts as a galactogogue.

ADMINISTERED AS: extract, infusion, tincture, liquid extract.

Eryngo *Eryngicum campestre.* COMMON NAME: Sea holly, eringo, sea hulver, sea holme.

OCCURRENCE: found on sandy soils and seashores around England and the rest of Europe's coastline, but rare in Scotland.

PARTS USED: the root.

MEDICINAL USES: diaphoretic, diuretic, aromatic, stimulant, expectorant. It is good in dealing with coughs, consumption, paralysis and chronic nervous diseases. It has effective results against all diseases of the bladder, scorbutic complaints, jaundice and liver problems.

ADMINISTERED AS: decoction.

Eucalyptus *Eucalyptus globulus.* COMMON NAME: Blue gum tree, stringy bark tree.

OCCURRENCE: native to Australia and Tasmania; now introduced into North and South Africa, India and southern Europe.

PARTS USED: the oil distilled from the leaves. The oil contains eucalyptol, which is the important medically-active chemical.

MEDICINAL USES: antiseptic, antispasmodic, stimulant, aromatic. The oil is used as an antiseptic and stimulant gargle; it increases the action of the heart and is said to have some antimalarial properties. It is taken internally in pulmonary tuberculosis, scarlet, typhoid and intermittent fevers. The oil is used as an inhalant to clear catarrh and used externally to ease croup and throat troubles. However, in large doses it can irritate the kidneys, depress the nervous system and possibly stop respiration and breathing. Despite its harmless appearance, care should be used when administering the drug internally.

ADMINISTERED AS: distilled oil, emulsion.

Euphorbia *Euphorbia hirta.* COMMON NAME: Asthma-weed, catshair, *Euphorbia pilulifera.*

OCCURRENCE: grows in India and other tropical countries.

PARTS USED: the herb.

MEDICINAL USES: anti-asthmatic, pectoral. It is highly effective in treating paroxysmal asthma, coughs and bronchial and pulmonary disorders. In India it is used against syphilis.

ADMINISTERED AS: tincture, liquid extract.

Evening primrose *Oenothera biennis*. COMMON NAME: Tree primrose, sun drop.

OCCURRENCE: native to North America but has been naturalized to British and European gardens.

PARTS USED: the bark and leaves.

MEDICINAL USES: astringent, sedative. The drug from this herb is not extensively used but has been of benefit in treating gastro-intestinal disorders, dyspepsia, liver torpor and in female problems in association with pelvic illness. It has also been successfully used in whooping cough and spasmodic asthma.

ADMINISTERED AS: liquid extract.

Eyebright *Euphrasia officinalis*. COMMON NAME: Euphrasia.

OCCURRENCE: a wild plant growing in meadows and grasslands in England and Europe.

PARTS USED: the herb. This plant contains various chemicals including euphrasia-tannin, mannite and glucose.

MEDICINAL USES: slightly tonic and astringent. As its name suggests, eyebright is recommended in treating diseases of the sight, weak eyes, etc. It is generally used as an infusion in water or milk and is combined in a lotion with GOLDEN SEAL, the pairing said to be highly effective.

ADMINISTERED AS: infusion, ointment or expressed juice.

Fennel *Foeniculum vulgare*. COMMON NAME: Hinojo, fenkel, sweet fennel, wild fennel.

OCCURRENCE: found wild in most areas of temperate Europe and generally considered indigenous to the shores of the Mediterranean. It is cultivated for medicinal benefit in France, Russia, India and Persia.

PARTS USED: the seeds, leaves and roots. The roots are rarely used in herbal medicine today. The essential oil is separated by distillation with water. Fennel oil varies widely in quality and composition dependent upon where and under what conditions the fennel was grown.

MEDICINAL USES: aromatic, stimulant, carminative and stomachic. The herb is principally used with purgatives to allay their tendency to griping, and the seeds form an ingredient of the compound liquorice powder. Fennel water also acts in a similar manner to DILL water in correcting infant flatulence.

ADMINISTERED AS: fluid extract, distilled water, essential oil.

Fenugreek *Trigonella foenum-graecum*. COMMON NAME: Bird's foot, Greek hay-seed.

OCCURRENCE: indigenous to eastern Mediterranean countries, but is cultivated in India, Africa and England.

PARTS USED: the seeds. These contain mucilage, two alkaloids trigonelline and choline—phosphates, lecithin and nucleoalbumin.

MEDICINAL USES: a preparation where seeds are soaked in water until they swell and form a thick paste is used to prevent fevers, is comforting to the stomach and has been utilized for diabetes. Alcoholic tinctures are used to prepare emollient cream, ointments and plasters while the mucilage is used externally as a poultice for skin infections such as abscesses, boils and carbuncles. It is also good at relieving rickets, anaemia and scrofula, while, combined with the normal dosage of conventional medicine e.g insulin, it is helpful in gout, diabetes and neurasthenia. It is widely used as a flavouring for both human and cattle feed.

ADMINISTERED AS: poultice, ointment, infusion or tincture.

Feverfew *Chrysanthemum parthenium*. COMMON NAME: Featherfew, featherfoil, flirtwort, bachelor's buttons, pyrethrum parthenium.

OCCURRENCE: a wild hedgerow plant found in many areas of Europe and Great Britain.

PARTS USED: the herb.

MEDICINAL USES: aperient, carminative, bitter, stimulant, emmenagogue. It is employed in hysterical complaints, nervousness and low spirits as a general tonic. A decoction is made and is useful in easing coughs, wheezing and difficult breathing. Earache was relieved by a cold infusion while a tincture of feverfew eased the pain and swelling caused after insect or vermin bites. The herb was planted around dwellings to purify the atmosphere and ward off disease. Today, it is used to prevent or ease migraines or headaches.

ADMINISTERED AS: warm or cold infusion, poultice, tincture, decoction.

Fig *Ficus carica*. COMMON NAME: Common fig.

OCCURRENCE: indigenous to Persia, Asia minor and Syria, but cultivated in most of the Mediterranean countries and England.

PARTS USED: the fleshy inflorescence (so-called fruit).

MEDICINAL USES: nutritive, emollient, demulcent, laxative. It is normally utilized in laxative confections and syrups with SENNA and carminatives. Demulcent decoctions are prepared from figs and are used in treating catarrhal afflictions of the nose and throat. Roasted figs, when split open, are used as a poultice to gumboils, dental abscesses, boils and carbuncles. The fruit is used both fresh and dried.

ADMINISTERED AS: poultice, syrup, decoction.

Figwort *Scrophularia nodosa*. COMMON NAME: Rose noble, throatwort, carpenter's square, kernelwort, scrofula plant.

OCCURRENCE: a wild plant of Great Britain and Europe.

PARTS USED: the herb.

MEDICINAL USES: diuretic, anodyne, depurative. Due to this herb's beneficial action on skin abscesses, eruptions and wounds, it has been termed the scrofula plant. The fresh leaves are used as a poultice on sprains, swellings, inflammation, wounds, gangrene and scrofulous sores to great effect.

ADMINISTERED AS: decoction, fresh leaves, dried herb, ointment and fluid extract.

Fireweed *Erechtites hieracifolia* or *Cineraria caradensis*. COMMON NAME: *Senecio hieracifolius*.

OCCURRENCE: a common weed found in Newfoundland and Canada and south to South America.

PARTS USED: the herb, and the oil of erechtites distilled from the herb. The oil is composed of various terpene chemicals.

MEDICINAL USES: astringent, alterative, tonic, cathartic, emetic. Taken internally, it is good for eczema, diarrhoea, haemorrhages and sore throats. It has also been used for colic, spasms, hiccoughs, dysentery and haemorrhoids. When used externally, the oil gives great relief to gout, rheumatism and sciatica.

ADMINISTERED AS: distilled oil in capsules or emulsion, tincture.

Flax *Linum usitatissimum*. COMMON NAME: Linseed.

OCCURRENCE: grows in most temperate and tropical countries.

PARTS USED: the seeds and oil expressed from the seeds, a cake remains which can be ground up to form linseed meal.

MEDICINAL USES: emollient, demulcent, pectoral. A poultice of linseed meal, either alone or with mustard, is effective in relieving pain and irritation from boils, ulcers, inflamed areas and abscesses. Flax is normally utilized as an addition to cough medicines, while linseed oil is sometimes given as a laxative or to remove gravel and stones. When mixed with lime water the oil is excellent on burns and scalds.

administered as: essential oil, ground seed

coats (meal), infusion, syrup and poultice.

Foxglove *Digitalis purpurea*. COMMON NAME: Witch's gloves, dead men's bells, fairy's glove, gloves of Our Lady, bloody fingers, virgin's glove, fairy caps, folk's glove, fairy thimbles, fair women's plant.

OCCURRENCE: indigenous and widely distributed throughout Great Britain and Europe.

PARTS USED: the leaves, which contain four important glucosides—digitoxin, digitalin, digitalein and digitonin—of which the first three listed are cardiac stimulants.

MEDICINAL USES: cardiac tonic, sedative, diuretic. Administering digitalis increases the activity of all forms of muscle tissue, particularly the heart and arterioles. It causes a very high rise in blood pressure and the pulse is slowed and becomes regular. Digitalis causes the heart to contract in size, allowing increased blood flow and nutrient delivery to the organ. It also acts on the kidneys and is a good remedy for dropsy, particularly when it is connected with cardiac problems. The drug has benefits in treating internal haemorrhage, epilepsy, inflammatory diseases and delirium tremens. Digitalis has a cumulative action whereby it is liable to accumulate in the body and then have poisonous effects. It should only be used under medical advice. Digitalis is an excellent antidote in aconite poisoning when given as a hypodermic injection.

ADMINISTERED AS: tincture, infusion, powdered leaves, solid extract, injection.

Fringe tree *Chionanthus virginica*. COMMON NAME: old man's beard, snowdrop tree, poison ash, fringe tree bark, chionanthus.

OCCURRENCE: a small tree, native to the southern United States.

PARTS USED: the dried bark of the root which is thought to contain saponin and a glucoside.

MEDICINAL USES: aperient, diuretic, alterative, tonic. The root is used in typhoid, intermittent or bilious fevers, in liver complaints, jaundice and gallstones. It is taken in conjunction with ANEMONE PULSATILLA and other herbs for women's complaints. Also used as a poultice on wounds and inflammations.

ADMINISTERED AS: infusion, fluid extract.

Frostwort *Helianthemum canadense*. COMMON NAME: Cistus, frostweed, frostplant, rock rose, *Cistus canadensis, Lechea Major, Canadisches Sonnenroschen, Helianthemum ramultoflorum, H. rosmarinifolium, H. michauxii, H. Coprymbosum, Hetraneris canadensis.*

OCCURRENCE: grows in the eastern United States, Great Britain and Europe.

PARTS USED: the dried herb. The main chemical components are a volatile oil, wax, tannin, fatty oil, chlorophyll, gum, inorganic salts and a glucoside.

MEDICINAL USES: antiscrofulous, astringent, alterative, tonic. The herb has a long history of use for diarrhoea, ulcerations, eye complaints, secondary syphilis and any conditions arising from scrofula. It has been beneficial as a poultice for tumours and ulcers and as a gargle in scarlatina. An overdose of the drug is possible and causes nausea and vomiting.

ADMINISTERED AS: liquid extract.

Fumitory *Fumaria officinalis.* COMMON NAME: Earth smoke, beggary, fumus, vapor, nidor, fumus terrae, fumiterry, scheiteregi, taubenkropp, kaphnos, wax dolls.

OCCURRENCE: a common weed plant in Great Britain and Europe, which has been naturalized into North America; originally from Asia and Greece.

PARTS USED: the herb and the expressed juice and fluid extract derived from it.

MEDICINAL USES: weak tonic, diaphoretic, diuretic, aperient. This herb is valuable in all internal obstructions, particularly those of the liver and stomach and is also of benefit in scorbutic afflictions and skin eruptions including leprosy. It is the preferred herb to purify the blood in France and Germany, and in some areas it is smoked as tobacco. It was said to aid removal of skin blemishes and freckles and was also used to ease dyspepsia and headaches.

ADMINISTERED AS: expressed juice, essence, syrup, distilled water, decoction, dried herb, several different tinctures, powdered seed.

Gale, Sweet *Myrica gale.* COMMON NAME: bayberry, English bog myrtle, dutch myrtle, gale palustris.

OCCURRENCE: a bushy shrub found in higher latitudes of the northern hemisphere; abundant in Scottish moors and bogs.

PARTS USED: the shrub.

MEDICINAL USES: aromatic, astringent. The leaves have been used as an emmenagogue and an abortifacient (induces abortion or miscarriage).

ADMINISTERED AS: dried leaves and infusion.

Garlic *Allium sativum.* COMMON NAME: Poor man's treacle.

OCCURRENCE: cultivated throughout Europe since antiquity.

PARTS USED: the bulb.

MEDICINAL USES: antiseptic, diaphoretic, diuretic, expectorant, stimulant. It may be externally applied as ointment, lotion, antiseptic or as a poultice. Syrup of garlic is very good for asthma, coughs, difficulty in breathing and chronic bronchitis, while fresh juice has been used to ease tubercular consumption. The essential oil is commonly taken as a supplement in the form of gelatine capsules. Several species of wild garlic are utilized for both medicinal and dietary purposes.

ADMINISTERED AS: expressed juice, syrup, tincture, essential oil, poultice, lotion and ointment.

Gelsemium *Gelsemium sempervirens.* COMMON NAME: Yellow jasmine, *Gelsemium nitridum*, false jasmine, wild woodbine, Carolina jasmine.

OCCURRENCE: a native North American plant found along the sea coast from Virginia, to southern Florida and Mexico.

PARTS USED: the root which contains two alkaloids — gelsemium and gelsemine, as well as gelsemic acid, a volatile oil, resin and starch.

MEDICINAL USES: antispasmodic, arterial sedative, diaphoretic, febrifuge. Used in small doses to treat neuralgic pains, muscular irritability, nervous excitement and hysteria while its antispasmodic qualities aid asthma, whooping cough, croup and convulsions with great success. It relaxes all muscles and acts on the whole body to remove all sense of pain. The root is very good against bowel inflammation, diarrhoea, dysentery, toothache, chorea, epilepsy, insomnia and headaches due to sickness or alcohol consumption. The drug also benefits acute rheumatism, pleurisy, pneumonia, bronchitis, typhoid fever and pelvic disorders in women. This drug is poisonous and so should be administered in small doses, with very careful monitoring of the patient. Death occurs due to the action of the drug on nervous control of the respiratory system, and can occur very quickly after taking the drug — between one and seven hours after ingestion. Treatment of gelsemium poisoning must be rapid with evacuation of the stomach, artificial respiration and the use of atropine, BELLADONNA (*Atropa belladonna*); strychnine, NUX VOMICA (*Strychnos nux-vomica*); or digitalis, FOXGLOVE (*Digitalis purpurea*) to maintain action of the heart being recommended.

ADMINISTERED AS: tincture, solid extract, infusion.

Gentian, Yellow *Gentiana lutea.*
OCCURRENCE: native to alpine regions of central and southern Europe
PARTS USED: the root. The dried root contains gentian, gentiamarin, bitter glucosides, gentianic acid and various sugars. The fresh root also contains gentiopicrin, another bitter glucoside.
MEDICINAL USES: bitter tonic, stomachic, febrifuge, emmenagogue, anthelmintic and antiseptic. This drug is probably the most effective bitter tonic of use in exhaustion from chronic disease, general debility, weakness of the digestive organs and lack of appetite. It acts to strengthen the whole body and is a very good tonic to combine with purgative drugs in order to temper their debilitating effects. Yellow gentian is useful in many dyspeptic complaints, hysteria, female weakness, intermittent fevers and jaundice. The roots have also been used to make an alcoholic beverage in Germany and Switzerland.
ADMINISTERED AS: infusion, tincture, solid extract, fluid extract.

Germander, Wall *Teucrium chamaedys.* COMMON NAME: Petit chêne, chasse fièvre.
OCCURRENCE: a native of many parts of Europe, the Greek Islands and Syria but is an escape from garden cultivation in England.
PARTS USED: the whole herb, dried.
MEDICINAL USES: stimulant, tonic, diaphoretic, diuretic, aperient. Germander has a reputation as a specific cure for gout, dating back to the sixteenth century. It has been used as a tonic in treating intermittent fevers and uterine obstructions and a decoction of the fresh herb is good against asthmatic afflictions and coughs. The expressed juice is taken for obstructions of the viscera, while the herb has also been used for jaundice, as a vermifuge, ulcers, continual headache and cramps.
ADMINISTERED AS: expressed juice, poultice, decoction, powdered seeds.

Ginger *Zingiber officinale.*
OCCURRENCE: a native of Asia, it is now cultivated in the West Indies, Jamaica and Africa.
PARTS USED: the root, which contains volatile oil, two resins, gum, starch, lignin, acetic acid and asmazone as well as several unidentified compounds.
MEDICINAL USES: stimulant, carminative, expectorant. A valuable herb in dyspepsia, flatulent colic, alcoholic gastritis and diarrhoea. Ginger tea is taken to relieve the effects of cold

temperatures including triggering normal menstruation patterns in women. Ginger is also used to flavour bitter infusions, cough mixtures or syrups.
ADMINISTERED AS: infusion, fluid extract, tincture and syrup.

Ginseng *Panax quinquefolium.* COMMON NAME: *Aralia quinquefolia,* five fingers, tartar root, red berry, man's health, panax, pannag.
OCCURRENCE: native to certain areas of China, eastern Asia and North America. It is largely cultivated in China, Korea and Japan.
PARTS USED: the root which contains a large quantity of gum, resin, volatile oil and the peculiar sweetish compound, panaquilon.
MEDICINAL USES: mild stomachic, tonic, stimulant. The generic name, *panax,* is derived from the Greek for panacea meaning "all-healing." The name ginseng is said to mean "the wonder of the world" and the Chinese consider this herb a sovereign remedy in all diseases. It is good in dyspepsia, vomiting and nervous disorders, consumption and exhaustion. In the West, it is used to treat loss of appetite, stomach and digestive problems, possibly arising from nervous and mental exhaustion. Ginseng is considered to work well against fatigue, old age and its infirmities and to help convalescents recover their health. In healthy people, the drug is said to increase vitality, cure pulmonary complaints and tumours and increase life expectancy. It was also used by the native American Indians for similar problems.
ADMINISTERED AS: tincture, decoction, capsules.

Gladwyn *Iris foetidissina.* COMMON NAME: Stinking gladwyn, gladwin, gladwine, stinking gladdon, spurgewort, spurge plant, roast beef plant.
OCCURRENCE: found in woods and shady parts in southern England.
PARTS USED: the root.
MEDICINAL USES: antispasmodic, cathartic, anodyne. A decoction acts as a strong purge; has been used as an emmenagogue and for removing eruptions. The dried powdered root can be of benefit in hysterical disorders, fainting, nervous problems and to relieve cramps and pain. Taken both internally and as an external poultice, this is an excellent herb to remedy scrofula. The use of this herbal remedy can be dated back to the fourth century before Christ.
ADMINISTERED AS: decoction, dried root, infusion.

Globe flower *Trollius europaeus.* COMMON NAME:

Globe trollius, boule d'or, European globe flower, globe rananculus, globe crow-foot, luchen-gowans.

OCCURRENCE: a native European plant found in moist woods and mountain pastures.

PARTS USED: the whole plant, fresh.

MEDICINAL USES: currently this plant is not used to treat many diseases and it has properties which would benefit from further investigation. It has been used in Russia to treat obstinate scorbutic disorders.

Golden rod *Solidago virgaurea*. COMMON NAME: Verge d'or, solidago, goldruthe, woundwort, Aaron's rod.

OCCURRENCE: normally found wild in woods in Britain, Europe, central Asia and North America but it is also a common garden plant.

PARTS USED: the leaves contain tannin, with some bitter and astringent chemicals which are unknown.

MEDICINAL USES: aromatic, stimulant, carminative. This herb is astringent and diuretic and is highly effective in curing gravel and urinary stones. It aids weak digestion, stops sickness and is very good against diphtheria. As a warm infusion it is a good diaphoretic drug and is used as such to help painful menstruation and amenorrhoea (absence or stopping of menstrual periods).

ADMINISTERED AS: fluid extract, infusion, spray.

Golden seal *Hydrastis canadensis*. COMMON NAME: Orange root, yellow root, yellow puccoon, ground raspberry, wild curcuma, tumeric root, Indian root, eyebalm, Indian paint, jaundice root, warnera, eye root.

OCCURRENCE: a native plant of Canada and the eastern United States.

PARTS USED: the rhizome which contains the alkaloids berberine, hydastine and canadine, as well as resin, albumin, starch, fatty matter, sugar, lignin and volatile oil.

MEDICINAL USES: tonic, stomachic, laxative, alterative, detergent. Native American Indians use this plant as a source of yellow dye for clothing and weapons and also as a remedy for sore eyes, general ulceration and disordered digestion. The herb has a special action on the mucous membranes of the body, making it an excellent remedy for catarrh, dyspepsia, gastric catarrh, loss of appetite and liver problems. Given as a tonic, the root is highly effective in easing constipation and is very good at stopping sickness and vomiting. chronic inflammation of the colon and rectum can be treated by an injection of golden seal, as can haemorrhoids. When taken as an infusion, it may cure night-sweats and passive bleeding from the pelvic tissues. In large doses, *Hydrastis* is very poisonous.

ADMINISTERED AS: injection, infusion, tincture, lotion, fluid extract, dried powdered root, solid extract.

Gooseberry *Ribes grossularia*. COMMON NAME: Fea, feverberry, feabes, carberry, groseille, groset, groser, krusbaar, dewberries, goosegogs, honeyblobs, feaberry.

OCCURRENCE: a well-known shrub native to central and northern Europe, especially Great Britain.

PARTS USED: the fruit and leaves, which contain citric acid, sugar, various minerals and pectose.

MEDICINAL USES: the expressed juice is said to be a cure for all inflammations. The acid red fruit is made into a light jelly which is good for sedentary and bilious complaints as well as in cases of excess body fluid. An infusion of dried leaves is effective in treating gravel and is a useful tonic for menstruating young girls. In the Highlands of Scotland, the prickles were used as charms to remove warts and styes.

ADMINISTERED AS: an infusion, expressed juice, dietary item.

Goutwort *Aegopodium podagraria*. COMMON NAME: Goutweed, goutherb, ashweed, Jack-jump-about, herb gerard, English masterwort, pigweed, eltroot, ground elder, bishops elder, white ash, ground ash, weyl ash, bishopsweed.

OCCURRENCE: a weed plant of Europe, Great Britain and Russian Asia.

PARTS USED: the herb

MEDICINAL USES: diuretic and sedative. Taken internally for aching joints, gouty and sciatic pain and as an external poultice for inflamed areas. It was thought that carrying some of the herb in a pocket would prevent an attack of gout developing.

ADMINISTERED AS: poultice, liquid extract.

Groundsel *Senecio vulgaris*. COMMON NAME: Common groundsel, grundy, swallow, ground glutton, simson, sention, grounsel.

OCCURRENCE: very common weed throughout Europe and Russian Asia.

PARTS USED: the whole herb and fresh plant. The plant contains senecin and seniocine.

MEDICINAL USES: diaphoretic, anti scorbutic, purgative, diuretic, anthelmintic. It is good for sickness of the stomach, used as a purgative in a weak infusion and as an emetic when in a strong infusion. This infusion removes bilious trouble and lowers body temperature. A poultice of groundsel is used warm on boils but nursing mothers have cold poultices as a coolant on swollen, inflamed or hardened breasts. If boiling water is poured on to the fresh plant, the resulting liquid is a pleasant swab for the skin and helps soften chapped hands

ADMINISTERED AS: infusion, poultice lotion.

Guarana *Paullinia cupara*. COMMON NAME: Paullina, guarana bread, Brazilian cocoa, uabano, uaranzeiro, *Paullina sorbilis*.

OCCURRENCE: native to Brazil and Uruguay.

PARTS USED: the prepared seed, crushed. The seeds are shelled, roasted for six hours and shaken until their outer shell comes off. They are ground to a fine powder, made into a dough with water and formed into cylinders which are dried in the sun or over a fire. The seed preparation is eaten with water by the native people. The roasted seeds contain caffeine, tannic acid, catechutannic acid, starch and a fixed oil.

MEDICINAL USES: nervine, tonic, stimulant, aphrodisiac, febrifuge, slightly narcotic. It is used in mild forms of diarrhoea or leucorrhoea and also for headaches, in particular those linked to the menstrual cycle. Guarana stimulates the brain after mental exertion, or after fatigue or exhaustion due to hot temperatures. It may also have diuretic effects where it can help rheumatism, lumbago and bowel complaints. The drug is similar to that of COCA or COFFEE.

ADMINISTERED AS: powder, fluid extract, tincture.

Hair-cap moss *Polytrichium juniperum*. COMMON NAME: Bear's bed, robin's eye, ground moss, golden maidenhair, female fern herb, robinsrye, rockbrake herb.

OCCURRENCE: found in woods and hedges across Europe and Britain.

PARTS USED: the whole plant.

MEDICINAL USES: powerful diuretic. It is a very important remedy in dropsy, urinary obstructions, gravel and suppression of urine. The herb does not cause nausea and is frequently combined with BROOM or CARROT for best effects.

ADMINISTERED AS: infusion.

Hawthorn *Crataegus oxyacantha*. COMMON NAME: May, mayblossom, quick, thorn, whitethorn, haw, hazels, gazels, halves, hagthorn, ladies meat, bread and cheese tree, maybush.

OCCURRENCE: a familiar tree in Great Britain, Europe, North Africa and Western Asia.

PARTS USED: the dried fruits which contain the chemical amyddalin.

MEDICINAL USES: cardiac, diuretic, astringent, tonic. Mainly used as a cardiac tonic in organic and functional heart problems, e.g. hypertrophy, dyspnoea, heart oppression. A decoction of the flowers and berries is good at curing sore throats, and is utilized as a diuretic in dropsy and kidney disorders.

ADMINISTERED AS: liquid extract, decoction.

Heartease *Viola tricolor*. COMMON NAME: Wild pansy, love-lies-bleeding, loving idol, call-me-to-you, three-faces-under-a-hood, godfathers and godmothers, pink-eyed-John, flower o'luce, Jack-jump-up-and-kiss-me.

OCCURRENCE: abundant all over Great Britain, in cornfields, gardens, waste ground and hedge banks. It is also distributed through Arctic Europe, North Africa, Siberia and North India.

PARTS USED: the whole herb, fresh and dried. The active chemicals within the plant include violine, mucilage, resin, salicylic acid and sugar.

MEDICINAL USES: diaphoretic and diuretic. It was formerly held in high regard as a remedy for epilepsy, asthma and catarrhal infections. It has been utilized in blood disorders and heart diseases, while a decoction of the flowers was recommended for skin diseases. In America, they use heartease as an ointment or poultice in eczema, and it is taken internally for bronchitis. People on the continent have used *Viola tricolor* for its mucilaginous, demulcent and expectorant qualities.

ADMINISTERED AS: decoction, ointment, poultice and tincture.

Hedge-hyssop *Gratiola officinalis*

OCCURRENCE: a perennial plant, native to southern Europe and found wild in damp areas in Great Britain.

PARTS USED: the root and herb. The plant contains the glucosides gratiolin and gratiosolin.

MEDICINAL USES: diuretic, cathartic, emetic. Recommended in scrofula, chronic liver complaints and enlargement of the spleen. It is also utilized in relieving dropsy and as a vermifuge.

ADMINISTERED AS: an infusion of powdered root.

Hellebore, Black *Helleborus niger*. COMMON NAME: Christe herbe, Christmas rose, melampodium.

OCCURRENCE: a native of the mountains in central and southern Europe, Greece and Asia minor, but found in Britain as a garden plant.

PARTS USED: the rhizome and root. The plant has

two glucosides within it, helleborin and helleborcin, both of which are powerful poisons.

MEDICINAL USES: the drug has drastic purgative, emmenagogue and anthelmintic properties, but is a violent narcotic. It is of value in treating nervous disorders, hysteria and melancholia and was previously used in dropsy and amenorrhoea. Given externally, the fresh root is violently irritant. The drug must be administered with great care.

ADMINISTERED AS: fluid extract, tincture, solid extract, powdered root or decoction.

Hemlock *Conium maculatum.* COMMON NAME: Herb bennet, spotted conebane, musquash root, beaver poison, poison hemlock, poison parsley, spotted hemlock, vex, vecksies.

OCCURRENCE: common in hedges, meadows, waste ground and stream banks throughout Europe and is also found in temperate Asia and North Africa.

PARTS USED: the leaves, fruits and seeds. The most important constituent of hemlock leaves is the alkaloid coniine, which is poisonous, with a disagreeable odour. Other alkaloids in the plant include methyl-coniine, conhydrine, pseudoconhydrine, ethyl piperidine.

MEDICINAL USES: sedative, antispasmodic, anodyne. The drug acts on the centres of motion and causes paralysis and so it is used to remedy undue nervous motor excitability, e.g. teething, cramp and muscle spasms of the larynx and gullet. When inhaled, hemlock is said to be good in relieving coughs, bronchitis, whooping cough and asthma. The method of action of *Conium* means it is directly antagonistic to the effects of strychnine, from NUX VOMICA (*Strychnos nux-vomica*), and hence it is used as an antidote to strychnine poisoning and similar poisons. Hemlock has to be administered with care as narcotic poisoning may result from internal application and overdoses induce paralysis, with loss of speech and depression of respiratory function leading to death. Antidotes to hemlock poisoning are tannic acid, stimulants, e.g. COFFEE, MUSTARD and CASTOR OIL.

ADMINISTERED AS: powdered leaves, fluid extract, tincture, expressed juice of the leaves and solid extract.

Henbane *Hyoscyamus niger.* COMMON NAME: Hyoscyamus, hog's bean, Jupiter's-bean, symphonica, cassilata, cassilago, deus caballinus.

OCCURRENCE: native to central and southern Europe and western Asia and was introduced to Great Britain, North America and Brazil where it is found on waste ground, ditches and near old buildings.

PARTS USED: the fresh leaves and flowering tops. The chief constituents of henbane leaves are the alkaloids hyoscyamine, atropine and hyoscine. The leaves also contain a bitter principle called hyoscytricin, choline, mucilage, calcium oxalate, potassium nitrate and fixed oil.

MEDICINAL USES: antispasmodic, hypnotic, mild diuretic, mydriatic, anodyne, sedative. The herb has a milder narcotic effect than BELLADONNA or STRAMONIUM and is utilized to lessen muscle spasms, reduce pain and can stop nervous irritation. It is used in cystitis, irritable bladder, hysteria, irritable cough, asthma, gastric ulcers and chronic gastric catarrh. When taken in small doses repeated over time, Henbane tranquillizes people affected by severe nervous irritability, enabling them to sleep without adversely affecting the digestive organs or causing headaches, which opium has the tendency to do. Thus, henbane is given to people with insomnia and to children, to which opium cannot be given. The fresh leaves of henbane can be used as a poultice to relieve local pain from gout, neuralgia, cancerous ulcers, sores and swellings. The solid extract of the drug is used to produce suppositories which are used to relieve the pain of haemorrhoids. Henbane is poisonous and should never be used except under medical advice.

ADMINISTERED AS: powdered leaves, tincture, fluid extract, expressed juice, solid extract, suppositories.

Holly *Ilex aquifolium.* COMMON NAME: Holm, hulver bush, hulm, holme chase, holy tree, Christ's thorn.

OCCURRENCE: native to central and southern Europe and grows freely in Great Britain

PARTS USED: the leaves, berries and bark

MEDICINAL USES: diaphoretic, febrifuge, cathartic, tonic. Infused holly leaves are used in catarrh, pleurisy and formerly against smallpox. Also in intermittent fevers and rheumatism where the alkaloid ilicin works to good effect. Juice expressed from fresh holly leaves is effective against jaundice. The berries have different properties and are violently emetic and purgative, but they have been utilized in dropsy and as a powder to check bleeding. Holly leaves have been utilized as a tea substitute.

ADMINISTERED AS: infusion of leaves, juice, whole or powdered berries.

Honeysuckle *Lonicera caprifolium*. COMMON NAME: Dutch honeysuckle, goat's leaf, perfoliate honeysuckle.

OCCURRENCE: grows freely in Europe, Great Britain and through the northern temperate zone.

PARTS USED: the dried flowers and leaves

MEDICINAL USES: expectorant, laxative. A syrup made of the flowers is used for respiratory diseases and asthma. A decoction of the leaves is laxative and is also good against diseases of the liver and spleen, and in gargles.

ADMINISTERED AS: syrup, decoction.

Hops *Humulus lupulus*.

OCCURRENCE: a native British plant, found wild in hedges and woods from Yorkshire southward. It is considered an introduced species to Scotland but is also found in most countries of the northern temperate zone.

PARTS USED: the flowers, which contain a volatile oil, two bitter principles — lupamaric acid, lupalinic acid and tannin.

MEDICINAL USES: tonic, nervine, diuretic, anodyne, aromatic. The volatile oil has sedative and soporific effects while the bitter principles are stomachic and tonic. Hops are used to promote the appetite and enhance sleep. An infusion is very effective in heart disease, fits, neuralgia, indigestion, jaundice, nervous disorders and stomach or liver problems. Hop juice is a blood cleanser and is very effective in remedying calculus problems. As an external application, hops are used with CHAMOMILE heads as an infusion to reduce painful swellings or inflammation and bruises. This combination may also be used as a poultice.

ADMINISTERED AS: an infusion, tincture, poultice, expressed juice or tea.

Horehound *Marrubium vulgare*. COMMON NAME: Hoarhound, white horehound.

OCCURRENCE: indigenous to Britain and found all over Europe.

PARTS USED: the herb, which contains the bitter principle marrubium, volatile oil, tannin sugar and resin.

MEDICINAL USES: tonic, expectorant, pectoral, diuretic. It is probably the most popular pectoral herbal remedy. Very valuable in coughs, asthma, consumption and pulmonary complaints. For children, it is given as a syrup to ease croup, stomach upsets and as a tonic.

Taken in large doses, Horehound is a gentle purgative and the powdered leaves have been used as a vermifuge. A tea of the herb is excellent for colds. A sweetmeat candy and an ale is also made from horehound.

ADMINISTERED AS: syrup, infusion, tea, powdered leaves, ointment, expressed juice.

Horsemint, American *Monarda punctata*

OCCURRENCE: native to North America and was introduced into England in 1714.

PARTS USED: the herb produces a volatile oil which is composed of thymol and higher oxygenated compounds.

MEDICINAL USES: rubefacient, stimulant, carminative, diuretic. It is used as an infusion for flatulent colic, sickness and urinary disorders and has diaphoretic and emmenagogue actions also. It is principally used externally wherever a rubefacient is required, e.g. chronic rheumatism.

ADMINISTERED AS: a volatile oil.

Horseradish *Cochlearia armoracia*. COMMON NAME: Mountain radish, great raifort, red cole, *Armoracia rusticara*.

OCCURRENCE: cultivated in the British Isles for centuries. The place of origin is unknown.

PARTS USED: the root which contains the glucoside sinigrin, vitamin C, aspargin and resin.

MEDICINAL USES: stimulant, aperient, rubefacient, diuretic, antiseptic, diaphoretic. Horseradish is a powerful stimulant of the digestive organs, and it acts on lung and urinary infections clearing them away. The herb is a very strong diuretic and as such is used to ease dropsy, gravel and calculus, as well as being taken internally for gout and rheumatism. A poultice can be made from the fresh root and applied to rheumatic joints, chilblains and to ease facial neuralgia. Horseradish juice, when diluted with vinegar and glycerine, was used in children's whooping cough and to relieve hoarseness of the throat. An infusion of the root in urine was stimulating to the entire nervous system and promoted perspiration, while it was also used to expel worms in children. Care should be taken when using this herb because over-use of horseradish can blister the skin and is not suitable for people with thyroid troubles.

ADMINISTERED AS: infusion, syrup, expressed juice, fluid extract.

Horsetail *Equisetum arvense*. COMMON NAME: Mare's tail, shave-grass, bottlebrush, paddock-pipes, Dutch rushes, pewterwort.

OCCURRENCE: native to Great Britain and distributed through the temperate northern regions.

PARTS USED: the herb which is composed of silica, saponin, flavonoids, tannin and traces of alkaloids — nicotine, palustrine and palustrinine.

MEDICINAL USES: diuretic, astringent. Due to the herb's rich store of minerals, horsetail is given for anaemia and general debility and can also work to encourage the absorption and efficient use of calcium by the body, helping prevent fatty deposits forming in the arteries (arteriosclerosis). It helps stop bleeding and hence is good for stomach ulcers and haemorrhage as well as easing dropsy, gravel, cystitis and inflamed prostate glands due to its astringent qualities. The herb can be of benefit in the treatment of bed-wetting in children.

ADMINISTERED AS: infusion, dried herb, syrup.

Hound's tongue *Cynoglossum officinale.* COMMON NAME: dog's tongue, *Lindefolia spectabilis.*

OCCURRENCE: a common plant in Switzerland and Germany; occasionally found in Great Britain.

PARTS USED: the herb.

MEDICINAL USES: anodyne, demulcent, astringent. Used as pills or as a decoction for colds, coughs, catarrh, diarrhoea and dysentery. Administered both internally and externally to soothe the digestive organs and haemorrhoids.

ADMINISTERED AS: decoction, pills, ointment.

Houseleek *Sempervivum tectorum.* COMMON NAME: Jupiter's eye, Thor's beard, bullock's eye, sengreen, ayron, ayegreen.

OCCURRENCE: native to the mountains of central and southern Europe and the Greek islands but introduced to Britain many centuries ago.

PARTS USED: the fresh leaves.

MEDICINAL USES: refrigerant, astringent, diuretic. The bruised fresh leaves or its expressed juice are often applied as a poultice to burns, scalds, bumps, scrofulous ulcers and general skin inflammation. The juice is a cure for warts and corns. In large doses, houseleek juice is emetic and purgative. The plant was supposed to guard where it grew against fire, lightning and sorcery, hence it was grown on house roofs.

Hydrangea *Hydrangea aborescens.* COMMON NAME: Wild hydrangea, seven barks, common hydrangea, *Hydrangea vulgaris.*

OCCURRENCE: native to the United States and is cultivated across the world as a garden plant.

PARTS USED: the root which contains two resins, gum, sugar, starch, sulphuric and phosphoric acids and a glucoside called hydrangin.

MEDICINAL USES: diuretic, cathartic, tonic, nephritic. This herb is very good at preventing and removing stones in the urinary system, and relieving the pain due to urinary gravel. The fluid extract is also used to correct alkaline urine, chronic vaginal discharges and irritation of the bladder in older people. This drug was used by native American Indians and its benefits were passed on to European settlers.

ADMINISTERED AS: fluid extract, decoction, syrup.

Iceland moss *Cetraria islandica.* COMMON NAME: Iceland lichen, cetraria.

OCCURRENCE: indigenous to a wide area of the northern hemisphere.

PARTS USED: the dried whole lichen. The moss contains a large quantity of starchy mater called lichenin as well as fumaric acid, oxalic acid and iodine.

MEDICINAL USES: demulcent, tonic, nutritive. The lichen has antibiotic properties and used to be given for tuberculosis as it was reputed to kill the tubercle bacillus, and clear phlegm from the lungs. It is used today for asthma, other respiratory problems and to soothe the digestive tract, stopping nausea. It is also used as a food, once the bitter principles are removed by boiling.

ADMINISTERED AS: decoction, dietary item.

Ipecacuanha *Cephaelis ipecacuanha.* COMMON NAME: *Psychotria ipecacuanha.*

OCCURRENCE: native to Brazil, Bolivia and parts of South America and was introduced into Europe in the seventeenth century.

PARTS USED: the chief constituents of the root are the alkaloids emetrine, cephaelin and psychotrine, as well as two glucosides, choline, resin, calcium oxalate and a volatile oil among other compounds.

MEDICINAL USES: diaphoretic, emetic, expectorant, stimulant. The effects of the drug on the body are entirely dependent on the dose given. In very small doses, ipecacuanha stimulates the stomach, liver and intestine aiding digestion and increasing appetite while in slightly larger doses it has diaphoretic and expectorant properties which are good for colds, coughs and dysentery. Large doses of the drug are emetic. There is a lot of historical use of this drug against amoebic (or tropical) dysentery where rapid cures can occur. Care should be taken in utilizing this drug as emetine can have a toxic effect on the heart, blood vessels, lungs and intestines and cause severe illness.

ADMINISTERED AS: powdered root, fluid extract, tincture, syrup.

Irish moss *Chondrus crispus*. COMMON NAME: Carrageen, chondrus, carrahan, carragheen.
OCCURRENCE: common at low tide on all shores of the North Atlantic.
PARTS USED: the dried plant which contains mucilage and sulphur compounds.
MEDICINAL USES: demulcent, pectoral, emollient; nutritive. A popular remedy which is made into a jelly for pulmonary complaints, kidney and bladder diseases. It is widely used as a culinary article.
ADMINISTERED AS: dietary item.

Ivy *Hedera helix*. COMMON NAME: Common ivy.
OCCURRENCE: native to many parts of Europe and northern and central Asia.
PARTS USED: the leaves and berries.
MEDICINAL USES: stimulating, diaphoretic, cathartic. The leaves have been used as poultices on enlarged glands, ulcers and abscesses and the berries ease fevers and were used extensively during the Great Plague of London.
ADMINISTERED AS: poultice, infusion.

Ivy, Ground *Glechoma Hederacea*. COMMON NAME: alehoof, gill-go-over-the-ground, haymaids, tun-hoof, hedgemaids, coltsfoot, robin-run-in-the-hedge.
OCCURRENCE: very common on hedges and waste ground all over Britain.
PARTS USED: the whole herb
MEDICINAL USES: diuretic, astringent, tonic and gently stimulant. It is good in relieving kidney diseases and indigestion. Ground ivy tea is useful in pectoral complaints and in weakness of the digestive organs. The expressed juice, when sniffed up the nose, is said to successfully cure a headache and can be administered externally to ease bruises and black eyes. It also has antiscorbutic qualities.
ADMINISTERED AS: fluid extract, expressed juice and infusion.

Ivy, Poison *Rhus toxicodendron*. COMMON NAME: Poison oak, poison vine.
OCCURRENCE: native to the United States of America.
PARTS USED: the fresh leaves which contain a resin called toxicodendron as the active principle.
MEDICINAL USES: irritant, rubefacient, stimulant, narcotic. This herb is successful in treating obstinate skin eruptions, palsy, paralysis, acute rheumatism and joint stiffness. It has also been good in treating ringworm, allergic rashes and urinary incontinence. In small doses, poison ivy is a very good sedative for the nervous system, but care must be taken in its use as it can trigger gastric and intestinal irritation, drowsiness, stupor and delirium.
ADMINISTERED AS: tincture, fluid extract, infusion.

Jaborandi *Pilocarpus microphyllus*. COMMON NAME: Arruda do mato, arruda brava, jamguarandi, juarandi.
OCCURRENCE: a native Brazilian plant.
PARTS USED: the dried leaves. The main constituents of the leaves are a volatile oil and three alkaloids—pilocarpine, isopilocarpine, pilocarpidine.
MEDICINAL USES: stimulant, diaphoretic, expectorant. This herb is used as the crude drug and as the purified alkaloid, pilocarpine. Jaborandi is used for psoriasis, deafness, baldness, chronic catarrh, tonsillitis, dropsy and catarrhal jaundice. It can also benefit fat removal from the heart in heart disease, pleurisy, chronic renal diseases and reducing thirst in fevered patients. The extracted alkaloid, Pilocarpine, has an antagonistic effect to atropine, from BELLADONNA, *Atropa belladonna* and other related plants, and causes contraction of the pupil of the eye. It is used as a fast and highly effective diaphoretic drug, increasing gland secretions and the flow of breast milk. Both the jaborandi and pilocarpine can irritate the stomach, causing vomiting even when given as an injection, so care should be advised upon using this drug.
ADMINISTERED AS: powdered leaves, tincture, injection, fluid extract.

Jacob's ladder *Polemonicum coeruleum*. COMMON NAME: Greek valerian, charity.
OCCURRENCE: found wild in ditches and streams across England and southern Scotland.
PARTS USED: the herb.
MEDICINAL USES: diaphoretic, astringent, alterative, expectorant. A useful drug in fevers and inflammatory diseases, pleurisy, etc. It induces copious perspiration and eases coughs, colds, bronchial and lung complaints.
ADMINISTERED AS: an infusion.

Jewelweed *Impatiens aurea, Impatiens biflora*. COMMON NAME: Wild balsam, balsamweed, pale-touch-me-not, slipperweed, silverweed, wild lady's slipper, speckled jewels, wild celandine, quick in the hand, *Impatiens pallida, I. fulva*.
OCCURRENCE: members of the genus *Impatiens* are found distributed across the northern temperate zone and South Africa; mostly natives

of mountainous regions in tropical Asia and Africa.

PARTS USED: the herb.

MEDICINAL USES: aperient, diuretic, emetic, cathartic. The diuretic qualities of the herb make it useful against dropsy and jaundice while the fresh juice is reputed to remove warts, corns and cure ringworm. The fresh herb was made into an ointment with lard and used for piles. Due to its acrid taste and strong action, jewelweed is rarely used in herbal medicine today.

ADMINISTERED AS: expressed juice, ointment.

Juniper *Juniperus communis*

OCCURRENCE: a common shrub native to Great Britain and widely distributed through many parts of the world.

PARTS USED: the berry and leaves.

MEDICINAL USES: the oil of juniper obtained from the ripe berries is stomachic, diuretic and carminative and is used to treat indigestion, flatulence as well as kidney and bladder diseases. The main use of juniper is in dropsy, and aiding other diuretic herbs to ease the disease.

ADMINISTERED AS: essential oil from berries, essential oil from wood, fluid extract, liquid extract, solid extract.

Kamala *Mallotus philippinensis*. COMMON NAME: Glandulae rottelerde, kamcela, spoonwood, *Röttlera tinctoria*, kameela.

OCCURRENCE: native to India, Abyssinia, southern Arabia, China and Australia.

PARTS USED: the powder removed from the capsular fruit, composed of hairs and glands.

MEDICINAL USES: taeniafuge, purgative. The powder kills and expels tapeworms from the body. The worm is usually removed whole. It is a quick and active purgative drug, causing griping and nausea. It is used externally for cutaneous complaints including scabies and herpetic ringworm.

ADMINISTERED AS: powdered kamala, fluid extract.

Kava-kava *Piper methysticum*. COMMON NAME: Ava, ava pepper, kava, intoxicating pepper.

OCCURRENCE: indigenous to Polynesia, Sandwich Islands, South Sea Islands and Australian colonies.

PARTS USED: the peeled, dried rhizome. The plant contains two resins, one called kavine, a volatile oil, starch and an alkaloid termed kavaine methysticcum yangonin.

MEDICINAL USES: tonic, stimulant, diuretic. There

is a long history of use against gonorrhoea, vaginitis, leucorrhoea, nocturnal incontinence and other problems of the urinary-genital tract. As a strong diuretic, kava is good for gout, rheumatism, bronchial problems and heart trouble. Kava acts on the nerve centres in a stimulating, then depressing manner, and has been used as a local anaesthetic as it causes paralysis of the respiratory centre. It relieves pain and has an aphrodisiac effect.

ADMINISTERED AS: powdered root, fluid extract, solid extract.

Knapweed, Greater *Centaurea scabiosa*.

COMMON NAME: Hardhead, ironhead, hard irons, churls head, logger head, horse knops, mat fellon, bottleweed, bullweed, cowede, bottsede.

OCCURRENCE: a perennial plant frequently seen in field borders and waste ground in England, but rare in Scotland.

PARTS USED: the root and seeds.

MEDICINAL USES: diuretic, diaphoretic and tonic. Formerly greatly appreciated as a vulnerary herb and used to cure loss of appetite. When taken as a decoction, it is good for catarrh; as an ointment for wounds, bruises and sores, etc.

ADMINISTERED AS: decoction and ointment.

Knotgrass *Polyganum ariculare*. COMMON NAME: Centuriode, ninety-knot, nine-joints, allseed, bird's tongue, sparrow tongue, red robin, armstrong, cowgrass, hogweed, pigrush, swynel grass, swine's grass.

OCCURRENCE: native around the globe; abundant on arable land, waste ground and roadside verges.

PARTS USED: the whole herb.

MEDICINAL USES: astringent, diuretic, anthelmintic, vulnerary and styptic. An infusion of the herb was used in diarrhoea, bleeding haemorrhoids and all haemorrhages. As a diuretic, it was said to expel stones and also parasitic worms. The fresh juice stops nosebleeds, if squirted up the nose and applied to the temples. As an ointment, it heals sores very well.

ADMINISTERED AS: expressed juice, infusion, decoction and ointment.

Kola nuts *Kola vera*. COMMON NAME: Guru nut, cola, kola seeds, gurru nuts, bissy nuts, cola seeds, *Cola acuminata*, *Sterculia acuminata*.

OCCURRENCE: native to Sierra Leone and North Ashanti and cultivated in tropical western Africa, West Indies, Brazil and Java.

PARTS USED: the seeds.

MEDICINAL USES: nerve stimulant, diuretic, cardiac tonic. This drug is a good overall tonic, largely due to the caffeine it contains. It has been used as a remedy for diarrhoea and for those with an alcoholic habit.

ADMINISTERED AS: powdered seeds, tincture, fluid and solid extract.

Laburnum *Cytisus laburnam*. COMMON NAME: Yellow laburnum.

OCCURRENCE: indigenous to high mountain regions of Europe and widely cultivated across the globe as a garden plant.

PARTS USED: the alkaloid, obtained from the plant, called cytisine.

MEDICINAL USES: all parts of the laburnum are thought to be poisonous, particularly the seeds. The alkaloid has been recommended in whooping cough and asthma, and also as an insecticide, but it has not been used due to the very poisonous nature of the compound. Laburnum poisoning symptoms include intense sleepiness, vomiting, convulsive movements, coma and unequally dilated pupils. Laburnum is also poisonous to cattle and horses and deaths of both livestock and humans have resulted from ingestion of this plant.

Lady's mantle *Alchemilla vulgaris*. COMMON NAME: Lion's foot, bear's foot, nine hooks, stellaria.

OCCURRENCE: native to mountainous districts of Britain and widely distributed over northern or Arctic Europe, Asia and greenland.

PARTS USED: the herb.

MEDICINAL USES: astringent, styptic, vulnerary. Herbalists used to say that lady's mantle was one of the best herbs for wounds. In modern times, it is used as a cure for excessive menstruation as an infusion or injection. The root is very good for stopping all bleeding and may also act as a violent purge. The herb is also said to promote quiet sleep.

ADMINISTERED AS: decoction, infusion, injection, tincture, fluid extract, dried root.

Larch *Pinus larix*. COMMON NAME: *Larix europaea*, *Abies larix*, *Larix decidua*, *Laricus cortex*, European larch, Venice turpentine.

OCCURRENCE: indigenous to hilly regions of central Europe, but was introduced into Britain in 1639.

PARTS USED: the inner bark which contains tannic acid, larixinic acid and turpentine.

MEDICINAL USES: stimulant, diuretic, astringent, balsamic and expectorant. It is very useful as an external application for eczema and psoria-

sis. However, it is mainly used as a stimulant expectorant in chronic bronchitis, internal haemorrhage and cystitis. Larch turpentine has also been suggested as an antidote in cyanide or opium poisoning and has been used as a hospital disinfectant.

ADMINISTERED AS: fluid extract or syrup.

Larkspur *Delphinicum consolida*. COMMON NAME: Field larkspur, lark's chaw, lark's heel, knight's spur.

OCCURRENCE: found wild in fields through Europe and Great Britain.

PARTS USED: the seeds. The active principle in the plant is delphinine, an irritant poison also found in STAVESACRE.

MEDICINAL USES: parasiticide, insecticide. The tincture of the seeds is used to destroy lice and nits in the hair and given internally in spasmodic asthma and dropsy. The expressed juice from the leaves was applied to bleeding piles and an infusion of the whole plant was said to benefit colic.

ADMINISTERED AS: infusion, tincture, expressed juice.

Laurel *Laurus nobilis*. COMMON NAME: bay, sweet bay, true laurel, laurier d'apollon, roman laurel, noble laurel, lorbeer, laurier sauce, daphne.

OCCURRENCE: native to the shores of the Mediterranean and cultivated in Britain.

PARTS USED: the leaves, fruit and essential oil. The volatile oil contains pinene, geraniol, eugenol, cineol, bitter principles and tannin.

MEDICINAL USES: stomachic, narcotic, diaphoretic, emetic. In ancient times, laurel was highly valued as a medicine but now laurel is only selectively utilized. The leaves were formerly used in hysteria, flatulent colic and in treating the absence of menstrual periods, but now are only used to stimulate the digestion. The oil of bays is also used for earache, sprains and bruises and rheumatism.

ADMINISTERED AS: essential oil, infusion.

Lavender, English *Lavandula vera*

OCCURRENCE: indigenous to mountainous regions in the western Mediterranean and is cultivated extensively in France, Italy, England and Norway.

PARTS USED: the flowers and the essential oil which contains linalool, linalyl acetate, cineol, pinene, limonene and tannin

MEDICINAL USES: aromatic, carminative, stimulant, nervine. It is mainly used as a flavouring agent for disagreeable odours in ointments or syrups. The essential oil when taken internally is restorative and a tonic against faintness, heart palpitations, giddiness and colic. It raises the spirits, promotes the appetite and dispels flatulence. When applied externally, the oil relieves toothache, neuralgia, sprains and rheumatism. The oil is utilized widely in aromatherapy, often to very beneficial effects.

ADMINISTERED AS: fluid extract, tincture, essential oil, spirit, infusion, tea, poultice, distilled water.

Lemon *Citrus limonica*. COMMON NAME: Limon, *Citrus medica*, *Citrus Limonum*, citronnier, neemoo, leemoo, limoun, limone.

OCCURRENCE: indigenous to northern India and widely cultivated in Mediterranean countries.

PARTS USED: the fruit, rind, juice and oil. Lemon peel contains an essential oil and a bitter principle, while lemon juice is rich in citric acid, sugar and gum. Oil of lemon contains the aldehyde, citral and the oils pinene and citronella.

MEDICINAL USES: antiscorbutic, tonic, refrigerant, cooling. Lemon juice is the best preventative drug for scurvy and is also very valuable in fevers and for allaying thirst. It is recommended in acute rheumatism and may be given to counteract narcotic poisons such as opium. It is used as an astringent gargle in sore throats, for uterine haemorrhage after childbirth, as a lotion in sunburn and as a cure for severe hiccoughs. The juice is also good for jaundice and heart palpitations. A decoction of lemon is a good antiperiodic drug and can be used to replace quinine in malarial injections, or to reduce the temperature in typhoid fever. Lemon oil is a strong external rubefacient and also has stomachic and carminative qualities.

ADMINISTERED AS: syrup, decoction, fresh juice, tincture, essential oil, dietary item.

Lettuce, Wild *Lactuca virosa*. COMMON NAME: Lachicarium, strong-scented lettuce, green endive, lettuce opium, acrid lettuce, laitue vireuse.

OCCURRENCE: found in western and southern Europe, including Great Britain.

PARTS USED: the leaves, dried milk juice — lactuarium. Lactuarium is obtained by cutting the stem in sections and collecting the latex juice. It turns reddish-brown in colour when dried.

MEDICINAL USES: anodyne, sedative, narcotic, mild diaphoretic, diuretic. The drug resembles a weak opium, without opium's tendency to upset the digestive system. It is used to allay irritable coughs and as a sedative and narcotic, but only infrequently. It is also used for dropsy, inducing sleep and easing colic.

ADMINISTERED AS: powder, tincture, fluid extract, syrup, alcoholic extract.

Lilac *Syringa vulgaris*. COMMON NAME: Common lilac.

OCCURRENCE: a shrub native to Persia and the mountains of eastern Europe.

PARTS USED: the leaves and fruit.

MEDICINAL USES: as a vermifuge, tonic, antiperiodic and febrifuge. It may be used as a substitute for ALOES (*Aloe vera*/*Aloe perryi*) and in the treatment of malaria.

ADMINISTERED AS: an infusion.

Lily, Madonna *Lilium candidum*. COMMON NAME: White lily, meadow lily.

OCCURRENCE: a southern European native which has been cultivated in Great Britain and America for centuries.

PARTS USED: the bulb.

MEDICINAL USES: demulcent, astringent, mucilaginous. The bulb is mainly used as an emollient poultice for ulcers, tumours and external inflammation. When made into an ointment, Madonna lily removes corns and eliminates pain and inflammation from burns and scalds, reducing scarring. When used in combination with life root (*Senecio aureus*), Madonnna lily is of great value in treating leucorrhoea, prolapse of the womb and other female complaints. The bulb is very often eaten as food in Japan.

ADMINISTERED AS: poultice, ointment, decoction.

Lily of the valley *Convallaria magalis*. COMMON NAME: May lily, convarraria, Our Lady's tears, conval-lily, lily constancy, ladder to heaven, Jacob's ladder.

OCCURRENCE: native to Europe and distributed over North America and northern Asia. It is a very localized plant in England and Scotland.

PARTS USED: the flowers, leaves and whole herb. The chief constituents are two glucosides — convallamarin (the active principle) and convallarin, as well as tannin and mineral salts.

MEDICINAL USES: cardiac tonic, diuretic. A similar drug to digitalis, from the FOXGLOVE, although it is less powerful. Strongly recommended in valvular heart disease, cardiac debility, dropsy and it slows the action of a weak, irritated heart. Lily of the valley does not have accumulatory effects and can be taken in full and frequent doses without harm. A decoction of the flowers is good at removing obstructions in the urinary canal.

ADMINISTERED AS: fluid extracts, decoction tincture, powdered flowers.

Lime fruit *Citrus medica* var. *acida*. COMMON NAME: *Citrus acris*, *Citrus acida*, limettae fructus.

OCCURRENCE: a native Asian tree which is cultivated in many warm countries including the West Indies and Italy.

PARTS USED: the fruit and juice.

MEDICINAL USES: refrigerant, antiscorbutic. The juice of the lime contains citric acid and is a popular beverage, sweetened as a syrup. It is used to treat dyspepsia.

ADMINISTERED AS: fresh juice, syrup

Lime tree *Tilia europoea*. COMMON NAME: Linden flowers, linn flowers, common lime, tilleul, flores tiliae, *Tilia vulgaris*, *T. intermedia*, *T. cordata*, *T. platyphylla*.

OCCURRENCE: native to the British Isles and the northern temperate zone.

PARTS USED: the lime flowers, bark, powdered charcoal. The flowers contain volatile oil, flavonid glucosides, saponins, condensed tannins and mucilage.

MEDICINAL USES: nervine, stimulant, tonic. An infusion of the flowers is good for indigestion, hysteria, nervous vomiting, colds, 'flu and catarrh. They can also help calm overactive children and relax the nervous system. Lime flower tea eases headaches and insomnia. The flowers are said to lower blood pressure (possibly due to the bioflavonoids they contain) and are said to remedy arteriosclerosis. The inner bark of the lime has a diuretic effect and is utilized for gout and kidney stones as well as treating coronary artery disease by dilating the coronary arteries. The powdered charcoal was used in gastric and dyspeptic disorders and applied to burnt or sore areas.

ADMINISTERED AS: infusion, powdered charcoal, dried inner bark, tea.

Liquorice *Glycyrrhiza glabra*. COMMON NAME: Licorice, lycorys, *Liquiriha officinalis*.

OCCURRENCE: a shrub native to south-east Europe and south-west Asia and cultivated in the British Isles.

PARTS USED: the root. The chief compound in the root is glycyrrhizin along with sugar, starch, gum, asparagus, tannin and resin.

MEDICINAL USES: demulcent, pectoral, emollient. A very popular and well-known remedy for coughs, consumption and chest complaints. Liquorice extract is included in cough lozenges and pastilles, with sedatives and expectorants. An infusion of bruised root and FLAX (linseed) is good for irritable coughs, sore throats and laryngitis. Liquorice is used to a greater extent as a medicine in China and other eastern countries. The herb is used by brewers to give colour to porter and stout and is employed in the manufacture of chewing or smoking tobacco.

ADMINISTERED AS: powdered root, fluid extract, infusion, solid extract.

Liverwort, English *Peltigera canina*. COMMON NAME: Lichen caninus, lichen cinereus terrestris, ash-coloured ground liverwort, liverleaf, *Hepatica triloba*.

OCCURRENCE: grows in moist, shady places in Britain and Europe.

PARTS USED: the whole lichen.

MEDICINAL USES: deobstruent, slightly purgative, *Peltigera canina* is held in esteem as a cure for liver complaints and was formerly regarded as a remedy for hydrophobia.

ADMINISTERED AS: infusion and fluid extract.

Lobelia *Lobelia inflata*. COMMON NAME: Indian tobacco, asthma weed, pukeweed, jagroot, vomitwort, bladderpod, *Rapuntium inflatum*.

OCCURRENCE: native to North America and grown in British gardens for many years.

PARTS USED: the herb, which contains the alkaloids, lobeline, isolobeline, lobelanidine and lobinaline along with fixed oil, gum, resin and lignin.

MEDICINAL USES: expectorant, emetic, diaphoretic, anti-asthmatic, stimulant. The use of this plant was passed to Europeans from native American Indians and it has been used as a major relaxant remedy used to treat pain caused by muscle spasms. Thus it is highly effective against asthma, bronchial complaints and lung problems. Lobelia may be given to ease convulsive and inflammatory disorders such as epilepsy, tonsillitis, diphtheria and tetanus. Externally, the herb is used for eye complaints, insect bites, POISON IVY irritation, ringworm, sprains, bruises and muscle spasms. The use of lobelia as an emetic is debatable as to whether it would benefit the patient, and its use is encouraged or discouraged by different herbals. Lobelia is a very important herbal remedy in modern usage.

ADMINISTERED AS: tincture, infusion, powdered bark, syrup and fluid extract.

Loosestrife *Lysimachia vulgaris*. COMMON NAME: Yellow loosestrife, yellow willow herb, herb willow, willow-wort, wood pimpernel.

OCCURRENCE: grows in shady banks and riversides in England.

PARTS USED: the herb.

MEDICINAL USES: astringent, expectorant. This herb is good at stopping bleeding of any kind, particularly of the mouth, nose and wounds. It is also used to restrain profuse menstrual bleeding and calm severe diarrhoea. Distilled water made with loosestrife was utilized to clean ulcers and reduce inflammation and to clear spots, marks and scabs from the skin. An infusion was used as a gargle in relaxed throat and quinsy.

ADMINISTERED AS: distilled water, dried herb, infusion and ointment.

Lovage *Levisticum officinale.* COMMON NAME: *Ligusticum levisticum*, old English lovage, Italian lovage, Cornish lovage, Chinese tang kui, man-mu.

OCCURRENCE: one of the old English herbs which was very generally cultivated; it was not indigenous to Great Britain but native to the Mediterranean region.

PARTS USED: the root, leaves, young stems and seeds. The plant contains a volatile oil, angelic acid, a bitter extract and resin.

MEDICINAL USES: the young stems are used in a similar manner to ANGELICA for flavouring and confectionery. The roots and fruits are aromatic, stimulant, diuretic and carminative in action. They are generally used in stomach disorders, and feverish attacks including those with colic and flatulence. The fresh leaves are eaten as a salad and when dried are infused into a pleasant tea with emmenagogue properties. An infusion of the root was recommended by old herbalists for gravel, jaundice and urinary problems and the sudorific nature of the roots and seeds meant they were highly favoured in treating "pestilential disorders".

ADMINISTERED AS: infusion of leaves and root infusion.

Lucerne *Medicago sativa.* COMMON NAME: Purple medick, cultivated lucern, alfalfa, purple medicle.

OCCURRENCE: an ancient herb, of unknown origin. It has been cultivated in Europe, Great Britain, Peru and Persia for hundreds of years.

PARTS USED: the herb.

MEDICINAL USES: this herb is used, as an infusion, to encourage weight gain and flesh development. It has also been used to feed cattle and horses.

ADMINISTERED AS: infusion.

Lungwort *Sticta pulmonaria.* COMMON NAME: Jerusalem cowslip, oak lungs, lung moss.

OCCURRENCE: found in Europe, but uncommon in woods in Britain.

PARTS USED: the whole lichen.

MEDICINAL USES: astringent, mucilaginous, pectoral, healing. It is very valuable in treating coughs, lung complaints and asthma. It is also good at reducing inflammation and pain.

ADMINISTERED AS: liquid extract, infusion.

Lupin, White *Lupinus albus.* COMMON NAME: Lupine, wolfsbohne.

OCCURRENCE: native to southern Europe and parts of Asia and is now extensively cultivated in Italy.

PARTS USED: the seeds, herb. The main compounds within the plant are the glucoside, lupinin; the alkaloids lupinidine and luparine.

MEDICINAL USES: anthelmintic, diuretic, emmenagogue. The bruised seeds, when soaked in water, are applied to ulcers and sores and when taken internally the seeds kill parasitic worms and excite the menstrual discharge. It was used by the Romans as food and can also be used for fibres to make cloth, paper and adhesive.

ADMINISTERED AS: poultice, infusion.

Mace *Myristica fragrans.* COMMON NAME: Macis, muscadier, *Arillus myristicae*, *Myristica officinalis*, *Myristica moschata*.

OCCURRENCE: native to the Molucca Islands, New Guinea, bondy Islands and introduced into Sri Lanka and the West Indies.

PARTS USED: the growth outside the shell of the nutmeg seed—called the arillus. The main constituents of mace are a volatile oil, protein, gum, resins, sugars and two fixed oils. The volatile oil contains a lot of pinene and some myristicin.

MEDICINAL USES: stimulant, tonic, carminative, flavouring agent. This herb is used to help digestion and stomach weakness and increase the blood circulation and body temperature. Mace has been used against putrid and pestilential fevers and, combined with other herbs, intermittent fevers.

ADMINISTERED AS: powdered herb.

Magnolia *Magnolia Virginiana.* COMMON NAME: Cucumber tree, blue magnolia, swamp sassfras, *Magnolia glauca*, *M. acuminata*, *M. tripetata*.

OCCURRENCE: native to the USA but is cultivated in Great Britain.

PARTS USED: the bark of stem and root.

MEDICINAL USES: mild, diaphoretic, tonic, aromatic, stimulant. The bark is used against rheumatism and malaria, and the cones of the tree are steeped in spirit to make a tonic tincture. A warm infusion of bark is laxative and sudorific while a cold infusion is antiperiodic and tonic in effect.

ADMINISTERED AS: tincture, infusion, fluid extract.

Maidenhair *Adiantum capillus-veneris*. COMMON NAME: True maidenhair, hair of venus, rock fern, capillaire common or capillaire de montpellier.

OCCURRENCE: this grows wild in southern Europe and southern and central Britain.

PARTS USED: the herb, which contains tannin and mucilage but has not yet been fully investigated.

MEDICINAL USES: pectoral, expectorant, mucilaginous. The fern has been used as a remedy in chest complaints, coughs and throat problems. It is an ingredient of cough mixtures, its flavour masked by sugar and ORANGE-FLOWER water. Maidenhair is good at easing pulmonary catarrh and is used in Europe as an emmenagogue.

ADMINISTERED AS: infusion, syrup.

Male fern *Dryopteris felix-mas*. COMMON NAME: *Aspidium felix-mas*, male shield fern.

OCCURRENCE: grows in all areas of Europe, temperate Asia, North India, North and South Africa, the temperate areas of the United States and the South American Andes.

PARTS USED: the root and the oil extracted from it. The oil is extracted using ether and contains the acid, filmaron, filicic acid, tannin, resin and sugar.

MEDICINAL USES: anthelmintic, vermifuge, taeniafuge. It is probably the best drug against tapeworm, and it is normally given at night after several hours of fasting. When followed by a purgative drug in the morning, e.g. CASTOR OIL very good results are obtained. The size of the dose administered must be carefully assessed as male fern is an irritant poison in too large a dose, causing muscle weakness, coma and possible damage to the eyesight.

ADMINISTERED AS: powdered root, fluid extract, oil of male fern.

Mandrake *Atropa mandragora*. COMMON NAME: Mandragora, satan's Apple.

OCCURRENCE: a plant native to southern Europe but it can be cultivated in Great Britain.

PARTS USED: the herb and root.

MEDICINAL USES: emetic, purgative, cooling, anodyne, hypnotic. The fresh root is a very powerful emetic and purgative drug and the dried bark of the root also shares the purgative qualities. Ancient herbalists used mandrake to kill pain and to give rest and sleep to patients, as well as using it for melancholy, convulsions, rheumatic pain and scrofulous tumours. They administered the drug as the bark of the root, expressed juice or as an infusion of the root. In large doses, mandrake was said to cause delirium and madness. The herb was used as an anaesthetic in ancient Greek medicine.

ADMINISTERED AS: infusion, fresh root, powdered bark, expressed juice.

Maple, Red *Acer rubrum*. COMMON NAME: Swamp maple, curled maple.

OCCURRENCE: a native American tree, introduced into Britain in 1656 as an ornamental tree.

PARTS USED: the bark.

MEDICINAL USES: astringent. The native American Indians used an infusion of the bark as an application for sore eyes.

ADMINISTERED AS: an infusion.

Mare's Tail *Hippuris vulgaris*. COMMON NAME: Female horsetail, marsh barren horsetail.

OCCURRENCE: a native British aquatic flowering plant found in shallow ponds, rivers, ditches and lake margins.

PARTS USED: the herb.

MEDICINAL USES: vulnerary. Old herbalists viewed mare's tail as good for stopping bleeding, be it internal or external. It was said to be used to heal ulcers, green wounds in children, ruptures and urinary stones. The herb was also used to strengthen the intestinal system, for head colds and as a warm poultice on skin eruptions and inflammations.

ADMINISTERED AS: poultice, decoction.

Marigold *Calendula officinalis*. COMMON NAME: *Caltha officinalis*, golds, ruddes, marg gowles, oculus Christi, marygold, garden marigold, solis sponsa.

OCCURRENCE: a native of southern Europe and a common garden plant in Great Britain.

PARTS USED: the petals and herb. Only the deep orange-flowered variety is of medicinal use.

MEDICINAL USES: stimulant, diaphoretic. Mainly used as a local remedy. Taken internally, an infusion of the herb prevents pus formation and externally is good in cleaning chronic ulcers and varicose veins. Formerly considered to be of benefit as an aperient and detergent to clear visceral obstructions and jaundice. A marigold flower, when rubbed onto a bee or wasp sting, was known to relieve pain and reduce swelling, while a lotion from the flowers was good for inflamed and sore eyes. The expressed juice of the plant was used to clear headaches and remove warts.

ADMINISTERED AS: infusion, distilled water and lotion.

Marjoram *Origanum vulgare*

OCCURRENCE: generally distributed over Asia, Europe and North Africa and also found freely in England.

PARTS USED: the herb and volatile oil.

MEDICINAL USES: the oil has stimulant, carminative, diaphoretic, mildly tonic and emmenagogue qualities. As a warm infusion, it is used to produce perspiration and bring out the spots of measles as well as giving relief from spasms, colic and dyspeptic pain. The oil has been used externally as a rubefacient and liniment, and on cotton wool placed next to an aching tooth, it relieves the pain. The dried herb may be utilized as a hot poultice for swellings, rheumatism and colic, while an infusion of the fresh plant will ease a nervous headache.

ADMINISTERED AS: essential oil, poultice and infusion.

Marjoram, Sweet *Origanum marjorana*. COMMON NAME: knotted marjoram, *Majorana hortensis*.

OCCURRENCE: native to Portugal and grown as an annual plant through the rest of Europe and Great Britain.

PARTS USED: the herb and leaves. The plant contains tannic acid, mucilage, bitter substances and an essential oil.

MEDICINAL USES: tonic, stimulant, emmenagogue. The essential oil, oleum majoranae, when extracted from the leaves, makes a good external application for sprains and bruises, and acts as an emmenagogue when taken internally. Sweet marjoram is widely used in cookery and aids digestion of food.

ADMINISTERED AS: essential oil, dried or fresh leaves.

Marshmallow *Althaea officinalis*. COMMON NAME: Mallards, mauls, schloss tea, cheeses, mortification, root, guimauve.

OCCURRENCE: a native of Europe, found in salt marshes, meadows, ditches and riverbanks. It is locally distributed in England and has been introduced to Scotland.

PARTS USED: the leaves, root and flowers. Marshmallow contains starch, mucilage, pectin, oil, sugar, asparagin, glutinous matter and cellulose.

MEDICINAL USES: demulcent, emollient. Very useful in inflammation and irritation of the alimentary canal and the urinary and respiratory organs. A decoction of the root is effective against sprains, bruises and muscle aches. When boiled in milk or wine marshmallow relieves diseases of the chest, e.g. coughs, bronchitis or whooping cough and it eases the bowels after dysentery without any astringent effects. It is frequently given as a syrup to infants and children.

ADMINISTERED AS: infusion, decoction, syrup, fluid extract.

Masterwort *Imperatoria ostruthium*

OCCURRENCE: native to central Europe and alpine regions; cultivated in Great Britain for many years.

PARTS USED: the rhizome.

MEDICINAL USES: stimulant, antispasmodic, carminative. Masterwort has been used in asthma, stroke, dyspepsia and menstrual problems. A decoction of the herb in urine was considered beneficial against dropsy, cramp, epilepsy, flatulence, gout, and kidney and uterine problems.

ADMINISTERED AS: distilled water, decoction, fluid extract.

Mastic *Pistacia lentiscus*. COMMON NAME: Mastich, Lentisk.

OCCURRENCE: indigenous to the Mediterranean regions of Spain, Portugal, France, Greece, Turkey, tropical Africa and the Canary Islands.

PARTS USED: the resin, which contains a volatile oil, an alcohol-insoluble resin and an alcohol-soluble resin.

MEDICINAL USES: stimulant, diuretic. Similar to TURPENTINE in effect, but its use in medicine has declined. In some areas it is used for diarrhoea in children, or chewed to sweeten the breath. Today, mastic is mainly used as a filling for carious teeth.

ADMINISTERED AS: resin.

Matico *Piper angustifolium*. COMMON NAME: Soldier's herb, thoho-thoho, moho-moho, *Artanthe elongata*, *Stephensia elongata*, *Piper granulosium*, matica.

OCCURRENCE: native to Peru and spread over much of tropical America. It has been grown in England.

PARTS USED: the dried leaves which contain a volatile oil, artanthic acid, tannin and resin.

MEDICINAL USES: astringent, stimulant, styptic, diuretic. It is recommended for chronic mucous discharges, leucorrhoea, haemorrhoids, diarrhoea, dysentery and urinary and genital complaints. The leaves stop bleeding from most sites, and are used as an application to slight wounds, ulcers, bites from leeches or after teeth extraction.

ADMINISTERED AS: dried leaves, fluid extract.

Mayweed *Anthemis cotula*. COMMON NAME: Maroute, cotula, dog chamomile, wild chamomile, foetid or stinking chamomile (or mayweed), dog's fennel, maithes, mathor, *Maruta cotula, Maruta foetida, Manzilla loca, Camomille puante.*

OCCURRENCE: frequently grows in fields and wild places in Great Britain and Europe.

PARTS USED: the flowers and leaves. The flowers contain volatile oil, oxalic, valeric and tannic acids, a bitter extractive and salts of iron, potassium, calcium and magnesium.

MEDICINAL USES: tonic, antispasmodic, emmenagogue and emetic. The smell of the flowers is still repulsive, but it is less offensive than that of the rest of the plant, so the flowers are mainly used in medicine. It is used in hysteria, as a poultice for haemorrhoids and as an infusion in the bath. The flowers have also been used in sick headaches, menstrual problems, scrofula, gastric troubles and dysentery; to induce sleep in asthma sufferers and in convalescence after fevers.

ADMINISTERED AS: fluid extract, poultice, infusion, decoction.

Meadowsweet *Spiraea ulmaria*. COMMON NAME: Meadsweet, dolloff, queen of the meadow, bridewort, lady of the meadow.

OCCURRENCE: common in the British Isles in meadows or woods.

PARTS USED: the herb.

MEDICINAL USES: aromatic, astringent, diuretic, alterative. This herb is good against diarrhoea, stomach complaints and blood disorders. It is highly recommended for children's diarrhoea and dropsy and was used as a decoction in wine to reduce fevers. Meadowsweet makes a pleasant everyday drink when infused and sweetened with honey. It is also included in many herb beers.

ADMINISTERED AS: infusion, decoction.

Melilot *Melilotus officinalis, Melilotus alba, Melilotus arvensis*. COMMON NAME: King's clover, king's chafer, yellow melilot, white melilot, corn melilot, sweet clover, plaster clover, sweet lucerne, wild laburnham hart's tree.

OCCURRENCE: naturalized in all parts of the British Isles.

PARTS USED: the dried herb containing coumarin, hydrocoumaric acid, orthocoumaric acid and melilotic anhydride.

MEDICINAL USES: aromatic, emollient, carminative. When applied as a plaster, ointment or poultice, the herb is good at relieving abdominal or rheumatic pain. It is taken internally to relieve flatulence. The herb was formerly used for clearing the eyesight, headaches, wounds, ulcers and inflammation.

ADMINISTERED AS: poultice, expressed juice, infusion.

Mercury, Dog's *Mercurialis perennis*.

OCCURRENCE: a common plant in woods and shady places in Europe and Russian Asia.

PARTS USED: the herb.

MEDICINAL USES: purgative. Recommended for use externally to treat sore, watery eyes, deafness, pains in the ear, ague, jaundice and women's diseases. The fresh juice of the plant is used to remove warts and to cleanse inflammatory and discharging sores and swellings. A lotion is made for antiseptic external dressings while the juice is used as a nasal douche for catarrh.

ADMINISTERED AS: expressed juice, lotion, fresh herb.

Mescal buttons *Anhalonicum lewinii*. COMMON NAME: *Lopophora lewinii, Analonium williamsii, Echinacactus lewinii, Echinocactus williamsii*, pellote, muscal buttons.

OCCURRENCE: Mexico and Texas.

PARTS USED: the tops of the cacti plant. The drug contains four alkaloids—anhalonine, mescaline, anhalonidine and lophophorine—as well as the chemicals pellotine and anhalamine.

MEDICINAL USES: cardiac, tonic, narcotic, emetic. The drug is useful in head injuries, hysteria, asthma, gout, neuralgia and rheumatism. The extracted compound pellotine has been used to induce sleep in people with insanity as it has no undesirable reactions. Large doses of mescal buttons produce an odd cerebral excitement, with visual disturbances. The physical effects include muscular relaxation, wakefulness, nausea, vomiting and dilation of the pupil. The ancient Aztec Indians believed mescal buttons to have divine properties and included its use to produce exaltation in their religious ceremonies.

ADMINISTERED AS: fluid extract, tincture, extracted alkaloid.

Mezereon *Daphne mezereum*. COMMON NAME: Spurge olive, spurge laurel, camolea, wolt schjeluke, kellernals, dwarf bay, flowering spurge, wild pepper, *Mezerei cortex*, *Mezerei officinarum*, *Laureole gentille*.

OCCURRENCE: indigenous to Britain, Europe and Siberia and was naturalized into the United States and Canada.

PARTS USED: the root, berries, the bark of the stem and root. The bark tastes acrid and this is due to a resin called mezeen. The other active chemicals are a fixed oil, a bitter glucoside called daphnin and a substance similar to euphorbone.

MEDICINAL USES: alterative, diuretic, stimulant, vesicant. An ointment of the bark is used to promote discharge from indolent ulcers, and it is also used for snake and other venomous bites. It is taken internally for chronic rheumatism, scrofula, syphilis, skin diseases and dropsy. The tincture is used to ease neuralgic pain and toothache. In large doses, it acts as an irritant poison and purgative drug causing vomiting, so care should be taken in monitoring the dose used.

ADMINISTERED AS: infusion, tincture, ointment.

Mistletoe *Viscum album*. COMMON NAME: European mistletoe, bird lime mistletoe, herbe de la croix, mystyldene, lignum crucis.

OCCURRENCE: an evergreen, true parasitic plant found on several tree species including fruit and oak trees. It is found throughout Europe and Britain except in Scotland, where it is very rare.

PARTS USED: the leaves and young twigs. They contain mucilage, sugar, fixed oil, tannin and viscin, the active part of the plant.

MEDICINAL USES: nervine, antispasmodic, tonic and narcotic. It is highly recommended for epilepsy and other convulsive disorders, along with stopping internal haemorrhage. It has also been used in delirium, hysteria, neuralgia, nervous debility, urinary disorders and many other complaints arising from a weakened state of the nervous system. The berries are taken to cure severe stitches in the side, and the plant produces a sticky substance called bird-lime which is applied to ulcers and sores. Mistletoe is excellent for reducing blood pressure and has been indicated to be a successful cure for chronic arthritis and in treating malignant tumours in the body.

ADMINISTERED AS: tincture, powdered leaves, infusion, fluid extract.

Motherwort *Leonurus cardiaca*. COMMON NAME: Lion's ear, lion's tail.

OCCURRENCE: a native plant in many parts of Europe, but only rarely found in the wild in Britain.

PARTS USED: the dried herb which contains the alkaloids leonurinine and stachydrine; the bitter glucosides leonurine and leonuridin, tannins and a volatile oil.

MEDICINAL USES: diaphoretic, antispasmodic, tonic, nervine, emmenagogue, sedative. An important use of the herb is in easing the anxiety after childbirth or at the menopause by lowering the blood pressure. It is excellent for female complaints by allaying nervous irritability, regulating menstruation and treating functional infertility. As a tonic, the herb acts well and is effective in treating fevers and allowing good recovery from them. Throughout history, Motherwort has been used to treat palpitations and rapid heart beat, particularly when they develop from anxiety or hysteria. As the name suggests, motherwort acts on the uterine system and the alkaloid stachydrine has the effect of hastening childbirth so this herb should not be used by pregnant women. It is beneficial, however, in causing the uterus to contract after delivery and in this manner is more effective than ERGOT.

ADMINISTERED AS: powdered herb, infusion, decoction, conserve.

Mountain flax *Linum catharticum*. COMMON NAME: Purging flax, dwarf flax, fairy flax, mill mountain.

OCCURRENCE: a common plant in meadows and pastures across Europe and Great Britain.

PARTS USED: the herb which contains a bitter resin and a crystalline principle called linin.

MEDICINAL USES: purgative, laxative, cathartic. It is a gentle cathartic drug with a laxative action preferred to SENNA. As an infusion, the dried herb has been used internally to treat muscular rheumatism and catarrhal infections. It can also be beneficial in liver complaints and jaundice.

ADMINISTERED AS: infusion, dried herb.

Mugwort *Artemisia vulgaris*. COMMON NAME: Felon herb, St. John's plant, moxa, cirigulum Sancti Johannis.

OCCURRENCE: this grows wild in Great Britain on roadsides and hedgerows.

PARTS USED: the leaves, which contain volatile oil, flavonoids, tannin and a bitter principle called absinthin; the roots.

MEDICINAL USES: emmenagogue, stimulant, tonic, nervine, diuretic, diaphoretic. As a nervine, this herb is good in palsy, fits, epilepsy and for people with a feeble constitution. An infusion of the herb is used for intermittent fevers and the ague and given as a tonic. Mugwort's main use is as an emmenagogue to provoke delayed or absent periods and therefore it should not be used during pregnancy, except under the guidance of a qualified herbal practitioner. However, it does help during and after childbirth in speeding up the birth process and to expel the afterbirth. Mugwort acts on the digestive process and stimulates the liver and is used to treat gout and rheumatism. In China, the dried herb is burnt on or near the skin to stop rheumatic pain caused by damp and cold conditions. In China, mugwort is taken during pregnancy to prevent miscarriage, differing from the Western viewpoint.

ADMINISTERED AS: dried herb, fluid extract.

Mulberry *Monus nigra.* COMMON NAME: Common mulberry, black mulberry, purple mulberry.

OCCURRENCE: a native of Turkey, Armenia, Persia and is cultivated throughout Europe and Britain.

PARTS USED: the fruit which contains glucose, protein, pectin, tartaric and malic acids and ash.

MEDICINAL USES: laxative, refrigerant, nutritive. The fruit juice is a beneficial drink for convalescent people, as it checks the thirst and cools the blood after fevers. The fruits are made into wine, jam and conserve. The bark of the tree has a purgative and vermifuge effect on the body.

ADMINISTERED AS: syrup, expressed juice, infusion of bark.

Mullein *Verbascum thapsus.* COMMON NAME: Blanket herb, beggar's blanket, Aaron's rod, lady's foxglove, donkey's ears, torches, candlewick plant, wild ice leaf, Jupiter's staff, clown's lungwort, velvet plant, clot.

OCCURRENCE: widely distributed through Europe, temperate Asia, North America, Ireland and Great Britain.

PARTS USED: the leaves and flowers. The plant contains saponins, mucilage, gum volatile oil, flavonoids and glucosides.

MEDICINAL USES: demulcent, emollient, astringent, sedative, narcotic. This herb is very useful in pectoral complaints, hoarseness, bronchitis, asthma, whooping-cough, wasting diseases and bleeding of the lungs and bowels. It can also be good for diarrhoea, mild catarrh,

colic, inflammation of the urinary system, and as a poultice for boils and sores. The dried leaves may be smoked to remove irritation of the mucous membranes, the cough associated with consumption and spasmodic coughs in general. After placing bruised mullein leaves in olive oil and leaving it for a period, the oil can be used for relieving pain from bruises, frostbite and earache. Water distilled from the flowers was recommended for gout, burns and the condition called erysipelas, where the skin and tissue is infected with the bacterium *Streptococcus pyogenes* and the affected areas are red and swollen.

ADMINISTERED AS: fluid extract, distilled water, poultice, tincture, decoction.

Musk seed *Hibiscus abelmoschus.* COMMON NAME: Ambretta, Egyptian alcée, bisornkorner, target-leaved hibiscus, galu gastrin, *Abelmoschus moschatus.*

OCCURRENCE: native to India and grown in Egypt and the East and West Indies.

PARTS USED: the seeds. They contain fixed oil, a resin and a volatile body.

MEDICINAL USES: antispasmodic, aromatic, stomachic, nervine, aphrodisiac, insecticide. An emulsion of the seeds is regarded as antispasmodic and the seeds were chewed to benefit the nerves and stomach. The seeds are dusted over woollens to protect the fibre from moths.

ADMINISTERED AS: whole seeds, emulsion.

Mustard, Black *Brassica nigra, Siriapis nigra.* COMMON NAME: *Brassica sinapioides.*

OCCURRENCE: it grows wild throughout Europe, South Siberia, Turkey and North Africa and is cultivated in England, Italy, Germany and the Netherlands as a condiment.

PARTS USED: the seeds which contain an acrid, volatile oil, an active principle, the glucoside sinigrin and the enzyme myrosin. When the seeds are crushed with water, these latter two chemicals come into contact and form oil of mustard.

MEDICINAL USES: irritant, stimulant, diuretic and emetic. Mainly used as a poultice to relieve acute local pain, e.g. pneumonia, bronchitis and other respiratory organ diseases. The herb draws blood to the skin surface, easing congestion of the organs, headaches, neuralgia and spasms. The oil of mustard is a powerful irritant and rubefacient when undiluted, but is very useful when dissolved in spirit for chilblains, rheumatism and colic. A hot infusion of the seed is a stimulating footbath and aids removal of colds or headaches. Mustard flour, when taken internally, can act as an emetic, aperient and alterative herb and may also cure hiccups. It is also a very good antiseptic and sterilizing agent and deodorizer.

ADMINISTERED AS: poultice, infusion, essential oil, seed flour, leaves.

Myrrh *Commiphora molmol.* COMMON NAME: *Balsamodendron myrrha, Commiphora myrrha* var. *molmol*, mira, morr.

OCCURRENCE: obtained from bushes in North-East Africa and in Arabia.

PARTS USED: the oleo-gum-resin which contains volatile oil, resins and gum.

MEDICINAL USES: stimulant, tonic, healing, antiseptic, astringent, expectorant, emmenagogue. Myrrh has a long history of use in countering poisons and putrid tissues throughout the body. It is used in leucorrhoea, chronic catarrh, thrush, athlete's foot, absence of menstrual periods, ulcers and as a vermifuge. The resin acts as a tonic in dyspepsia, stimulates the circulation, appetite and the production of gastric juices. It makes a very good gargle or mouthwash for an inflamed sore throat, spongy gums and mouth ulcers.

ADMINISTERED AS: fluid extract, tincture, pills.

Nettle *Urtica dioica, Urtica urens.* COMMON NAME: Common nettle, stinging nettle.

OCCURRENCE: widely distributed throughout temperate Europe and Asia, Japan, South Africa and Australia.

PARTS USED: the whole herb, which contains formic acid, mucilage, mineral salts, ammonia and carbonic acid.

MEDICINAL USES: astringent, stimulating, diuretic, tonic. The herb is anti-asthmatic and the juice of the nettle will relieve bronchial and asthmatic troubles, as will the dried leaves when burnt and inhaled. The seeds are taken as an infusion or in wine to ease consumption or ague. Nettles are used widely as a food source and can be made into puddings, tea, beer, juice and used as a vegetable. A hair tonic or lotion can also be made from the nettle. In the Highlands of Scotland, they were chopped, added to egg white and applied to the temples as a cure for insomnia.

ADMINISTERED AS: expressed juice, infusion, decoction, seeds, dried herb, dietary item.

Nightshade, Black *Solarum nignum.* COMMON NAME: garden nightshade, petty morel.

OCCURRENCE: a common plant in south England,

seen less frequently in northern England and Scotland.

PARTS USED: the whole plant, fresh leaves. Both contain the active principle, solanine which is found in variable quantities within the plant, throughout the year.

MEDICINAL USES: the bruised fresh leaves are used external to the body to ease pain and reduce inflammation. Juice of the leaves has been used for ringworm, gout and earache and is supposed to make a good gargle or mouthwash when mixed with vinegar. This species of plant is reputed to be very poisonous, narcotic and sudorific, so is only utilized in very small doses, under careful supervision.

ADMINISTERED AS: infusion, expressed juice and fresh leaves.

Nutmeg *Myristica fragrans.* COMMON NAME: Nux moschata, *Myristica officinalis, M. aromata*, myristica

OCCURRENCE: native to the Banda Islands, Malayan Archipelago and the Molucca Islands. It is cultivated in Java, West Indies, Sumatra and French Guiana.

PARTS USED: the dried kernel of the seed which contains a volatile and a fixed oil, starch, gum, various acids and terpenes.

MEDICINAL USES: carminative, stomachic, stimulant. The grated or powdered kernel is used to relieve flatulence, vomiting and nausea. It is mainly used as an ingredient of various medicines and as a culinary spice. Nutmeg has similar properties to MACE but mace has a stronger flavour. Large doses of nutmeg can be toxic, producing disorientation, double vision and convulsions.

ADMINISTERED AS: expressed oil, powdered kernel.

Nux vomica *Strychnos Nux-vomica.* COMMON NAME: Poison nut, semen strychnox, Quaker buttons.

OCCURRENCE: a tree indigenous to India and now grown in Burma, China, Australia and the Malay Archipelago.

PARTS USED: the dried ripe seeds. They contain the alkaloids, strychnine, brucine and strychnicine, fatty matter, caffeotannic acid and the glucoside, loganin.

MEDICINAL USES: tonic, bitter, stimulant. Nux vomica is utilized as a general tonic, mainly when combined with other herbal remedies, to treat neuralgia, dyspepsia, impotence, chronic constipation and general debility. This drug can also be of benefit in cardiac failure, surgical shock or poisoning by chloroform where it raises blood pressure and increases pulse rate, but it can also cause violent convulsions. *Nux vomica* should only be used in limited circumstances and under strict control as strychnine is very poisonous.

ADMINISTERED AS: fluid extract, tincture.

Oak *Quercus robur*. COMMON NAME: Common oak, tanner's bark.

OCCURRENCE: a tree widely dispersed over Europe.

PARTS USED: the bark.

MEDICINAL USES: slightly tonic, strongly astringent, antiseptic. It is very good in chronic diarrhoea, dysentery as a decoction and used as a gargle for sore throats. May also be used as an injection for leucorrhoea and applied locally for piles and bleeding gums. Water distilled from the oak buds was said to be good on any kind of inflammation.

ADMINISTERED AS: fluid extract, infusion, tincture, injection.

Oats *Avena sativa*. COMMON NAME: Groats, oatmeal.

OCCURRENCE: distributed across Europe, Britain and the USA.

PARTS USED: the seeds which are made up of starch, gluten, albumen and other proteins, sugar, gum oil and salts.

MEDICINAL USES: nervine, stimulant, antispasmodic, *Avena* forms a nutritious and easily digested food for convalescent patients and for exhaustion after fevers. It can be made into a demulcent enema, or a good emollient poultice. Oat extract or tincture is useful as a nerve and uterine tonic.

ADMINISTERED AS: fluid extract, tincture, enema, dietary item.

Olive *Olea Europea*. COMMON NAME: *Olea oleaster, Olea larcifolia, Olea gallica,* oliver.

OCCURRENCE: native to the Mediterranean countries, Syria and Turkey. Now cultivated in Chile, Peru and Australia.

PARTS USED: the oil expressed from the ripe fruit, the leaves.

MEDICINAL USES: the oil is emollient, demulcent, laxative and aperient. It is a good substitute for CASTOR OIL when given to children, but its value in clearing parasitic worms or gallstones is unsure. The oil is a good ingredient in liniments or ointment and is used for bruises, sprains, cutaneous injuries and rheumatic problems. It is also utilized externally in joint, kidney and chest complaints or for chills, typhoid

and scarlet fevers, plague and dropsy. When combined with alcohol, the oil is good as a hair tonic. Olive leaves have astringent and antiseptic properties, and an infusion of these leaves has proved beneficial in obstinate fevers.

ADMINISTERED AS: expressed oil, infusion, ointment.

Onion *Allium cepa*.

OCCURRENCE: originally native to south-west Asia and now cultivated around the globe.

PARTS USED: the bulb.

MEDICINAL USES: diuretic, expectorant, antiseptic. Although onions are extensively used in cookery, they also have medicinal uses. A roasted onion is applied to tumours or earache to remove the pain and onions steeped in gin produce a fluid extract which is given for gravel and dropsy. A homoeopathic remedy is made from red onions and is useful in neuralgic pain, colds, hay fever, toothache and in the early stages of laryngitis with hoarseness.

ADMINISTERED AS: poultice, tincture.

Orange, Bitter *Citrus aurantium* subsp. *amara*.
Orange, Sweet *Citrus vulgaris*. COMMON NAME: (bitter orange) *Citrus bigaradia, Citrus vulgaris, Bi garadier,* bigarade orange, Seville orange, naranja. (sweet orange) Portugal orange, China orange, *Citrus dulcis*.

OCCURRENCE: the bitter orange originated from northern India but is now grown in Mediterranean countries. The sweet orange is grown in Sicily, Africa and the West Indies.

PARTS USED: the fruit, peel and flowers. Oil is extracted from the peel of both types of orange—bitter orange produces oil of bigarde and the sweet orange oil is oil of Portugal. Distillation of the bitter orange flowers with water produces orange flower water and an essential oil called neroli.

MEDICINAL USES: tonic, stomachic, carminative, aromatic. Both sweet and bitter orange oils are used as flavouring agents for medicinal compounds but may be used in a similar manner to oil of TURPENTINE in treating chronic bronchitis. An infusion of dried flowers can be taken as a mild nervous stimulant and a tonic may be given of bitter orange peel, either on its own or as an infusion. In China, the dried peel of the sweet orange is used as a diuretic and to aid digestion. Oil of neroli is used in aromatherapy for treating anxiety and nervous depression.

ADMINISTERED AS: infusion, dried peel, essential oil, distilled water.

Orris *Iris florentina* (and other species). COMMON NAME: Florentine orris, orris root.

OCCURRENCE: grown in Italy and Morocco and to a smaller extent in England.

PARTS USED: the root, which contains oil of orris, fat, resin, starch, mucilage, a glucoside called iridin and a bitter extractive substance.

MEDICINAL USES: Orris root is rarely used in medicine today. The fresh root has emetic, diuretic and cathartic properties and was formerly used against congested headache, dropsy, bronchitis and chronic diarrhoea. It is more generally used in perfumery, as it strengthens the odour of other fragrant herbs and acts as a fixative in perfumes and pot pourri. It is also part of dusting powders, toilet powders and tooth powders.

Paraguay Tea *Ilex paraguayensis*. COMMON NAME: Paraguay herb, maté, yerba maté, jesuit's tea, Brazil tea, gón gouha, ilex maté, houx maté.

OCCURRENCE: largely cultivated in South America.

PARTS USED: the leaves, which contain caffeine, tannin ash and insoluble matter.

MEDICINAL USES: tonic, diuretic, diaphoretic, powerful stimulant. The leaves are infused in a similar manner to TEA and drunk with lemon juice and sugar by the local people in South America. There is a huge consumption of this herb as it is taken at every meal. In large doses, it can cause purging and vomiting.

ADMINISTERED AS: infusion.

Paris, Herb *Paris quadrifolia*. COMMON NAME: herba Paris, true love, one berry, *Solarum quadrifolium, Aconitum pardalianches*.

OCCURRENCE: found in Europe, Russian Asia and locally distributed in Great Britain.

PARTS USED: the whole plant, picked as it is just coming into bloom.

MEDICINAL USES: narcotic. In large doses, the herb induces nausea, vertigo, vomiting, profuse sweating, delirium, dry throat and convulsions. Overdoses can be fatal, particularly in children. If administered in small doses, the herb can relieve spasmodic cough, rheumatism, bronchitis, cramp, heart palpitation and colic. Juice expressed from the leaves is good for green wounds, tumours and inflammation while the juice from the berries eases inflammation of the eyes. In Russia, the leaves are proposed to ease madness and its effects. As it has a similar set of qualities to opium, it has been used as an aphrodisiac. Herb Paris has also been utilized as an antidote against mercury and arsenic poisoning.

ADMINISTERED AS: tincture, expressed juice of leaves, expressed juice of berries, ointment, powdered root, decoction.

Parsley *Carum petroselinum*. COMMON NAME: *Apium petroselinum, Petroselinum lativum*, petersylinge, persely, persele.

OCCURRENCE: this was first cultivated in Britain in 1548, now completely naturalized through England and Scotland.

PARTS USED: the root, seeds and leaves. The root is slightly aromatic and contains starch mucilage, sugar, volatile oil and apiin. Parsley seeds contain more volatile oil, which consists of terpenes and apiol, an allyl compound.

MEDICINAL USES: carminative, tonic, aperient, diuretic. A strong decoction of the root is used in gravel, stone, kidney congestion, jaundice and dropsy. Bruised parsley seeds used to be given against plague and intermittent fevers, while the external application of the leaves may help to dispel tumours. A poultice of the leaves is effective against bites and stings of poisonous insects.

ADMINISTERED AS: fluid extract, essential oil, infusion, ointment and poultice.

Parsley piert *Alchemilla arvensis*. COMMON NAME: Parsley breakstone, parsley piercestone, field lady's mantle.

OCCURRENCE: common across Great Britain, Europe and North Africa and was introduced into North America.

PARTS USED: the herb.

MEDICINAL USES: diuretic, demulcent, refrigerant. This herb is mainly employed in gravel, stone, dropsy and in bladder and kidney problems. It can effect results even in seemingly incurable cases. It can also help jaundice and clearing obstructions of the liver. To limit its irritancy, it is sometimes combined with demulcent or diuretic herbs for best effect, e.g. BROOM, JUNIPER, CARROT, COMFREY or MARSHMALLOW.

ADMINISTERED AS: fresh herb or infusion.

Parsnip *Pastinaca sativa*. COMMON NAME: Le panais, die pastinake.

OCCURRENCE: native European, cultivated commercially as food.

PARTS USED: the root.

MEDICINAL USES: nutritive. The parsnip exceeds almost all other vegetables in terms of food value (except potatoes) and is very nourishing for humans and animals alike. They are preferred to carrots for fattening pigs and given to cattle. Some old herbalists saw parsnips as a cure for asthma, cancer and consumption and used bruised parsnip roots as an application on bruises. In many areas, parsnips were made into a preserve, a beer or wine. They are also used extensively in salads, soups, as a vegetable and in cakes.

Passionflower *Passiflora incarnata.* COMMON NAME: passion vine, granadilla, maracoc, maypops.

OCCURRENCE: a native of Virginia in the United States.

PARTS USED: the flower and the dried vine. The plant contains flavonoids, sugars, sterols and gum as well as the alkaloids harmone, harmol, harmaline, harmine and harmalol.

MEDICINAL USES: antispasmodic, sedative, narcotic. This drug relaxes the nervous system and the sedative effects are good as well. It is non-addictive. It is a very good remedy for anxiety, tension, insomnia, diarrhoea, dysentery, neuralgia and painful menstruation. The alkaloids have tranquillizing effects and it is used to reduce high blood pressure.

ADMINISTERED AS: fluid extract.

Peach *Prunus persica.* COMMON NAME: *Persica vulgaris, Amygdalus persica.*

OCCURRENCE: cultivated in Asia for centuries and introduced into Europe from Persia.

PARTS USED: the bark, leaves and the oil expressed from the seeds.

MEDICINAL USES: demulcent, sedative, diuretic, expectorant. The leaves or bark, when used as an infusion, are almost a specific for irritation and congestion of the gastric surfaces. The infusion is also good for chronic bronchitis, whooping cough and ordinary coughs. A syrup or infusion made of the peach flowers was thought to be a mild acting purgative for children, as well as good for jaundice and giving health to a poorly child. The kernel oil was thought to induce sleep and rest if rubbed on to the temples. The oil is also used as a substitute for the more expensive ALMOND oil.

ADMINISTERED AS: infusion, fresh leaves, powdered leaves, oil.

Pellitory *Anacyclus pyrethrum.* COMMON NAME: Roman pellitory, pellitory of Spain, Spanish chamomile, pyrethre, *Matricaria pyrethrum, Anthemis pyrethrum, Pyrethrum officinarum, Pyrethri radix.*

OCCURRENCE: cultivated in Spain, Algeria and other Mediterranean countries.

PARTS USED: the root, which contains two oils, a brown resin thought to contain peletonin, tannin, gum, lignin and various mineral salts. The alkaloid, pyrethrine is the active chemical.

MEDICINAL USES: local irritant, rubefacient. The main use of this herb is to relieve toothache and promoting the flow of saliva. This eases conditions such as dryness of the throat and partial paralysis of the lips and tongue. The powdered root is used as snuff to clear chronic catarrh of the head, exciting the flow of nasal mucous and tears. The herb is added to many dental toothpowders.

ADMINISTERED AS: powdered root, infusion, tincture.

Pellitory-of-the-wall *Parietaria officinalis.* COMMON NAME: Parietaria diffusa, lichwort, paritary.

OCCURRENCE: a common wild plant in Europe and Great Britain.

PARTS USED: the herb, which contains a bitter glucoside, tannin, sulphur, mucilage and flavones among its chemical constituents.

MEDICINAL USES: diuretic, laxative, refrigerant, demulcent. It is given as an infusion or decoction to treat urine retention, cystitis, nephritis, dropsy, prostate inflammation, urinary stones and gravel. In the form of an ointment, this herb was used for haemorrhoids, gout and fistulas. The fresh herb is more effective than the dried herb.

ADMINISTERED AS: infusion, syrup, poultice, decoction.

Pennyroyal *Mentha pulegium.* COMMON NAME: Pulegium, run-by-the-ground, pudding grass, lurk-in-the-ditch, piliolerial.

OCCURRENCE: a native plant of most of Europe and parts of Asia and commonly grown in gardens.

PARTS USED: the herb and the oil distilled from the herb called oil of pulegiam.

MEDICINAL USES: carminative, diaphoretic, stimulant, emmenagogue. The herb is mainly used to bring on menstruation which has been obstructed by cold or chills. It is also beneficial in spasms, flatulence, hysteria, sickness, colds, headaches and is a blood purifying herb. Pennyroyal is supposed to encourage sleep and was hung in bedrooms for that purpose. The oil has been used to prevent mosquito and gnat bites for many years. If taken internally, the oil can be highly toxic and death can result. This herb should not be taken by pregnant women as it promotes menstruation and may cause haemorrhage and death.

ADMINISTERED AS: dried herb, infusion, distilled oil.

Peony *Paeonia officinalis*. COMMON NAME: Paeony, paeonia, common peony, piney, *Paeonia lactifloria*, *Paeonia corrallina*.

OCCURRENCE: introduced into Great Britain some centuries ago.

PARTS USED: the root, which contains benzoic acid, asparagin, an alkaloid and an essential oil.

MEDICINAL USES: antispasmodic, tonic. In the past, peony has been used successfully in spasmodic nervous problems such as epilepsy and spasms as well as lunacy. An infusion of the powdered root is recommended for liver obstructions, and helps kidney and gall bladder diseases. Since this plant is poisonous, it is rarely utilized in modern herbal medicine.

ADMINISTERED AS: infusion.

Pepper *Piper nigrum*. COMMON NAME: Black pepper, piper.

OCCURRENCE: grows wild in South India and Cechin-China; now cultivated in the East and West Indies, Malay Archipelago, the Philippines, Java, Sumatra and Borneo.

PARTS USED: the dried unripe fruits. White pepper comes from the same plant, except that the pericarp of the fruit has been removed prior to drying. The active chemicals in black or white pepper are piperine, volatile oil, starch, cellulose and a resin called chavicin.

MEDICINAL USES: aromatic, stimulant, carminative, febrifuge. The herb is useful in treating constipation, gonorrhoea, prolapsed rectum, paralysis of the tongue and acts on the urinary organs. The stimulant properties of pepper work on the gastro-intestinal system to aid digestion, ease dyspepsia, torbid stomach conditions, and relieve flatulence and nausea. Pepper has also been recommended in diarrhoea, cholera, scarlatina, vertigo and paralytic and arthritic disorders. Peppercorns, as the dried fruit is known, are used both whole and ground in many culinary dishes and are used as a condiment. In the Siege of Rome in 408 AD, pepper was so highly priced that it was used as a form of currency.

ADMINISTERED AS: powdered dried fruits, gargle.

Peppermint *Mentha piperita*. COMMON NAME: Brandy mint, curled mint, balm mint.

OCCURRENCE: found across Europe, was introduced into Britain and grows widely in damp places and waste ground.

PARTS USED: the herb and distilled oil. The plant contains peppermint oil, which is composed of menthol, menthyl acetate and isovalerate, menthone, cineol, pinene and limonene. The medicinal qualities are found in the alcoholic chemicals.

MEDICINAL USES: stimulant, antispasmodic, carminative, stomachic, oil of peppermint is extensively used in both medicine and commerce. It is good in dyspepsia, flatulence, colic and abdominal cramps. The oil allays sickness and nausea, is used for chorea and diarrhoea but is normally used with other medicines to disguise unpalatable tastes and effects. Peppermint water is in most general use and is used to raise body temperature and induce perspiration. Peppermint tea can help ward off colds and influenza at an early stage, can calm heart palpitations and is used to reduce the appetite.

ADMINISTERED AS: infusion, distilled water, spirit, essential oil and fluid extract.

Pimpernel, Scarlet *Anagallis arvensis*. COMMON NAME: Shepherd's barometer, poor man's weatherglass, adder's eyes, bipinella.

OCCURRENCE: a very widely distributed plant found in all the temperate regions, in both hemispheres.

PARTS USED: the whole herb, of which little is known of the active chemicals within it. It does contain the compound, saponin.

MEDICINAL USES: diuretic, diaphoretic, expectorant. This plant has an ancient reputation for healing, particularly dealing with diseases of the brain and mental illness. It is considered beneficial in dropsy, liver obstruction, disorders of the spleen, gravel, rheumatic complaints and gout, but caution should be taken as in experiments extracts from this plant have been found to be poisonous to animals and its full effects on humans are not yet known.

ADMINISTERED AS: infusion, dried herb, tincture, fluid extract.

Pine oils there are several kinds: **Siberian pine oil**, from *Abies Sibirica*; **Pumilio pine oil**, from *Pinus muge*; **Sylvestris pine oil**, from *Pinus sylvestris*.

PARTS USED: the oil produced from when pine wood is distilled using steam under pressure.

MEDICINAL USES: rubefacient, aromatic. These oils are mainly used as inhalants for bronchitis or laryngitis or as liniment plasters.

ADMINISTERED AS: distilled oil.

Pine, White *Pinus strobus*. COMMON NAME: Weymouth pine, pin du lord, *Pinus alba*, deal pine.

OCCURRENCE: widely distributed in the northern hemisphere, especially in North America.

PARTS USED: the bark.

MEDICINAL USES: expectorant, diuretic, demulcent. Used for the relief of coughs, colds and chest diseases. It has a beneficial effect on the bladder and kidney systems. A compound syrup is the most commonly administered form of the drug, but it contains morphine so care must be taken that morphine dependence does not develop.

ADMINISTERED AS: compound syrup and fluid extract.

Pink root *Spigelia marylandica.* COMMON NAME: Indian pink, wormgrass, carolina pink, Maryland pink, American wormroot, starbloom.

OCCURRENCE: grows in the southern states of the United States of America.

PARTS USED: the whole plant or the root. This plant contains a poisonous alkaloid called spigeline, volatile oil, resin, mucilage, lignin, a bitter principle and salts of calcium potassium and sodium.

MEDICINAL USES: very active vermifuge. This plant has very beneficial effects on removing tapeworms and roundworms, and is safe enough to give to children as long as a saline aperient is given after pinkroot, to temper the unpleasant side effects. These side effects include disturbed vision, muscular spasms, increased heart action and dizziness and are increased in severity as the dose given rises. This can lead to convulsions and death if care is not taken with this drug.

ADMINISTERED AS: fluid extract, powdered root.

Pipsissewa *Chinaphila umbellata.* COMMON NAME: Winter green, butter winter, prince's pine, king's cure, ground holly, love in winter, rheumatism weed, *Pyrola umbellata.*

OCCURRENCE: grows in Europe, Asia, the United States and Siberia.

PARTS USED: the leaves, which contain chinaphilin, arbutin gum, resin, pectic acid, starch, chlorophyll, tannic acids and several mineral salts.

MEDICINAL USES: diuretic, astringent, tonic, alterative. A decoction of the leaves is good for fluid retention, chronic gonorrhoea, dropsy and catarrh of the bladder. Applied to the skin, it acts as a rubefacient and vesicant which is good in kidney and cardiac diseases, scrofular and chronic rheumatism. It is also of value in skin diseases and may be a effective against diabetes.

ADMINISTERED AS: fresh leaves, decoction, fluid extract, syrup.

Plantain, Common *Plantago major.* COMMON NAME: broad-leaved plantain, ripple grass, waybread, snakeweed, cuckoo's bread, Englishman's foot, white man's foot, waybroad.

OCCURRENCE: a familiar weed all over Europe, Great Britain and other parts of the world.

parts used: the root, leaves and flowers.

MEDICINAL USES: refrigerant, diuretic, deobstruent, astringent, cooling, alterative. The plant has been used in inflammation of the skin, malignant ulcers, intermittent fever, applied to sores and as a vulnerary. The fresh leaves can stop bleeding of minor wounds, relieve the pain of insect stings, nettles, burns and scalds.

ADMINISTERED AS: expressed juice, poultice, infusion, fresh leaves, fluid extract, decoction, ointment.

Pleurisy root *Asclepias tuberose.* COMMON NAME: butterfly-weed, swallow-wort, tuber root, wind root, colic root, orange milkweed, white root, flux root, Canada root.

OCCURRENCE: native to North America.

PARTS USED: the root which contains several resins, volatile oil, fatty matter, glucosides including asclepiadin and cardiac glycosides.

MEDICINAL USES: antispasmodic, diaphoretic, expectorant, tonic, carminative, mildly cathartic. One of the most important indigenous North American herbs which has a specific action on the lungs, reducing inflammation, helping expectoration and delivering a mild tonic effect to the pulmonary system. It is of great benefit in pleurisy, pulmonary catarrh and difficult breathing as it relieves the pain. The root also helps in acute and chronic rheumatism, eczema, flatulent colic, indigestion, dysentery and diarrhoea. It is often combined with other herbs, e.g. angelica to best effect. In large doses, pleurisy root can be emetic and purgative in effect.

ADMINISTERED AS: decoction, fluid extract, infusion.

Poke root *Phytolacca decandra.* COMMON NAME: Garget, pigeon berry, bear's grape, red-ink plant, American spinach, skoke, crowberry, cancer-root, pocan, coakum, poke berry, herbe de la laque, *Phytolaccae radix, Phytolacca vulgaris, P. americana, Blitun americanum.*

OCCURRENCE: indigenous to North America and is grown in most Mediterranean countries.

PARTS USED: dried root and berries. The root is made up of triterpenoid saponins, phytolaccine (an alkaloid), resins, phytolaccic acid and tannin.

MEDICINAL USES: emetic, cathartic, alterative, narcotic. The root is used for conjunctivitis, chronic rheumatism, skin diseases and paralysis of the bowels. It is said to stimulate the lymphatic system and so is good for tonsillitis, swollen glands and mumps. Herbalists disagree as to whether poke root is effective against cancer. It may be effective, when used both as a poultice and taken internally, against breast cancer and mastitis and has been used in cases of uterine cancer. The berries are thought to have a milder action on the body than the root. The use of the root as an emetic is not recommended and the fresh root is poisonous so this drug should only be prescribed by a qualified herbal practitioner.

ADMINISTERED AS: infusion, ointment, tincture, fluid extract.

Polypody root *Polypodium vulgare.* COMMON NAME: Rock polypody, polypody of the oak, wall fern, brake root, rock brake, oak fern, rock of polypody.

OCCURRENCE: a common fern growing in sheltered places, hedge-banks, old walls and tree stumps in Great Britain and Europe.

PARTS USED: the root.

MEDICINAL USES: alterative, tonic, expectorant, pectoral. This herb is used as a laxative; as a tonic in dyspepsia and loss of appetite. It is also good for skin diseases, coughs and catarrh, consumption, hepatic complaints and some types of parasitic worm. The action of this drug is such that it may cause the formation of a rash, but these spots should disappear after a short period of time with no after effects. This fern is still used as a cure for whooping cough in many rural areas.

ADMINISTERED AS: fresh root, decoction, powdered root, fluid extract.

Poplar *Populus tremuloides.* COMMON NAME: White poplar, American aspen, quaking aspen.

OCCURRENCE: native to North America and commonly grown in Great Britain.

PARTS USED: the bark, which is thought to contain salicin and populin.

MEDICINAL USES: febrifuge, diuretic, stimulant, tonic. This drug is very useful against fevers, particularly those of an intermittent nature. It is often used as a substitute for Peruvian bark or quinine, as it lacks dangerous long-term side effects. Poplar bark is helpful in treating chronic diarrhoea, debility, hysteria, indiges-

tion and faintness as well as acting as a diuretic in gleet, gonorrhoea and urinary complaints. This drug could be considered a 'universal tonic'.

ADMINISTERED AS: infusion, fluid extract.

Poppy, Red *Papaver rhoeas.* COMMON NAME: Headache, corn poppy, corn rose, flores rhoeados.

OCCURRENCE: a common flowering plant in fields and waste ground across Europe and Great Britain.

PARTS USED: flowers and petals. The fresh petals contain rhoeadic and papaveric acids, which give the flowers their colour, and the alkaloid rhoeadine. The amount and quantity of active ingredients in the plant is uncertain so its action is open to debate.

MEDICINAL USES: very slightly narcotic, anodyne, expectorant. The petals can be made into a syrup which is used to ease pain. It may be used for chest complaints, e.g. pleurisy.

ADMINISTERED AS: syrup, infusion, distilled water.

Poppy, White *Papaver somniferum.* COMMON NAME: Opium poppy, mawseed.

OCCURRENCE: indigenous to Turkey and Asia, cultivated in Europe, Great Britain, Persia, India and China for opium production.

PARTS USED: the capsules and flowers. The white poppy contains twenty one different alkaloids of which morphine, narcotine, codeine, codamine and thebaine are the most important.

MEDICINAL USES: hypnotic, sedative, astringent, expectorant, diaphoretic, antispasmodic, anodyne. The use of this drug dates back to Greek and Roman times. It is the best possible hypnotic and sedative drug, frequently used to relieve pain and calm excitement. It has also been used in diarrhoea, dysentery and some forms of cough. The tincture of opium is commonly called laudanum, and when applied externally with soap liniment it provides quick pain relief.

ADMINISTERED AS: syrup, tincture, decoction and poultice.

Primrose *Primula vulgaris.*

OCCURRENCE: a common wild flower found in woods, hedgerows and pastures throughout Great Britain.

PARTS USED: the root and whole herb. Both parts of the plant contain a fragrant oil called primulin and the active principle saponin.

MEDICINAL USES: astringent, antispasmodic, vermifuge, emetic. It was formerly considered to be an important remedy in muscular rheumatism, paralysis and gout. A tincture of the whole plant has sedative effects and is used successfully in extreme sensitivity, restlessness and insomnia. Nervous headaches can be eased by treatment with an infusion of the root, while the powdered dry root serves as an emetic. An infusion of primrose flowers is excellent in nervous headaches and an ointment can be made out of the leaves to heal and salve wounds and cuts.

ADMINISTERED AS: infusion, tincture, powdered root and ointment.

Puffball *Lycoperdon bovista.* COMMON NAME: *Lycoperdon giganteum.*

OCCURRENCE: grows wild throughout Great Britain and Europe.

PARTS USED: the lower section of the fungi.

MEDICINAL USES: haemostatic. This fungi grows completely enclosing its spores in fungal tissue (peridium), and then matures so that the colour changes from yellow-white to brown and then the peridium ruptures and the spores are released. When young, the spongy fungal tissue makes an excellent food and is consumed with relish by people in many European areas, including the Gaelic community in the Highlands of Scotland. Once matured, it is not edible but it can then be used to stop bleeding from wounds. It is a highly effective cure. Puffballs were also used as tinder many years ago and are burnt, producing smoke which stupefies bees so that honey can be collected safely.

ADMINISTERED AS: dried or fresh fungal tissue and spores.

Pumpkin *Cucurbita maxima.* COMMON NAME: Pumpkin seed, melon pumpkin, pompion.

OCCURRENCE: a plant grown for food and animal fodder in the United States and common in gardens in Great Britain.

PARTS USED: the seeds. They contain a fixed oil, a volatile oil, sugar, starch and an acrid resin which may be the active component.

MEDICINAL USES: taeniacide, diuretic, demulcent. This fruit has long been used as a vermifuge, removing parasitic worms including tapeworm. A mixture of the seeds, sugar, milk or water is mixed up and taken over six hours after which CASTOR OIL is given, a few hours after the final dose of pumpkin. The vermifuge effects are thought to come from the mechanical effects of the seeds. A basic infusion of the seeds in water is used in urinary complaints.

ADMINISTERED AS: infusion.

Purslane, Golden *Portulaca sativa.* COMMON NAME: Garden purslane, pigweed.

OCCURRENCE: an herbaceous annual plant which is distributed all over the world. It is not indigenous to Great Britain.

PARTS USED: the herb, expressed juice and seeds.

MEDICINAL USES: Purslane is a herb with a great history of use for medical complaints. The expressed juice of the herb was good for strangury, dry coughs, shortness of breath, hot agues, headaches, haemorrhages and as an external application to sores and inflammation. When combined with oil of ROSES, the juice was used for sore mouths, swollen gums and to fasten loose teeth. The bruised seeds were made into a decoction with wine and used to expel worms from children. The bruised herb was used as a poultice to remove heat from the head and temples and to reduce eye inflammation. It was also used on cramps or gouty areas.

ADMINISTERED AS: poultice, decoction, expressed juice.

Pyrethrum, Dalmatian *Chrysanthemum cinerariaefolium.* COMMON NAME: Insect flowers.

OCCURRENCE: the Dalmatian coast and Japan.

PARTS USED: the closed flowers.

MEDICINAL USES: insecticide, vermin killer. A powder of ground flowers is used in powder, lotions and fumigation materials to kill insects. The active ingredient is pyrethrin. The powder is not toxic to mammals.

ADMINISTERED AS: ground flowers.

Quince *Cydonia oblongata.* COMMON NAME: Quince seed, *Cydonica vulgaris.*

OCCURRENCE: grown in England for its fruit but is native to Persia.

PARTS USED: the fruit and seeds.

MEDICINAL USES: astringent, mucilaginous, demulcent. The fruit is used to prepare a syrup which is added to drinks when ill, as it restrains looseness of the bowels and helps relieve dysentery and diarrhoea. The soaked seeds form a mucilaginous mass similar to that produced by FLAX. A decoction of the seeds is used against gonorrhoea, thrush and in irritable conditions of the mucous membranes. The liquid is also used as a skin lotion or cream and administered in eye diseases as a soothing lotion.

ADMINISTERED AS: syrup, decoction or lotion.

Radish *Raphanus satinus*

OCCURRENCE: a native plant of China, Japan and cochin-China and widely cultivated in Europe, Great Britain and temperate Asia.

PARTS USED: the root which has been found to contain a volatile oil, an amylclytic enzyme and a chemical called phenyl-ethyl isothiocyanite.

MEDICINAL USES: antiscorbutic, diuretic. This plant is a very good food remedy for scurvy, gravel and stone. The juice has been beneficial in preventing the formation of gallstones.

ADMINISTERED AS: expressed juice, fresh root, dietary item.

Ragwort *Senecio jacobaea*. COMMON NAME: St. James's wort, stinking nanny, staggerwort, ragweed, dog standard, cankerwort, stammerwort, fireweed.

OCCURRENCE: an abundant wild plant, widely distributed over Great Britain, Europe, Siberia and north-west India.

PARTS USED: the herb.

MEDICINAL USES: diaphoretic, detergent, emollient, cooling, astringent. The leaves were used as emollient poultices, while the expressed juice of the herb was utilized as a wash in burns, eye inflammation, sores and cancerous ulcers. It has been successful in relieving rheumatism, sciatica, gout and in reducing inflammation and swelling of joints when applied as a poultice. Ragwort makes a good gargle for ulcerated throats and mouths and a decoction of its root is said to help internal bruising and wounds. The herb was previously thought to be able to prevent infection. This plant is poisonous to cattle and should be removed from their pastures. The alkaloids in the ragwort have cumulative effects in the cattle and low doses of the chemical eaten over a period of time can build up to a critical level, where the cattle show obvious symptoms and death then results. It is uncertain if sheep are also susceptible to this chemical.

ADMINISTERED AS: poultice, infusion and decoction.

Raspberry *Rubus idaeus*. COMMON NAME: American raspberry, raspbis, hindberry, bramble of Mount Ida, *Rubus strigosus*.

OCCURRENCE: found wild in Great Britain and cultivated in many parts of Europe.

PARTS USED: the leaves and fruit. The fruit contains fruit sugar, a volatile oil, pectin, mineral salts and citric and malic acids.

MEDICINAL USES: astringent and stimulant. Tea made of raspberry leaves is employed as a gargle for sore mouths, canker of the throat and as a wash for wounds and ulcers. It was also reckoned to give strength to pregnant women

and encourage fast and safe delivery of the child. The leaves make a good poultice for cleaning wounds and promoting healing. Raspberry vinegar made with fruit juice, sugar and white wine vinegar makes a very good cooling drink when added to water, and is beneficial in fevers and as a gargle for sore throats. The infusion of raspberry leaves is also good in extreme laxity of the bowels and in stomach complaints of children.

ADMINISTERED AS: infusion, poultice, tea and liquid extract.

Red root *Ceanothus americanus*. COMMON NAME: New Jersey tea, wild snowball.

OCCURRENCE: a shrub indigenous to the United States.

PARTS USED: the root, which contains tannin, a resin, a bitter extract, gum, lignin, a volatile substance and a principle called ceanothine.

MEDICINAL USES: antispasmodic, astringent, expectorant, sedative, anti-syphilis drug. It is very good in chronic bronchitis, whooping cough, consumption, asthma, dysentery and pulmonary complaints. The decoction is an excellent mouth wash or gargle for sores or ulcers. The herb is also used as an injection for gonorrhoea, gleet and leucorrhoea.

ADMINISTERED AS: fluid extract, decoction, injection.

Rest-harrow *Ononis arvensis*. COMMON NAME: Wild liquorice, cammock, stinking tommy, ground furze, land whin, *Ononis spinosa*.

OCCURRENCE: a weed found on arable and waste land in Britain.

PARTS USED: the root.

MEDICINAL USES: diuretic. This herb was taken internally for dropsy, jaundice, gout, rheumatism and bladder stones. When made into a decoction, it was used as a wash for ulcers, fluid accumulation in tissues and enlarged glands. It was also proposed to subdue delirium. The young shoots were used as a vegetable or pickled, when they were said to refresh the breath and remove the smell of alcohol from the breath.

ADMINISTERED AS: decoction, dietary item.

Rhubarb, English *Rheum rhaponticum*. COMMON NAME: Garden rhubarb, bastard rhubarb, sweet round-leaved dock, *Rheum officinale*.

OCCURRENCE: its cultivation started in England around 1777 and spread throughout Great Britain. It is found growing wild or near dwellings.

PARTS USED: the rhizome and root. The stem and

leaves of the plant contain potassium oxalate in quantity and some people are more sensitive to these salts and should avoid eating the plant. People with gout or those subject to urinary irritation should avoid the plant as well.

MEDICINAL USES: stomachic, aperient, astringent, purgative. This plant has a milder action than its relative, Turkey rhubarb (*Rheum palmatum*). It has a milder purgative effect and is particularly useful for stomach troubles in infants and looseness of the bowels. In large doses, rhubarb has a laxative effect. A decoction of the seed is proposed to ease stomach pain and increase the appetite. Rhubarb leaves were formerly used as a vegetable in the nineteenth century, and several fatal cases of poisoning were recorded.

ADMINISTERED AS: decoction and powdered root.

Rice *Oryza sativa*. COMMON NAME: Nivona, dhan, bras, paddy, *Oryza montana, O. setegera, O. latifolia.*

OCCURRENCE: native to China and India; now cultivated in most sub-tropical countries.

PARTS USED: the seeds.

MEDICINAL USES: nutritive, demulcent, refrigerant. Boiled rice is good in treating upset digestion, bowel problems and diarrhoea. Rice-water, made from a decoction of the seeds, is an excellent demulcent and refrigerant drink in febrile and inflammatory diseases of the intestines, painful urination and other related conditions. It may be given as an enema for best results. Finely powdered rice flour can be used for burns, scalds and erysipelas or rice starch can be utilized in the same manner as wheat starch.

ADMINISTERED AS: poultice, decoction, dietary item, enema.

Rose, pale *Rosa centifolia*. COMMON NAME: cabbage rose, hundred-leaved rose.

OCCURRENCE: cultivated in southern Europe and grown as a garden plant in many countries.

PARTS USED: the petals, which contain an acid red colouring matter, the glucoside quercitrin, gallic acid, tannic acid, sugar, gum and fat. Also the leaves.

MEDICINAL USES: aperient, laxative, astringent. The petals of this pink rose are rarely taken internally in modern herbal medicine, although they do have aperient properties. These flowers are mainly used for the preparation of rose-water, which is used as an eye lotion and as a carrier medium for other medicines. Cold cream is also made from rose-water and it is used on the skin of the hand and face to soothe abrasions and lesions. Rose leaves are laxative and astringent and were used to heal wounds.

ADMINISTERED AS: distilled water, ointment.

Rose, red *Rosa gallica*. COMMON NAME: Rose flowers, Provence rose, provins rose.

OCCURRENCE: a native plant of southern Europe and grown in gardens all over the world.

PARTS USED: the petals. Their composition is the same as that of the PALE ROSE, except they do not contain tannic acid.

MEDICINAL USES: tonic, astringent. Today, the petals are not normally taken internally. The petals are prepared in three manners which are then used. A confection is made of petals and sugar and this is utilized in making pills. The fluid extract is prepared using powdered rose petals, glycerine and dilute alcohol while an acid infusion is made with dried rose petals, sulphuric acid, sugar and boiling water. The infusion may be used as a flavouring for other medicines, as a lotion for eye complaints and for the treatment of night sweats relating to depression. Syrup of roses, honey of rose and rose vinegar are also preparations used medicinally in various countries around Europe. The petals are also used as flavour enhancers in two alcoholic liqueurs. *Rosa gallica* petals are used in aromatherapy.

ADMINISTERED AS: pills, lotion, infusion, poultice, syrup, fluid extract.

Rosemary *Rosmarinus officinalis*. COMMON NAME: Polar plant, compass-weed, compass plant, romero, *Rosmarinus coronarium.*

OCCURRENCE: native to the dry hills of the Mediterranean, from Spain westward to Turkey. A common garden plant in Britain, having been cultivated prior to the Norman Conquest.

PARTS USED: the herb and root. Oil of rosemary is distilled from the plant tops and used medicinally. Rosemary contains tannic acid, a bitter principle, resin and a volatile oil.

MEDICINAL USES: tonic, astringent, diaphoretic, stimulant. The essential oil is also stomachic, nervine and carminative and cures many types of headache. It is mainly applied externally as a hair lotion which is said to prevent baldness and the formation of dandruff. The oil is used externally as a rubefacient and is added to liniments for fragrance and stimulant properties. Rosemary tea can remove headache, colic, colds and nervous diseases and may also lift nervous depression.

ADMINISTERED AS: infusion, essential oil and lotion.

Rosinweed *Silphium paciniatum*. COMMON NAME: Compass plant, compass-weed, polar plant.

OCCURRENCE: native to the western United States, especially Ohio. This plant is closely related to *Silphium laciniatum* and is often confused with it.

PARTS USED: the root, which yields a resinous secretion very similar to MASTIC.

MEDICINAL USES: tonic, diaphoretic, alterative, emetic, diuretic, antispasmodic, expectorant. The root is used in dry, stubborn coughs, asthma and other pulmonary diseases. The decoction of the root is said to be emetic and has cured intermittent fevers. A strong infusion is good against enlarged spleen, internal bruising, liver problems and digestive ulcers. The resin has diuretic qualities and taints the urine, giving it a strong odour.

ADMINISTERED AS: fluid extract, decoction, infusion.

Rowan tree *Pyrus aucuparia*. COMMON NAME: Mountain ash, *Sorbus aucuparia*, *Mespilus aucuparia*.

OCCURRENCE: generally distributed over Great Britain and Europe, especially at high altitudes.

PARTS USED: the bark and fruit. The fruit may contain tartaric, citric or malic acids dependent upon its stage of ripeness. It also contains sorbitol, sorbin, sorbit, parascorbic acid and bitter, acrid colouring matters. The bark contains amygdalin.

MEDICINAL USES: astringent, antiscorbutic. A decoction of Rowan bark is given for diarrhoea and as a vaginal injection for leucorrhoea. The berries are made into an acid gargle to ease sore throats and inflamed tonsils. An infusion of the fruit is administered to ease haemorrhoids. The berries may also be made into jelly, flour, cider, ale or an alcoholic spirit. The rowan tree planted next to a house was said to protect the house against witchcraft.

ADMINISTERED AS: decoction, injection, infusion and dietary item.

Rue *Ruta graveolens*. COMMON NAME: Herb of grace, garden rue, herbygrass, ave-grace.

OCCURRENCE: indigenous to southern Europe and was introduced into Great Britain by the Romans.

PARTS USED: the herb. The herb is covered by glands which contain a volatile oil. The oil is composed of methylnonylketone, limonene, cineole, a crystalline substance called rutin and

several acids. The plant also contains several alkaloids including fagarine and arborinine as well as coumarins.

MEDICINAL USES: stimulant, antispasmodic, emmenagogue, irritant, rubefacient. This is a very powerful herb and the dose administered should be kept low. It is useful in treating coughs, croup, colic, flatulence, hysteria and it is particularly good against strained eyes and headaches caused by eyestrain. An infusion of the herb is good for nervous indigestion, heart palpitations, nervous headaches and to expel worms. The chemical, rutin, strengthens weak blood vessels and aids varicose veins. In Chinese medicine, rue is a specific for insect and snake bites. When made into an ointment, rue is effective in gouty and rheumatic pains, sprained and bruised tendons and chilblains. The bruised leaves irritate and blister the skin and so can ease sciatica. This herb should not be used in pregnancy as the volatile oil, alkaloids and coumarins in the plant all stimulate the uterus and strongly promote menstrual bleeding. When a fresh leaf is chewed, it flavours the mouth and relieves headache, giddiness or any hysterical spasms quickly.

ADMINISTERED AS: fresh leaf, volatile oil, ointment, infusion, decoction, tea, expressed juice.

Rupturewort *Herniara glabra*. COMMON NAME: Herniary, breastwort.

OCCURRENCE: found in temperate and southern Europe and Russian Asia. It is a British native plant, particularly in southern and central England.

PARTS USED: the herb, which contains the alkaloid paronychine, and a crystalline principle called herniarne.

MEDICINAL USES: astringent, diuretic. This is a very active drug which has been successful in treating catarrhal infections of the bladder and oedema of cardiac or kidney origins.

ADMINISTERED AS: infusion.

Sabadilla *Veratrum sabadilla* or *Veratrum officinale*. COMMON NAME: Cevadilla, sabadillermer, caustic barley, *Schoenocaulon officinale*, *Melanthian sabadilla*, *Helonias officinalis*, *Sabadilla officinarum*, *Asagraea officinalis*.

OCCURRENCE: grows in southern North America, guatemala, Venezuela and Mexico.

PARTS USED: the seeds. They contain several alkaloids including veratrine, sabadillie, sabadine, sabadinine and cevadine, which hydrolyzes to cevine. They also contain voatric acid, cevadic acid, resin and fat.

MEDICINAL USES: drastic emetic and cathartic, vermifuge. The powdered seeds have been used to expel parasitic worms and to kill and remove parasitic mites or other vermin from the hair. An extract called veratria is derived from the seeds and despite it being highly poisonous, it is occasionally taken internally in minute doses. When taken internally, it can ease acute rheumatic pain and gout and also help some inflammatory diseases. Veratria is more commonly used as an ointment for neuralgia and rheumatism. This drug has a powerful action on the heart causing it to slow and eventually stop beating entirely.

ADMINISTERED AS: powdered seeds, ointment.

Saffron *Crocus sativus*. COMMON NAME: Croccus, karcom, Alicante saffron, valencia saffron, krokos, gatinais, saffron, hay saffron, saffron crocus.

OCCURRENCE: grown from Persia and Kurdistan in the east to most European countries including Great Britain.

PARTS USED: the dried flower pistils. These parts contain an essential oil composed of terpenes, terepene alcohols and esters, a coloured glycoside called crocin and a bitter glucoside, called picrocrocin.

MEDICINAL USES: carminative, diaphoretic, emmenagogue. This herb is used as a diaphoretic drug for children and can also benefit female hysteria, absent or painful menstruation and stop chronic haemorrhage of the uterus in adults.

ADMINISTERED AS: tincture, powdered saffron.

Saffron, Meadow *Colchicum autumnale*. COMMON NAME: Colchicum, naked ladies.

OCCURRENCE: grows wild in North Africa and Europe and is found in meadows and limestone areas in the British Isles.

PARTS USED: the root and seeds.

MEDICINAL USES: cathartic, emetic, anti-rheumatic. This herb is very useful for acute rheumatic and gouty ailments, and it is normally taken along with an alkaline diuretic for best results. The active chemical in the plant is colchinine, an alkaline substance which is very poisonous. It has sedative effects and particularly acts on the bowels and kidneys. It acts as an irritant poison in large doses, and can cause undue depression. As such, care should be used when utilizing this herb.

ADMINISTERED AS: fluid extract, powdered root, tincture, solid extract.

Sage, Common *Salvia officinalis*. COMMON NAME: garden sage, red sage, saurge, broad-leaved white sage, *Salvia salvatrix*.

OCCURRENCE: native to the northern Mediterranean and cultivated through Britain, France and Germany.

PARTS USED: the leaves, whole herb. The herb contains a volatile oil, tannin and resin and is distilled to produce sage oil. This is made up of salvene, pinene, cineol, vorneol, thujone and some esters.

MEDICINAL USES: stimulant, astringent, tonic, carminative, aromatic. Sage makes an excellent gargle for relaxed throat and tonsils, bleeding gums, laryngitis and ulcerated throat. Sage tea is valuable against delirium of fevers, nervous excitement and accompanying brain and nervous diseases; as a stimulant tonic in stomach and nervous system complaints and in weak digestion. It also works as an emmenagogue, in treating typhoid fever, bilious and liver problems, kidney troubles and lung or stomach haemorrhages. The infusion is used in head colds, quinsy, measles, painful joints, lethargy, palsy and nervous headaches. Fresh leaves are rubbed on the teeth to cleanse them and strengthen gums—even today sage is included in toothpowders. The oil of sage was used to remove mucus collections from the respiratory organs and is included in embrocations for rheumatism. The herb is also applied warm as a poultice.

ADMINISTERED AS: infusion, essential oil, tea and poultice.

Salep: early purple orchid, *Orchis mascula*; **spotted orchid**, *Orchis maculata*; **marsh orchid**, *Orchis latifolia*. COMMON NAME: Saloop, schlep, satrion, Levant salep.

OCCURRENCE: *Orchis mascula* is found in woods throughout England. *O. maculata* grows wild on heaths and commons; *O. latifolia* is found growing in marshes and damp pastures across Great Britain.

PARTS USED: the tuberous root, which contains mucilage, sugar, starch and volatile oil.

MEDICINAL USES: very nutritive, demulcent. This herb is used as a food item for convalescent people and children, made with milk or water and flavoured. It is prepared in a similar way to arrowroot. A decoction with sugar, spice or wine was given to invalids to build them up. The root is used to stop irritation of the gastro-intestinal canal and for invalids suffering from bilious fevers or chronic diarrhoea. In the old sailing ships, salep was carried and used as an emergency food source. It was sold on street corners in London as a hot drink, before COFFEE replaced its use as a beverage.

ADMINISTERED AS: decoction, dietary item.

Samphire *Crithmum maritimum*. COMMON NAME: Sea fennel, crest marine, sampier, rock fennel, rock samphire.

OCCURRENCE: found on rocks or salt marshes around the west or south of England but rare in the North and Scotland.

PARTS USED: the herb.

MEDICINAL USES: an infusion of samphire has a diuretic effect and acts on the kidneys. It is reputed to be an excellent treatment for obesity. It is eaten as a condiment, as a salad ingredient or pickled.

ADMINISTERED AS: infusion.

Sandalwood *Santalum album*. COMMON NAME: Santalwood, sanders-wood.

OCCURRENCE: a tree native to India and the Malay Archipelago.

PARTS USED: the wood oil.

MEDICINAL USES: aromatic, antiseptic, diuretic. The oil is given internally for chronic mucous conditions, e.g. bronchitis, inflammation of the bladder. It is also used in chronic cystitis, gleet and gonorrhoea. The oil is used in aromatherapy to lessen tension and anxiety and it was also considered a sexual stimulant in folk traditions. The fluid extract of sandalwood may be better tolerated by some people than the oil.

ADMINISTERED AS: wood oil, fluid extract.

Sarsaparilla, Jamaica, *Smilax ornata*. COMMON NAME: red-bearded sarsaparilla, *Smilax medica*, *Smilax officinalis*.

OCCURRENCE: a perennial climbing plant which grows in central America, primarily Costa Rica. It is termed Jamaican sarsaparilla as the plant was exported to Europe through Jamaica.

PARTS USED: the root, which is composed of starch, sarsapic acid, the glucoside sarsaponin and palmitic, stearic, behenic, oleic and linoleic fatty acids. The active principle is a crystalline compound called porillin or smilacin.

MEDICINAL USES: alterative, tonic, diaphoretic, diuretic. This root was introduced into Europe in 1563 as a remedy for syphilis. It is used in other chronic diseases, particularly rheumatism or skin diseases. It is still considered an excellent blood purifier, often given in conjunction with SASSAFRAS or BURDOCK. When smoked,

Jamaican sarsaparilla was recommended for asthma.

ADMINISTERED AS: powdered root, fluid extract, solid extract.

Sassafras *Sassafras officinale*. COMMON NAME: Laurus sassafras, sassafrax, *Sassafras radix*, *Sassafras varifolium*.

OCCURRENCE: native to the eastern United States and Canada then south to Mexico.

PARTS USED: the root-bark, root and pith. The root-bark contains a heavy and light volatile oil, resin, wax, tannic acid, lignin, starch and camphorous matter. The pith is made up of mucilage which is used as a demulcent. The bark yields an oil, which is mainly safrol. This is a heavy volatile oil associated with sassafras camphor when cold.

MEDICINAL USES: aromatic, stimulant, diaphoretic, alterative, diuretic. This herb is usually given in combination with other herbs, e.g. sarsaparilla, to treat chronic rheumatism, skin diseases or syphilis. The oil relieves pain after childbirth and due to obstructed menstruation and also benefits gonorrhoea and gleet. A decoction of the pith is used as an eye wash in eye complaints and in general inflammations. Safrol, when taken internally, can produce narcotic poisoning, but when used externally it can be used for rheumatic pains and as a dental disinfectant.

ADMINISTERED AS: oil of sassafras, fluid extract, decoction.

Sassy bark *Erythrophloeum guineense*. COMMON NAME: maneona bark, casca bark, doom bark, ordeal bark, saucy bark, red water bark, nkasa, *Cortex erythrophei*.

OCCURRENCE: a large tree native to the west coast of Africa in Upper Guinea, Senegal, Gambia and Sudan.

PARTS USED: the bark, which contains the poisonous chemical erythrophleine, tannin and resin.

MEDICINAL USES: narcotic, astringent, anodyne, laxative. It has been used successfully in dysentery, diarrhoea and passive haemorrhages. The chemical erythrophleine acts on the pulse rate, peristalsis and the nerve centres to cause relief from pain, purging and vomiting. It needs more research to see if erythrophleine would make a good anaesthetic drug. Since it is very poisonous and has severe effects on the body, it is rarely used in modern herbal medicine. In native West African cultures, this drug is given as an ordeal in trials of witchcraft and sorcery to determine the truth.

ADMINISTERED AS: fluid extract, powdered bark.

Savory, Summer *Saturcia hortensis*. COMMON NAME: Garden savory.

OCCURRENCE: a shrub native to the Mediterranean region and introduced into Great Britain.

PARTS USED: the herb.

MEDICINAL USES: aromatic, carminative. This herb is mainly used in cookery, as a pot-herb or flavouring. In medicine, it is added to remedies to flavour and add warmth. It was formerly used for colic, flatulence and was considered a good expectorant. A sprig of summer savory rubbed on a wasp or bee sting relieves the pain quickly.

ADMINISTERED AS: fresh or dried herb.

Savine *Juniperus sabina*. COMMON NAME: Savin, savine tops.

OCCURRENCE: indigenous to the northern states in the USA and middle and southern Europe, e.g. Switzerland, Italy and Austria.

PARTS USED: the tops of the herb. It contains gallic acid, resin, chlorophyll, a volatile oil, lilgnin, calcium salts, gum and a fixed oil.

MEDICINAL USES: emmenagogue, diuretic, anthelmintic. This herb is rarely given internally as it is an irritant herb and also poisonous, whose use can be fatal if not properly managed. It is a powerful emmenagogue which can induce abortion when given in large doses — should never be taken when pregnant. It used to be administered with TANSY, PENNY ROYAL and HEMLOCK. As a vermifuge, it has been used for worms along with PINK ROOT and SENNA. Mainly used externally as an ointment for skin eruptions, blisters and syphilitic warts. It is said to remove warts from the hands.

ADMINISTERED AS: powdered herb, tincture, fluid extract.

Saw palmetto *Sarenoa serrulata*. COMMON NAME: Sabal, *Sabal serrulata*.

OCCURRENCE: native to the North Atlantic coast of the United States and southern California.

PARTS USED: the ripe fruit, which contains volatile oil, glucose and a fixed oil.

MEDICINAL USES: nutritive, tonic, diuretic, sedative. This herb affects the mucous membranes of the respiratory system to ease many diseases linked to chronic catarrh. Saw palmetto is a tissue-building herb which aids atony of the testicles or breasts. It reduces catarrhal irritation in the body and can ease catarrh of the bladder and urethra.

ADMINISTERED AS: solid extract, powdered fruit, fluid extract.

Saxifrage, Burnet *Pimpinella saxifraga*. COMMON NAME: Lesser burnet, saxifrage.

OCCURRENCE: found on dry, chalky pastures throughout the British Isles.

PARTS USED: the root and the herb.

MEDICINAL USES: resolvent, diaphoretic, diuretic, stomachic, aromatic, carminative. This herb is prescribed for flatulent indigestion, toothache, paralysis of the tongue, asthma and dropsy. A decoction is used as a gargle in throat infections and hoarseness. The herb was added to casks of beer or wine to impart its aromatic flavour to the drink.

ADMINISTERED AS: fresh root, decoction dried root.

Scullcap, Virginian *Scutellaria lateriflora*. COMMON NAME: Mad-dog scullcap, helmet flower, madweed, mad-dog weed, skullcap, Quaker bonnet.

OCCURRENCE: native to the United States of America.

PARTS USED: the herb, which contains a volatile oil called scutellonin, flavonoid glucosides including scutellonin and scutellanein, some bitter principle, sugar, cellulose, tannin and fat.

MEDICINAL USES: strong tonic, nervine, antispasmodic, astringent. This herb is an invaluable tonic for the nervous system, treating nervous headaches, anxiety, depression, insomnia and neuralgia. It is most beneficial in hysteria, convulsions, rickets, epilepsy and Speakman's chorea where it soothes nervous excitement and induces sleep without any unpleasant side effects. The bitter taste of the herb stimulates and strengthens the digestion. It is said that many cases of hydrophobia have been cured by the use of this herb alone. The European species, *Scutellaria galericulata*, was once used for malaria and it shares the nervine qualities of Virginian scullcap. This herb may be difficult to obtain as most commercial supplies of it are adulterated with wood sage (*Teucrium scorodonia*).

ADMINISTERED AS: fluid extract, infusion, decoction, powdered herb.

Scurvy grass *Cochlearia officinalis*. COMMON NAME: Spoonwort.

OCCURRENCE: native to the coastline of Scotland, Ireland and England; also found in the sea coasts of northern and western Europe, the Arctic Circle and at altitude on the mountain chains of Europe.

PARTS USED: the herb.

MEDICINAL USES: stimulant, aperient, diuretic, antiscorbutic. It was formerly used on sea voyages to prevent scurvy. The essential oil from the herb is beneficial in cases of rheumatism or paralysis. When made into scurvy grass ale it was drunk as a tonic.

ADMINISTERED AS: infusion, essential oil.

Self-heal *Prunella vulgaris.* COMMON NAME: Prunella, all-heal, hook-heal, slough-heal, brunella, heart of the Earth, blue curls, siclewort.

OCCURRENCE: a very abundant wild plant in woods and fields all over Europe and Great Britain.

PARTS USED: the whole herb, containing a volatile oil, a bitter principle, tannin, sugar and cellulose.

MEDICINAL USES: astringent, styptic and tonic. An infusion of the herb is taken internally for sore throats, internal bleeding, leucorrhoea and as a general strengthener.

ADMINISTERED AS: infusion, injection and decoction.

Senega *Polygala senega.* COMMON NAME: Snake root, seneca, milkwort, mountain flax, rattlesnake root, senega snakeroot, seneka, *Senegae radix, Polygala virginiana, Plantula marilandica, Senega officinalis.*

OCCURRENCE: grows wild throughout central and western North America.

PARTS USED: the dried root, which contains polygalic acid, virgineic acid, pectic and tannic acids, fixed oil, albumen, sugar and various mineral salts. The active chemical is called senegin which is almost identical to the saponin chemical found in SOAPWORT (*Saponaria officinale*).

MEDICINAL USES: stimulant, expectorant, diaphoretic, diuretic, emmenagogue. It is highly effective in treating acute bronchial catarrh, chronic pneumonia or bronchitis and kidney-related dropsy. Senega is also of benefit for croup, whooping cough and rheumatism. The ancient herbalists of Greek or Roman times considered senega of identical action with IPECACUANHA (*Cephaelis ipecacuanha*). In large doses senega is an emetic and cathartic drug, and overdoses are possible.

ADMINISTERED AS: powder, fluid extract, syrup, tincture, infusion.

Senna, Alexandrian *Cassia acutifolia*; **Senna, East Indian** *Cassia angustifolia.* COMMON NAME: Nubian senna, Egyptian senna, tinnevelly senna, *Cassia senna, Cassia lenitiva,*

Cassia lanceolata, Cassia officinalis, Cassia aethiopica, Senna acutifolia.

OCCURRENCE: *C. acutifolia* is native to the upper and middle Nile in Egypt and Sudan. *C. angustifolia* is indigenous to southern Arabia and is cultivated in southern and eastern India.

PARTS USED: the dried leaflets and pods. The active principles of senna can be extracted using water or dilute alcohol. The drug contains anthraquinone derivatives and their glucosides, as well as cathartic acid as its active chemicals.

MEDICINAL USES: laxative, purgative, cathartic. This drug acts primarily on the lower bowel, acts locally upon the intestinal wall, increasing the peristaltic movements of the colon. The taste is nauseating and prone to cause sickness and griping pains. It is generally combined with aromatics, e.g. GINGER or CINNAMON and stimulants to modify senna's deleterious effects. When the problems are overcome, senna is a very good medicine for children, delicate women and elderly persons. Senna pods have milder effects than the leaves and lack their griping effects.

ADMINISTERED AS: infusion, powdered leaves, syrup, fluid extract, tincture, dried pods.

Sheep's sorrel *Rumex acetosella.* COMMON NAME: Field sorrel.

OCCURRENCE: this grows in pastures and dry places around the globe, except in the tropics and is abundant in the British Isles.

PARTS USED: the herb.

MEDICINAL USES: diaphoretic, diuretic, refrigerant. The fresh juice of the herb is used for kidney and urinary diseases. Less active than SORREL (*Rumex acetosa*).

ADMINISTERED AS: expressed juice.

Shepherd's purse *Capsella bursa-pastoris.* COMMON NAME: Shepherd's bag, shepherd's scrip, lady's purse, witches' pouches, case-weed, pick-pocket, blindweed, pepper and salt, sanguinary, mother's heart, poor man's parmacettie, clappedepouch.

OCCURRENCE: native to Europe and found all over the world outside tropical zones.

PARTS USED: the whole plant which contains various chemicals which have not yet been entirely analyzed but they include an organic acid, a volatile oil, a fixed oil, a tannate, an alkaloid and a resin.

MEDICINAL USES: haemostatic, antiscorbutic, diuretic, stimulant. As an infusion of the dried plant, shepherd's purse is one of the best specifics for arresting bleeding of all kinds, particularly from the kidneys, uterus, stomach or lungs. It is said to be as effective as ergot or golden seal. It has been used for diarrhoea, haemorrhoids, dysentery, dropsy and kidney complaints. Shepherd's purse is an important remedy in catarrhal infections of the bladder and ureter and in ulcerated and abscess of the bladder where it increases the flow of urine and provides relief. Externally, the bruised herb is used as a poultice on bruised and strained areas, rheumatic joints and some skin problems. Since the herb tastes slightly unpleasant it is normally taken internally with other herbs to disguise the flavour, e.g. couch grass, juniper, pellitory-of-the-wall.

ADMINISTERED AS: fluid extract, poultice, decoction, infusion.

Silverweed *Potentilla anserina*. COMMON NAME: Trailing tansy, wild tansy, goosewort, silvery cinquefoil, goose grey, goose tansy, wild agrimony, moor grass, prince's feathers.

OCCURRENCE: very abundant in Great Britain and across temperate regions from Lapland to the Azores. It also grows in New Zealand, Chile, Armenia and China.

PARTS USED: the herb, which contains tannin.

MEDICINAL USES: astringent, tonic. an infusion is used as a lotion for bleeding haemorrhoids, as a gargle for sore throats and for cramps in the abdomen, stomach or heart. The infusion may also be used as a compress. A tea of Silverweed has been good for tetanus infections, for malarial infections, in gravel and as a specific in jaundice. A decoction of silverweed is useful for mouth ulcers, spongy gums, fixing loose teeth, toothache and preserving gums from scurvy. A distilled water made from the herb was used as a cosmetic to remove freckles, spots and pimples and to reduce the skin damage after sunburn.

ADMINISTERED AS: decoction, infusion, poultice, distilled water.

Simaruba *Simaruba amara*. COMMON NAME: Dysentery bark, mountain damson, slave wood, maruba, sumaruppa, bitter damson, quassia simaruba.

OCCURRENCE: native to French Guiana, Brazil, Florida and the islands of Dominica, Martinique, St. Lucia, St. Vincent and Barbados.

PARTS USED: the bark, which contains a volatile oil, malic and gallic acids, lignin, resinous matter, various mineral salts and a bitter principle very similar to quassin.

MEDICINAL USES: bitter tonic. It was used successfully against dysentery in France from 1718 onwards. The drug restores lost tone of the intestines and encourages the patient to sleep. It is also useful in loss of appetite, weakened digestion and when convalescing after a fever. In large doses, simaruba can cause sickness and vomiting, so care should be taken when using this drug. It is seldom used in herbal medicine today.

ADMINISTERED AS: infusion, fluid extract.

Skunk cabbage *Symplocarpus foetidus*. COMMON NAME: dracontium, skunkweed, meadow cabbage, polecat weed, *Dracontium foetidum*, *Spathyema foetida*, *Ictodes foetidus*.

OCCURRENCE: grows in moist places across the middle and northern United States of America.

PARTS USED: the root, which contains resin, silica, iron, manganese, an acrid principle and a volatile oil.

MEDICINAL USES: antispasmodic, diaphoretic, expectorant, narcotic, sedative. This plant is so-named as it has an unpleasant odour when bruised. The root has been used for asthma, chronic rheumatism, chorea, dropsy, hysteria and chronic catarrh. It is good for tightness of the chest, irritant coughs and other spasmodic respiratory disorders. The herb is also believed to be effective against epilepsy and convulsions which can occur during pregnancy or labour. It has a diuretic action and can be used to calm the nervous system. Skunk-cabbage forms an ingredient in well-known herbal ointments and powders.

ADMINISTERED AS: powdered root, tincture, fluid extract.

Slippery elm *Ulmus fulva*. COMMON NAME: Red elm, moose elm, Indian elm.

OCCURRENCE: the United States and Canada.

PARTS USED: the inner bark of the tree, which contains mucilage similar to that of flax, starch and calcium oxalate.

MEDICINAL USES: demulcent, emollient, expectorant, diuretic, nutritive, pectoral. This is one of the most valuable remedies in herbal practice. Finely powdered bark makes very good gruel or food which can be used in all cases of weakness, stomach inflammation, bronchitis, etc. It has a soothing and healing action on all the parts it comes into contact with. A drink of the powder and water called Slippery elm food is excellent in cases of irritation of the mucous membrane of the stomach and intestines, induces sleep and gives very good results in gastritis, colitis and enteritis and gastric catarrh. May also be employed as a heart and lung remedy and is used in typhoid fever.

The coarse powdered bark is the finest available poultice for all inflamed areas, ulcers, wounds, burns, boils, skin diseases, etc. It is utilized by various methods in treating many disorders of the bowel and urinary systems. It is also used to remove worms and is an ingredient in many specialist preparations, e.g. poultices, ointments, etc.

ADMINISTERED AS: infusion, injection, poultice, ointment and dietary item.

Smartweed *Polygonum hydropiper.* COMMON NAME: Water pepper, pepper plant, smartass, ciderage, red knees, culrage, biting persicaria, bloodwort, arsesmart.

OCCURRENCE: a native plant of most parts of Europe and Russian Asia up to the Arctic regions. Also seen in Great Britain and Ireland, although rarer in Scotland. It mainly grows in areas that are under water in the winter period.

PARTS USED: the whole herb and the leaves. The active principle is called polygonic acid but its action is not fully understood. It is destroyed by heat or drying.

MEDICINAL USES: stimulant, diuretic, diaphoretic, emmenagogue. As a cold water infusion, this herb is used for amenorrhoea, gravel, coughs and colds and gout. It is also of benefit in dysentery, sore mouths, bowel complaints, jaundice and dropsy. After simmering with water and vinegar, the herb has been utilized on gangrenous or dead tissue, applied to chronic ulcers and haemorrhoidal tumours. In poultice form, smartweed has been used in chronic erysipelas infections, flatulent colic, cholera and rheumatism. There is a tradition which is mentioned in old herbals, that if a handful of the plant is placed under the saddle of a horse then it will be able to travel for some time before requiring feeding or watering. This belief dates back to the Ancient Greek period.

ADMINISTERED AS: infusion, tincture, fluid extract.

Snapdragon *Antirrhinum magus.* COMMON NAME: Calves, snout, lyons snap.

OCCURRENCE: naturalized in Great Britain and is a garden plant.

PARTS USED: the leaves.

MEDICINAL USES: bitter, stimulant. The fresh leaves have been applied as a poultice to tumours an ulcers. In old herbals, it is mentioned that the herb protects against witchcraft and that it makes the wearer "look gracious in the sight of people."

ADMINISTERED AS: poultice.

Soap tree *Quillaja saponia.* COMMON NAME: Quillaia, soap bark, cullay, Panama bark.

OCCURRENCE: native to Chile and Peru in South America.

PARTS USED: the dried inner bark, which contains calcium exalate, can sugar and saponin which is made from a mixture of two glucosides—guillaic acid and guillaia—sapotoxin. The active principles are the same as those found in SENEGA.

MEDICINAL USES: alterative, expectorant, detergent, diuretic, stimulating, sternutatory. This bark can be used in aortic hypertrophy. Since Saponin is a powerful irritant and muscular poison, it can be fatal if used in too large doses and is only occasionally used today. The bark has been used to produce a foam head on beverages and for washing clothes and hair.

ADMINISTERED AS: injection, tincture, powdered bark.

Soapwort *Saponaria officinalis.* COMMON NAME: Latherwort, soaproot, bruisewort, fuller's herb, crow soap, sweet betty, wild sweet william, bouncing bet.

OCCURRENCE: a common garden plant in Great Britain and it also grows wild in central and southern Europe.

PARTS USED: the dried root and leaves. The root contains gum, resin, woody fibre, mucilage and saponin.

MEDICINAL USES: alterative, detergent, tonic, sternutatory. This herb has been used for scrofula and other skin complaints and in jaundice and other visceral obstructions. It is also good for venereal diseases and in rheumatism or skin eruptions due to infection with syphilis. This drug should be very carefully administered due to the very poisonous nature of saponin. In large doses, soapwort is strongly purgative so should only be given by a qualified herbalist. Soapwort is also used to clean clothes, skin and hair and is an ingredient of most herbal shampoo.

ADMINISTERED AS: decoction, expressed juice from fresh root, fluid extract.

Solomon's seal *Polygonatum multiflorum.* COMMON NAME: Lady's seals, St. Mary's seal, sigillum sanctae Mariae.

OCCURRENCE: a native plant of northern Europe and Siberia. It is found wild in some localities in England but naturalized in Scotland and Ireland.

PARTS USED: the rhizome which contains asparagin, gum, sugar, starch, pectin and convallarin, one of the active chemicals in LILY OF THE VALLEY.

MEDICINAL USES: astringent, demulcent, tonic. When combined with other herbs, it is good for bleeding of the lungs and pulmonary complaints. It is used on its own in female complaints and as a poultice for tumours, inflammations, bruises and haemorrhoids. As it is mucilaginous, it makes a very good healing and restorative tonic for inflammation of the bowels and stomach, haemorrhoids and chronic dysentery. A decoction was used to cure erysipelas and was taken by people with broken bones, as Solomon's Seal was supposed to 'encourage the bones to knit'. A distilled water prepared from the root was used as a cosmetic to remove spots, freckles and marks from the skin.

ADMINISTERED AS: decoction, infusion, poultice, distilled water.

Sorrel *Rumex acetosa.* COMMON NAME: Garden sorrel, green sauce, sour grabs, sour suds, cuckoo sorrow, cuckoo's meate, gowke-meat. OCCURRENCE: indigenous to Britain and found in moist meadows throughout Europe.

PARTS USED: the leaves, dried and fresh.

MEDICINAL USES: refrigerant, diuretic, antiscorbutic. Sorrel is given as a cooling drink in all febrile conditions and can help correct scrofulous deposits. Its astringent qualities meant it was formerly used to stop haemorrhages and was applied as a poultice on cutaneous tumours. Sorrel juice and vinegar are said to cure ringworm, while a decoction was made to cure jaundice, ulcerated bowel, and gravel and stone in the kidneys.

ADMINISTERED AS: expressed juice, decoction, poultice and dried leaves.

Spearmint *Mentha viridis.* COMMON NAME: Mackerel mint, Our Lady's mint, green mint, spire mint, sage of Bethlehem, fish mint, lamb mint, menthe de Notre Dame, erba Santa Maria, *Mentha spicata, Mentha crispa,* yerba buena. OCCURRENCE: originally a Mediterranean native and was introduced into the British Isles by the Romans.

PARTS USED: the herb and essential oil. The main component of the essential oil is carvone along with phellandrine, limonene and dihydrocarveol acetate. The oil also has the esters of acetic, butyric and caproic acids within it.

MEDICINAL USES: antispasmodic, aromatic, carminative, stimulant. This herb is very similar to peppermint, but it seems to be less powerful. It is more suited to children's remedies. A distilled water from spearmint is used to relieve hiccoughs, flatulence and indigestion while the infusion is good for fevers, inflammatory diseases and all infantile troubles. Spearmint is considered a specific in stopping nausea and vomiting and in easing the pain due to colic. As a homoeopathic remedy, spearmint has been used for strangury, gravel and as a local application for painful haemorrhoids.

ADMINISTERED AS: distilled water, infusion, tincture, fluid extract.

Spearwort, Lesser *Ranunculus flammula.* OCCURRENCE: a very common plant throughout Britain, growing in wet and boggy heaths and commons.

PARTS USED: the whole plant.

MEDICINAL USES: rubefacient, emetic. The bruised leaves have a long history of use on the Isle of Skye and in the Highlands of Scotland in raising blisters. A distilled water from the plant is used as a painless emetic drug while a tincture is good at curing ulcers.

ADMINISTERED AS: distilled water, tincture, poultice.

Speedwell, Common *Veronica officinalis.* COMMON NAME: bird's-eye, cat's-eye. OCCURRENCE: a common wild plant in Europe and Great Britain.

PARTS USED: the herb.

MEDICINAL USES: diaphoretic, alterative, expectorant, astringent, diuretic, tonic. Lesser spearwort was formerly used in pectoral and nephritic complaints, haemorrhages, skin diseases and in treating wounds. An infusion of the dried herb is good for catarrh, coughs and most skin problems. May promote menstruation.

ADMINISTERED AS: infusion and dried herb.

Sphagnum moss *Sphagnum cymbifolium.* COMMON NAME: Bog moss. OCCURRENCE: found in wet and boggy land, normally on peat soils on mountains and moors in Scotland, England, Ireland and parts of western Europe.

PARTS USED: the moss, which is made up of plant cells which are penetrated with a system of tubes and air spaces. This capillary tube system makes the moss resemble a very fine sponge and allows the plant to absorb huge quantities of water.

MEDICINAL USES: wound dressing. The use of sphagnum as a dressing for wounds can be dated back to the Battle of Flodden. There is a long history of use in Lapland where the dried moss is used as a mattress and blankets for infants. The moss has many advantages over other surgical dressings, e.g. cotton wool. Prepared moss can retain twice as much moisture as cotton; a 2oz dressing can absorb up to 2lb of liquid. This means that dressings need to be changed less frequently with less disturbance to the patient. In many times of war sphagnum was prepared in gauze bags, often in association with GARLIC for its antiseptic qualities. Sphagnum moss also has an antibiotic action due to micro-organisms associated with the plant which aids healing. The moss has also been used as bedding in stables and for hanging baskets and other gardening applications.

Spinach *Spinacio oleracea.*

OCCURRENCE: originally native to Persia and Asia and was introduced into Europe in the fifteenth century.

PARTS USED: the leaves, which contain iron, nitrogenous substances, hydrocarbons, chlorophyll and vitamins A and D.

MEDICINAL USES: nutritive, antiscorbutic. Spinach is primarily used as a food source as it is a good source of iron and vitamins. Experiments have shown the benefit of eating spinach on people weakened by illness.

ADMINISTERED AS: expressed juice, dietary item.

Spindle tree *Euonymus atropurpureus.*

Euonymus europoeus. COMMON NAME: Indian arrowroot, burning bush, wahoo, gatten, pigwood, dogwood, skewerwood, prickwood, gadrose, fusanum, fusoria.

OCCURRENCE: *Euonymus europoeus* is found in copses and hedges across Great Britain. *E. atropurpureus* is commonly found in the eastern United States and is the variety normally used in herbal medicine.

PARTS USED: the root, bark and berries. The chief constituents of the plant include an intensely bitter principle called euonymin resin, euonic acid, asparagin, resins, fat, dulcitol and a crystalline glucoside.

MEDICINAL USES: alterative, cholagogue, laxative, hepatic stimulant, tonic. This drug is particularly good in liver complaints which follow or accompany fever, and in stimulating the liver and producing a free flow of bile. Depending on the dose given euonymin has different effects on the digestive system. In large doses it irritates the intestine and has cathartic effects, but in smaller doses it can stimulate the appetite and the flow of gastric juices. The herb is normally administered with other tonic or laxative herbs for best results.

ADMINISTERED AS: pills, powdered root or bark, decoction, fluid extract.

St. John's wort *Hypericum perforatum.*

OCCURRENCE: found in woods, hedges, roadsides and meadows across Britain, Europe and Asia.

PARTS USED: the herb and flowers.

MEDICINAL USES: aromatic, astringent, resolvent, expectorant, diuretic and nervine. It is generally utilized in all pulmonary complaints, bladder trouble, suppression of urine, dysentery, diarrhoea and jaundice. It is good against hysteria, nervous depression, haemorrhages, coughing up blood and dispelling worms from the body. If children have a problem with night incontinence, an infusion of St. John's wort taken before bed will stop the problem. The herb is used externally to break up hard tissues, e.g. tumours, bruising. and swollen, hard breasts when feeding infants.

ADMINISTERED AS: an infusion and poultice.

Stavesacre *Delphinium staphisagria.* COMMON NAME: Starvesacre, staphisagris, lousewort.

OCCURRENCE: indigenous to southern Europe and Asia Minor, and is now cultivated in France and Italy.

PARTS USED: the dried ripe seeds. The main components of the seeds are alkaloid compounds including the poisonous delphinine, delphisine, delphinoidine, staphisagroine and staphisagrine, which may make up twenty five per cent of the seeds.

MEDICINAL USES: vermifuge, vermin-destroying, violent emetic and cathartic. The seeds are so very poisonous that they are rarely taken internally. Occasionally, the powdered seeds may be used as a purge in treating dropsy, with the dose monitored very carefully. The seeds are used externally as a parasiticide to kill lice of the genus *Pediculus*, and as a poultice or decoction compress on some skin eruptions and scrofula. The extracted alkaloid delphinine has been used both internally and externally to ease neuralgia. It resembles ACONITE in its action, slowing the pulse and respiration rates, paralysing the spinal cord and leading to death by asphyxia when taken in large doses. It can be used as an antidote to poisoning by strychnine.

ADMINISTERED AS: ointment, expressed oil, powdered seeds, decoction, poultice, fluid extract.

Stockholm tar *Pinus sylvestris* (and other species). COMMON NAME: Tar, *Pix liquida.*

OCCURRENCE: obtained from various *Pinus* species grown across the northern hemisphere in Sweden, Russia, North America and Switzerland.

PARTS USED: the tar is an impure turpentine obtained from the stems and roots of *Pinus* species by destructive distillation.

MEDICINAL USES: antiseptic, diuretic, diaphoretic, expectorant, stimulant. It may be used for chronic coughs and consumption but is mainly used externally as a cutaneous stimulant and as an ointment for eczema. It is mainly used in veterinary practices.

ADMINISTERED AS: ointment, fluid extract.

Stramonium *Datura stramonium.* COMMON NAME: Thornapple, jimsonweed, Jamestown-weed, devil's apple, devil's trumpet, datura, mad apple, stinkweed, apple of Peru.

OCCURRENCE: a plant of unknown origin that is currently found throughout the world except in cold or Arctic areas.

PARTS USED: the whole plant has medicinal qualities but it is the leaves and seeds that are most commonly used today. The leaves contain the same alkaloids as belladonna, but in slightly smaller amounts. The alkaloids include lyoscyamine, atropine, lyoscine along with malic acid, volatile oil, gum, resin and starch. The seeds are made up of fixed oil and the same alkaloids as the leaves, but the fixed oil makes the alkaloids difficult to extract so the leaves are the most extensively utilized.

MEDICINAL USES: antispasmodic, anodyne, narcotic. A herb which acts in a very similar manner to belladonna except it does not cause constipation. An extract of the seeds is given in pill form to stop coughing in spasmodic bronchial asthma, to ease whooping cough and spasm of the bladder. It is considered a better cough remedy than opium, but is used with extreme care as it can act as a narcotic poison in overdoses. When smoked with tobacco, alone or with other herbs, e.g. sage and belladonna, stramonium can ease asthma by relaxing spasms of the bronchioles during an attack. Taken in this form, it can also help control the spasms that occur in Parkinson's disease. The herb can relieve the pain of sciatica and rheumatism when used externally in the form of an ointment. Signs of an overdose of stramonium include dryness of the throat and mouth and an overdose can cause double vision, thirst, palpitations, restlessness, confusion and hallucinations. This drug is highly toxic and should only be used under the guidance of a herbal medicine practitioner or doctor. In India, thieves and assassins used to give their victims stramonium in order to make them insensible while history states that the herb was taken by the priests of Apollo at Delphi, in Ancient Greece, to assist them in their prophecies. Stramonium was considered to be a plant which aided witches in their ill-doing, and during the time of the witch and wizard hunt in England, it was exceedingly dangerous to grow stramonium in your garden as it was said to confirm the supernatural powers of the householder. Many people were sentenced to death purely because stramonium was found in their garden.

ADMINISTERED AS: powdered leaves, powdered seeds, fluid extract, tincture and ointment.

Strawberry *Fragaria vesca.*

OCCURRENCE: found through the whole of the northern hemisphere, excluding the tropics.

PARTS USED: the leaves, which contain cissotanic, malic and citric acids, sugar, mucilage and a volatile aromatic chemical which is, as yet, unidentified.

MEDICINAL USES: laxative, diuretic, astringent. The berries are of great benefit for rheumatic gout while the root is good against diarrhoea. The leaves have similar properties and are used to stop dysentery. Fresh strawberries remove discolouration of the teeth if the juice is left on for about five minutes and then the teeth are cleaned with warm water, to which a pinch of bicarbonate of soda has been added. Sunburn could be relieved by rubbing a cut strawberry over a freshly washed face.

ADMINISTERED AS: infusion, fresh berries.

Strophanthus *Strophanthus kombé.* COMMON NAME: Kombe seeds, *Strophanthus hispidus, S. semina.*

OCCURRENCE: native to tropical East Africa.

PARTS USED: the seeds. These contain the glucoside strophanthus, the alkaloid inoeine and a fixed oil.

MEDICINAL USES: cardiac tonic. This drug has a large influence on the circulatory system. It is used in chronic heart weakness, muscular debility of the heart and in cardiac pains with difficult or laboured breathing. It acts in the same way as digitalis (FOXGLOVE, *Digitalis purpurea*), but with increased digestive disturbance and strophanthus does not have a cumulative poisoning effect. Strophanthus has diuretic powers and is beneficial in dropsy, particularly when related to heart problems. In urgent cases, the intravenous injection of strophanthus can be used to increase circulation. The strength and power of the seeds are highly variable, and the seeds are so highly poisonous that they should only be used under medical supervision. In Africa, strophanthus is used as an arrow poison.

ADMINISTERED AS: liquid extract, tincture, solid extract.

Sumbul *Ferula sumbul.* COMMON NAME: Musk root, ouchi, ofnokgi, racine de sumbul, sumbulwurzel, moschuswurzel, jatamarsi, *Sumbul radix.*

OCCURRENCE: thought to be native to Turkestan, northern India and Russia.

PARTS USED: the root and rhizome. They contain two balsamic resins (thought to cause the strong musk-like odour), wax, gum, a bitter substance, a volatile oil, starch and angelic and valeric acids.

MEDICINAL USES: nerve stimulant, antispasmodic, tonic. Sumbul resembles VALERIAN in action and is very good for various hysterical conditions. It is thought to have a specific action on the pelvic organs and is used for dysmenorrhoea and similar female problems. Sumbul acts as a stimulant of the mucous membranes easing chronic diarrhoea and dysentery as well as pneumonia, chronic bronchitis and asthma. The side effects of the drug can occur producing narcotic symptoms, confusion, tingling feelings and a strong odour on the breath which may take two days to disappear.

ADMINISTERED AS: solid extract, tincture, fluid extract.

Sundew *Drosera rotundifolia.* COMMON NAME: Roundleaved sundew, dew plant, red rot, youthwort, rosa solis, herba rosellae, rosée du soleil.

OCCURRENCE: an insectivorous plant found in bogs, wet places and river edges throughout Britain, Europe, India, China, North and South America and Russian Asia.

PARTS USED: the air-dried flowering plant.

MEDICINAL USES: pectoral, expectorant, demulcent, anti-asthmatic. In small doses sundew is a specific in dry, spasmodic, tickling coughs and is considered very good in whooping cough, for which it may also be used as a prophylactic drug. The fresh juice is used to remove corns and warts. In America, the sundew

has been advocated as a cure for old age and has been used with colloidal silicates in cases of thickening of arteries due to old age, or calcium or fat deposition.

ADMINISTERED AS: fluid extract, expressed juice, solid extract.

Sunflower *Helicanthus annuus.* COMMON NAME: Helianthus, marigold of Peru, *Sola indianus, Chrysanthemum peruvianum, Corona solis.*

OCCURRENCE: native to Peru and Mexico and was introduced into America, Europe and Great Britain as a garden plant.

PARTS USED: the seeds. These contain a vegetable oil, carbonate of potash, tannin and vitamins B1, B3 and B6. The oil is expressed from the crushed seeds and, according to the range of temperature to which the seeds are heated, several grades of oil are obtained.

MEDICINAL USES: diuretic, expectorant. It has been used successfully in treating pulmonary, bronchial and laryngeal afflictions as well as whooping cough, colds and coughs. The leaves are used, in some parts of the world, to treat malaria and the tincture may replace quinine in easing intermittent fevers and the ague. Sunflowers produce the seed cake which is used as cattle food; the fresh leaves are given to poultry; the plants can be used as a vegetable; the stems are used as bedding for ducks; the plant used for silage, fuel, manure, textiles and as a soil improver.

ADMINISTERED AS: sunflower oil, tincture, decoction, poultice.

Tag alder *Alnus semulata.* COMMON NAME: Smooth alder, red alder, common alder, *Alnus rubra.*

OCCURRENCE: a common tree found in Europe, Great Britain and the United States of America.

PARTS USED: the bark and cones.

MEDICINAL USES: tonic, alterative, emetic, astringent. This plant is good for scrofula, diarrhoea, dyspepsia, indigestion, secondary syphilis and debility of the stomach. A decoction of the cones was said to be astringent in effect and of use in all types of haemorrhages. The bark was also of benefit to some cutaneous diseases and intermittent fevers.

ADMINISTERED AS: infusion, decoction, fluid extract.

Tansy *Tanacetum vulgare.* COMMON NAME: Buttons.

OCCURRENCE: a hardy perennial plant, commonly seen in heathland and on waste ground all over Europe and Great Britain.

PARTS USED: the herb. It contains the chemicals tanacetin, tannic acid, a volatile oil, thujone, sugar and a colouring matter.

MEDICINAL USES: anthelmintic, tonic, emmenagogue, stimulant. Tansy is largely used for expelling worms from children. It is good in female disorders, like hysteria and nausea and in kidney weakness. The herb is also used for slight fevers, for allaying spasms and as a nervine drug. In large doses, the herb is violently irritant and induces venous congestion of the abdominal organs. In Scotland, an infusion was administered to cure gout. Tansy essential oil, when given in small doses, has helped in epilepsy and has also been used externally to help some eruptive diseases of the skin. Bruised fresh leaves can reduce swelling and relieve sprains, as can a hot infusion used as a poultice.

ADMINISTERED AS: essential oil, infusion, poultice, fresh leaves, solid extract.

Tarragon *Artemisia dracunculus*. COMMON NAME: Mugwort, little dragon.

OCCURRENCE: cultivated in kitchen gardens across Europe and Great Britain. Tarragon originally arose from both Siberia and southern Europe to form the French and Russian tarragon we know today.

PARTS USED: the leaves, which contain an essential volatile oil which is lost on drying.

MEDICINAL USES: today there are few medicinal uses for tarragon but it has been used previously to stimulate the appetite and to cure toothache. Tarragon is mostly used in cooking—particularly on the European continent. It is used for dressings, salads, vinegar and pickles.

ADMINISTERED AS: fresh root, fresh herb.

Tea *Camellia thea*. COMMON NAME: *Camellia theifera*, *Thea sinensis*, *Thea veridis*, *Thea bohea*, *Thea stricta jassamica*.

OCCURRENCE: native to Assam in India, and the plant has spread to Sri Lanka, Java, China and Japan.

PARTS USED: the dried leaves.

MEDICINAL USES: stimulant, astringent. The infusion of the leaves has a stimulating effect on the nervous system, producing a feeling of comfort. It may also act as a nerve sedative where it can relieve headaches. When drunk in excessive quantities, tea can produce unpleasant nervous symptoms, dyspepsia and unnatural wakefulness.

ADMINISTERED AS: infusion.

Thistle, Holy *Carbenia benedicta*. COMMON NAME: Blessed thistle, *Cnicus benedictus*, *Carduus benedictus*.

OCCURRENCE: a native of southern Europe and has been cultivated in Britain for hundreds of years.

PARTS USED: the whole herb which contains a volatile oil, a bitter crystalline compound called cnicin which is said to be similar to salicin in its properties.

MEDICINAL USES: tonic, stimulant, diaphoretic, emetic and emmenagogue. Very useful as an infusion to weak and debilitating stomach conditions, creating appetite and preventing sickness. It is said to be good in all fevers, as a purifier of the blood and circulation and its main modern day use is for bringing on a proper supply of milk in nursing mothers. In large doses, however, holy thistle is a strong emetic, producing vomiting. It may be used as a vermifuge.

ADMINISTERED AS: infusion and fluid extract.

Thistle, Scotch *Onopordon acanthium*. COMMON NAME: Woolly thistle, cotton thistle.

OCCURRENCE: a common plant in all of Great Britain, found in waste ground and roadsides.

PARTS USED: the leaves and root.

MEDICINAL USES: ancient herbalists believed that the Scotch thistle was a specific against cancer and even today the expressed juice of the plant has been used to good effect on cancers and ulcers. A decoction of thistles was thought to restore a healthy, growing head of hair when applied to a bald head, while a root decoction has astringent effects and reduces production from mucous membranes. Thistles were also supposed to be effective against rickets in children, a crick in the neck and nervous complaints.

ADMINISTERED AS: expressed juice, decoction.

Thyme *Thymus vulgaris*. COMMON NAME: Garden or common thyme, tomillo.

OCCURRENCE: cultivated in temperate countries in northern Europe.

PARTS USED: the herb. Thyme gives rise to oil of thyme after distillation of the fresh leaves. This oil contains the phenols, thymol and carvacrol, as well as cymene, pinene and borneol.

MEDICINAL USES: antiseptic, antispasmodic, tonic, carminative. The fresh herb, in syrup, forms a safe cure for whooping cough, as is an infusion of the dried herb. The infusion or tea is beneficial for catarrh, sore throat, wind spasms, colic and in allaying fevers and colds.

Thyme is generally used in conjunction with other remedies in herbal medicine.

ADMINISTERED AS: fluid extract, essential oil and infusion.

Tobacco *Nicotiana tabacum, N. acuminata, N. rustica* and other varieties. COMMON NAME: Leaf tobacco, tabacca.

OCCURRENCE: native to America and cultivated in many sub-tropical countries including China, Greece, France and Turkey.

PARTS USED: the cured and dried leaves, which contain five alkaloids including nicotine. Upon smoking, nicotine decomposes into various chemicals—the very poisonous carbon monoxide, pyridine and hydrogen cyanide.

MEDICINAL USES: narcotic, sedative, diuretic, expectorant, emetic. Medicinally, tobacco has been used internally for hernias, constipation, tetanus, retention of urine, worms and hysterical convulsions. It is best utilized externally as a plaster or poultice to ease cutaneous diseases, haemorrhoids and facial neuralgia. A combination of tobacco leaves along with the leaves of stramonium or belladonna make a very good treatment for spasmodic afflictions, painful tumours and obstinate ulcers. Tobacco is a local irritant and the nicotine within it is very poisonous, causing heart palpitations and irregularity and disturbing the digestive and circulatory organs. The use of tobacco as a medicine is unusual in today's western herbal medicine, although it is still used in some native societies. The poisonous nature of the alkaloids within the plant have discouraged its use as use of tobacco, even within small doses, can cause depression, convulsions and even death.

ADMINISTERED AS: poultice, ointment, suppositories, smoking herb.

Tree of heaven *Ailanthus glandulosa*. COMMON NAME: ailanto, vernis de Japan, Chinese sumach.

OCCURRENCE: indigenous to China and India, and is now cultivated through Europe and the United State.

PARTS USED: the root and the inner bark of the tree. The bark contains chlorophyll, pectin, lignin, volatile oil, resin, quassin, tannin and various mineral salts.

MEDICINAL USES: astringent, antispasmodic, cardiac depressant. Despite this herb's unpleasant and nauseating action on patients, it has been successful against diarrhoea, dysentery, leucorrhoea, prolapse of the rectum and for tapeworms. A tincture prepared from the root bark of the tree has been good for epilepsy, asthma and cardiac palpitations.

ADMINISTERED AS: infusion, tincture.

Turpentine oil distilled from *Pinus palustris*, *Pinus maritima* and other species.

MEDICINAL USES: rubefacient, irritant, diuretic. When taken internally, turpentine forms a valuable remedy in bladder, kidney, and rheumatic problems and diseases of the mucous membranes. The oil is also used for respiratory complaints and externally as a liniment, an embrocation and an inhalant for rheumatism and chest problems. Turpentine may be combined with other aromatic oils as a remedy.

ADMINISTERED AS: essential oil.

Valerian *Valeriana officinalis*. COMMON NAME: all-heal, great wild valerian, amantilla, setwall, sete-wale, capon's tail.

OCCURRENCE: found throughout Europe and northern Asia. It is common in England in marshy thickets, riverbanks and ditches.

PARTS USED: the root, which contains a volatile oil, two alkaloids called chatarine and valerianine as well as several unidentified compounds.

MEDICINAL USES: powerful nervine, stimulant, carminative anodyne and antispasmodic herb. It may be given in all cases of nervous debility and irritation as it is not narcotic. The expressed juice of the fresh root has been used as a narcotic in insomnia and as an anticonvulsant in epilepsy. The oil of valerian is of use against cholera and in strengthening the eyesight. A herbal compound containing valerian was given to civilians during the Second World War, to reduce the effects of stress caused by repeated air raids and to minimize damage to health.

ADMINISTERED AS: fluid and solid extract, tincture, oil, expressed juice.

Verbena, Lemon *Lippia citriodora*. COMMON NAME: Herb louisa, lemon-scented verbena, *Verveine citronelle* or *odorante*, *Verbena triphylla, Lippia triphylla, Aloysia citriodora*.

OCCURRENCE: originally from Peru and Chile, it was introduced into England in 1784 and is now a common garden plant.

PARTS USED: the leaves and flowering tops.

MEDICINAL USES: febrifuge, sedative. This herb has similar uses to BALM, PEPPERMINT, ORANGE flowers and SPEARMINT in relieving flatulence, indigestion and dyspepsia through its antispasmodic and stomachic actions. It is commonly made into a refreshing tisane. The leaves of lemon verbena were once used in finger bowls at banquets and the essential oil distilled from the herb was used to impart a strong lemon scent to cosmetics and soaps.

ADMINISTERED AS: tea.

Vervain *Verbena officinalis*. COMMON NAME: Herb of grace, herbe sacrée, herba veneris, *Verbena hastrata*.

OCCURRENCE: grows across Europe, China, Japan and Barbary. Also found in England by roadsides and in sunny pastures.

PARTS USED: the herb. Vervain contains a peculiar tannin, which has not yet been fully investigated.

MEDICINAL USES: nervine, tonic, emetic, sudorific, astringent, diaphoretic, antispasmodic. This herb is recommended in many complaints including intermittent fevers, ulcers, pleurisy, ophthalmic disorders and is said to be a good galactogogue. May also be administered as a poultice to ease headache, ear neuralgia, rheumatism and taken as a decoction to ease bowel pain during purging. Vervain is often applied externally for piles.

ADMINISTERED AS: fluid extract, decoction.

Vine *Vitis vinifera*. COMMON NAME: Grape vine.

OCCURRENCE: a very ancient plant, frequently mentioned in the Bible after the Great Flood. It now grows in Asia, central and southern Europe, Africa, Australia, Greece, California and South America.

PARTS USED: the fruit, leaves and juice. The wine sold commercially is made from fermented fruit juice. This juice, which is called 'must', contains malic acid, gum, sugar, inorganic salts and potassium bicarbonate. The leaves contain tartaric acid, tannin, malic acid, gum, quercetine, quercitrin, potassium bitartrate, cane sugar and glucose.

MEDICINAL USES: the leaves and seeds have an astringent action, with the leaves previously used to stop haemorrhages and bleeding. Ripe grapes, when eaten in some quantity, increase the flow of urine and can be of great benefit in exhaustion, anaemia, smallpox, sleeplessness and neuralgia. They are also eaten for poor biliary function and torpid liver. Grape sugar is chemically different to other sugars, as the saliva has no enzymatic effect on it. Thus it acts faster to warm up the body and build tissues, to increase strength and repair the body after illness. Raisins, have demulcent, nutritive and slightly laxative effects on the body.

ADMINISTERED AS: fermented fruit juice, fresh or dried leaves, fresh or dried fruits.

Violet *Viola adorata*. COMMON NAME: Blue violet, sweet violet, sweet-scented violet.

OCCURRENCE: native to Great Britain and found widely over Europe, northern Asia and North America.

PARTS USED: the dried flowers and leaves and whole plant when fresh.

MEDICINAL USES: antiseptic, expectorant, laxative. The herb is mainly taken as syrup of violets which has been used to cure the ague, epilepsy, eye inflammation, pleurisy, jaundice and sleeplessness which are some of the many other complaints that benefit from treatment with this herb. The flowers possess expectorant properties and have long been used to treat coughs. The flowers may also be crystallized as a sweetmeat or added to salads. The rhizome is strongly emetic and purgative and has violent effects when administered. The seeds also have purgative and diuretic effects and are beneficial in treating urinary complaints and gravel. In the early part of this century, violet preparations were used to great effect against cancer. Fresh violet leaves are made into an infusion which was drunk regularly, and a poultice of the leaves was applied to the affected area. The herb has been used successfully to both allay pain and perhaps cure the cancer. It is said to be particularly good against throat cancer.

ADMINISTERED AS: infusion, poultice, injection, ointment, syrup and powdered root.

Walnut *Juglans nigra*. COMMON NAME: Carya, Jupiter's nuts, *Juglans regia*.

OCCURRENCE: cultivated throughout Europe and was probably native to Persia.

PARTS USED: the bark and leaves. The active principle of the walnut tree is nucin or juglon, while the kernels also contain oil, mucilage, albumin, cellulose, mineral matter and water.

MEDICINAL USES: alterative, laxative, detergent, astringent. The bark and leaves are used in skin problems, e.g. scrofulous diseases, herpes, eczema and for healing indolent ulcers. A strong infusion of the powdered bark has purgative effects, while the walnut has various properties dependent upon its stage of ripeness. Green walnuts are anthelminthic and vermifuge in action and are pickled in vinegar, which is then used as a gargle for sore and ulcerated throats. The wood is used for furniture, gun-stocks and for cabinets. Walnut oil expressed from the kernels is used in wood polishing, painting and is used as butter or frying oil.

ADMINISTERED AS: fluid extract, infusion, expressed oil, whole fruit.

Water betony *Scrophularia aquatica.* COMMON NAME: Water figwort, brownwort, bishop's leaves, crowdy kit, fiddlewood, fiddler, *Betonica aquatica.*

OCCURRENCE: found growing wild in damp places, on the banks of rivers and ponds throughout Great Britain and Europe.

PARTS USED: the leaves, fresh and dried.

MEDICINAL USES: detergent, vulnerary. The leaves are used as a poultice, or as an ointment for wounds, sores, haemorrhoids, ulcers and scrofulous glands in the neck. It was also used to expel nightmares, cure toothache and as a cosmetic for blemished or sunburnt skin.

ADMINISTERED AS: decoction, poultice, ointment.

Watercress *Nasturtium officinale*

OCCURRENCE: a perennial creeping plant often growing near springs and running water across Great Britain and Europe.

PARTS USED: the stem and leaves, which contain nicotinamide, volatile oil, a glucoside, gluconasturtin and vitamins A, C and E.

MEDICINAL USES: stimulant, expectorant, nutritive, antiscorbutic, diuretic. Watercress was proposed as a specific in tuberculosis and has a very long history of medical use. It is used to treat bronchitis and coughs as well as boosting digestion, lowering blood sugar and helping the body to remove toxic wastes from the blood and tissues. The herb is of value nutritionally as it contains many vitamins and mineral salts which help during convalescence and general debility. It can be bruised and made into a poultice for arthritis and gout, and is chewed raw to strengthen gums.

ADMINISTERED AS: expressed juice, poultice, dietary item.

Water dock *Rumex aquaticus.* COMMON NAME: Red Dock, bloodwort.

OCCURRENCE: found frequently in fields, meadows, pools and ditches throughout Europe and Great Britain and is particularly common in the northern latitudes.

PARTS USED: the root.

MEDICINAL USES: alterative, deobstruent, detergent. It has a tonic action and is used externally to clean ulcers in afflictions of the mouth. It is applied to eruptive and scorbutic diseases, skin ulcers and sores. As a powder, Water dock has a cleansing and detergent effect upon the teeth.

ADMINISTERED AS: fluid extract and infusion.

Willow, White *Salix alba.* COMMON NAME: European willow.

OCCURRENCE: a large tree growing in moist places and running streams around Great Britain and Europe.

PARTS USED: the bark and leaves. The bark contains tannin and salicin.

MEDICINAL USES: tonic, antiperiodic, astringent. The bark has been used in febrile diseases of rheumatic or gouty origin, diarrhoea and dysentery. It has been used in dyspepsia connected with digestive organ disorders. The bark has also been of benefit in convalescence after acute diseases and against parasitic worms.

ADMINISTERED AS: decoction, powdered root.

Wintergreen *Gaultheria procumbens.* COMMON NAME: Mountain tea, teaberry, boxberry, thé du Canada, aromatic wintergreen, partridge berry, deerberry, checkerberry.

OCCURRENCE: native to the northern United States and Canada from Georgia northwards.

PARTS USED: the leaves, which produce a volatile oil upon distillation. The oil is made up of methyl salicylate, gaultherilene, an aldehyde, a secondary alcohol and an ester. The aromatic odour of the plant is due to the alcohol and the ester.

MEDICINAL USES: aromatic, tonic, stimulant, diuretic, emmenagogue, astringent, galactogogue. The oil is of great benefit in acute rheumatism, but must be given in the form of capsules so stomach inflammation does not occur. The true distilled oil when applied to the skin can give rise to an eruption and so the synthetic oil of wintergreen is recommended for external use as it still contains methyl salicylate, but with no deleterious effects. The synthetic oil is exceedingly valuable for all chronic joint and muscular troubles, lumbago, sciatica and rheumatism. The oil is also used as a flavouring for toothpowders and mouth washes, particularly when combined with menthol and EUCALYPTUS. The berries are a winter food for many animals and also produce a bitter tonic, after being steeped in brandy. The leaves are either used to flavour tea or as a substitute for tea itself.

ADMINISTERED AS: capsules, synthetic oil, infusion, tincture.

Witch hazel *Hamamelis virginiana.* COMMON NAME: Spotted alder, winterbloom, snapping hazelnut.

OCCURRENCE: native to the United States of America and Canada.

PARTS USED: the dried bark, both fresh and dried leaves. The leaves contain tannic and gallic acids, volatile oil and an unknown bitter principle. The bark contains tannin, gallic acid, a physterol, resin, fat and other bitter and odorous bodies.

MEDICINAL USES: astringent, tonic, sedative. Valuable in stopping internal and external haemorrhages and in treating piles. Mainly used for bruises, swelling, inflammation and tumours as a poultice. It may also be utilized for diarrhoea, dysentery and mucous discharges. A decoction is used against tuberculosis, gonorrhoea, menorrhagia and the debilitated state resulting from abortion. Tea made from the bark or leaves aids bleeding of the stomach, bowel complaints and may be given as an injection for bleeding piles. Witch hazel is used to treat varicose veins as a moist poultice, as an extract to ease burns, scalds and insect and mosquito bites, and to help inflammation of the eyelids.

ADMINISTERED AS: liquid extract, injection, tincture, lotion, ointment, suppositories, poultice, infusion and decoction.

Woodruff *Asperula odorata.* COMMON NAME: Wuderove, wood-rova, sweet woodruff, woodroof, waldmeister tea.

OCCURRENCE: grows in woods or shaded hedges in England.

PARTS USED: the herb, which contains coumarin, a fragrant crystalline chemical, citric, malic and rubichloric acids and tannic acid.

MEDICINAL USES: diuretic, tonic. The fresh leaves, when applied to wounds, were said to have a strong healing effect. A strong decoction of the fresh herb was used as a cordial and stomachic and is said to be useful in removing biliary obstructions of the liver.

ADMINISTERED AS: a poultice and decoction.

Wormseed, American *Chenopodium anthelminticum.* COMMON NAME: Mexican tea, jesuit's tea, herba Sancti Mariae, *Chenopodium ambrosioides.*

OCCURRENCE: indigenous to Mexico and South America, and naturalized in almost all areas of the eastern United States.

PARTS USED: the fruits and seeds. An oil is distilled from the crushed fruits called chenopodium oil. It is made up of ascaridole, an unstable substance, choline, betzine, sylvestrene and several other compounds.

MEDICINAL USES: anthelmintic, vermifuge. The herb is used to expel roundworms and hookworms, particularly in children. The drug should be given in one full dose, then fasting until an active purgative drug e.g. CASTOR OIL is given two hours later. The treatment should be repeated ten days later. The drug may be given as volatile oil, expressed juice of the fresh plant, the fluid extract, or the bruised fruit. Chenopodium oil has been of benefit in chorea, malaria, hysteria and similar nervous diseases and has been used as a pectoral drug in asthma and catarrh. Unfortunately the chenopodium oil on the market varies as to the quantity of ascaridole within it and care must be taken to prevent overdoses occurring. Toxic symptoms caused by this drug include temporary dizziness and vomiting.

ADMINISTERED AS: distilled oil, expressed juice, bruised fruit, fluid extract.

Wormwood *Artemisia absinthium.* COMMON NAME: Green ginger, old women, ajenjo.

OCCURRENCE: a plant found wild in many parts of the world including Siberia, Europe and the United States of America.

PARTS USED: the whole herb. The herb contains a volatile oil made up of thujone, pinene, cadinene and chamazulene, a bitter principle called absinthum, carotene, tannins and vitamin C.

MEDICINAL USES: bitter tonic, anthelmintic, febrifuge, stomachic. The liqueur, absinthe, was made using this plant as flavouring and it was banned in France in 1915 as excess intake caused irreversible damage to the nervous system. In modern herbal medicine, it is used as a bitter tonic to stimulate the appetite, the liver and gall bladder, production of digestive juices and peristalsis. Wormwood also expels parasitic worms, particularly roundworms and threadworms. The plant contains chemicals which have anti-inflammatory effects and help reduce fevers. Since ancient times this herb has been used by women to encourage menstruation, and it is applied as an external compress during labour to speed up the birth process. After labour, wormwood was taken both internally and externally to expel the afterbirth. This herb should not be used during pregnancy and should only be administered for short time periods.

ADMINISTERED AS: infusion, essential oil, fluid extract.

Woundwort *Stachys palustris.* COMMON NAME: all-heal, panay, opopanewort, clown's woundwort, rusticum vulna herba, downy woundwort, stinking marsh stachys.

OCCURRENCE: common to marshy meadows, riversides and ditches in most parts of Great Britain.

PARTS USED: the herb.

MEDICINAL USES: antiseptic, antispasmodic. The herb relieves cramp, gout, painful joints and vertigo, while bruised leaves will stop bleeding and encourage healing when applied to a wound. Woundwort had an excellent reputation as a vulnerary among all of the early herbalists. A syrup made of the fresh juice will stop haemorrhages and dysentery when taken internally. The tuberous roots are edible as are the young shoot which resemble ASPARAGUS.

ADMINISTERED AS: poultice or syrup.

Yam, wild *dioscorea villosa*. COMMON NAME: Dioscorea, colic root, rheumatism root, wilde yamwurzel.

OCCURRENCE: native to the southern United States and Canada.

PARTS USED: the roots and rhizome, which contain steroidal saponins, phytosterols, tannins, starch and various alkaloids including dioscorine.

MEDICINAL USES: antispasmodic, diuretic. This plant has a history of traditional use in relieving menstrual cramps and in stopping threatened miscarriage. It brings quick relief for bilious colic and flatulence, particularly in pregnant women. It is prescribed for the inflammatory stage of rheumatoid arthritis and in painful disorders of the urinary tract. Wild Yam is also beneficial for poor circulation, spasmodic hiccoughs, neuralgic complaints and spasmodic asthma. Prior to 1970, the wild yam was the only source of diosgenin, one of the starting materials used in commercial manufacturing of steroid hormones for the contraceptive pill.

ADMINISTERED AS: fluid extract, powdered bark, infusion.

Yerba santa *Eriodictyon glutinosum*. COMMON NAME: Mountain balm, gum bush, bear's weed, holy or sacred herb, consumptive's weed, *Eriodictyon californicum*.

OCCURRENCE: native to California and northern Mexico.

PARTS USED: the dried leaves which contain five phenolic chemicals, free acids including free formic acids, volatile oil, phytosterol, glucose, a resin and some glycerides of fatty acids.

MEDICINAL USES: bitter tonic, stimulant, expectorant, aromatic. This herb is recommended in laryngeal and bronchial problems, catarrh, hay fever, asthma and chronic lung afflictions. It is also used for catarrh of the bladder and haemorrhoids. Yerba santa is used as a bitter tonic upon the digestion and is highly effective in masking the unpleasant taste of quinine, when given as an aromatic syrup. The dried leaves are smoked to ease asthma.

ADMINISTERED AS: powdered leaves, fluid extract, syrup.

Yew *Taxus baccata*.

OCCURRENCE: found in Europe, North Africa and Western Asia. The tree has been closely associated with the history and legends of Europe.

PARTS USED: the leaves, seeds and fruit. The seeds and fruit are the most poisonous parts of the plant and contain an alkaloid toxine and another principle milrossin.

MEDICINAL USES: it has few medicinal uses due to its poisonous nature but the leaves were once used effectively in treating epilepsy. The wood was used for making longbows.

ADMINISTERED AS: powdered leaves.

Herb Action

alterative a term given to a substance that speeds up the renewal of the tissues so that they can carry out their functions more effectively.

anodyne a drug that eases and soothes pain.

anthelmintic a substance that causes the death or expulsion of parasitic worms.

antiperiodic a drug that prevents the return of recurring diseases, e.g. malaria.

antiscorbutic a substance that prevents scurvy and contains necessary vitamins, e.g. vitamin C.

antiseptic a substance that prevents the growth of disease-causing micro-organisms, e.g. bacteria, without causing damage to living tissue. It is applied to wounds to cleanse them and prevent infection.

antispasmodic a drug that diminishes muscle spasms.

aperient a medicine that produces a natural movement of the bowel.

aphrodisiac a compound that excites the sexual organs.

aromatic a substance that has an aroma.

astringent a substance that causes cells to contract by losing proteins from their surface. This causes localized contraction of blood vessels and tissues.

balsamic a substance that contains resins and benzoic acid and is used to alleviate colds and abrasions.

bitter a drug that is bitter-tasting and is used to stimulate the appetite.

cardiac compounds that have some effect on the heart.

carminative a preparation to relieve flatulence and any resultant griping.

cathartic a compound that produces an evacuation of the bowels.

cholagogue the name given to a substance that produces a flow of bile from the gall bladder.

cooling a substance that reduces the temperature and cools the skin.

demulcent a substance that soothes and protects the alimentary canal.

deobstruent a compound that is said to clear obstructions and open the natural passages of the body.

detergent a substance that has a cleansing action, either internally or on the skin.

diaphoretic a term given to drugs that promote perspiration.

diuretic a substance that stimulates the kidneys and increases urine and solute production.

emetic a drug that induces vomiting.

emmenagogue a compound that is able to excite the menstrual discharge.

emollient a substance that softens or soothes the skin.

expectorant a group of drugs that are taken to help in the removal of secretions from the lungs, bronchi and trachea.

febrifuge a substance that reduces fever.

galactogogue an agent that stimulates the production of breast milk or increases milk flow.

haemostatic a drug used to control bleeding.

hepatic a substance that acts upon the liver.

hydrogogue a substance that has the property of removing accumulations of water or serum.

hypnotic a drug or substance that induces sleep.

insecticide a substance that kills insects.

irritant a general term encompassing any agent that causes irritation of a tissue.

laxative a substance that is taken to evacuate the bowel or soften stools.

mydriatic a compound that causes dilation of the pupil.

narcotic a drug that leads to a stupor and complete loss of awareness.

nephritic a drug that has an action on the kidneys.

nervine a name given to drugs that are used to restore the nerves to their natural state.

nutritive a compounds that is nourishing to the body.

parasiticide a substance that destroys parasites internally and externally.

pectoral a term applied to drugs that are remedies in treating chest and lung complaints.

purgative the name given to drugs or other measures that produce evacuation of the bowels. They normally have a more severe effect than aperients or laxatives.

refrigerant a substance that relieves thirst and produces a feeling of coolness.

resolvent a substance that is applied to swellings to reduce them in size.

rubefacient a compound that causes the skin to

redden and peel off. It causes blisters and inflammation.

sedative a drug that lessens tension, anxiety and soothes over-excitement of the nervous system.

sternutatory the name given to a substance that irritates the mucous membrane and produces sneezing.

stimulant a drug or other agent that increases the activity of an organ or system within the body.

stomachic name given to drugs that treat stomach disorders.

styptic applications that check bleeding by blood vessel contraction or by causing rapid blood clotting.

sudorific a drug or agent that produces copious perspiration.

taeniacide drugs that are used to expel tapeworms from the body.

tonic substances that are traditionally thought to give strength and vigour to the body and that are said to produce a feeling of wellbeing.

vermifuge a substance that kills, or expels, worms from the intestines.

vesicant similar to a rubefacient, agent that causes blistering when applied to the skin.

vulnerary a drug that is said to be good at healing wounds.

Classification of Herbs by Action

alterative anemone pulsatilla, bethroot, betony (wood), bitter root, bittersweet, blue flag, brooklime, burdock, burr marigold, caroba, celandine, clivers, clover (red), cohosh (black), dock (yellow), dropwort (water), echinacea, elder, fireweed, fringe tree, frostwort, golden seal, Jacob's ladder, meadowsweet, mezeron, pipsissewa, plantain (common), poke root, polypody root, rosinweed, sarsaparilla (jamaica), sassafras, soap tree, soapwort, speedwell, spindle tree, tag alder, walnut.

anodyne aconite, camphor, chamomile, coca, figwort, gladwyn, henbane, hemlock, hops, hound's tongue, lettuce (wild), mandrake, poppy (red), poppy (white), sassy bark, stramonium, valerian.

anthelmintic aloes, balmony, camphor, cedar (yellow), cohosh (blue), gentian (yellow), groundsel, hellebore (black), knotgrass, lupin (white), male fern, savine, tansy, walnut, wormseed (American), wormwood.

antiperiodic lilac, willow (white).

antiscorbutic groundsel, lemon, lime fruit, radish, rowan tree, scurvy grass, shepherd's purse, sorrel, spinach, watercress.

antiseptic avens, barberry, beech, bergamot, bethroot, black root, camphor, cinnamon, costmary, echinacea, elecampane, eucalyptus, garlic, gentian (yellow), horseradish, myrrh, oak, olive, sandalwood, stockholm tar, thyme, violet, woundwort.

antispasmodic anemone pulsatilla, arrach, baneberry, belladonna, bergamot, camphor, chamomile, clover (red), cohosh (blue), cowslip, cramp bark, cumin, daisy (ox-eye), ephedra, eucalyptus, gelsemium, gladwyn, hemlock, henbane, masterwort, mayweed, mistletoe, motherwort, musk seed, oats, passionflower, peony, peppermint, pleurisy root, poppy (white), primrose, red root, rosinweed, rue, scullcap (Virginian), skunk-cabbage, spearmint, stramonium, sumbul, thyme, tree of heaven, valerian, vervain, woundwort, yam (wild).

aperient butcher's broom, clivers, club moss, costmary, couchgrass, dandelion, elder, feverfew, fringe tree, fumitory, germander (wall), horseradish, jewelweed, olive, parsley, rhubarb, rose (pale), scurvy grass.

aphrodisiac celery, coca, damiana, guarana, musk seed.

aromatic allspice, angelica, angostura, asarabacca, avens, basil, bergamot, betony (wood), birthwort, bugle, calamint, calamus, camphor, caraway, cardamom, cedar (yellow), cicely (sweet), cinnamon, cloves, coriander, dill, eryngo, eucalyptus, fennel, gale (sweet), golden rod, hops, lavender, lovage, magnolia, meadowsweet, melilot, musk seed, orange (bitter), orange (sweet), pepper, pine oils, sage (common), St. John's wort, sandalwood, sassafras, savory (summer), saxifrage (burnet), spearmint, wintergreen, yerba santa.

astringent agrimony, alder, apple, avens,

bayberry, bearberry, bethroot, betony (wood), birch, bistort, blackberry, bugle, burnet (greater), cassia, cedar (yellow), chestnut (horse), chestnut (sweet), cinnamon, cohosh (black), columbine, comfrey, costmary, cudweed, dog-rose, elder, elecampane, elm, evening primrose, eyebright, fireweed, frostwort, gale (sweet), golden rod, hawthorn, horsetail, hound's tongue, houseleek, ivy (ground), Jacob's ladder, knotgrass, lady's mantle, larch, lily (Madonna), loosestrife, lungwort, maple (red), matico, meadowsweet, mullein, myrrh, nettle, oak, olive, pipsissewa, plantain (common), poppy (white), primrose, quince, ragwort, raspberry, red root, rhubarb, rose (pale), rose (red), rosemary, rowan tree, rupturewort, sage (common), sassy bark, scullcap (Virginian), self-heal, St. John's wort, silverweed, solomon's seal, speedwell (common), strawberry, tag alder, tea, thistle (scotch), tree of heaven, vervain, vine, walnut, willow (white), wintergreen, witch hazel, balsamic larch.

bitter angostura, bugle, birch, calumba, feverfew, gentian (yellow), nux vomica, simaruba, snapdragon, wormwood, yerba santa.

cardiac asparagus, bitter root, butterbur, foxglove, hawthorn, kola nuts, lily of the valley, mescal buttons, strophanthus, tree of heaven.

carminative allspice, angelica, anise, balm, basil, bergamot, calamus, caraway, cardamom, cassia, catmint, cayenne, celery, cicely (sweet), cinnamon, cloves, coriander, cumin, dill, fennel, feverfew, ginger, golden rod, horsemint (American), juniper, lavender, lovage, mace, marjoram, masterwort, melilot, nutmeg, orange (bitter), orange (sweet), parsley, pennyroyal, pepper, peppermint, pleurisy root, saffron, sage (common), savory (summer), saxifrage (burnet), spearmint, thyme, valerian.

cathartic black root, bloodroot, blue flag, bogbean, broom, bryony (white), castor oil plant, croton, fireweed, gladwyn, hedge-hyssop, hydrangea, ivy, jewelweed, mountain flax, pleurisy root, poke root, sabadilla, saffron (meadow), senna, stavesacre.

cholagogue spindle tree.

cooling basil, cucumber, lemon, mandrake, plantain (common), ragwort, sorrel, witch hazel.

demulcent almonds, barley, borage, chickweed, coltsfoot, comfrey, couchgrass, elm, fig, flax, hound's tongue, Iceland moss, Irish moss, lily (Madonna), liquorice, marshmallow, mullein,

olive, parsley piert, peach, pellitory-of-the-wall, pine (white), pumpkin, quince, rice, salep, slippery elm, solomon's seal, sundew.

deobstruent agrimony, bladderwrack, bogbean, butcher's broom, carrot, liverwort (English), plantain (common), water dock.

depurative figwort.

detergent balmony, blackcurrant, golden seal, ragwort, soap tree, soapwort, walnut, water betony, water dock.

diaphoretic aconite, anemone pulsatilla, angelica, balm, blackcurrant, black root, boneset, box, buchu, burdock, burr marigold, butcher's broom, camphor, caroba, carrot, catmint, chicory, clematis, clivers, cohosh (blue), cuckoopint, dwarf elder, elder, elecampane, eryngo, fumitory, garlic, gelsemium, germander (wall), groundsel, heartease, hedge-hyssop, horehound, horsemint (American), horseradish, ipecacuanha, ivy, jaborandi, Jacob's ladder, knapweed (greater), laurel, lettuce (wild), lily of the valley, lobelia, lovage, marigold, marjoram, motherwort, mugwort, pennyroyal, pimpernel (scarlet), pine (white), pleurisy root, poppy (white), ragwort, rosemary, rosinweed, saffron, samphire, sarsaparilla (jamaica), sassafras, saxifrage (burnet), senega, sheep's sorrel, skunk-cabbage, slippery elm, smartweed, speedwell (common), stockholm tar, thistle (holy), turpentine, vervain, woodruff.

diuretic apple, arnica, asparagus, belladonna, bittersweet, blackcurrant, blue flag, bluebell, broom, buchu, burdock, burr marigold, butterbur, cacao, caroba, cedar (yellow), celandine, celery, clematis, club moss, coffee, cohosh (black), cohosh (blue), coolwort, couchgrass, cucumber, daisy (ox-eye), damiana, dandelion, dropwort (water), dwarf elder, elder, elm, eryngo, figwort, foxglove, fringe tree, fumitory, garlic, germander (wall), golden rod, groundsel, goutwort, hair cup moss, hawthorn, heartease, henbane, hops, horsemint (American), horseradish, horsetail, houseleek, hydrangea, ivy (ground), jewelweed, juniper, kava-kava, knotgrass, kola nuts, larch, lettuce (wild), lupin (white), mastic, matico, meadowsweet, mezeron, mugwort, mustard (black), nettle, parsley, parsley piert, peach, pellitory-of-the-wall, pimpernel (scarlet), pipsissewa, plantain (common), poplar, pumpkin, radish, rest-harrow, rosinweed, rupturewort, sandalwood, sarsaparilla (jamaica), sassafras, savine, saw palmetto, saxifrage (burnet), scurvy grass, senega, sheep's sorrel, shepherd's purse, smartweed, soap tree, sorrel, St. John's wort, stockholm tar, strawberry, sunflower, tobacco, vine, watercress, wintergreen, yam (wild).

emetic asarabacca, black root, bloodroot, daffodil, elder, fireweed, groundsel, hedge-hyssop, ipecacuanha, jewelweed, laurel, lobelia, mandrake, mayweed, mescal buttons, mustard (black), poke root, primrose, rosinweed, sabadilla, saffron (meadow), spearwort (lesser), stavesacre, tag alder, thistle (holy), tobacco, vervain.

emmenagogue aloes, arrach, bloodroot, cassia, catmint, cedar (yellow), cohosh (black), cohosh (blue), cornflower, cotton root, ergot, feverfew, gale (sweet), gentian (yellow), hellebore (black), horsemint (American), lupin (white), marjoram, marjoram (sweet), mayweed, motherwort, mugwort, myrrh, pennyroyal, rue, saffron, savine, senega, smartweed, tansy, thistle (holy), wintergreen.

emollient almonds, borage, cacao, cucumber, fenugreek, fig, flax, Irish moss, liquorice, marshmallow, melilot, mullein, olive, ragwort, slippery elm.

expectorant balsam of Peru, beech, bethroot, bloodroot, boneset, calamint, cedar (yellow), cicely (sweet), cohosh (black), coltsfoot, comfrey, cuckoopint, cup moss, dropwort (water), dwarf elder, elder, elecampane, eryngo, garlic, ginger, honeysuckle, horehound, ipecacuanha, jaborandi, Jacob's ladder, larch, lobelia, loosestrife, maidenhair, myrrh, peach, pimpernel (scarlet), pine (white), pleurisy root, polypody root, poppy (red), poppy (white), red root, rosinweed, St. John's wort, senega, skunk-cabbage, slippery elm, soap tree, speedwell (common), stockholm tar, sundew, sunflower, tobacco, violet, watercress, yerba santa.

febrifuge aconite, avens, balm, blackcurrant, bogbean, boneset, calumba, chestnut (horse), gelsemium, gentian (yellow), guarana, holly, lilac, pepper, poplar, verbena (lemon), wormwood.

galactogogue castor oil plant, vervain, wintergreen.

haemostatic puffballa, shepherd's purse.

hepatic dodder, spindle tree.

hydragogue bitter root, bryony (white).

hypnotic corkwood tree, henbane, mandrake, poppy (white).

insecticide laburnum, larkspur, musk weed,

pyrethrum (dalmatian).

irritant bryony (white), cedar (yellow), croton, ivy (poison), mustard (black), pellitory, rue, turpentine.

laxative almonds, asparagus, boneset, castor oil plant, chicory, dock (yellow), dodder, elder, fig, golden seal, honeysuckle, mountain flax, mulberry, olive, pellitory-of-the-wall, rose (pale), sassy bark, senna, spinidle tree, strawberry, violet, walnut.

mydriatic belladonna, corkwood tree, henbane.

narcotic belladonna, bittersweet, box, cherry laurel, chestnut (horse), guarana, hellebore (black), henbane, ivy (poison), laurel, lettuce (wild), mescal buttons, mistletoe, mullein, nightshade (black), paris (herb), passionflower, poke root, poppy (red), sassy bark, skunk-cabbage, stramonium, tobacco.

nephritic hydrangea.

nervine anemone pulsatilla, arrach, celery, club moss, cramp bark, guarana, kola nuts, hops, lavender, lime tree, mistletoe, motherwort, mugwort, musk seed, oats, scullcap (Virginian), St. John's wort, sumbul, valerian, vervain.

nutritive almonds, barley, cacao, fig, Iceland moss, Irish moss, mulberry, oats, parsnip, rice, salep, saw palmetto, slippery elm, spinach, watercress.

parasiticide balsam of Peru, larkspur.

pectoral anise, bethroot, dog-rose, euphorbia, flax, horehound, Irish moss, liquorice, lungwort, maidenhair, polypody root, slippery elm, sundew.

purgative aloes, angostura, asarabacca, barberry, bindweed (greater), castor oil plant, celandine, croton, cucumber, damiana, dodder, dwarf elder, elder, groundsel, hellebore (black), kamala, liverwort (English), mandrake, mercury (dog's), mountain flax, rhubarb, senna.

refrigerant blackcurrant, borage, catmint, chickweed, dog-rose, houseleek, lemon, lime fruit, mulberry, parsley piert, pellitory-of-the-wall, plantain (common), rice, sheep's sorrel, sorrel.

resolvent bittersweet, saxifrage (burnet), St. John's wort.

rubefacient bryony (black), buttercup (bulbous), cayenne, croton, horsemint (American), horseradish, ivy (poison), pellitory, pine oils, rue, spearwort (lesser), turpentine.

sedative aconite, asparagus, belladonna, box, camphor, cherry laurel, clover (red), corkwood tree, cowslip, cramp bark, ergot, evening primrose, foxglove, gelsemium, goutwort, hemlock, henbane, lettuce (wild), motherwort, mullein, passionflower, peach, poppy (white), red root, saw palmetto, skunk-cabbage, tobacco, verbena (lemon), witch hazel.

sternutatory asarabacca, soap tree, soapwort.

stimulant allspice, angelica, angostura, arnica, asarabacca, balsam of Peru, bayberry, beech, birthwort, blue flag, boneset, buchu, butterbur, cacao, calamus, caraway, cardamom, carrot, catmint, cayenne, celery, chives, cinnamon, cloves, coca, coffee, coriander, cornflower, cuckoopint, cumin, damiana, dill, elder, elecampane, ephedra, ergot, eryngo, eucalyptus, fennel, feverfew, garlic, germander (wall), ginger, ginseng, golden rod, guarana, horsemint (American), horseradish, ipecacuanha, ivy, ivy (ground), ivy (poison), jabarandi, kava-kava, kola nuts, larch, lavender, lime tree, lobelia, lovage, mace, magnolia, marigold, marjoram, marjoram (sweet), masterwort, mastic, matico, mezeron, mugwort, mustard (black), myrrh, nettle, nutmeg, nux vomica, oats, pennyroyal, pepper, peppermint, poplar, raspberry, rosemary, rue, sage (common), sassafras, scurvy grass, senega, shepherd's purse, smartweed, snapdragon, soap tree, spearmint, spindle tree, stockholm tar, sumbul, tansy, tea, thistle (holy), valerian, watercress, wintergreen, yerba santa.

stomachic angelica, avens, cassia, chamomile, cicely (sweet), dill, fennel, gentian (yellow), ginseng, golden seal, juniper, laurel, musk seed, nutmeg, orange (bitter), orange (sweet), peppermint, rhubarb, saxifrage (burnet), wormwood.

styptic avens, bluebell, knotgrass, lady's mantle, matico, self-heal.

sudorific avens, nightshade (black), vervain.

taeniacide cucumber, kamala, male fern, pumpkin.

tonic agrimony, alder, angelica, angostura, asarabacca, avens, balmony, barberry, bayberry, bergamot, bethroot, bitter root, black root, blackberry, bogbean, boneset, burnet (greater), butterbur, calamus, calumba, cassia, catmint, cayenne, celery, chamomile, chestnut (horse), chestnut (sweet), chicory, clivers, coca, coltsfoot, coolwort, cornflower, daisy (ox-eye), damiana, dandelion, dock (yellow), elecampane, elm, eyebright, fireweed, foxglove, fringe tree, frostwort, fumitory, gentian (yellow), germander (wall), ginseng, golden seal, guarana, hawthorn, holly, hops, horehound, hydrangea, Iceland moss, ivy (ground), kava-kava, knapweed (greater), kola nuts, lemon, lilac, lily of the valley, lime tree, mace, magnolia, marjoram, marjoram (sweet), mayweed, mescal buttons, mistletoe, motherwort, mugwort, myrrh, nettle, nux vomica, oak, orange (bitter), orange (sweet), parsley, peony, pipsissewa, pleurisy root, polypody root, poplar, rose (red), rosemary, rosinweed, sage (common), sarsaparilla (jamaica), saw palmetto, scullcap (Virginian), self-heal, silverweed, simaruba, soapwort, solomon's seal, speedwell (common), spindle tree, strophanthus, sumbul, tag alder, tansy, thistle (holy), thyme, vervain, willow (white), wintergreen, witch hazel, wormwood, woodruff, yerba santa.

vermifuge aloes, castor oil plant, cohosh (blue), lilac, male fern, pink root, primrose, sabadilla, stavesacre, walnut, wormseed (American).

vesicant mezereon.

vulnerary arnica, comfrey, knotgrass, mare's tail, water betony.

Chemical Glossary

acid a substance that can form hydrogen ions when dissolved in water. Aqueous solutions of acids typically have a sharp taste and turn litmus paper red. Most organic acids have the C(O)OH grouping but they may have other acid groups, e.g. the sulphonic group — S(O$_2$)OH. Acids can vary in strength according to the degree of ionization in solution.

alcohol an organic compound with one or more hydroxyl (-OH) groups attached directly to a carbon atom. This is a large assemblage of compounds that forms part of waxes, esters, aldehydes, ketones and volatile oils. Alcohols may be in the solid or liquid form depending on the size of the carbon chain.

aldehydes organic compounds with a carbonyl group joined directly to another carbon atom. Aldehydes may be either solids or colourless liquids.

alkali the name given to a substance that gives a solution in water with a pH of greater than seven. They may also be called a base.

alkaloid probably the most important chemicals found in plants, as they usually have a medical action. They are organic substances, found in association with organic acids in most plant groups, particularly the flowering plants. Alkaloids are alkaline and combine with acids to form crystalline salts which are water-soluble in most cases. The alkaloids themselves are generally insoluble in water but dissolve well in alcohol or ether. Alkaloids include a number of important drugs, e.g. morphine, caffeine, atropine, quinine and nicotine and many of these chemicals are very poisonous with characteristic physiological effects.

anthraquinones glycoside compounds present in some plants and that are used to prepare dyes and purgative drugs.

bitters the name given to herbs that have a bitter taste. It may be due to a combination of chemicals within the plant. The herbs include angostura, yellow gentian, nux vomica and wormwood and they can be used as appetite stimulants, relaxant drugs and for their anti-inflammatory action.

carbohydrates these compounds are formed in plants as a result of photosynthesis. They include sugars, starches and cellulose which all have an important nutritional value. A polysaccharide is made up of hundreds of sugar molecules linked together, and they form part of compounds such as mucilage or pectin which help protect the alimentary canal. Carbohydrates are one of the main classes of naturally-derived organic compounds.

coumarins glycoside compounds widely distributed in plants. They provide the distinctive smell of many grass species.

ester organic compounds produced when an acid and an alcohol react. They often have distinctive fruity odours and are found naturally in fruits. An ester is generally a volatile liquid but may exist in a solid form.

fatty acids an organic compound made up of a hydrocarbon chain and a terminal carboxyl group (-COOH). The chain can range in length from one to thirty carbon atoms and branches can occur in the compound. Fatty acids are classified as saturated or unsaturated depending on the presence of a double bond in the chain structure. In nature, fatty acids form part of glycerides, that make up part of many important tissues and are important in many energy-releasing processes in the body.

flavonoid glycosides compounds made up of glycoside sugars and a flavone compound. The flavones are a group of chemicals, that give a yellow pigmentation to plants. This group of compounds is widely distributed through the plant kingdom, and they can have diuretic antispasmodic or stimulating effects on the body.

glucoside a term given to glycoside chemicals that contain glucose as the sugar.

glycoside molecules made up of two sections, a sugar and another chemical group. This name is given to all compounds independent of the sugar within them. As a class, glycosides are colourless, crystalline and bitter and are very common in plants. There are various classes of glycosides including cardiac glycosides, e.g. foxglove/digitalis and purgative glycosides, e.g. the anthraquinone chemicals in senna and rhubarb.

gum complex polysaccharides, that contain several different sugar and acid groups. They are generally soluble in water and produce viscous solutions, that are sometimes called mucilages. They are normally insoluble in organic solvents and are found in variable quantities in plant tissues.

hydrocarbons compounds made up of carbon and hydrogen alone. There are various categories of compounds, depending upon the arrangement of carbon atoms in the molecule and the number of double bonds in the molecule.

isomer compounds can have the same chemical composition and molecular weight but differ in their physical structure and hence are termed isomers. These isomers can have different physical and physiological qualities. Isomers can differ in the order in which the atoms are joined together (structural isomers) or they differ in the spatial orientation of atoms in the molecule (stereo-isomerism). In plants, two isomeric forms of an active chemical may exist with one form having beneficial medical effects, and the other having no impact or a deleterious impact on the body. Care must be taken where several isomers of a chemical exist to utilize the correct form.

mucilage a gum-like substance found in the cell walls or seed coats of plants. They are polysaccharides that have a soothing effect on inflamed tissues, and they are used as an ingredient in some cosmetic preparations.

phenols slightly acidic compounds with at least one hydroxyl (-OH) group bonded to a carbon atom in an aromatic ring. They are widely found in natural plant constituents, e.g. tannins, anthocyanine glucoside pigments and salicylic acid. salicylic acid frequently combines with a sugar to form a glycoside that has antiseptic properties, e.g. in crampbark, meadowsweet and white willow.

resin a naturally-produced acidic polymer obtained from trees. It is thought to help protect the tree from physical or mechanical damage, and attack by fungi and insects, in a similar way to how gums or mucilage protect green plants. It is a high molecular weight class of compounds usually produced by coniferous trees.

saponins glycosides that form a lather when shaken with water. They are found in two groups; the steroidal saponins that mimic the precursors of female sex hormones and the tri-terpenoid saponins that mimic the adrenocorticotropic hormone ACTH. They occur in a wide variety of plant groups and also act as a poison affecting fish.

starch a complex polysaccharide carbohydrate made by green plants during photosynthesis and which forms one of the plants' main energy stores. It is composed of water-soluble amylose and amylopectin, which forms a mucilaginous paste in water. Starch grains formed in the plant vary in size and shape according to the plant that produced them. Starch is used in industry as a food thickener, an adhesive and for sizing paper and cloth.

sugars a group of water-soluble carbohydrates with a sweet taste. They can contain six or twelve carbon units in each molecule and the simple sugar units or monosaccharides can combine to form more complex sugar groups. It is a crystalline substance, found in many forms in plants.

tannins a group of complex organic chemicals found in the leaves, unripe fruits and bark of trees. They generally taste astringent and may be a protective mechanism against the grazing of some animals. They have commercial uses in treating cattle hides to produce leather, in producing ink and as mordants in the textile industry.

terpenes a group of unsaturated hydrocarbons, made up of multiples of isoprene units. The group includes vitamins A, E and K, carotene and other carotenoid pigments and squalene, the precursor to cholesterol. The terpenes are of great scientific and industrial importance. They are very reactive chemicals, with characteristic and pleasant odours that are used in perfumery.

volatile oil these compounds are formed from an alcohol and a hydrocarbon. They are found in many plants and can give a plant a characteristic taste and flavour. Many volatile oils have medicinal properties and are used as antifungal, antiseptic or aromatic oils taken internally or externally. They are very important oils in herbal medicine.

waxes fatty acid esters of alcohols with a high molecular weight. They are normally solid and have water-repellent properties. Waxes form a protective coating on animal skin, fur or feathers and also reduce water loss in leaves and fruits. The waxes are used for various commercial uses including polishes, textiles and pharmaceuticals.

Forms of Herbal Preparations

capsule this is a gelatine container for swallowing and holding oils or balsams that would otherwise be difficult to administer due to their unpleasant taste or smell. It is used for cod liver oil and castor oil.

decoction this is prepared using cut, bruised or ground bark and roots placed into a stainless

steel or enamel pan (not aluminium) with cold water poured on. The mixture is boiled for 20–30 minutes, cooled and strained. It is best drunk when warm.

herbal dressing this may be a compress or poultice. A compress is made of cloth or cotton wool soaked in cold or warm herbal decoctions or infusions while a poultice can be made with fresh or dried herbs. Bruised fresh herbs are applied directly to the affected area and dried herbs are made into a paste with water and placed on gauze on the required area. Both dressings are very effective in easing pain, swelling and inflammation of the skin and tissues.

infusion this liquid is made from ground or bruised roots, bark, herbs or seeds, by pouring boiling water onto the herb and leaving it to stand for 10-30 minutes, possibly stirring the mixture occasionally. The resultant liquid is strained and used. Cold infusions may be made if the active principles are yielded from the herb without heat. Today, infusions may be packaged into teabags for convenience.

liquid extract this preparation, if correctly made, is the most concentrated fluid form in which herbal drugs may be obtained and, as such, is very popular and convenient. Each herb is treated by various means dependent upon the individual properties of the herb, e.g. cold percolation, high pressure, evaporation by heat in a vacuum. These extracts are commonly held in a household stock of domestic remedies.

pessary similar to suppositories, but it is used in female complaints to apply a preparation to the walls of the vagina and cervix.

pill probably the best known and most widely used herbal preparation. It is normally composed of concentrated extracts and alkaloids, in combination with active crude drugs. The pill may be coated with sugar or another pleasant-tasting substance that is readily soluble in the stomach.

solid extract this type of preparation is prepared by evaporating the fresh juices or strong infusions of herbal drugs to the consistency of honey. It may also be prepared from an alcoholic tincture base. It is used mainly to produce pills, plasters, ointments and compressed tablets.

suppository this preparation is a small cone of a convenient and easily soluble base with herbal extracts added, which is used to apply medicines to the rectum. It is very effective in the treatment of piles, cancers, etc.

tablet this is made by compressing drugs into a small compass. It is more easily administered and has a quicker action as it dissolves more rapidly in the stomach.

tincture this is the most prescribed form of herbal medicine. It is based on alcohol and, as such, removes certain active principles from herbs that will not dissolve in water, or in the presence of heat. The tincture produced is long-lasting, highly concentrated and only needs to be taken in small doses for beneficial effects. The ground or chopped dried herb is placed in a container with 40 per cent alcohol such as gin or vodka and left for two weeks. The tincture is then decanted into a dark bottle and sealed before use.

Medical Glossary

amenorrhoea an absence of menstruation which is normal before puberty, during pregnancy and while breast-feeding is being carried out and following the menopause. Primary amenorrhoea describes the situation where the menstrual periods do not begin at puberty. This occurs if there is a chromosome abnormality (such as Turner's syndrome) or if some reproductive organs are absent. It can also occur where there is a failure or imbalance in the secretion of hormones. In secondary amenorrhoea, the menstrual periods stop when they would normally be expected to be present. There are a variety of causes including hormone deficiency, disorders of the hypothalamus, psychological and environmental stresses, during starvation, anorexia nervosa or depression.

arthritis inflammation of the joints or spine, the symptoms of which are pain and swelling, restriction of movement, redness and warmth of the skin. There are many different causes of arthritis including osteoarthritis, rheumatoid arthritis, tuberculosis and rheumatic fever.

asthma a condition characterized by breathing difficulties caused by narrowing of the airways (bronchi) of the lung. It is a distressing condition with breathlessness and a paroxysmal wheezing cough and the extent to which the bronchi narrow varies considerably. Asthma may occur at any age but usually begins in early childhood, and is a hypersensitive response that can be brought on by exposure to a variety of allergens, exercise, stress or infections. An asthma sufferer may have other hypersensitive conditions such as eczema and hay fever, and it may be prevalent within a family. It may or may not be possible for a person to avoid the allergen(s) responsible for an asthma attack. Treatment involves the use of drugs to dilate the airways (bronchodilators) and also inhaled corticosteroids.

atheroma a degenerative condition of the arteries. The inner and middle coats of the arterial walls become scarred and fatty deposits (cholesterol) are built up at these sites. The blood circulation is impaired and it may lead to such problems as angina pectoris, stroke and heart attack. The condition is associated with the western lifestyle. i.e. lack of exercise, smoking, obesity and too high an intake of animal fats.

atrophy wasting of a body part due to lack of use, malnutrition or as a result of ageing. The ovaries of women atrophy after the menopause and muscular atrophy accompanies certain diseases.

boil (or furuncle) a skin infection in a hair follicle or gland that produces inflammation and pus. The infection is often due to the bacterium *Staphylococcus*, but healing is generally quick upon release of the pus or administration of antibiotics. Frequent occurrence of boils is usually investigated to ensure the patient is not suffering from diabetes mellitus.

bronchitis occurring in two forms, acute and chronic, bronchitis is the inflammation of the bronchi. Bacteria or viruses cause the acute form that is typified by the symptoms of the common cold initially, but develops with painful coughing, wheezing, throat and chest pains and the production of purulent (pus-containing) mucus. If the infection spreads to the bronchioles (bronchiolitis) the consequences are even more serious as the body is deprived of oxygen. Antibiotics and expectorants can relieve the symptoms.

Chronic bronchitis is identified by an excessive production of mucus and may be due to recurrence of the acute form. It is a common cause of death among the elderly and there are several parameters of direct consequence to its cause: excessive smoking of cigarettes; cold, damp climate; obesity; respiratory infections. Damage to the bronchi and other complications may occur giving rise to constant breathlessness. Bronchodilator drugs are ineffective in treatment of the chronic form.

bruises injuries of, and leakage of blood into, the subcutaneous tissues, but without an open wound. In the simplest case minute vessels rupture and blood occupies the skin in the immediate area. A larger injury may be accompanied by swelling. A bruise begins as blue/black in colour, followed by brown and yellow as the blood pigment is reabsorbed.

burns burns and scalds show similar symptoms and require similar treatment, the former being caused by dry heat, the latter moist heat. Burns may also be due to electric currents and chemicals. Formerly burns were categorized by degrees (a system developed by Dupuytres, a French surgeon) but are now either superficial, where sufficient tissue remains to ensure skin regrows, or deep where grafting will be necessary.

Severe injuries can prove dangerous because of shock due to fluid loss at the burn. For minor burns and scalds, treatment involves holding the affected area under cold water. In more severe cases antiseptic dressings are normally applied and in very severe cases hospitalization is required. Morphine is usually administered to combat the pain. If the burns exceed nine per cent then a transfusion is required.

calculus stones formed within the body, particularly in the urinary tract (gravel) or gall bladder (see gallstones). They are formed from mineral salts, e.g. calcium oxalate and they generally cause pain as they may block the ureter or bile ducts. Treatment is by removing or crushing the stone surgically, by drugs and diet (in gallstones a low fat diet eases pain and prevents formation of more stones) and also by the use of herbal remedies.

cancer a widely-used term describing any form of malignant tumour. Characteristically, there is an uncontrolled and abnormal growth of cancer cells that invade surrounding tissues and destroy them. Cancer cells may spread throughout the body via the blood stream or lymphatic system, a process known as metastasis, and set up secondary growths elsewhere. There are known to be a number of different causes of cancer including cigarette smoking, radiation, ultraviolet light, some viruses and possibly the presence of cancer genes (oncogenes). Treatment depends upon the site of the cancer but involves radiotherapy, chemotherapy and surgery, and survival rates in affected people are showing encouraging improvements.

chilblain a round, itchy inflammation of the skin that usually occurs on the toes or fingers during cold weather, and is caused by a localized deficiency in the circulation. Chilblains may sometimes be an indication of poor health or inadequate clothing and nutrition. Keeping the feet and hands warm, paying attention to the diet and exercise to improve the circulation help to prevent chilblains.

cholera an infection of the small intestine caused by the bacterium *Vibrio cholerae*. It varies in degree from very mild cases to extremely severe illness and death. The disease originated in Asia but spread widely during the nineteenth century when there were great cholera epidemics in Britain and elsewhere. During epidemics of cholera, the death rate is over fifty per cent and these occur in conditions of poor sanitation and overcrowding. The disease is spread through contamination of drinking water by faeces of those affected by the disease, and also by flies landing on infected material and then crawling on food.

Epidemics are rare in conditions of good sanitation but when cholera is detected, extreme attention has to be paid to hygiene including treatment and scrupulous disposal of the body waste of the infected person. The incubation period for cholera is one to five days and then a person suffers from severe vomiting and diarrhoea (known as "cholera diarrhoea" or "rice water stools"). This results in severe dehydration and death may follow within twenty four hours. Treatment involves bed rest and the taking by mouth of salt solutions, or these may need to be given intravenously. Tetracycline or other sulphonamide drugs are given to kill the bacteria. The death rate is low (five per cent) in those given proper and prompt treatment but the risk is greater in children and the elderly. Vaccination against cholera can be given but it is only effective for about six months.

chorea a disorder of the nervous system characterized by the involuntary, jerky movements of the muscles mainly of the face, shoulders and hips. *Sydenham's chorea* or *St. Vitus' dance* is a disease that mainly affects children and is associated with acute rheumatism. About one third of affected children develop rheumatism elsewhere in the body, often involving the heart, and the disease is more common in girls than in boys. If the heart is affected there may be

problems in later life but treatment consists of rest and the giving of mild sedatives. The condition usually recovers over a period of a few months. *Huntington's chorea* is an inherited condition that does not appear until after the age of forty and is accompanied by dementia. *Senile chorea* afflicts some elderly people but there is no dementia.

cirrhosis a disease of the liver in which fibrous tissue resembling scar tissue is produced as a result of damage and death to the cells. The liver becomes yellow-coloured and nodular in appearance, and there are various types of the disease including alcoholic cirrhosis and postnecrotic cirrhosis caused by viral hepatitis. The cause of the cirrhosis is not always found (cryptogenic cirrhosis) but the progress of the condition can be halted if this can be identified and removed. This particularly is applicable in alcoholic cirrhosis where the consumption of alcohol has to cease.

cold (common cold) widespread and mild infection of the upper respiratory tract caused by a virus. There is inflammation of the mucous membranes and symptoms include feverishness, coughing, sneezing, runny nose, sore throat, headache and sometimes face ache due to catarrh in the sinuses. The disease is spread by coughing and sneezing and treatment is by means of bed rest and the taking of mild analgesics.

conjunctivitis inflammation of the mucous membrane (conjunctiva) that lines the inside of the eyelid and covers the front of the eye. The eyes become pink and watery and the condition is usually caused by an infection that may be bacterial, viral or the micro-organism *Chlamydia* may be responsible. Treatment depends upon cause but a number of drugs are used often in the form of eyedrops.

constipation the condition in which the bowels are opened too infrequently and the faeces become dry, hard and difficult and painful to pass. The frequency of normal bowel opening varies between people but when constipation becomes a problem, it is usually a result of inattention to this habit or to the diet. To correct the condition a change of lifestyle may be needed including taking more exercise, fluid and roughage in the diet. laxatives and enemas are also used to alleviate the condition. Constipation is also a symptom of the more serious condition of blockage of the bowel (by a tumour), but this is less common.

convulsions also known as fits, these are involuntary, alternate, rapid, muscular contractions and relaxations throwing the body and limbs into contortions. They are caused by a disturbance of brain function and in adults usually result from epilepsy. In babies and young children they occur quite commonly but, although alarming, are generally not serious. Causes include a high fever due to infection, brain diseases such as meningitis and breath-holding, that is quite common in infants and very young children. Convulsions are thought to be more common in the very young because the nervous system is immature. Unless they are caused by the presence of disease or infection that requires to be treated, they are rarely life-threatening.

cramp prolonged and painful spasmodic muscular contraction that often occurs in the limbs but can affect certain internal organs. Cramp may result from a salt imbalance as in heat cramp. Working in high temperatures causes excessive sweating and consequent loss of salt. It can be corrected and prevented by an increase of the salt intake. Occupational cramp results from continual repetitive use of particular muscles, e.g. writer's cramp. Night cramp occurs during sleep and is especially common among elderly people, diabetics and pregnant women. The cause is not known.

croup a group of diseases characterized by a swelling, partial obstruction and inflammation of the entrance to the larynx, occurring in young children. The breathing is harsh and strained producing a typical crowing sound, accompanied by coughing and feverishness. Diphtheria used to be the most common cause of croup but it now usually results from a viral infection of the respiratory tract (laryngotracheo bronchitis). The condition is relieved by inhaling steam and also by mild sedatives and/or pain killers. Rarely, the obstruction becomes dangerous and completely blocks the larynx in which case emergency tracheostomy or nasotracheal intubation may be required. Usually, the symptoms of croup subside and the child recovers, but then he or she may have a tendency towards attacks on future occasions.

delirium a mental disorder typified by confusion, agitation, fear, anxiety, illusions and sometimes hallucinations. The causal cerebral disfunction may be due to deficient nutrition, stress, toxic poisoning or mental shock.

depression a mental state of extreme sadness dominated by pessimism and in which normal behaviour patterns (sleep, appetite, etc.) are disturbed. Causes are varied: upsetting events, loss, etc. and treatment involves the use of therapy and drugs.

diarrhoea increased frequency and looseness of bowel movement, involving the passage of unusually soft faeces. Diarrhoea can be caused by food poisoning, colitis, irritable bowel syndrome, dysentery, etc. A severe case will result in the loss of water and salts that must be replaced and anti-diarrhoeal drugs are used in certain circumstances.

diphtheria a serious, infectious disease caused by the bacterium *Corynebacterium diphtheriae,* and commonest in children. The infection causes a membranous lining on the throat that can interfere with breathing and eating. The toxin produced by the bacterium damages heart tissue and the central nervous system and it can be fatal if not treated. The infection is countered by injection of the antitoxin with penicillin or erythromycin taken to kill the bacterium. Diphtheria can be immunized against.

dropsy old-fashioned name for oedema.

dysentery an infection and ulceration of the lower part of the bowels that causes severe diarrhoea with the passage of mucus and blood. There are two forms of dysentery caused by different organisms. Amoebic dysentery is due to *Entamoeba histolytica* that is spread via infected food or water and occurs mainly in the tropics and sub-tropics. The appearance of symptoms may be delayed but in addition to diarrhoea there is indigestion, anaemia and weight loss. Drugs are used in treatment.

Bacillary dysentery is caused by the bacterium *Shigella* and spreads by contact with a carrier or contaminated food. Symptoms appear from one to six days after infection and include diarrhoea, cramp, nausea, fever and the severity of the attack varies. Antibiotics may be given to kill the bacteria but recovery usually occurs within one to two weeks.

dysmenorrhoea painful menstruation. There are two main types, primary and secondary. Primary or spasmodic dysmenorrhoea is extremely common, but is normally mild and short-lived in duration. In a small proportion of women, the pain is severe enough to cause partial or total debility. The pain generally occurs in the lower abdomen or back and is cramping, often coming in waves that is due to uterine contractions. It is associated with dizziness, nausea, vomiting, headache, fainting and pale complexion with obvious distress. Secondary or congestive dysmenorrhoea is pain with a congested ache and cramps in the lower abdomen. It is generally due to specific pelvic conditions, e.g. chronic pelvic infection, endometriosis, fibroid tumours and the presence of an interuterine contraceptive device (IUCD).

eczema an inflammation of the skin that causes itching, a red rash and often small blisters that weep and become encrusted. This may be followed by the skin thickening and then peeling off in scales. There are several types of eczema, *atopic* being one of the most common. (Atopic is the hereditary tendency to form allergic reactions due to an antibody in the skin). A form of atopic eczema is infantile eczema that starts at three or four months and it is often the case that eczema, hay fever and asthma is found in the family history. However, many children improve markedly as they approach the age of ten or eleven. The treatment for such conditions usually involves the use of hydrocortisone and other steroid creams and ointments.

epilepsy a neurological disorder involving convulsions, seizures and loss of consciousness. There are many possible causes or associations of epilepsy, including cerebral trauma, brain tumour, cerebral haemorrhage and metabolic imbalances as in hypoglycaemia. Usually an epileptic attack occurs without warning, with complete unconsciousness and some muscle contraction and spasms. Some drugs are used in treatment although little can be done during the fit itself.

erysipelas an infectious disease, caused by *Streptococcus pyogenes*. It produces an inflammation of the skin with associated redness. Large areas of the body may be affected and other symptoms may include vesicles, fever and pain with a feeling of heat and a tingling sensation. In addition to being isolated, patients are given penicillin.

fistula an abnormal opening between two hollow organs or between such an organ or gland and the exterior. These may arise during development so that a baby may be born with a fistula. Alternatively, they can be produced by injury, infection or as a complication following surgery. A common example is an anal fistula, that may develop if an abscess present in the rectum bursts and produces a communica-

tion through the surface of the skin. An operation is normally required to correct a fistula, but healing is further complicated in the case of an anal fistula because of the passage of waste material through the bowels.

gallstones stones of varying composition, that form in the gall bladder. Their formation seems to be due to a change in bile composition rendering cholesterol less soluble. Stones may also form around a foreign body. There are three types of stone cholesterol, pigment and mixed, the latter being the most common. Calcium salts are usually found in varying proportions. Although gallstones may be present for years without symptoms, they can cause severe pain and may pass into the common bile duct to cause, by the resulting obstruction, jaundice.

gleet discharge due to chronic gonorrhoea.

gonorrhoea the most common venereal disease that is spread primarily by sexual intercourse but may be contracted through contact with infected discharge on clothing, towels, etc. The causative agent is the bacterium *Neisseria gonorrhoeae* and it affects the mucous membrane of the vagina, or in the male, the urethra. Symptoms develop approximately one week after infection and include pain on urinating with a discharge of pus. Inflammation of nearby organs may occur (testicle, prostate in men; uterus, Fallopian tubes and ovaries in women) and prolonged inflammation of the urethra may lead to formation of fibrous tissue causing stricture. Joints may also be affected and later complications include endocarditis, arthritis and conjunctivitis.

If a baby is born to a woman with the disease, the baby's eyes may become infected, until recently a major cause of blindness (called *Ophthalmia neonatorum*). Treatment is usually very effective through the administration of penicillin, sulphonamides or tetracycline.

gout a disorder caused by an imbalance of uric acid in the body. Uric acid is normally excreted by the kidneys but sufferers of gout have an excess in their bloodstream that is deposited in joints as salts (urates) of the acid. This causes inflammation of the affected joints and painful gouty arthritis with destruction of the joints. The kidneys may also be damaged, with formation of stones. Deposits of the salts (called *tophi*) may reach the stage where they prohibit further use of the joints, causing hands and feet to be set in a particular position. Treatment of gout is through drugs that increase the excretion of the urate salts or slow their formation.

gravel this name refers to small stones formed in the urinary tract. They normally are made up of calcareous material and crystalline matter and passage of stones from the kidneys is normally linked to severe pain and, possibly, the presence of blood in the urine.

haemorrhoids (piles) varicose and inflamed veins around the lower end of the bowel situated in the wall of the anus. They are classified as internal, external and mixed depending upon whether they appear beyond the anus. They are commonly caused by constipation or diarrhoea, especially in middle and older age, and may be exacerbated by a sedentary life style. They may also occur as a result of childbearing. Symptoms of haemorrhoids are bleeding and pain, and treatment is by means of creams, injections and suppositories. Attention to diet (to treat constipation) and regular exercise are important, but in severe cases, surgery to remove the haemorrhoids may be necessary.

hysteria a type of neurosis that is difficult to define and in which a range of symptoms may occur. These include paralysis, seizures and spasms of limbs, swelling of joints, mental disorders and amnesia. The person is vulnerable to suggestion. Two types are recognized, *conversion hysteria* that is characterized by physical symptoms and *dissociative hysteria* in which marked mental changes occur. *Mass hysteria* affects a group, especially those gathered together under conditions of emotional excitement. A number of people may suffer from giddiness, vomiting and fainting that runs through the whole crowd. Recovery occurs when those affected are separated from the others under calmer conditions. Treatment for hysteria is by means of psychotherapy, involving suggestion.

influenza a highly infectious disease caused by virus that affects the respiratory tract. Symptoms include headache, weakness and fever, appetite loss and general aches and pains. Sometimes there is the complication of a lung infection that requires immediate treatment. There are three main strains of influenza virus, designated A, B and C. The viruses quickly produce new strains which is why an attack of one is unlikely to provide protection against a later bout of the disease. Epidemics occur periodically and in Britain virus A is responsible for the majority of outbreaks.

jaundice a condition characterized by the unusual presence of bile pigment (bilirubin) in the blood. The bile produced in the liver passes into the blood instead of the intestines and because of this there is a yellowing of the skin and the whites of the eyes.

There are several types of jaundice: *obstructive* due to bile not reaching the intestine due to an obstruction e.g. a gallstone; *haemolytic* where red blood cells are destroyed by haemolysis; *hepatocellular* due to a liver disease such as hepatitis which results in the liver being unable to use the bilirubin. *Neonatal jaundice* is quite common in newborn infants when the liver is physiologically immature but it usually lasts only a few days. The infant can be exposed to blue light that converts bilirubin to biliverdin, another (harmless) bile pigment.

laryngitis inflammation of the mucous membrane that lines the larynx and vocal cords. It is due to viral infection in the main, but also bacteria, chemical irritants, heavy smoking or excessive use of the voice. *Acute* laryngitis accompanies infections of the upper respiratory tract and the symptoms include pain, a cough, difficulty in swallowing. *Chronic* laryngitis may be due to recurrence of the acute form, but is often attributable to excessive smoking worsened by alcohol. Changes occurring in the vocal cords are more permanent and the symptoms are as for the acute form, but longer lasting.

leucorrhea a discharge of white or yellow-coloured mucus from the vagina. It may be a normal condition, increasing before and after menstruation but a large discharge probably indicates an infection somewhere in the genital tract. A common cause is the infection called thrush but it may also be due to gonorrhoea in which case the treatment will differ.

malaria an infectious disease caused by the presence of minute parasitic organisms of the genus *Plasmodium* in the blood. The disease is characterized by recurrent bouts of fever and anaemia, the interval between the attacks depending upon the species. The parasite is transmitted to man by the *Anopheles* mosquito, (common in sub-tropical and tropical regions) being present in the salivary glands and passed into the bloodstream of a person when the insect bites. Similarly, the parasite is ingested by the mosquito when it takes a blood meal from an infected person. Efforts to control malaria have centred on destruction of the mosquito and its breeding sites. Once injected into the blood, the organisms concentrate in the liver where they multiply and then re-enter the bloodstream destroying red blood cells. This releases the parasites causing shivering, fever, sweating and anaemia. The process is then repeated, with hours or days between attacks. Drugs are used both to prevent infection, although these may not be totally effective, and to cure the disease once present.

nephritis inflammation of the kidney, that may be due to one of several causes. Types of nephritis include glomerulonephritis (when the glomerulus is affected), acute nephritis, hereditary nephritis, etc.

neuralgia strictly, pain in some part or the whole of a nerve (without any physical change in the nerve) but used more widely to encompass pain following the course of a nerve or its branches, whatever the cause. Neuralgia often occurs at the same time each day and is frequently an agonizing pain. It occurs in several forms and is named accordingly, e.g. sciatica, trigeminal neuralgia (affecting the face) and intercostal neuralgia (affecting the ribs). Treatment often involves the application of ointments, and the taking of pain-killing drugs. If such treatments do not bring relief, it is possible to freeze the nerve or destroy part of it by surgery.

oedema an accumulation of fluid in the body, possibly beneath the skin or in cavities or organs. With an injury the swelling may be localized or more general as in cases of kidney or heart failure. Fluid can collect in the chest cavity, abdomen or lung (pulmonary oedema). The causes are numerous, e.g. cirrhosis of the liver, heart or kidney failure, starvation, acute nephritis, allergies or drugs. To alleviate the symptom, the root cause has to be removed. Subcutaneous oedema commonly occurs in women before menstruation, as swollen legs or ankles, but does subside if the legs are rested in a raised position.

palsy the term used formerly for paralysis and retained for the names of some conditions.

pleurisy (*or* **pleuritis**) inflammation of the pleura resulting in pain from deep breathing, and resulting shortness of breath. There is a typical frictional rub heard through a stethoscope. Pleurisy is often due to pneumonia in the adjacent lung and is always associated with disease in the lung, diaphragm, chest wall or abdomen e.g. tuberculosis, abscesses, bronchial carcinoma, etc.

pneumonia a bacterial infection of the lungs resulting in inflammation and filling of the alveoli with pus and fluid. As a result the lung becomes solid and air cannot enter. The symptoms vary depending upon how much of the lung is unavailable for respiration, but commonly there will be chest pain, coughing, breathlessness, fever and possibly cyanosis. Pneumonia may be caused by several bacteria, viruses or fungi, but bacterial infection is commonest. Bronchopneumonia affects the bronchi and bronchioles; lobar pneumonia the whole lobes of the lung(s). Antibiotic treatment is usually effective although it helps to know which is the infecting organism, to provide the most specific treatment.

prolapse a moving down of an organ or tissue from its normal position due to the supporting tissues weakening. This may happen to the lower end of the bowel (in children) or the uterus and vagina in women who have sustained some sort of injury during childbirth. In the latter case prolapse may result in the uterus itself showing on the outside. Surgery can shorten the supporting ligaments and narrow the vaginal opening.

psoriasis a chronic skin disease for which the cause is unknown and the treatment is palliative. The affected skin appears as itchy, scaly red areas, starting usually around the elbows and knees. It often runs in families and may be associated with anxiety, commencing usually in childhood or adolescence. Treatment involves the use of ointments and creams

rheumatism a general term used to describe aches and pains in joints and muscles.

rickets a disease affecting children that involves a deficiency of vitamin D. Vitamin D can be manufactured in the skin in the presence of sunlight but dietary sources are important especially where sunlight is lacking. The disease is characterized by soft bones that bend out of shape and cause deformities.

Bones are hardened by the deposition of calcium salts and this cannot happen in the absence of vitamin D. Treatment consists of giving vitamin D, usually in the form of calciferol, and ensuring that there is an adequate amount in the child's future diet. Vitamin D deficiency in adults causes the condition called osteomalacia.

scarlet fever an infectious disease, mainly of childhood, caused by the bacterium *Streptococcus*. Symptoms show after a few days and include sickness, sore throat, fever and a scarlet rash that may be widespread. Antibiotics are effective and also prevent any complications e.g. inflammation of the kidneys.

sciatica pain in the sciatic nerve, and therefore felt in the back of the thigh, leg and foot. The commonest cause is a prolapsed intervertebral disc pressing on a nerve root, but it may also be due to ankylosing spondylitis and other conditions.

scurvy a deficiency disease caused by a lack of vitamin C (ascorbic acid) due to a dietary lack of fruit and vegetables. Symptoms begin with swollen, bleeding gums and then subcutaneous bleeding, bleeding into joints, ulcers, anaemia and then fainting, diarrhoea and trouble with major organs. Untreated, it is fatal, but nowadays it is easily prevented, or cured should it arise, through correct diet or administration of the vitamin.

smallpox a highly infectious viral disease that has nonetheless been eradicated. Infection results, after about two weeks, in a high fever, head and body aches and vomiting. Eventually red spots appear that change to water and then pus-filled vesicles that on drying out leave scars. The person stays infectious until all scabs are shed. Fever often returns, with delirium. Recovery is usual, but complications often ensue, e.g. pneumonia. The last naturally-occurring case was in 1977.

stone another name for calculus.

strangury the desire to pass water, that can only be done in a few drops and with accompanying pain. It is symptomatic of an irritation of the base of the bladder by a stone, cancer at this site, or cystitis or prostatitis.

syphilis an infectious, sexually-transmitted disease, caused by the bacterium *Treponema pallidum* that shows symptoms in three stages. Bacteria enter the body through mucous membranes during sexual intercourse and an ulcer appears in the first instance. Within a short time the lymph nodes locally and then all over the body enlarge and harden and this lasts several weeks.

Secondary symptoms appear about two months after infection and include fever, pains, enlarged lymph nodes and a faint rash that is usually noticed on the chest. The bacterium is found in enormous numbers in the primary sores and any skin lesions of the secondary stage. The final stage may not appear until many months or years after infection and comprises the formation of numerous tumour-like masses throughout the body (in skin, muscle, bone, brain, spinal cord and other organs such as the liver, stomach., etc.). This stage can cause serious damage to the heart, brain or spinal cord resulting in blindness, tabes dorsalis, and mental disability.

Congenital syphilis is much rarer than the former, *acquired*, type. It is contracted by a developing foetus from the mother, across the placenta and symptoms show a few weeks after birth. Treatment of syphilis is with penicillin, but it should be administered early in the development of the disease.

torpor a state of physical and mental sluggishness that accompanies various mental disorders, some kinds of poisoning and may be present in elderly people with arterial disease.

tuberculosis a group of infections caused by the bacillus (bacterium) *Mycobacterium tuberculosis* of which pulmonary tuberculosis of the lungs (consumption or phthisis) is the best known form. The pulmonary disease is acquired through inhalation of air containing the organism from an infected person, or dust laden with bacteria. People infected in this way can show no symptoms but still be carriers. In the lungs, the infection causes formation of a *primary tubercle* that spreads to lymph nodes to form the *primary complex.*

The disease may wax and wane for years as the body's natural immune system acts against the infection. If the infection is severe, symptoms include fever, wasting, night sweats and the coughing up of blood. The bacteria may enter the blood stream and spread throughout the body setting up numerous tubercles in other tissues (*Miliary tuberculosis*). The organism may also be acquired by eating contaminated food, especially milk, in which case the production of a primary complex in abdominal lymph nodes can lead to peritonitis. Rarely, the infection is acquired via a cut from contact with an infected person or animal. Tuberculosis affects people throughout the world (about six thousand new cases each year in England and Wales). Many people acquire the infection and recover without suspecting its presence and the disease is curable with antibiotics, e.g. streptomycin. In addition, BCG vaccination as a preventive measure is given to children in the U.K., in addition to X-ray screening to detect carriers.

ulcer a break on the skin surface or on the

mucous membrane lining within the body cavities that may be inflamed and fails to heal. Ulcers of the skin include bedsores and varicose ulcers (that are caused by defective circulation). Ulcers of the alimentary tract include duodenal ulcers, gastric ulcers and peptic ulcers.

varicose veins veins that have become stretched, distended and twisted. The superficial veins in the legs are often affected although it may occur elsewhere. Causes include congenitally defective valves, obesity, pregnancy and also thrombophlebitis (inflammation of the wall of a vein with secondary thrombosis in the affected part of the vein). Elastic support is a common treatment although alternatives are sclerotherapy and phlebectomy.

whooping cough (*pertussis*) an infectious disease caused by the bacterium *Bordetella pertussis*. The mucous membranes lining the air passages are affected and after a one to two week incubation period, fever, catarrh and a cough develop. The cough then becomes paroxysmal with a number of short coughs punctuated with the 'whooping' drawing in of breath. Nosebleeds and vomiting may follow a paroxysm. After about two weeks the symptoms abate but a cough may continue for some weeks. Whooping cough is not usually serious and immunization reduces the severity of an attack. However, a child may be susceptible to pneumonia and tuberculosis during the disease.

Homoeopathy

Introduction

The aim of homoeopathy is to cure an illness or disorder by treating the whole person rather than merely concentrating on a set of symptoms. Hence, in homoeopathy the approach is holistic, and the overall state of health of the patient, especially his or her emotional and psychological wellbeing, is regarded as being significant. A homoeopath notes the symptoms that the person wishes to have cured but also takes time to discover other signs or indications of disorder that the patient may regard as being less important. The reasoning behind this is that illness is a sign of disorder or imbalance within the body. It is believed that the whole 'make-up' of a person determines, to a great extent, the type of disorders to which that individual is prone and the symptoms likely to occur. A homoeopathic remedy must be suitable both for the symptoms and the characteristics and temperament of the patient. Hence, two patients with the same illness may be offered different remedies according to their individual natures. One remedy may also be used to treat different groups of symptoms or ailments.

Like cures like

Homoeopathic remedies are based on the concept that 'like cures like', an ancient philosophy that can be traced back to the 5th century BC, when it was formulated by Hippocrates. In the early 1800s, this idea awakened the interest of a German doctor, Samuel Hahnemann, who believed that the medical practices at the time were too harsh and tended to hinder rather than aid healing. Hahnemann observed that a treatment for malaria, based on an extract of cinchona bark (quinine), actually produced symptoms of this disease when taken in a small dose by a healthy person. Further extensive studies convinced him that the production of symptoms was the body's way of combating illness. Hence, to give a minute dose of a substance that stimulated the symptoms of an illness in a healthy person could be used to fight that illness in someone who was sick. Hahnemann conducted numerous trials (called 'provings'), giving minute doses of substances to healthy people and recording the symptoms produced. Eventually, these very dilute remedies were given to people with illnesses, often with encouraging results.

Modern homoeopathy is based on the work of Hahnemann, and the medicines derived from plant, mineral and animal sources are used in extremely dilute amounts. Indeed, it is believed that the curative properties are enhanced by each dilution because impurities that might cause unwanted side effects are lost. Substances used in homoeopathy are first soaked in alcohol to extract their essential ingredients. This initial solution, called the 'mother tincture', is diluted successively either by factors of ten (called the 'decimal scale' and designated X) or 100 (the 'centesimal scale' and designated C). Each dilution is shaken vigorously before further ones are made, and this is thought to make the properties more powerful by adding energy at each stage while impurities are removed. The thorough shakings of each dilution are said to energize, or 'potentiate', the medicine. The remedies are made into tablets or may be used in the form of ointments, solutions, powders, suppositories, etc. High potency (i.e. more dilute) remedies are used for severe symptoms and lower potency (less dilute) for milder ones.

The homoeopathic view is that during the process of healing, symptoms are redirected from more important to less important body systems. It is also held that healing is from innermost to outermost parts of the body and that more recent symptoms disappear first, this being known as the 'law of direction of cure'. Occasionally, symptoms may worsen initially when a homoeopathic remedy is taken, but this is usually short-lived and is known as a 'healing crisis'. It is taken to indicate a change and that improvement is likely to follow. Usually, with a homoeopathic remedy, an improvement is noticed fairly quickly although this depends upon the nature of the ailment, health, age and wellbeing of the patient and potency of the remedy.

A first homoeopathic consultation is likely to last about one hour so that the specialist can obtain a full picture of the patient's medical history and personal circumstances. On the basis of this information, the homoeopathic doctor decides on an appropriate remedy and potency (which is usually 6C). Subsequent consultations are generally shorter, and full advice is given on how to store and take the medicine. It is widely accepted that homoeopathic remedies are safe and non-addictive, but they are covered by the legal requirements governing all medicines and should be obtained from a recognized source.

Potency table for homoeopathic medicines

The centesimal scale

1C =	1/100	$(1/100^1)$	of mother tincture
2C =	1/10 000	$(1/100^2)$	of mother tincture
3C =	1/1 000 000	$(1/100^3)$	of mother tincture
6C =	1/1 000 000 000 000	$(1/100^6)$	of mother tincture

The decimal scale

1X =	1/10	$(1/10^1)$	of mother tincture
2X =	1/100	$(1/10^2)$	of mother tincture
6X =	1/1 000 000	$(1/10^6)$	of mother tincture

The development of homoeopathy

The Greek physician Hippocrates, who lived several hundred years before the birth of Christ (460–370 BC), is regarded as the founding father of all medicine. The Hippocratic Oath taken by newly qualified doctors in orthodox medicine binds them to an ethical code of medical practice in honour of Hippocrates. Hippocrates believed that disease resulted from natural elements in the world in which people lived. This contrasted with the view that held sway for centuries that disease was some form of punishment from the gods or God. He believed that it was essential to observe and take account of the course and progress of a disease in each individual, and that any cure should encourage that person's own innate healing power. Hippocrates embraced the idea of 'like being able to cure like' and had many remedies that were based on this principle. Hence, in his practice and study of medicine he laid the foundations of the homoeopathic approach although this was not to be appreciated and developed for many centuries.

During the period of Roman civilization a greater knowledge and insight into the nature of the human body were developed. Many herbs and plants were used for healing by people throughout the world, and much knowledge was gained and handed down from generation to generation. The belief persisted, however, that diseases were caused by supernatural or divine forces. It was not until the early 1500s that a Swiss doctor, Paracelsus (1493–1541), put forward the view that disease resulted from external environmental forces. He also believed that plants and natural substances held the key to healing and embraced the 'like can cure like' principle. One of his ideas, known as the 'doctrine of signatures', was that the appearance of a plant, or the substances it contained, gave an idea of the disorders it could cure.

In the succeeding centuries, increased knowledge was gained about the healing properties of plants and the way the human body worked. In spite of this, the methods of medical practice were extremely harsh, and there is no doubt that many people suffered needlessly and died because of the treatment they received. It was against this background that Samuel Hahnemann (1755–1843), the founding father of modern homoeopathy, began his work as a doctor in the late 1700s. In his early writings, Hahnemann criticized the severe practices of medicine and advocated a healthy diet, clean living conditions and high standards of hygiene as a means of improving health and warding off disease. In 1790, he became interested in quinine, extracted from the bark of the cinchona tree, which was known to be an effective treatment for malaria. He tested the substance first on himself, and later on friends and close family members, and recorded the results. These 'provings' led him to conduct many further investigations and provings of other natural substances, during the course of which he rediscovered and established the principle of like being able to cure like.

By 1812, the principle and practice of homoeopathy had become established, and many other doctors adopted the homoeopathic approach. Hahnemann himself became a teacher in homoeopathy at the University of Leipzig and published many important writings—the results of his years of research. He continued to practise, teach and conduct research throughout his life, especially in producing more dilute remedies that were succussed, or shaken, at each stage and were found to be more potent. Although his work was not without its detractors, Hahnemann had attracted a considerable following by the 1830s. In 1831 there was a widespread cholera epidemic in central Europe for which Hahnemann recommended treatment with camphor. Many people were cured, including Dr Frederick Quin (1799–1878), a medical practitioner at that time. He went on to establish the first homoeopathic hospital in London in 1849. A later resurgence of cholera in Britain enabled the effectiveness of camphor to be established beyond doubt, as the numbers of people cured at the homoeopathic hospital were far greater than those treated at other hospitals.

In the United States of America, homoeopathy became firmly established in the early part of the 19th century, and there were several eminent practitioners who further enhanced knowledge and practice. These included Dr Constantine Hering (1800–80), who formulated the 'laws of cure', explaining how symptoms affect organ systems and move from one part of the body to another as a cure occurs. Dr James Tyler Kent (1849–1916) introduced the idea of constitutional types, which is now the basis of classical homoeopathy, and advocated the use of high potency remedies.

In the later years of the 19th century, a fundamental split occurred in the practice of homoeopathy, which was brought about by Dr Richard Hughes (1836-1902), who worked in London and Brighton. He insisted that physical symptoms and the nature of the disease itself was the important factor rather than the holistic approach based on the make-up of the whole individual person. Hughes rejected the concept of constitutional types and advocated the use of low potency remedies. Although he worked as a homoeopath, his approach was to attempt to make homoeopathy more scientific and to bring it closer to the practices of conventional medicine. Some other homoeopathic doctors followed the approach of Hughes, and the split led to a collapse in faith in the whole practice of homoeopathy during the earlier part of the 20th century. As the 20th century advanced, however, homoeopathy regained its following and respect. Conventional medicine and homoeopathy have continued to advance, and there is now a greater sympathy and understanding between the practitioners in both these important disciplines.

Homoeopathic Remedies in Common Use

Aconitum napellus
Aconite, monkshood, wolfsbane, friar's cap, mousebane

Aconitum is a native plant of Switzerland and other mountainous regions of Europe, where it grows in the damp conditions of alpine meadows. Attractive purple/dark blue flowers are borne on tall, upright stems produced from tubers developed from the root system. Aconite is highly poisonous, and its sap was used by ancient hunters on the ends of their arrows. 'Wolfsbane' refers to this use, and *Aconitum* is derived from the Latin word *acon*, meaning 'dart'. This was one of the homoeopathic remedies extensively tested and proved by Hahnemann. He used it for the acute infections and fevers, accompanied by severe pain, that were usually treated by blood-letting by the physicians of his day. This remains its main use in modern homoeopathy, and the whole plant is used to produce the remedy.

Aconite is a valuable treatment for acute illnesses of rapid onset in people who have previously been healthy and well. These often occur after the person has been out in cold wet weather. It is used especially at the start of feverish respiratory infections, such as colds and influenza and those affecting the eyes and ears. The person usually experiences restlessness, a hot, flushed face and pains and disturbed sleep but may be pale when first getting up. It is also used to treat the menopausal symptoms of hot flushes. It is an effective remedy for some mental symptoms, including extreme anxiety and fear, palpitations and attacks of panic, especially the belief that death is imminent during illness. The remedy encourages sweating and is sometimes used in conjunction with BELLADONNA. Symptoms are made worse by cold, draughts, tobacco smoke, stuffy, airless, warm rooms, listening to music, at midnight and by lying on the painful part. They improve out in the fresh air and with warmth. The people who benefit from Aconite are typically strong, solid or well-built, high-coloured and usually enjoy good health but have a poor opinion of themselves. Because of this, they tend to have a constant need to prove their own worth, to the point of insensitivity or unkindness to others. When in good health, Aconite people have a need for the company of others. However, they also have fears that they keep concealed and may be frightened of going out or of being in a crowd. When ill, they are inclined to be morbid and to believe that death is imminent, and they cope badly with any kind of shock.

Actea racemosa
Actea rac.; cimic, *Cimifuga racemosa*, black snakeroot, rattleroot, bugbane, rattleweed, squawroot

This plant is a native of woodlands in North America and was used by the American Indian peoples as a remedy for the bite of the rattlesnake. It was also used as a tranquillizer and for pain relief in labour and menstruation. An infusion made from the plant was sprinkled in the home to protect against supernatural forces and evil spirits. The plant has a dark, woody underground stem (rhizome) and roots, and produces feathery, tall stems of white flowers. The fresh rhizomes and roots are used in homoeopathy, being collected, cut and dried in the autumn after the stems and leaves have died down and the fruit has been formed. The rhizome has a faint, unpleasant smell and the taste is acrid and bitter. The remedy was extensively tested and proved by the English homoeopath Dr Richard Hughes, who used it in the treatment of a stiff neck and associated headache. It is used for this purpose in modern homoeopathy and also to treat pain in the lower back and between the shoulder blades. Also for rheumatic pain and swelling of joints or muscles and other sudden, sharp pains. Actea rac. is considered to be of great value in the treatment of menstrual problems with cramps, bloatedness, and pain and symptoms of pregnancy, e.g. morning sickness and abdominal discomfort. It is also of value for postnatal depression and menopausal symptoms. Emotional symptoms that accompany these periods of hormonal change, such as weepiness, anxiety and irritability, are also eased by this remedy. Symptoms are made worse by exposure to cold, wet, draughty conditions, by any sudden change in the weather, on drinking alcohol and with excitement. They improve with keeping warm, with gentle exercise and in the fresh, open air. A person suitable for this remedy is often a woman. She may be a bubbly, extrovert, talkative person or withdrawn, depressed and sad, heaving great sighs. The woman is usually emotionally intense with a fear of dying and madness. These fears are at their height in a woman going through the menopause.

Allium

Allium cepa; Spanish onion

The onion has been cultivated and used for many centuries, both for culinary and medicinal purposes, and was important in the ancient Egyptian civilization. The volatile oil released when an onion is sliced stimulates the tear glands of the eyes and mucous membranes of the nose, throat and air passages. Hence, in homoeopathy the onion is used to treat ailments with symptoms of a streaming nose and watering eyes. The red Spanish onion, which is cultivated throughout the world, is used to make the homoeopathic remedy. It is used to treat allergic conditions, such as hay fever, colds and pains or symptoms that go from one side to the other. It is useful for shooting, stabbing or burning pains associated with neuralgia, which may alternate from side to side, frontal headaches, painful molar teeth and earache in children. The symptoms are made worse by cold, damp conditions and improve in fresh air and cool, dry surroundings.

Apis mellifica

Apis; *Apis mellifera*, the honey bee

The source of the medicine is the entire body of the honey bee, which is crushed or ground to prepare the remedy. It is used particularly to treat inflammation, redness, swelling and itching of the skin, which is sensitive to touch, and with stinging hot pains. There is usually feverishness and thirst and the pains are worsened by heat and relieved by cold. The remedy is used for insect stings, nettle rash, allergic conditions, blisters, whitlow (an abscess on the fingertip) and infections of the urinary tract, including cystitis, with stabbing hot pains. Also for urinary incontinence in elderly

persons, fluid retention causing swelling of the eyelids or other areas, allergic conditions that cause sore throat and swallowing difficulty, and tonsillitis. The person often experiences hot, stabbing headaches and has dry skin. Apis is additionally valued as a remedy for swollen, painful inflammation of the joints as in arthritic conditions and for peritonitis and pleurisy. The symptoms are made worse by heat and touch, stuffy airless rooms following sleep and in the early evening. They improve in the fresh, cool open air, after taking a cold bath, or any cold application. A person suitable for the Apis remedy tends to expect high standards and may be rather irritable and hard to please. He (or she) likes to organize others and is jealous of his own domain, tending to be resentful of anyone new. Apis types may seem to be rushing around and working hard but may achieve very little as a result.

Argenticum nitricum

Argent. nit; silver nitrate, devil's stone, lunar caustic, hellstone

Silver nitrate is obtained from the mineral acanthite, which is a natural ore of silver. White silver nitrate crystals are derived from a chemical solution of the mineral ore and these are used to make the homoeopathic remedy. Silver nitrate is poisonous in large doses and has antiseptic and caustic properties. In the past it was used to clean out wounds and prevent infection. In homoeopathy, it is used to treat states of great anxiety, panic, fear or apprehension about a forthcoming event, e.g. taking an examination, having to perform a public role (speech-making, chairing a public meeting, acting, singing, going for an interview) or any activity involving scrutiny and criticism by others. It was also used as a remedy for digestive complaints including indigestion, abdominal pain, wind, nausea and headache. Often, there is a longing for sweet 'comfort' or other types of food. Argent. nit. may be given for laryngitis, sore throat and hoarseness, eye inflammation such as conjunctivitis, and period pains. Other types of pain, asthma and warts may benefit from Argent. nit.

Often, a person experiences symptoms mainly on the left side, and these are worse with heat and at night. Also, they are made worse by anxiety and overwork, emotional tension and resting on the left side. Pains are made worse with talking and movement. Symptoms improve in cold or cool fresh air and are relieved by belching. Pains are helped by applying pressure to the painful part. People suitable for Argent nit. are quick-witted and rapid in thought and action. They may appear outgoing and happy but are prey to worry, anxiety and ungrounded fears that make them tense. All the emotions are quick to surface, and Argent nit. people are able to put on an impressive performance. They enjoy a wide variety of foods, particularly salty and sweet things although these may upset the digestion. They have a fear of heights, crowds, of being burgled and of failure and arriving late for an appointment. Also, of serious illness, dying and madness. Argent. nit. people are generally slim and full of restless energy and tension. They may have deeply etched features and lines on the skin that make them appear older than their real age.

Arnica montana

Arnica; leopard's bane, sneezewort, mountain tobacco

Arnica is a native plant of woodland and mountainous regions of central Europe and Siberia. It has a dark brown root system from which a central stem arises, producing pairs of elongated green leaves and bright yellow flowers. If the flowers are crushed or bruised and a person then inhales the scent, this causes sneezing. All the fresh parts of the flowering plant are used to prepare the homoeopathic remedy. It is a commonly used first aid remedy for symptoms relating to injury or trauma of any kind, e.g. bruising, swelling, pain and bleeding. It is also used to treat physical and mental shock. It is helpful following surgery, childbirth or tooth extraction, promoting healing, and also for gout, rheumatic joints with pain, heat and inflammation, sore sprained or strained muscles, concussion, and osteoarthritis. Taken internally, it is a remedy for black eyes, eye strain, skin conditions such as eczema and boils. Arnica is helpful in the treatment of whooping cough in children and also wetting the bed when the cause is nightmares. Symptoms are made worse with heat, touch and continued movement, and also with heat and resting for a long period. The symptoms improve when the person first begins to move and with lying down with the head at a lower level than the feet. A person suitable for this remedy tends to be solemn, fatalistic and subject to morbid fears. Arnica types usually deny the existence of any illness, even when

obviously not well, and do not seek medical help, preferring to manage on their own.

Arsenicum album

Arsen. alb.; white arsenic trioxide

This is a widely used homoeopathic remedy, the source being white arsenic trioxide derived from arsenopyrite, a metallic mineral ore of arsenic. Arsenic has been known for centuries as a poison and was once used as a treatment for syphilis. White arsenic trioxide used to be given to improve muscles and skin in animals such as horses. It is used to treat acute conditions of the digestive system and chest and mental symptoms of anxiety and fear. Hence it is a remedy for diarrhoea and vomiting caused by eating the wrong kinds of food, or food poisoning or overindulgence in alcohol. Also, for dehydration in children following gastroenteritis or feverish illness. It is a remedy for asthma and breathing difficulty, mouth ulcers, carbuncle (a collection of boils), dry, cracked lips, burning skin, inflamed, watering stinging eyes and psoriasis. Also, for sciatica, shingles, sore throat and painful swallowing, candidiasis (fungal infection) of the mouth and motion sickness. There may be oedema (retention of fluid) showing as a puffiness around the ankles.

An ill person who benefits from Arsen. alb. experiences burning pains but also feels cold. The skin may be either hot or cold to the touch. The symptoms are worse with cold in any form, including cold food and drink, and between midnight and 3 a.m. They are worse on the right side and if the person is near the coast. Symptoms improve with warmth, including warm drinks, gentle movement and lying down with the head raised. People suitable for Arsen. alb. are precise, meticulous and ambitious and loathe any form of disorder. They are always immaculately dressed and everything in their life is neat and tidy. However, they tend to have great worries, especially about their financial security and their own health and that of their family. They fear illness and dying, loss of financial and personal status, being burgled, darkness and the supernatural. Arsen. alb. people have strongly held views and do not readily tolerate contrary opinions or those with a more relaxed or disordered lifestyle. They enjoy a variety of different foods, coffee and alcoholic drinks. They are usually thin, with delicate, fine features and pale skin that may show worry lines. Their movements tend to be rapid and their manner serious and somewhat restless, although always polite.

Atropa belladonna

Belladonna, deadly nightshade, black cherry, devil's cherries, naughty man's cherries, devil's herb

Belladonna is a native plant of most of Europe although it is uncommon in Scotland. The plant is extremely poisonous, and many children have died as a result of being tempted to eat the shiny black berries of deadly nightshade. It is a stout, stocky plant with light brown roots, growing to about four feet high, with green oval leaves and pale purple, bell-shaped flowers. In medieval times, the plant had its place in the potions of witchcraft. Italian women used extracts of the plant as eye drops to widen the pupils of the eye and make them more beautiful (hence *bella donna*, which means 'beautiful woman'). The plant contains atropine, an alkaloid substance that induces paralysis of nerves and is used in orthodox medicine to relieve painful spasms and in ophthalmic (eye) procedures.

In homoeopathy, the remedy is obtained from the pulped leaves and flowers. It was investigated and proved by Hahnemann as a treatment for scarlet fever. Belladonna is used to treat acute conditions that arise suddenly in which there is a throbbing, pulsing headache and red, flushed skin, high fever and staring wide eyes. The skin around the mouth and lips may be pale, but the tongue is a fiery red and the hands and feet are cold. It is used as a remedy for infectious diseases such as influenza, scarlet fever, measles, whooping cough, chicken pox, mumps and the early stages of pneumonia. Also for boils, earache (particularly on the right side and worse when the head is cold or wet), cystitis, boils, conjunctivitis, tonsillitis, inflammation of the kidneys, neuralgia (sharp pain along the course of a nerve) and sore throat. Other conditions that benefit from this remedy include labour pains, soreness of the breasts in breast-feeding, fever and teething in children, with broken sleep and whitlow (an infection of a fingernail). The symptoms are worse at night and with lying down, and occur more intensely on the right side. Also, they are exacerbated by loud noises, bright lights, jarring of the body, touch or pressure and with cool surroundings.

They improve with sitting upright or standing and keeping warm or warm applications to the painful area. People suitable for belladonna usually enjoy good health, being fit, energetic and ready to tackle any task. They are amusing, sociable and popular when in good health. However, if they become ill the reverse is often true and they may be restless, irritable and possibly even violent.

Aurum metallicum

Aurum met.; gold

Gold was highly prized by Arabian physicians in the early Middle Ages who used it to treat heart disorders. In the early part of this century, it was used in the treatment of tuberculosis. Gold is now used in conventional medicine for some cancer treatments and for rheumatic and arthritic complaints. In homoeopathy, pure gold is ground down to produce a fine powder, and it is used to treat both physical and mental symptoms. It is used as a remedy for congestive circulatory disorders and heart diseases including angina pectoris. The symptoms include a throbbing, pulsing headache, chest pain, breathlessness and palpitations. It is also used to treat liver disorders with symptoms of jaundice, painful conditions of bones and joints (especially the hip and knee), inflammation of the testes and an undescended testicle in small boys (especially if the right side is affected). It is a remedy for sinusitis and severe mental symptoms of despair, depression and thoughts of suicide. The person who is suitable for this remedy tends to drive himself very hard to the point of being a workaholic. He (or she) is excessively conscientious but usually feels that he has not done enough and is oversensitive to the criticism of other people. The person may come to regard himself as a failure and become severely clinically depressed or even suicidal. Symptoms are made worse by mental effort and concentration, or physical exercise, especially in the evening or night and by emotional upheaval. They improve with cold bathing, walking in the fresh air and with rest and quiet.

Bryonia alba

Bryonia, European white bryony, black-berried white bryony, wild hops

Bryony is a native plant of many parts of Europe and grows in England, although it is rarely found in Scotland. It has large, white, branched roots with swollen, expanded portions that are highly poisonous. The smell given off is unpleasant and, if eaten, the taste is very bitter and death soon follows. The tall stems of the plant climb up supports by means of corkscrew tendrils and round black berries are produced in the autumn. Bryony was used by the physicians of ancient Greece and Rome and was described by Hippocrates. The homoeopathic remedy is made from the fresh pulped root of the plant, and is mainly used for conditions producing acute stitch-like pains, which are made worse by even slight movement and relieved by rest. These ailments usually develop slowly and accompanying symptoms include dry skin, mouth and eyes with great thirst. It is used as a remedy for inflammation of the lining of joints in arthritic and rheumatic disorders with swelling, heat and pains. Also, for chest inflammation, pleurisy, chesty bronchitis and pneumonia with severe pain and dry, hacking cough. Digestive problems that are eased by Bryonia include indigestion, colic, constipation, nausea, vomiting and diarrhoea. Breast inflammation because of breast-feeding, colic in babies, gout and lumbago may be helped by Bryonia. The symptoms are made worse by movement and bending and improve with rest and pressure applied to the painful area. People suitable for Bryonia are hard-working, conscientious and reliable but have a dread of poverty. They tend to measure success in life in financial or materialistic terms. They cope badly with any threat to their security or lifestyle, becoming extremely worried, fretful and depressed.

Calcarea carbonica
Calc. carb.; calcium carbonate

This important homoeopathic remedy is made from powdered mother-of-pearl, the beautiful, translucent inner layer of oyster shells. Calcium is an essential mineral in the body, being especially important for the healthy development of bones and teeth. The Calc. carb. remedy is used to treat a number of different disorders, especially those relating to bones and teeth, and also certain skin conditions and symptoms relating to the female reproductive system. It is a remedy for weak or slow growth of bones and teeth and fractures that take a long time to heal. Also, for teething problems in children, pains in bones, teeth and joints, headaches and eye inflammations affecting the right side, and ear infections with an unpleasant-smelling discharge. Premenstrual syndrome, heavy periods and menopausal disorders are helped by Calc. carb., and also chapped skin and eczema.

Calc. carb. may be used as a remedy for verruca (a type of wart) and thrush infections. People who benefit from Calc. carb. are very sensitive to the cold, particularly in the hands and feet and tend to sweat profusely. They suffer from fatigue and anxiety, and body secretions (sweat and urine) smell unpleasant. Children who benefit from Calc. carb. have recurrent ear, nose and throat infections, especially tonsillitis and glue ear. Symptoms are made worse by draughts and cold, damp weather and also at night. They are worse when the person first wakens up in the morning and for physical exercise and sweating. In women, symptoms are worse premenstrually. They improve in warm, dry weather and are better later on in the morning and after the person has eaten breakfast. People suitable for Calc. carb. are often overweight or even obese with a pale complexion. They are shy and very sensitive, quiet in company and always worried about what other people think of them. Calc. carb. people are hard-working, conscientious and reliable and easily upset by the suffering of others. They need constant reassurance from friends and family and tend to feel that they are a failure. Usually, Calc. carb. people enjoy good health but have a tendency for skeletal weakness. They enjoy a wide variety of different foods and tend to overeat, but are upset by coffee and milk. They are afraid of dying and serious illness, the supernatural, madness, being a failure and becoming poor, and they tend to be claustrophobic.

Calcarea fluorica
Calc. fluor.; fluorite, calcium fluoride, fluoride of lime

This homoeopathic remedy is one of the Schussler tissue salts (see GLOSSARY). Calcium fluoride occurs naturally in the body in the enamel of the teeth, bones, skin and connective tissue. It is used to treat disorders of these body tissues or to maintain their elasticity. It is used to treat chronic lumbago, scars, and to prevent the formation of adhesions after operations, gout and arthritic nodules. Also, for rickets, slow growth of bones in children, enlarged adenoids that become stony because of persistent, recurrent respiratory tract infections and cataracts. It is used to strengthen weak tooth enamel and strained and stretched ligaments and muscles, e.g. around a joint. People suitable for Calc. fluor. are intelligent and punctual but tend to make mistakes through lack of planning. They benefit from the guidance of others to work efficiently and fear poverty and illness. They are often prone to piles, varicose veins, swollen glands and muscle and ligament strain. The manner of walking may be rapid with jerking of the limbs. Symptoms are made worse on beginning movement and in cold, damp, draughty conditions. They improve with warmth and heat and for continual gentle movement.

Calcarea phosphorica

Calc. phos., phosphate of lime, calcium
  phosphate

This homoeopathic remedy is a SCHUSSLER TISSUE SALT (*see* Glossary) and calcium phosphate is the mineral that gives hardness to bones and teeth. It is obtained by a chemical reaction between dilute phosphoric acid and calcium hydroxide, when a white precipitate of calcium phosphate is formed. Since calcium phosphate is an essential mineral in the normal, healthy development of bones and teeth, it is used to treat disorders in these tissues. It is particularly helpful as a remedy for painful bones, difficult fractures that are slow to heal, teeth prone to decay, problems of bone growth and teething in children and 'growing pains'. Also, it is beneficial during convalescence when a person is weakened and tired after an illness, and for digestive problems including diarrhoea, stomach pains and indigestion. It may be used as a remedy for tonsillitis, sore throats and swollen glands. Children who benefit from this remedy tend to be thin, pale, miserable and fail to thrive, and are prone to sickness and headaches. They are often fretful and demanding. Adults are also unhappy and discontented with their circumstances, although endeavour to be friendly towards others. They are restless and need plenty of different activities and stimulation, hating routine and needing a good reason to get out of bed in the morning. Symptoms are made worse by any change in the weather, and in cold, wet conditions, e.g. thawing snow. Also for worry or grief and too much physical activity. Symptoms improve when the weather is warm and dry, in summer, and from taking a hot bath.

Calendula officinalis

Calendula, marigold, garden marigold,
  marygold

This is a familiar garden plant that grows well in all parts of the United Kingdom, having light green leaves and bright orange flowers. The plant has been known for centuries for its healing properties and was used in the treatment of various ailments. The parts used in homoeopathy are the leaves and flowers, and the remedy is of value in first aid for its antiseptic and anti-inflammatory activity. It is used in the treatment of boils, stings, cuts and wounds, and to stem bleeding, often in the form of an ointment that can be applied to broken skin. It is helpful when applied to skin tears following childbirth. It is used in the form of an antiseptic tincture as a mouth wash and gargle after tooth extraction, for mouth ulcers or a septic sore throat. When taken internally it prevents suppuration (pus formation) and may be used for persistent chronic ulcers and varicose ulcers, fever and jaundice. It is a useful remedy in the treatment of children's ailments. The symptoms are made worse in damp, draughty conditions and cloudy weather and after eating. They improve with walking about and lying absolutely still.

Cantharis vesicatoria

Cantharis, Spanish fly

This remedy is derived from the body and wings of a bright green iridescent beetle that is found mainly in the southern parts of Spain and France. The beetle, *Cantharis vesicatoria*, secretes a substance called canthardin, which has irritant properties, is also poisonous and is an ancient remedy to cure warts. It was also used as an aphrodisiac, reputedly by the notorious Maquis de Sade. The beetles are dried and ground to produce a powder that is then used in homoeopathy. It is an irritant, blistering agent acting externally on the part of the body to which it is applied and internally on the bladder, urinary tract and genital organs. Hence it is used to treat conditions in which there are stinging and burning pains. An accompanying symptom is often a great thirst but a reluctance to drink. It is used to treat cystitis with cutting hot pains on passing urine, urinary frequency with pain and other urinary infections. Also, certain inflammations of the digestive system in which there is abdominal distension and burning pains and diarrhoea. In general it is used as a remedy for conditions that worsen rapidly. It is a remedy for burns and scalds of the skin, including sunburn, insect stings, and rashes with spots that contain pus. Some mental symptoms are eased by Cantharis, including angry and irritable or violent behaviour, extreme anxiety and excessive sexual appetite. Symptoms are made worse with movement, touch and after drinking coffee or chilled water. They improve when gastro-intestinal wind is eliminated and with warmth, at night time and with very light massage.

Carbo vegetabilis

Carbo veg., vegetable charcoal

The homoeopathic remedy Carbo veg. is made from charcoal, which itself is obtained from heating or partially burning wood without oxygen. The charcoal is hard and black or dark grey, and is a form of carbon that is present in all living things. Charcoal has been made for centuries, and usually silver birch, beech or poplar trees are the source of wood that is used. The homoeopathic remedy is used to treat a person who is run down, weak or exhausted, especially after a debilitating illness or operation. It is also used for postoperative shock, when there is a clammy, cold, pale skin but the person feels a sensation of heat or burning inside. It is helpful as a remedy for ailments of poor circulation such as varicose veins. Again, the skin tends to be pale, clammy and chilly with a bluish colour and the extremities feel cold. The legs may be puffy, and additional symptoms include hoarseness and laryngitis and lack of energy. Carbo veg. is a useful remedy for digestive problems, and carbon is also used for this purpose in orthodox medicine. Symptoms are those of indigestion, heartburn and flatulence with a sour taste in the mouth. Morning headaches with accompanying symptoms of nausea and giddiness or fainting may be relieved by Carbo veg., particularly if the cause is a large, heavy meal the night before. People suitable for this remedy often complain of a lack of energy and may indeed be physically and mentally exhausted, with poor powers of concentration and lapses of memory. They usually have fixed attitudes, with a lack of interest in news of the wider world. They do not like the night and are fearful of the supernatural. Symptoms are made worse by warm, moist weather, in the evening and night, and with lying down. They are also exacerbated after eating meals of fatty foods, coffee and milk and drinks of wine. They improve with burping and with circulating cool, fresh air.

Chamomilla

Camomile, common camomile, double camomile

A creeping and trailing plant that produces daisy-like flowers in summer and prefers dry, sandy soils. Camomiles are native to Britain and others part of northern Europe and have been used in medicine since ancient times, being described by Hippocrates. When walked on, it gives off an aromatic perfume and was gathered and strewn on the floor in medieval dwellings to counter unpleasant odours. It is prized for its many medicinal uses, the flowers and leaves both being used for a number of different ailments. Herbalists use camomile to treat skin conditions such as eczema, and for asthma and disturbed sleep. In homoeopathy, it is used for its soothing and sedative effect on all conditions producing restlessness, irritability and pains. It is a useful remedy for children's complaints such as teething where the child is fretful and cries if put down, colicky pains and disturbed sleep. Also, for toothache, when one cheek is red and the other white, that is exacerbated by heat and relieved by cold. It is used to treat a blocked ear and earache, painful, heavy periods and soreness and inflammation associated with breast-feeding. People suitable for this remedy are very sensitive to pain, which causes sweating or fainting, especially in children and women. They are irritable and fretful when ill. Symptoms are made worse if the person becomes angry or in cold winds and the open air. They improve if the person fasts for a time and if the weather is wet and warm. People who are suitable for camomile are noisy sleepers, in that they frequently cry out or talk while dreaming. If woken suddenly from sleep they are extremely irritable and they like to poke their feet out from the bed covers to keep them cool.

Chincona officinalis

Cinchona succirubra; china, Peruvian bark, Jesuit's bark

This homoeopathic remedy, known as china, is obtained from the dried bark of the cinchona tree and contains quinine. The attractive evergreen cinchona, with its red bark, is a native of the hot tropical forests of South America, but it is also cultivated in India, Sri Lanka and southeast Asia. A preparation of powdered bark was used to treat a feverish illness suffered by the Countess of Cinchon, wife of the viceroy of Peru in 1638. After her recovery she publicized the remedy, and the tree was called cinchona from this time. The value of the bark as a cure for malaria had long been known and used by Jesuit priests. This was the first homoeopathic substance tested and proved by Hahnemann on himself.

In modern homoeopathy it is used mainly as a remedy for nervous and physical exhaustion resulting from chronic debilitating illnesses. It is used for weakness because of dehydration, sweating, chills and fever, and headaches that are relieved if firm pressure is applied. The person wants drinks during periods of chills and shivering rather than when feverish and hot. He or she usually has a washed-out unhealthy complexion with very sensitive skin. China is also used as a remedy for neuralgia, muscles that twitch because of extreme fatigue, bleeding, including nosebleeds, and tinnitus (noises in the ears). It has a helpful effect on the digestion and is used to treat gastro-intestinal wind, gall bladder disorders and digestive upset. Some mental symptoms are helped by this remedy, including irritability and tetchy behaviour that is out of character, apathy and loss of concentration and sleeplessness.

People who are suitable for this remedy tend to be artistic, imaginative and highly strung. They find it easier to empathize with the natural world rather than with the people around them. They are intense and dislike trivial conversation and fatty foods such as butter, but have a liking for alcoholic drinks. Their nature makes them prone to irritability and depression, and they tend to draw up grand schemes at night that are later abandoned. Symptoms are made better by warmth and plenty of sleep and by the application of steady continuous pressure to a painful area. They are made worse by cold, draughty weather, particularly in the autumn, and in the evening and night.

Citrullus colocynthis
Colocynth; bitter cucumber, bitter apple

The plant *Citrullus colocynthis* is a native of Turkey and is also found in parts of Asia and Africa, flourishing in dry, arid conditions. It produces yellow flowers and then yellow-orange smooth fruits, about the size of a large apple, which contain many seeds embedded in a whitish pulp. The homoeopathic remedy colocynth is obtained from the dried fruits from which the seeds have been removed. This is then ground down to produce a powder. The fruit itself is poisonous, having a violent irritant effect on the digestive tract, causing severe, cramp-like pains, inflammation and bleeding. This is caused by the presence of a

substance called colocynthin. According to tradition, Elisha, the Old Testament prophet, is said to have performed a miraculous transformation of the fruit during the famine in Gilgal, making it fit for the people to eat. In homoeopathy, colocynth is used to treat colicky abdominal pains that may be accompanied by sickness and diarrhoea (including colic in young babies). Also, for neuralgia, especially of the face, sciatica, ovarian or kidney pain because of nerves, rheumatic disorders and headache.

People who are helped by colocynth are often reserved, with a tendency to bottle up anger. They have strong opinions about what is right and wrong, and may become quite agitated if someone else has a contrary viewpoint. Physical symptoms of colicky pains or neuralgia and upset stomach may follow on from becoming upset or angry. The symptoms are made worse when the person becomes irritated or angry and in cold, damp weather conditions. Also, eating meals and drinking exacerbate the symptoms. They are relieved by warmth and pressure on the painful part and drinking coffee. Abdominal flatulence also relieves the symptoms.

Cuprum metallicum
Cuprum met.; copper

Copper ore, which is found in rocks in many parts of the world, has been mined and used for many centuries in the manufacture of weapons, utensils and jewellery, etc. In earlier times, physicians made an ointment from the ground metal and this was applied to raw wounds to aid healing. Copper is poisonous in large doses affecting the nervous system and causing convulsions, paralysis and possibly death because of its effects upon respiratory muscles. Toxic effects were recognized in those who worked with the metal and who developed wasting because of poor absorption of food, coughs and respiratory symptoms, and colicky pains. The ruddy, gold-coloured metal is ground to produce a fine red powder that is used in homoeopathy to treat cramping, colicky pains in the abdomen, and muscular spasms in the calves of the legs, feet and ankles. It is also used as a remedy for epilepsy and problems of breathing and respiration such as asthma, croup and whooping cough in which there are spasms. The person may turn blue because of the effort of breathing.

The symptoms are made worse by touch, hot,

sunny weather and for keeping emotions bottled up. They improve with sweating and drinking cold fluids. People who benefit from Cuprum met. have mood swings that alternate from stubbornness to passivity, weepiness and depression. They tend to be serious people who judge themselves severely and keep their emotions very much suppressed. As babies or toddlers, they may be breath-holders who turn blue with anger or as a result of a tantrum. As children, some are destructive and others are loners who dislike the company of others.

Daphne mezereum

Daphne, spurge laurel, wild pepper, spurge olive, flowering spurge, dwarf bay

This poisonous plant is native to upland areas of Europe and is cultivated in the United Kingdom. It produces cheerful bright-red flowers and dark green leaves, and the bark is the part used in homoeopathy. It is used to treat skin conditions characterized by blistering, especially erysipelas, shingles and varicose ulcers. Also, for any condition in which there is a persistent, dry cough and tightness around the chest and a mucus discharge from the nose. There may be burning pains that are worse at night.

Drosera rotundifolia

Drosera, sundew, youthwort, red rot, moor grass

This small, carnivorous (insect-eating) plant is found widely throughout Europe and in Britain, where it grows in the poor, acidic soils of bogs, damp uplands, moorlands and woodlands. It is a small plant growing close to the ground, and needs to trap insects for extra nutrients as the soil in which it grows is so poor. It is remarkable for its leaves, which are covered with long red hairs, each with a small, fluid-containing gland at the top. When the sun shines on the leaves it resembles dew, hence the name sundew. An insect landing on the leaf is trapped because this curls over and inwards, and the sticky fluid secreted by the hairs holds it fast. The secretion contains enzymes that digest the body and the nutrients are absorbed by the plant. The small, white flowers of sundew are fully open in the early morning but close up when the sun is shining strongly. In medieval times, the plant was used to treat tuberculosis and the plague, and it was employed as a remedy for skin disorders in early Asian medicine. It was noticed that sheep who inadvertently cropped sundew developed a parox-

ysmal type of cough like whooping cough. It was investigated and proved as a remedy for this illness in homoeopathy, and the whole plant is used to prepare the medicine. Any condition in which there is a violent, dry, persistent barking cough of a spasmodic nature, as in whooping cough, benefits from the use of sundew, which has a particular action on the upper respiratory tract. Accompanying symptoms are gagging, sickness, sweating and nosebleeds. It is also used to treat bronchitis, asthma, corns and warts, growing pains and pains in the bones.

People who benefit from this remedy are restless and fearful of being alone when they are ill, and they tend to be stubborn and lack concentration. They are suspicious and may feel that others are talking about them or concealing bad news. They are sensitive to the supernatural and are afraid of ghosts. The symptoms are worse for being too warm in bed, after midnight, with crying, lying down, laughing, singing and talking. Also, for meals of cold food and drinks. Symptoms improve out in the fresh air, with walking or gentle exercise, sitting propped up in bed, with pressure applied to the painful part and in quiet surroundings.

Euphrasia officinalis

Euphrasia, eyebright

Eyebright is an attractive wild flower that is variable in size and grows widely throughout Europe, including Britain, and in North America. It has been known since medieval times as a remedy for inflammation of the eyes, and this remains its main use in homoeopathy. The plant flourishes on well-drained, chalky soils and may be between two and eight inches in height, depending upon conditions. It is partly parasitic, deriving some nourishment from the roots of grass, and produces pretty white, purple-veined flowers with yellow centres. The whole plant and flowers are used in homoeopathy, and the remedy is used to treat eye disorders characterized by redness, inflammation, watering, burning, stinging or itching. These include conjunctivitis, blepharitis (inflammation of eyelids), injuries to the eye and dry eyes. It is also used as a remedy for allergic conditions such as hay fever, in which the eyes are very much affected, and colds producing eye symptoms. It is a remedy for the early stages of measles, headaches, some menstrual problems and inflammation of the prostate gland in men. Symptoms are worse in the evening, in windy and warm weather and for being inside. They improve in subdued light, with drinking a cup of coffee and with cold applications.

Ferrum phosphoricum

Ferrum phos.; ferric phosphate of iron, iron phosphate

Ferrum phos. is one of the SCHUSSLER TISSUE SALTS (*see* GLOSSARY), and the iron phosphate powder is obtained by chemical reaction between sodium phosphate, sodium acetate and iron sulphate. Iron is a very important substance in the body, being found in the haemoglobin pigment of red blood cells that transports oxygen to all the tissues and organs. The homoeopathic remedy is used to treat the early stages of infections, inflammations and feverish conditions, before any other particular symptoms occur. It is used to treat colds and coughs in which there may be a slowly developing fever, headache, nosebleeds, bronchitis, hoarseness and loss of the voice, earache and rheumatic pains. Digestive symptoms such as sour indigestion, inflammation of the stomach (gastritis), and vomiting and some disorders of menstruation are helped by this remedy. It is also used to treat the early symptoms of dysentery. The person tends to be pale but is prone to flushing, and feels cold in the early afternoon. There may be a rapid weak pulse. Symptoms are worse at night and in the early morning between 4 a.m. and 6 a.m. Also, they are worse for heat and hot sun, movement and jarring of the body, pressure and touch and resting on the right side and suppressing sweating by the use of deodorants, etc. Symptoms improve for cold applications and with gentle movements. People who are suitable for Ferrum phos. tend to be thin and pale but may be liable to flush easily. They are intelligent and quick to absorb new concepts, having plenty of original ideas of their own. They may be prone to digestive and respiratory complaints, stomach upsets and coughs and colds.

Gelsemium sempervirens

Gelsemium, yellow jasmine, false jasmine, Carolina jasmine, wild woodbine

This attractive climbing plant is a native of the southern United States and parts of Mexico. It has a woody stem that twists around any available tree trunk, and grows on stream banks and on the sea coast. It produces attractive, large, bell-shaped, perfumed yellow flowers in the early spring, which belie the poisonous nature of the plant. It has an underground stem, or rhizome, from which arise a tangle of yellow roots that have an aromatic smell. The root is the part used in homoeopathy and, if eaten in significant amounts, it affects the central nervous system, causing paralysis and possible death through failure of the nerves and muscles of the respiratory system. In homoeopathy it is used to treat both physical and mental symptoms. The physical ailments treated mainly involve the nervous and respiratory systems. These include headaches that are worsened with bright light and movement, multiple sclerosis, eye pain, especially on the right side, sore throat and influenza-like symptoms, earache and feverish muscular pains. Accompanying symptoms include chills and shivering, flushed face and malaise. It is used to treat some menstrual problems including pain. Mental symptoms that are helped by Gelsemium include fears and phobias with symptoms of fatigue, weakness, trembling and apprehension. These fears may arise before an examination, interview or public performance (stage fright). Excitement or fear that causes the heart to skip a beat and extreme anxiety causing sleeplessness are helped by Gelsemium. Symptoms are made worse in the sun and in warm, moist, humid weather or damp and fog. They are also worse with smoking and for excitement, anticipation, stress or bad news. Symptoms improve with movement in the fresh air and after sweating and drinking alcohol or a stimulant drink. They improve after urinating—a large quantity of pale urine is usually passed. People suitable for Gelsemium tend to be well-built with a blue-tinged skin and often complain of feeling weak and tired. They are beset by fears, and may be cowardly and too fearful to lead or enjoy a normal active life.

Graphites

Graphite; black pencil lead

Graphite is a form of carbon that is the basis of all life. It is found in older igneous or metamorphic rocks, such as granite and marble, and is mined for its industrial uses, e.g. in batteries, motors, pencil leads, cleaning and lubricating fluids. It was investigated and proved by Hahnemann after he learned that it was being used by some factory workers to heal cold sores. The powder used in homoeopathy is ground graphite, and it is mainly used for skin disorders that may be caused by metabolic imbalances and stomach ulcers. It is a remedy for eczema, psoriasis, acne, rough, dry skin conditions with pustules or blisters, scarring and thickened cracked nails and cold sores. Also, for stomach ulcers caused by a thinning or weakness in the lining of the stomach wall, problems caused by excessive catarrh, loss of hair, and cramping pains or numbing of the feet and hands. In women it is used to treat some menstrual problems. The symptoms are worse in draughty, cold and damp conditions and for eating sweet meals or sea foods. Also, the use of steroids for skin complaints and, in women, during menstruation. Symptoms are often worse on the left side. They improve with warmth as long as the air is fresh and it is not stuffy, when it is dark and for eating and sleep. People suitable for Graphites are usually well-built and may be overweight, often having dark hair. They like to eat well but lack physical fitness, and sweat or flush with slight exertion. They are prone to dry, flaky skin conditions that may affect the scalp. Graphites people are usually lethargic and may be irritable, lacking in concentration for intellectual activities. They are prone to mood swings and subject to bouts of weeping, especially when listening to music. A Graphites person feels that he or she is unlucky and is inclined to self-pity, often feeling fearful and timid.

Guaiacum officinale

Guaiac, resin of lignum vitae

This attractive evergreen tree is a native of the West Indies and the northern coastal regions of South America. The tree grows to a height of 40-60 feet and produces striking, deep blue flowers. The part used in homoeopathy is a resin obtained from the wood. The wood is unusual in being very dense, which means that it sinks in water, and this property caused much interest when it was first discovered in the Middle Ages. The resin is obtained by firing the cut log, and the melted resin then flows out of a hole made in the wood and is collected. This is allowed to cool and harden, and it is usually exported in large blocks that split readily into glassy fragments. The remedy is used to treat inflammation of the pharynx (pharyngitis) and tonsillitis, being very helpful in relieving painful soreness of the throat. It is particularly indicated where there is foul-smelling sputum and sweating. It is also a remedy for gout and rheumatic conditions with severe and stabbing joint pains. The symptoms are

made worse by extremes of heat and cold and damp weather, and also with movement. They may be relieved by rest and keeping warm.

Hamamelis virginiana

Hamamelis, witch hazel, spotted alder, snapping hazelnut, winterbloom

This plant is a native of the eastern United States and Canada but it is also grown in Europe. It is a shrub with grey-green leaves and yellow flowers that appear in the autumn. The part used in homoeopathy is the bark of stems and twigs and the outer part of the fresh root. This has the effect of causing body tissues, especially blood vessels, to contract, and it is used to arrest bleeding. Its curative properties were known to the native North American Indians, and it was first investigated and proved in homoeopathy by Dr Hering. Its main effect is on the blood circulation of the veins, particularly when the walls of the vessels are inflamed and weakened, and bleeding does not stop easily. It is used as a remedy for haemorrhoids, or piles with bleeding, varicose veins and ulcers, phlebitis (inflamed veins), nosebleeds, heavy periods, internal bleeding and pain associated with bruising or bleeding. Some headaches are helped by Hamamelis and, also, mental symptoms of depression, irritability and impatience. The symptoms are made worse by warmth and moisture and with physical activity. They improve out in the fresh air and for concentrating on a particular task or event and for conversation, thinking and reading.

Hepar sulphuris calcareum

Hepar sulph.; sulphide of calcium

This remedy is impure calcium sulphide, which is obtained by heating crushed and powdered oyster shells with flowers of sulphur. This is an old remedy that was, at one time, applied externally to treat swellings caused by tuberculosis, gout, rheumatism and thyroid disorders (goitre) and also itching skin. It was investigated and proved by Hahnemann as a remedy for the toxic effects of mercury, which was widely used by contemporary physicians. It is now used to treat infections and any condition where there is a discharge of foul-smelling pus. It is used to treat skin conditions where the skin is highly sensitive to touch, such as boils and acne, and also, tonsillitis, sinusitis, earache, sore throat, hoarseness and laryngitis, mouth ulcers and cold sores. A wheezing, croup-like type of cough or chesty cough that may develop into a cold or influenza is helped by Hepar sulph. This remedy helps those who, when ill, tend to produce bodily secretions that have an unpleasant sour smell. During illness, those who benefit from this remedy are irritable, difficult to please and easily offended. They are difficult patients who make unreasonable demands and hate noise or disturbance, being touched or cold air. Symptoms are worse for cold and for getting chilled when undressing during winter and for touch. They improve with warmth and warm applications and for covering the head and for eating a meal. People suitable for Hepar sulph. tend to be overweight, lethargic, with pale skin and often depressed. They feel that life has dealt with them harshly and feel the symptoms of illness and pain acutely. They may appear to be calm but tend to be anxious and restless.

Hypericum perforatum

Hypericum, St John's wort

A perennial herbaceous plant that is a native of Britain, Europe and Asia, but is cultivated throughout the world. It grows between one and three feet in height, producing elongated, oval dark green leaves that appear to be covered in minute spots or holes (hence *perforatum*, or perforate). In fact, these are minute oil-secreting glands that secrete a bright red solution. The large, bright yellow flowers appear in June, July and August and have small black dots around the edges of the petals. The crushed flowers produce a blood-coloured juice that was used, in early times, to treat raw wounds. It was also believed that the plant could be hung up to ward off evil spirits (the name *Hypericum* being derived from the Greek, meaning 'over an apparition'). There are two traditions associated with the common name, St John's wort. One links the plant with 29 August, believed to be the anniversary of the execution of St John the Baptist. The other is that the plant is named after an ancient order of knights going back to the time of the Crusades, the knights of St John of Jerusalem.

The whole fresh green plant and flowers are used in homoeopathy to produce the mother tincture. It is mainly used to treat damage to nerves and nerve pain following accidental injury. Typically, there are shooting, stabbing pains that radiate upwards, and it is indicated especially where there are many nerve endings concentrated in a particular part of the body, e.g. the fingers and toes. It is very effective in pains associated with the spinal nerves and spinal cord, concussion, head or eye injuries. It is also a remedy for wounds and lacerations producing stabbing pains indicating nerve damage, and accidental crushing injuries. It is useful for bites, stings, splinters and puncture wounds, toothache and pain following dental extractions. In addition, it is a treatment for asthma and some digestive complaints of indigestion, sickness and diarrhoea. It is sometimes helpful in the treatment of piles, or haemorrhoids, and some menstrual problems with accompanying headache. The symptoms are made worse by cold, damp or foggy weather, before a storm and getting chilled when undressing. Also for touch and for a close, stuffy atmosphere. Symptoms improve when the person remains still and tilts the head backwards.

Ignatia amara

Agnate; *Strychnos ignatii*, St Ignatius' bean

Ignatia amara is a large tree that is native to the Philippine Islands, China and the East Indies. The tree has many branches and twining stems and produces stalked white flowers. Later, seed pods are produced, each containing ten to twenty large, oval seeds, that are about one inch long and are embedded in pulp. The seeds are highly poisonous and contain strychnine, which affects the central nervous system. Similar active constituents and properties are found in nux vomica. The tree is named after the founder of the Jesuits, Ignatius Loyola (1491-1556), and Spanish priests belonging to this order brought the seeds to Europe during the 1600s. The homoeopathic remedy is made from the powdered seeds and is used especially for emotional symptoms. It is used for grief, bereavement, shock and loss, particularly when a person is having difficulty coming to terms with his or her feelings and is inclined to suppress the natural responses. Accompanying symptoms include sleeplessness, anger and hysteria. Similar emotional and psychological problems are helped by this remedy, including anxiety and fear, especially of appearing too forward to others, a tendency to burst into fits of crying, self-doubt, pity and blame, and depression. Nervous tension headaches and digestive upsets, feverish symptoms, chills and pains in the abdomen may be helped by Ignatia. Some problems associated with menstruation, especially sharp pains or absence of periods are relieved by this remedy, as are conditions with changeable symptoms. These are worse in cold weather or conditions, with emotional trauma, being touched, for smoking and drinking coffee. They improve with warmth, moving about, eating, lying on the side or area that is painful and after passing urine.

The person for whom Ignatia is suitable is usually female and with a tendency towards harsh, self criticism and blame; she is usually a creative artistic person, highly sensitive but with a tendency to suppress the emotions. She is perceptive and intelligent but inclined to be hysterical and subject to erratic swings of mood. Typically, the person expects a high standard in those she loves. The person enjoys dairy products, bread and sour foods but sweets, alcoholic drinks and fruit upset her system. She is afraid of crowds, tends to be claustrophobic, and fears being burgled. Also, she is afraid of being hurt emotionally, and is very sensitive to pain. The person is usually dark-haired and of slim build with a worried expression and prone to sighing, yawning and excessive blinking.

Ipecacuanha

Ipecac.; *Cephaelis ipecacuanha, Psychotria ipecacuanha*, the ipecac plant

This plant is a native of South America, particularly Brazil, Bolivia and New Grenada. The plant contains the alkaloids emetine and cephaeline, and different varieties contain differing proportions of these alkaloids. The root is the part used in homoeopathy, and the preparations may be in a number of different forms. It is used to treat conditions where the main symptoms are nausea and vomiting, which are intractable and persistent, e.g. motion sickness and morning sickness. It is also used as a remedy for bronchitis, breathlessness because of the presence of fluid in the lung, whooping cough and heart failure. The symptoms are made worse by cold weather and lying down, and after a meal of pork or veal. They improve in the fresh open air and while resting with the eyes shut.

Kalium bichromicum

Kali bich.; potassium dichromate, potassium bichromate

This substance has several uses in industry (e.g. in the preparations of dyes and in batteries) as well as its medicinal purposes. The crystals of potassium dichromate are bright orange and are prepared from a chemical reaction involving the addition of a solution of potassium chromate to an acid. It is used for discharges of mucus and disorders of the mucous membranes, particularly involving the vagina and genital and urinary tracts, throat, nose and stomach. The remedy is useful for catarrhal colds and sinusitis, feelings of fullness and pressure, headache, migraine and glue ear. Also, for joint and rheumatic disorders with pains that may move about or even disappear. People who benefit from this remedy are highly sensitive to cold and chills when ill, but also experience a worsening of symptoms in hot, sunny conditions. They tend to be people who adhere very closely to a regular routine and may be somewhat rigid and inflexible. They like everything to be done properly down to the smallest detail and are law-abiding, moral and conformist. Symptoms are worse during the summer and also in wet and chilly conditions. They are at their height in the early hours of the morning between 3 and 5 a.m., and also on first waking up. Drinking alcohol and becoming chilled while taking off clothes exacerbates the symptoms. They improve with moving around and after eating a meal. Also, symptoms improve with warmth and heat (but not hot sun) and after vomiting.

Kalium iodatum

Kali iod.; *Kali hydriodicum*, potassium iodide

This is prepared by chemical reaction from potassium hydroxide and iodine and is an old remedy for syphilis. It is recommended that potassium iodide should be added to animal feed concentrates and table salt to prevent deficiency in iodine. The homoeopathic remedy is used to relieve catarrh in those who are prone to chesty conditions. It is also used to treat swollen glands, sore throats, sinusitis, hay fever and influenza-type infections. It is used to treat male prostate gland disorders. The symptoms tend to improve with movement and from being out in the fresh air. They are made worse by heat and touch and are at their most severe between two and five in the early morning. People who suit this remedy tend to be dogmatic, knowing exactly what they think about a particular subject. They may be irritable or bad-tempered and not easy to get along with. They have a preference for cool rather than warm or hot weather.

Kalium phosphoricum

Kali phos.; potassium phosphate, phosphate of potash

This remedy is one of the SCHUSSLER TISSUE SALTS (*see* GLOSSARY), and it is obtained from a chemical reaction between dilute phosphoric acid and solution of potassium carbonate. Potassium carbonate is derived from potash, the white powder that is left when wood is burnt completely. Potassium is an essential element in the body, vital for the healthy functioning of nerve tissue. Kali phos. is used to treat mental and physical exhaustion and depression, particularly in young persons in whom it may have been caused by too much work or studying. Accompanying symptoms include jumping at noise or interruption and a desire to be alone. Also, there may be a pus-containing discharge from the bladder, vagina, bowels or lungs and extreme muscular fatigue. They may suffer from gnawing hunger pains, anxiety, insomnia, tremor and have a tendency to perspire on the face when excited or after a meal. People who are suitable for Kali phos. are usually extrovert, hold clearly formed ideas and are easily exhausted. They become distressed by bad news, including that which does not affect them directly, such as a disaster in another country. They tend to crave sweet foods and dislike bread. Symptoms are made worse by any anxiety, in cold, dry weather and in winter and on drinking cold drinks. Also, they are exacerbated by noise, conversation, touch and physical activity. Symptoms improve with heat, gentle exercise, in cloudy conditions and after eating.

Lachesis

Trigonocephalus lachesis, Lachesis muta,
venom of the bushmaster or surukuku snake
This South African snake produces a deadly venom that may prove instantly fatal because of its effects upon the heart. The venom causes the blood to thin and flow more freely, hence increasing the likelihood of haemorrhage. Even a slight bite bleeds copiously with a risk of blood poisoning or septicaemia. The snake is a ferocious hunter, and its African name, surukuku, describes the sound it makes while in pursuit of prey. The properties of the venom were investigated by the eminent American homoeopathic doctor Constantine Hering during the 1800s. He tested and proved the remedy on himself. It is effective in treating a variety of disorders, particularly those relating to the blood circulation and where there is a risk of blood poisoning, or septicaemia. It is used to treat varicose veins and problems of the circulation indicated by a bluish tinge to the skin. The remedy is useful for those suf-

fering from a weak heart or angina, palpitations and an irregular, fast or weak pulse. There may be symptoms of chest pain and breathing difficulty. It is of great benefit in treating uterine problems, particularly premenstrual congestion and pain that is relieved once the period starts. It is also an excellent remedy for menopausal symptoms, especially hot flushes, and for infections of the bladder and rectum. It is used to treat conditions and infections where symptoms are mainly on the left side, such as headache or stroke. Also, as a treatment for sore throats and throat infections, tonsillitis, lung abscess, boils, ulcers, wounds that heal slowly, vomiting because of appendicitis and digestive disorders, fevers with chills and shivering, nosebleeds and bleeding piles.

It is used to treat severe symptoms of measles and serious infections including scarlet fever and smallpox. Symptoms are made worse by touch and after sleep and by tight clothing. They are worse for hot drinks and baths, exposure to hot sun or direct heat in any form. For women, symptoms are worse during the menopause. They improve for being out in the fresh air and drinking cold drinks and for release of normal bodily discharges. People suitable for Lachesis tend to be intelligent, creative, intense and ambitious. They have strong views about politics and world affairs and may be impatient of the views of others. They may be somewhat self-centred, possessive and jealous, which can cause problems in close relationships with others. They dislike being tied down and so may be reluctant to commit themselves to a relationship. Lachesis people have a liking for sour pickled foods, bread, rice and oysters and alcoholic drinks. They like coffee, but hot drinks and wheat-based food tends to upset them. They have a fear of water, people they do not know, being burgled and of dying or being suffocated. Lachesis people may be somewhat overweight and are sometimes red-haired and freckled. Alternatively, they may be thin and dark-haired, pale and with a lot of energy. Children tend to be somewhat jealous of others and possessive of their friends, which can lead to naughty or trying behaviour.

Ledum palustre

Ledum; marsh tea, wild rosemary
Wild rosemary is an evergreen shrub that grows in the bogs and cold upland conditions of the northern United States, Canada and northern Europe, especially Scandinavia, Ireland and

parts of Asia. The bush produces elongated, dark green leaves, about one or two inches long, that are smooth and shiny on the upper surface but underneath are covered with brown woolly hairs. ('Ledum' is derived from the Greek word *ledos*, meaning 'woolly robe'). The leaves contain a volatile, aromatic oil like camphor, and the plant has been used for centuries by Scandinavian people to repel insects, moths and mice. The plant produces attractive white flowers and is valued for its antiseptic properties. The fresh parts of the plant are gathered, dried and ground to make a powder used in homoeopathy, and it is a valuable first aid remedy. It is taken internally for animal bites, insect stings, lacerations and wounds in which there is bruising and sharp stabbing pains. There is usually inflammation, redness, swelling and throbbing accompanied by feverish symptoms of chills and shivering. It is additionally used as a remedy for gout in the big toe, rheumatic pains in the feet that radiate upwards, hot, painful, stiff joints and tendons but with cold skin. People who benefit from this remedy tend to get hot and sweaty at night when ill, and usually throw off the bed coverings. They often have itchy skin on the feet and ankles and have a tendency to sprain their ankles. When ill, they are irritable and hard to please or may be withdrawn, and do not want the company of others. The symptoms are made worse by warmth or heat, touch and at night. They improve with cold applications to the painful part and for cool conditions.

Lycopodium clavatum

Lycopodium; club moss, wolf's claw,
vegetable sulphur, stag's-horn moss, running pine

This plant is found throughout the northern hemisphere, in high moorlands, forests and mountains. The plant produces spore cases on the end of upright forked stalks, which contain the spores. These produce yellow dust or powder that is resistant to water and was once used as a coating on pills and tablets to keep them separate from one another. The powder was also used as a constituent of fireworks. It has been used medicinally for many centuries, as a remedy for digestive disorders and kidney stones in Arabian countries and in the treatment of gout. The powder and spores are collected by shaking the fresh, flowering stalks of the plant, and its main use in homoeopathy is for digestive and kidney disorders. It is used to treat indigestion, heartburn, the effects of eating a large meal late at night, sickness, nausea, wind, bloatedness and constipation. Also, in men, for kidney stones, with the production of a red-coloured urine containing a sand-like sediment and enlarged prostate gland. It is used in the treatment of some problems of male impotence and bleeding haemorrhoids, or piles. Symptoms that occur on the right side are helped by Lycopodium, and the patient additionally tends to crave sweet, comfort foods. Nettle rash, psoriasis affecting the hands, fatigue because of illness and ME (myalgic encephalomyelitis), some types of headache, cough and sore throat are relieved by this remedy. It is used to relieve emotional states of anxiety, fear and apprehension caused by chronic insecurity or relating to forthcoming events, such as taking an examination or appearing in public (stage fright). Also, night terrors, sleeplessness, shouting or talking in the sleep and being frightened on first waking up can all benefit from this treatment.

The symptoms are worse between 4 p.m. and 8 p.m. and in warm, stuffy rooms and with wearing clothes that are too tight. They are also worse in the early morning between 4 a.m. and 8 a.m., for eating too much and during the spring. They improve outside in cool fresh air, after a hot meal or drink and with loosening tight clothing, with light exercise and at night. People suitable for Lycopodium tend to be serious, hard-working and intelligent, often in professional positions. They seem to be self-possessed and confident but are in reality rather insecure with a low self-opinion. They are impatient of what they perceive as being weakness and are not tolerant or sympathetic of illness. Lycopodium people are sociable but may keep their distance and not get involved; they may be sexually promiscuous. They have a great liking for sweet foods of all kinds and enjoy hot meals and drinks. They are easily filled but may carry on eating regardless of this and usually complain of symptoms on the right side. Lycopodium people are afraid of being left on their own, of failure in life, of crowds, darkness and the supernatural, and tend to be claustrophobic. They are often tall, thin and pale with receding hair or hair that turns grey early in life. They may be bald, with a forehead lined with worry lines and a serious appearance. They tend to have weak muscles and are easily tired after physical exercise. They may have a tendency to unconsciously twitch the muscles of the face and to flare the nostrils.

Mercurius solubilis

Merc. sol.; quicksilver

The mineral cinnabar, which is found in volcanic crystalline rocks, is an important ore of mercury and is extracted for a variety of uses, including dental fillings and in thermometers. Mercury is toxic in large doses, and an affected person produces great quantities of saliva and suffers repeated bouts of vomiting. Mercury has been used since ancient times and was once given as a remedy for syphilis. A powder of precipitate of mercury is obtained from dissolving liquid mercury in a dilute solution of nitric acid, and this is the source of the remedy used in homoeopathy. It is used as a remedy for conditions that produce copious bodily secretions that often smell unpleasant, with accompanying symptoms of heat or burning and a great sensitivity to temperature. It is used as a remedy for fevers with profuse, unpleasant sweating, bad breath, inflammation of the gums, mouth ulcers, candidiasis (fungal infection) of the mouth, infected painful teeth and gums, and excessive production of saliva. Also, for a sore infected throat, tonsillitis, mumps, discharging infected ear, and a congested severe headache and pains in the joints. It is good for eye complaints, including severe conjunctivitis, allergic conditions with a running nose, skin complaints that produce pus-filled pustules, spots, and ulcers, including varicose ulcers. The symptoms are made worse by extremes of heat and cold and also by wet and rapidly changing weather. They are worse at night and for sweating and being too hot in bed.

Symptoms improve with rest and in comfortable temperatures where the person is neither too hot nor too cold. People suitable for Merc. sol. tend to be very insecure although they have an outwardly calm appearance. They are cautious and reserved with other people and consider what they are about to say before speaking so that conversation may seem laboured. Merc. sol. types do not like criticism of any kind and may suddenly become angry if someone disagrees with their point of view. They tend to be introverted, but their innermost thoughts may be in turmoil. They tend to be hungry and enjoy bread and butter, milk and other cold drinks but dislike alcohol with the exception of beer. They usually do not eat meat and do not have a sweet tooth. They dislike coffee and salt. Merc. sol. people often have fair hair with fine, unlined skin and an air of detachment. They are afraid of dying and of mental illness leading to insanity, and worry about the wellbeing of their family. They fear being burgled and are afraid or fearful during a thunderstorm.

Natrum muriaticum

Natrum mur.; common salt, sodium chloride

Salt has long been prized for its seasoning and preservative qualities, and Roman soldiers were once paid in salt, such was its value (the word 'salary' comes from the Latin word *salarium*, which refers to this practice). Sodium and chlorine are essential chemicals in the body, being needed for many metabolic processes, particularly the functioning of nerve tissue. In fact, there is seldom a need to add salt to food as usually enough is present naturally in a healthy, well-balanced diet. (An exception is when people are working very hard physically in a hot climate and losing a lot of salt in sweat). However, people and many other mammals frequently have a great liking for salt. If the salt/water balance in the body is disturbed, a person soon becomes very ill and may even die.

In ancient times, salt was usually obtained by boiling sea water, but natural evaporation around the shallow edges of salt lakes results in deposits of rock salt being formed. Rock salt is the usual source of table salt and also of the remedy used in homoeopathy. This remedy has an effect on the functioning of the kidneys and the salt/water balance of body fluids, and is used to treat both mental and physical symptoms. Emotional symptoms that benefit from Natrum mur. include sensitivity and irritability, tearfulness and depression, suppressed grief and premenstrual tension. Physical ailments that respond to this remedy are often those in which there is a thin, watery discharge of mucus and in which symptoms are made worse by heat. Hence Natrum mur. is used in the treatment of colds with a runny nose or other catarrhal problems. Also, for some menstrual and vaginal problems, headaches and migraines, cold sores, candidiasis (fungal infection) of the mouth, mouth ulcers, inflamed and infected gums and bad breath. Some skin disorders are helped by Natrum mur., including verruca (a wart on the foot), warts, spots and boils, and cracked, dry lips. It may be used in the treatment of fluid retention with puffiness around the face, eyelids and abdomen, etc, urine retention, constipation, anal fissure, indigestion, anaemia and thyroid disorders (goitre). When ill, people who benefit from this remedy feel cold and shivery, but their symptoms are made worse, or even brought on, by heat. Heat, whether from hot sun and fire or a warm, stuffy room, exacerbate the symptoms, which also are made worse by cold and thundery weather. They are worse on the coast from the sea breeze, and in the morning between 9 and 11 o'clock. Too much physical activity and the sympathy of others exacerbate the symptoms. They improve in the fresh, open air and for cold applications or a cold bath or swim. Also, sleeping on a hard bed and sweating and fasting make the symptoms better. People suitable for Natrum mur. are often women who are highly sensitive, serious-minded, intelligent and reliable. They have high ideals and feel things very deeply, being easily hurt and stung by slights and criticism. They need the company of other people but, being so sensitive, can actually shun them for fear of being hurt. They are afraid of mental illness leading to loss of self-control and insanity, and of dying. Also, they fear the dark, failure in work, crowds, being burgled and have a tendency to be claustrophobic. They worry about being late and are fearful during a thunderstorm. Merc. sol. people tend to become introverted and react badly to the criticism of others. They are highly sensitive to the influence of music, which easily moves them to tears. Natrum mur. people are usually of squat or solid build with dark or fairish hair. They are prone to reddened, watery eyes as though they have been crying, and a cracked lower lip. The face may appear puffy and shiny with an air of stoicism.

Nux vomica

Strychnos nux vomica; poison nut, Quaker buttons

The Strychnos nux vomica tree is a native of India but also grows in Burma, Thailand, China and Australia. It produces small, greenish-white flowers and, later, apple-sized fruits, containing small, flat, circular pale seeds covered in fine hair. The seeds, bark and leaves are highly poisonous, containing strychnine, and have been used in medicine for many centuries. In medieval times, the seeds were used as a treatment for the plague. Strychnine has severe effects upon the nervous system but in minute amounts can help increase urination and aid digestion. The seeds are cleaned and dried and used to produce the homoeopathic remedy. Nux vomica is used in the treatment of a variety of digestive complaints, including cramping, colicky abdominal pains, indigestion, nausea and vomiting, diarrhoea and constipation. Also, indigestion or stomach upset caused by overindulgence in alcohol or rich food and piles, which cause painful contractions of the rectum. Sometimes these complaints are brought on by a tendency to keep emotions, particularly anger, suppressed and not allowing it to show or be expressed outwardly. Nux vomica is a remedy for irritability, headache and migraine, colds, coughs and influenza-like symptoms of fever, aching bones and muscles and chills and shivering. It is a useful remedy for women who experience heavy, painful periods that may cause fainting, morning sickness during pregnancy and pain in labour. It is also used to treat urinary frequency and cystitis.

The type of person who benefits from this remedy is frequently under stress and experiences a periodic flare-up of symptoms. The person may be prone to indigestion and heartburn, gastritis and stomach ulcer, and piles, or haemorrhoids. The person usually has a tendency to keep everything bottled up but has a passionate nature and is liable to outbursts of anger. Nux vomica people are very ambitious and competitive, demanding a high standard of themselves and others and intolerant of anything less than perfection. They enjoy challenges and using their wits to keep one step ahead. Often they are to be found as managers, company directors, scientists, etc, at the cutting edge of their particular occupation. They are ungracious and irritable when ill and cannot abide the criticism of others. This type of person is afraid of being a failure at work and fears or dislikes crowded public places. He or she is afraid of dying. The person enjoys rich, fattening foods containing cholesterol and spicy meals, alcohol and coffee, although these upset the digestive system. Symptoms are worse in cold, windy, dry weather and in winter and in the early morning between 3 and 4 a.m. They are aggravated by certain noises, music, bright lights and touch, eating (especially spicy meals) and overwork of mental faculties. Nux vomica people usually look serious, tense and are thin with a worried expression. They have sallow skin and tend to have dark shadows beneath the eyes.

Phosphorus

Phos; white phosphorus

Phosphorus is an essential mineral in the body found in the genetic material (DNA), bones and teeth. White phosphorus is extremely flammable and poisonous and was once used in the manufacture of matches and fireworks. As it tends to catch fire spontaneously when exposed to air, it is stored under water. In the past it has been used to treat a number of disorders and infectious diseases such as measles. In homoeopathy, the remedy is used to treat nervous tension caused by stress and worry, with symptoms of sleeplessness, exhaustion and digestive upset. Often there are pains of a burning nature in the chest or abdomen. It is a remedy for vomiting and nausea, heartburn, acid indigestion, stomach ulcer and gastroenteritis. It is also used to treat bleeding, e.g. from minor wounds, the gums, nosebleeds, gastric and profuse menstrual bleeding.

Severe coughs, which may be accompanied by retching, vomiting and production of a blood-tinged phlegm, are treated with Phos. as well as some other severe respiratory complaints. These include pneumonia, bronchitis, asthma and laryngitis. Styes that tend to recur and poor circulation may be helped by Phos. Symptoms are worse in the evening and morning and before or during a thunderstorm. They are also made worse for too much physical activity, hot food and drink and lying on the left side. Symptoms improve in the fresh open air and with lying on the back or right side. They are better after sleep or when the person is touched or stroked. People who need Phos. do not like to be alone when ill and improve with the sympathy and attention of others. They are warm, kind, affectionate people who are highly creative, imaginative and artistic. They enjoy the company of other people and need stimulation to give impetus to their ideas. Phos. people have an optimistic outlook, are full of enthusiasm but sometimes promise much and deliver little. They are very tactile and like to be touched or stroked and offered sympathy when unhappy or unwell. They enjoy a variety of different foods but tend to suffer from digestive upsets. Phos. people are usually tall, slim and may be dark or fair-haired, with an attractive, open appearance. They like to wear brightly coloured clothes and are usually popular. They have a fear of illness, especially cancer, and of dying and also of the dark and supernatural forces. They are apprehensive of water and fear being a failure in their work. Thunderstorms make them nervous.

Pulsatilla nigricans

Pulsatilla, *Anemone pratensis*, meadow anemone

This attractive plant closely resembles *Anemone pulsatilla*, the pasqueflower, which is used in herbal medicine but has smaller flowers. *Anemone pratensis* is a native of Germany, Denmark and Scandinavia and has been used medicinally for hundreds of years. The plant produces beautiful deep purple flowers with orange centres and both leaves and flowers are covered with fine, silky hairs. The whole fresh plant is gathered and made into a pulp, and liquid is extracted to make the homoeopathic remedy. It is used to treat a wide variety of disorders with both physical and mental symptoms. It is useful for ailments in which there is a greenish, yellowish discharge. Hence it is used for colds and coughs and sinusitis with the production of profuse catarrh or phlegm. Also, eye infections with discharge such as styes and conjunctivitis. Digestive disorders are helped by it, particularly indigestion, heartburn, nausea and sickness caused by eating too much fatty or rich food. The remedy is helpful for female disorders in which there are a variety of physical and emotional symptoms. These include premenstrual tension, menstrual problems, menopausal symptoms and cystitis, with accompanying symptoms of mood swings, depression and tearfulness. It is a remedy for headaches and migraine, swollen glands, inflammation and pain in the bones and joints as in rheumatic and arthritic disorders, nosebleeds, varicose veins, mumps, measles, toothache, acne, frequent urination and incontinence.

Symptoms are worse at night or when it is hot, and after eating heavy, rich food. Symptoms improve out in the cool fresh air and for gentle exercise such as walking. The person feels better after crying and being treated sympathetically by others. Pulsatilla people are usually women who have a mild, passive nature and are kind, gentle and loving. They are easily moved to tears by the plight of others and love animals and people alike. The person yields easily to the requests and demands of others and is a peacemaker who likes to avoid a scene. An outburst of anger is very much out of character, and a Pulsatilla person usually has many friends. The person likes rich and sweet foods, although these may upset the digestion, and dislikes spicy meals. Pulsatilla people may fear darkness, being left alone, dying and any illness leading to insanity. They are fearful of crowds, the supernatural and tend to be claustrophobic. Usually, they are fair and blue-eyed with clear, delicate skin that blushes readily. They are attractive and slightly overweight or plump.

Rhus toxicodendron

Rhus tox.; *Rhus radicaris*, American poison ivy, poison oak, poison vine.

This large bush or small tree is a native species of the United States and Canada. Its leaves are extremely irritant to the touch, causing an inflamed and painful rash, swelling and ulceration. Often the person experiences malaise, swollen glands, headache, feverishness and a lack of appetite. The plant produces white flowers with a green or yellow tinge in June, followed later by clusters of berries. The fresh leaves are gathered and pulped to make the remedy used in homoeopathy. It is used especially as a treatment for skin rashes and lesions with hot, burning sensations and also for inflammation of muscles and joints. Hence it is used to treat eczema, chilblains, cold sores, shingles, nappy rash and other conditions in which there is a dry, scaling or blistered skin. Also, for rheumatism, sciatica, lumbago, gout, synovitis (inflammation of the synovial membranes surrounding joints), osteoarthritis, ligament and tendon strains. Feverish symptoms caused by viral infections, such as high temperature, chills and shivering, swollen, watering eyes, aching joints, nausea and vomiting, may be helped by Rhus tox. Some menstrual problems, including heavy bleeding and abdominal pains that are relieved by lying down, benefit from this remedy. People who are helped by Rhus tox tend to be depressed and miserable when ill, with a tendency to burst into tears, and are highly susceptible to cold, damp weather. Usually they have a dry, irritating cough and thirst and are irritable, anxious and restless. The symptoms are made worse in stormy, wet, windy weather and at night, and when the person moves after a period of rest. Also, for becoming chilled when undressing. Warm, dry conditions and gentle exercise im-

prove and lessen the symptoms. Rhus tox people may be initially shy in company, but when they lose this are charming, entertaining and lively and make friends easily. They are usually conscientious and highly motivated and serious about their work to the extent of being somewhat workaholic. Rhus tox people often have an inner restlessness and become depressed and moody when affected by illness. They may be prone to carry out small compulsive rituals in order to function.

Ruta graveolens

Ruta grav.; rue, garden rue, herbygrass, avegrace, herb-of-grace, bitter herb

This hardy, evergreen plant is a native of southern Europe but has been cultivated in Britain for centuries, having been first brought here by the Romans. It thrives in poor soil in a dry and partially shaded situation, producing yellow-green flowers. The whole plant has a distinctive, pungent, unpleasant smell and was once used to repel insects, pestilence and infections. It has been used medicinally throughout history to treat ailments in both animals and people, and was used to guard against the plague. It was believed to be effective in guarding against witchcraft, and Hippocrates recommended it as an antidote to poisoning. Rue was believed to have beneficial effects on sight and was used by the great artists, such as Michelangelo, to keep vision sharp. In the Catholic High Mass, brushes made from rue were once used to sprinkle the holy water, hence the name herb-of-grace. Taken internally in large doses, rue has toxic effects causing vomiting, a swollen tongue, fits and delirium.

The homoeopathic remedy is prepared from the sap of the green parts of the plant before the flowers open. It is indicated especially for bone and joint injuries and disorders, and those affecting tendons, ligaments and muscles where there is severe, deep, tearing pain. Hence it is used for synovitis (inflammation of the synovial membranes lining joints), rheumatism, sprains, strains, bruising, fractures and dislocations and also sciatica. Also, it is a useful remedy for eyestrain with tired, aching eyes, redness and inflammation and headache. Chest problems may be relieved by Ruta grav., particularly painful deep coughs, and some problems affecting the rectum, such as prolapse. Pain and infection in the socket of a tooth after dental extraction may be helped by this remedy. A person who is ill and who benefits from

Ruta grav. tends to feel low, anxious, depressed and dissatisfied both with himself (or herself) and others. The symptoms are usually worse in cold, damp weather, for resting and lying down and for exercise out of doors. They improve with heat and gentle movement indoors.

Sepia officinalis
Sepia; ink of the cuttlefish

Cuttlefish ink has been used since ancient times, both for medicinal purposes and as a colour in artists' paint. The cuttlefish has the ability to change colour to blend in with its surroundings and squirts out the dark brown-black ink when threatened by predators. Sepia was known to Roman physicians who used it as a cure for baldness. In homoeopathy it is mainly used as an excellent remedy for women experiencing menstrual and menopausal problems. It was investigated and proved by Hahnemann in 1834. It is used to treat premenstrual tension, menstrual pain and heavy bleeding, infrequent or suppressed periods, menopausal symptoms such as hot flushes, and postnatal depression. Physical and emotional symptoms caused by an imbalance of hormones are helped by Sepia. Also, conditions in which there is extreme fatigue or exhaustion with muscular aches and pains. Digestive complaints, including nausea and sickness, abdominal pain and wind, caused by eating dairy products, and headaches with giddiness and nausea are relieved by Sepia. Also, it is a remedy for incontinence, hot, sweaty feet and verruca (a wart on the foot). A woman often experiences pelvic, dragging pains frequently associated with prolapse of the womb. Disorders of the circulation, especially varicose veins and cold extremities, benefit from sepia.

Symptoms are worse in cold weather and before a thunderstorm, and in the late afternoon, evening and early in the morning. Also, before a period in women and if the person receives sympathy from others. The symptoms are better with heat and warmth, quick vigorous movements, having plenty to do and out in the fresh open air. People suitable for Sepia are usually, but not exclusively, women. They tend to be tall, thin and with a yellowish complexion, and are rather self-contained and indifferent to others. Sepia people may become easily cross, especially with family and close friends, and harbour resentment. In company, they make a great effort to appear outgoing and love to dance. A woman may be either an ex-ternally hard, successful career person or someone who constantly feels unable to cope, especially with looking after the home and family. Sepia people have strongly held beliefs and cannot stand others taking a contrary opinion. When ill, they hate to be fussed over or have the sympathy of others. They like both sour and sweet foods and alcoholic drinks but are upset by milk products and fatty meals. They harbour deep insecurity and fear being left alone, illness resulting in madness, and loss of their material possessions and wealth. One physical attribute is that they often have a brown mark in the shape of a saddle across the bridge of the nose.

Silicea terra
Silicea; silica

Silica is one of the main rock-forming minerals and is also found in living things, where its main function is to confer strength and resilience. In homoeopathy, it is used to treat disorders of the skin, nails and bones and recurring inflammations and infections, especially those that occur because the person is somewhat rundown or has an inadequate diet. Also, some disorders of the nervous system are relieved by Silicea. The homoeopathic remedy used to be derived from ground flint or quartz but is now prepared by chemical reaction. The remedy is used for catarrhal infections such as colds, influenza, sinusitis, ear infections including glue ear. Also, for inflammations producing pus, such as a boil, carbuncle, abscess, stye, whitlow (infection of the fingernail) and peritonsillar abscess. It is beneficial in helping the natural expulsion of a foreign body, such as a splinter in the skin. It is a remedy for a headache beginning at the back of the head and radiating forwards over the right eye, and for stress-related conditions of overwork and sleeplessness.

Symptoms are worse for cold, wet weather, especially when clothing is inadequate, draughts, swimming and bathing, becoming chilled after removing clothes and in the morning. They are better for warmth and heat, summer weather, warm clothing, particularly a hat or head covering, and not lying on the left side. People who are suitable for Silicea tend to be thin with a fine build and pale skin. They often have thin straight hair. They are prone to dry, cracked skin and nails and may suffer from skin infections. Silicea people are usually unassuming, and lacking in confidence and physical stamina. They are conscientious and hard-working to the point of working too hard once a task has been undertaken. However, they may hesitate to commit themselves through lack of confidence and fear of responsibility. Silicea people are tidy and obsessive about small details. They may feel 'put upon' but lack the courage to speak out, and may take this out on others who are not responsible for the situation. They fear failure and dislike exercise because of physical weakness, often feeling mentally and physically exhausted. They enjoy cold foods and drinks.

Sulphur

Sulphur, flowers of sulphur, brimstone

Sulphur has a long history of use in medicine going back to very ancient times. Sulphur gives off sulphur dioxide when burnt, which smells unpleasant ('rotten eggs' odour) but acts as a disinfectant. This was used in mediaeval times to limit the spread of infectious diseases. Sulphur is deposited around the edges of hot springs and geysers and where there is volcanic activity. Flowers of sulphur, which is a bright yellow powder, is obtained from the natural mineral deposit and is used to make the homoeopathic remedy. Sulphur is found naturally in all body tissues, and in both orthodox medicine and homoeopathy is used to treat skin disorders. It is a useful remedy for dermatitis, eczema, psoriasis and a dry, flaky, itchy skin or scalp. Some digestive disorders benefit from it, especially a tendency for food to rise back up to the mouth and indigestion caused by drinking milk. Sulphur is helpful in the treatment of haemorrhoids, or piles, premenstrual and menopausal symptoms, eye inflammations such as conjunctivitis, pain in the lower part of the back, catarrhal colds and coughs, migraine headaches and feverish symptoms. Some mental symptoms are helped by this remedy, particularly those brought about by stress or worry, including depression, irritability, insomnia and lethargy. When ill, people who benefit from sulphur feel thirsty rather than hungry and are upset by unpleasant smells. The person soon becomes exhausted and usually sleeps poorly at night and is tired through the day. The symptoms are worse in cold, damp conditions, in the middle of the morning around 11 a.m., and in stuffy, hot, airless rooms. Also, for becoming too hot at night in bed and for wearing too many layers of clothes. Long periods of standing and sitting aggravate the symptoms, and they are worse if the person drinks alcohol or has a wash. Symptoms improve in dry, clear, warm weather and for taking exercise. They are better if the person lies on the right side.

Sulphur people tend to look rather untidy and have dry, flaky skin and coarse, rough hair. They may be thin, round-shouldered and inclined to slouch or be overweight, round and red-faced. Sulphur people have lively, intelligent minds full of schemes and inventions, but are often useless on a practical level. They may be somewhat self-centred with a need to be praised, and fussy over small unimportant details. They enjoy intellectual discussion on subjects that they find interesting and may become quite heated although the anger soon subsides. Sulphur people are often warm and generous with their time and money. They enjoy a wide range of foods but are upset by milk and eggs. They have a fear of being a failure in their work, of heights and the supernatural.

Tarentula cubensis

Tarentula cub.; Cuban tarantula

The bite of the Cuban tarantula spider produces a delayed response in the victim. About 24 hours after a bite, the site becomes inflamed and red, and swelling, fever and abscess follow. The homoeopathic remedy, made from the poison of the spider, is used to treat similar septic conditions, such as an abscess, boil, carbuncle or whitlow (an infection of the fingernail) and genital itching. Also, it is a remedy for anthrax and shock, and is of value as a last-resort treatment in severe conditions. The infected areas are often tinged blue, and there may be burning sensations of pain that are especially severe at night. It is of particular value in the treatment of recurring boils or carbuncles. The symptoms tend to improve with smoking and are made worse by physical activity and consuming cold drinks.

Thuja occidentalis

Thuja; tree of life, yellow cedar, arbor vitae, false white cedar

This coniferous, evergreen tree is a native species of the northern United States and Canada and grows to a height of about 30 feet. It has feathery green leaves with a strong, aromatic smell resembling that of camphor. The leaves and twigs were used by the Indian peoples to treat a variety of infections and disorders, and the plant has long been used in herbal medicine. It is an important remedy in aromatherapy. The fresh green leaves and twigs are used to prepare the homoeopathic remedy, which is especially valuable in the treatment of warts and wartlike tumours on any part of the body. It is a useful remedy for shingles and also has an effect on the genital and urinary tracts. Hence it is used to treat inflammations and infections such as cystitis and urethritis and also pain on ovulation. It may be given as a remedy for infections of the mouth, teeth and gums, catarrh and for tension headaches.

People who benefit from Thuja tend to sweat profusely, and it helps to alleviate this symptom. They tend to suffer from insomnia and when they do manage to sleep, may talk or cry out. They are prone to severe left-sided frontal headaches that may be present on waking in the morning. Symptoms are worse at night, from being too hot in bed and after breakfast. Also, at 3 a.m. and 3 p.m. and in weather that is cold and wet. Symptoms are felt more severely on the left side. Symptoms improve for movement and stretching of the limbs, massage and after sweating. People suitable for Thuja tend to be insecure and unsure about themselves. They try hard to please others but are very sensitive to criticism and soon become depressed. This may lead them to neglect their appearance. Thuja people are often thin and pale and tend to have greasy skin and perspire easily.

Urtica urens
Urtica; stinging nettle
One of the few plants that is familiar to all and that, for hundreds of years, has been valued for its medicinal and culinary uses. Nettles have always been used as a source of food both for people and animals, the young leaves being a nutritious vegetable with a high content of vitamin C. Nettles were thought to purify the blood, and an ancient cure for rheumatism and muscular weakness was the practice of 'urtication', or lashing the body with stinging nettles. The hairs covering the leaves of the nettle release a volatile liquid when touched, which causes the familiar skin reaction of painful, white bumps to appear. The fresh, green parts of the plant are used to prepare the homoeopathic remedy, which is used as a treatment for burning and stinging of the skin. Hence it is used to treat allergic reactions of the skin, urticaria, or nettle rash, insect bites and stings and skin lesions caused by burns and scalds. Also, for eczema, chicken pox, nerve inflammation and pain (neuritis and neuralgia), shingles, rheumatism, gout and cystitis in which there are burning, stinging pains. The person who benefits from this remedy is prone to inflamed, itching and irritated skin complaints and may be fretful, impatient and restless. Symptoms are made worse by touch and in cold, wet weather, snow and for contact with water. Allergic skin reactions may occur if the person eats shellfish such as prawns. The symptoms improve if the affected skin is rubbed and also if the person rests and lies down.

Minor Homoeopathic Remedies

Aethusa cynapium

Aethusa; fool's parsley, dog parsley, dog
  poison, lesser hemlock

This plant is a common weed that grows throughout most of Europe, including Great Britain. It resembles hemlock but is smaller and has three to five long, thin, leaflike bands that hang down beneath each flower head of small, white flowers. The leaves have an unpleasant smell although this is less strong than that of hemlock and is quite different from that of garden parsley. The plant is poisonous, although less potent than hemlock, and has effects on the digestive organs and nervous system. The green parts of the flowering plant are used in homoeopathy, and it is used especially to treat bouts of violent vomiting, particularly in babies with an allergy to milk. Accompanying symptoms include abdominal pains and diarrhoea. It is used to treat summer diarrhoea in children and also severe mental symptoms of confusion, fits and delirium. (These symptoms are produced in cases of poisoning with fool's parsley). It is used to help alleviate mental weakness and fatigue and inability to concentrate. Symptoms are made worse by heat, summer weather, in the evening and between 3 and 4 a.m. in the early morning. They improve out in the fresh open air and when the person has the company of others.

Agaricus muscarius

Agaricus; Amanita muscaria, common
  toadstool, fly agaric, bug agaric

This striking toadstool, with its bright red-orange cap studded with small white flakes, grows in damp, boggy, upland woods in Scotland, northern Europe, North America and Asia. It is deadly poisonous, and juice obtained from the fungus used to be extracted and used as a fly killer. It has effects on the mind and has been exploited for its hallucinogenic properties. These attributes mean that it must be handled with very great care and its use is banned in some countries. The whole fresh fungus is used to prepare the homoeopathic remedy, which is given for chilblains and itching, burning hot, swollen fingers and toes. Also, it is a remedy for epilepsy and disorders in which there are twitching, jerking spasms of muscles (chorea). It is given as a remedy for dizziness and unsteadiness, confusion, delirium tremens (alcoholism) and senile dementia. People who benefit from it feel the cold at all times but particularly acutely when not well. Symptoms are made worse by cold conditions or weather, thunderstorms and after a meal. They improve with gentle, slow movements.

Ailanthus olandulosa

Ailanthus; Ailanthus altissima, shade tree,
  Chinese sumach, copal tree, tree of heaven,
  tree of the gods, ailanto

A large, attractive tree that produces yellow-green flowers with a highly unpleasant smell. When inhaled, the scent causes digestive upset, and the fresh flowers are used to make the homoeopathic remedy. The tree is a native of China but was introduced into Britain during the 18th century as an ornamental species. It is used as a remedy for glandular fever in which there is a highly painful sore throat and swollen glands. The tonsils are red and inflamed and it is difficult to swallow. The person may have a severe headache and pains in the muscles. The symptoms are made worse by swallowing and bending the body forwards. Also, for lying down and during the morning, and for being exposed to light.

Aloe socotrina

Aloe; Aloe ferox, the common aloe

Aloes are succulent plants, and there are a number of species flourishing in the hotter climates of the world. Juice drained from the cut leaves is dried and made into a resin that is powdered to make the homoeopathic remedy. Aloe has been used in medicine for many centuries and was given by Greek and Roman physicians for digestive and abdominal disorders. In more recent times, it has been used as a medicine to purge the bowels.

Aloe was investigated and proved by Dr

Constantine Hering in the mid-1800s, and the remedy is used in homoeopathy for various congestive problems. These include headache, enlarged prostate gland in men, prolapsed uterus, haemorrhoids, or piles, diarrhoea and constipation and overindulgence in alcoholic drinks. Symptoms are made worse by heat and hot, dry summer weather. They are at their most severe in the very early morning and following meals and drinks. Symptoms improve in cold weather and for cold applications, and also for abdominal flatulence. People who are suitable for Aloe tend to be short-tempered and cross, feeling generally displeased with themselves and those around them. They frequently feel tired and unable to face up to their daily work, and symptoms are at their most severe when the person is constipated. Aloe types enjoy beer but it upsets their digestion.

Aluminium oxide

Alumina; oxide of aluminium

Aluminium is obtained from bauxite, a type of rock containing hydrated aluminium oxide. In conventional medicine, aluminium is used in indigestion remedies where there is an excess of stomach acid. The brain tissue of people suffering from Alzheimer's disease has been found to contain elevated levels of aluminium, and there is some concern that the metal may leach out from cooking utensils, especially when acid fruits are stewed. One of the main uses of the homoeopathic remedy is for the treatment of confusional states. It is also used to treat all ailments where there is a slowness or sluggishness in the system. The remedy is given for senile dementia, confusion and memory loss, constipation, poor co-ordination, and heaviness and deadness of the limbs, poor flow of urine, and giddiness when the eyes are closed. Symptoms are worse in the morning and for being out in the cold and also following meals that are high in carbohydrate and salt. People suitable for alumina are usually pale and thin with dry skin. They are pessimistic and gloomy, beset with feelings of impending disaster, and have a phobia about sharp, pointed objects such as knives. Alumina types may experience strange cravings for inappropriate substances to eat, but they do not like meat or beer.

Ammonium carbonicum

Ammon. carb.; ammonium carbonate, sal volatile

Ammonium carbonate was long in use in medi-

cine in the treatment of scarlet fever and as a constituent of smelling salts. The remedy was investigated and proved by Hahnemann in the 1800s and was found to be an effective treatment for a number of different disorders. The remedy is obtained from a chemical reaction between ammonium chloride and sodium carbonate. It is of particular value if the circulation is slow and if the heart is weak. It can be used to treat post-viral tiredness and ME (myalgic encephalomyelitis). The symptoms are made worse by prolonged exertion and cloudy, overcast weather. They improve in warm, dry weather and surroundings, by lying down with the feet higher than the head and by the application of pressure. People suitable for Ammon. carb. are usually of large build and soon feel tired. They tend to be short-tempered, irritable and are prone to forgetfulness and bouts of crying. They are especially sensitive to the effects of overcast, dull weather.

Ammonium muriaticum

Ammon. mur.; sal ammoniac, ammonium chloride

Ammonium chloride has been used since ancient times and was especially prized by alchemists. There used to be only one source of the substance, which was the Fire Mountain in central Asia, but it is now prepared by chemical reaction. Ammonium chloride is used in conventional medicine in remedies for colds and coughs, and it has several important industrial uses. It is a remedy for conditions in which there is a feeling of tightness and constriction. Ailments include coughs, bronchitis and pneumonia in which it feels as though there is a tight band around the chest, and with a sticky, thick mucus. Also for disorders affecting joints and tendons, backache, lumbago and sciatica with symptoms especially affecting the left side and being worse in the morning. Often the person experiences a frontal headache at the base of the nose and may have an irritated dry scalp and dandruff. Symptoms are worse in the early hours of the morning between 2 and 4 a.m. and also during the afternoon. They are better in the evening and night and improve for brisk exercise, especially out in the fresh air. The person who benefits from Ammon. mur. tends to be obese, although the limbs may appear to be thin, and has a puffy skin because of fluid retention. The metabolism is slow, and the circulation is sluggish and erratic, which may cause pains of a throbbing nature. Ammon. mur. people have a somewhat pessimistic outlook on life and cry easily, and tend to have a painful heel that may be caused by an ulcer. They may take an unreasonable dislike of some people and are afraid of the dark.

Amyl nitrosum

Amyl nitrate

This remedy is used for irregularities of heartbeat and anxiety. Symptoms include a racing heart (tachycardia), throbbing in the head and awareness of the heart rate with the sensation of the heart missing a beat and palpitations. There may be pain and numbness in the chest, which can spread to involve the arm and may be severe, as in angina. The person may experience hot flushes and sweats, especially if a woman going through the menopause. There is a feeling of fullness in the head and the person may flush easily.

Anacardium orientale

Anacard. or.; *Semecarpus anacardium*, cashew nut, marking nut

There are several products of the cashew nut tree that are useful to humans, and these have long been used for culinary and medicinal purposes. The nuts are gathered and eaten and used in cookery, and the fruits also are edible. The nut is surrounded by an inner and outer shell, and in between the two there is a thick, caustic, dark fluid that is the substance used in homoeopathy. This fluid causes blistering of the skin and has been used to treat warts, ulcers, corns, bunions and other lesions of the skin. The fluid was also used to make an indelible ink by mixing it with chalk, and this was employed to mark cloth (hence 'marking nut'). Arabian physicians used the juice for treating psychiatric and nervous system disorders, including convulsions, paralysis and dementia. The cashew nut tree has an attractive appearance, produces perfumed pink flowers, and is a native species of the East Indies and Asia. In homoeopathy, the remedy is used to treat symptoms of constriction, as though there are tight belts around the body. The person feels as though the digestive system is blocked by a plug, and there is pain, indigestion and constipation. Also, Anacard. or. is given for rheumatism and ulcers, and while symptoms are initially relieved by eating, they are worse once digestion is completed. Symptoms are worse late at night around midnight and for pressure and hot baths. They are relieved by fasting. People suitable for this remedy tend to be to-

tally lacking in self-confidence, feeling constantly inferior. They often have a poor memory and may be prone to mental disorders, particularly an inability to distinguish between reality and fantasy.

Antimonium tartaricum

Antim. tart.; tartar emetic, antimony potassium tartrate

This substance is important in the manufacture of textiles, being used to fix dyes used to colour materials. In orthodox medicine it has been used in cough remedies and as an emetic to cause vomiting. The homoeopathic remedy is obtained by means of a chemical reaction between potassium tartrate and antimony oxide. It is used in the treatment of bronchitis and conditions in which there is an accumulation of phlegm. Breathing is difficult and laboured, and the person has a wheezing cough that is ineffective in bringing up the accumulated fluid. It is useful for young children and elderly persons who are in a weakened condition and are not able to cough effectively. Also, it may be used as a remedy for a tension headache with a feeling of tight constriction around the head. The person generally does not feel thirsty and may have some puffiness of the skin because of fluid retention. The tongue appears to be thickly furred. Symptoms are made worse by exercise, lying flat, wet, cold conditions and in warm, stuffy, airless rooms. They are relieved by cold, dry air and resting by sitting propped up.

Apomorphia

Alkaloid of morphine

This is a remedy for severe and persistent vomiting accompanied by weakness, dizziness, fainting and sweating. Nausea may or may not be present. The vomiting may be the result of a number of different causes, such as the morning sickness of pregnancy. Additionally, it may be caused by overindulgence in alcohol or too much rich food or misuse of drugs.

Aranea diadema

Aranea diad.; *Aranea diadematus*, papal cross spider

This spider is widely found in many countries throughout the northern hemisphere. It has a spherical brown body marked with white spots on its back that form the shape of a crucifix. It is a web-spinning spider that paralyses its prey by biting and injecting a venom. The whole spider is used to prepare the homoeopathic remedy, which was first investigated and proved by von Grauvogl, a German doctor during the mid 1800s. He used it as a remedy for symptoms of cutting and burning neuralgic pains that are made worse by damp, cold conditions. It is used to treat any kind of neuralgic pains but especially those affecting the face. The pains usually arise suddenly and are intermittent and severe in nature, being hot and searing. There may also be sensations of numbness and symptoms are worsened by exposure to cold, damp conditions and any cold applications. They improve in warm, summer weather and with warm applications. Also, and most unusually, they are relieved by smoking.

Argentum metallicum
Argent. met.; silver

Silver is usually found in association with other metallic minerals in ore deposits in ancient rocks. It has been prized throughout human history and used to make jewellery, utensils, artistic ornamentation and has modern industrial uses, e.g. in photographic film. It is widely used in dentistry in fillings and is valued in conventional medicine for its antiseptic and astringent properties. The homoeopathic remedy is used for arthritic and rheumatic disorders, particularly those affecting the joints of the toes, ankles, fingers and wrists. The joints are painful, but usually the pain is intermittent in character and may disappear altogether for a time. Other types of pain from deep within the body may also be relieved by Argent. met. and also asthmatic and bronchitic symptoms and laryngitis. Symptoms are made worse for movement of the affected joints and also late in the morning towards midday. They improve with resting the affected part and being out in fresh clean air. Symptoms are better at night and for the application of gentle pressure.

Arsenicum iodatum
Arsen. iod.; iodide of arsenic

This homoeopathic remedy is obtained from a chemical reaction between iodine and metallic arsenic and was formerly used in the treatment of tuberculosis. It is used as a remedy for allergic conditions such as hay fever in which there is a copious watery discharge from the nose. Also, for bronchitis, psoriasis and eczema and hyperactivity in children. The symptoms are worse at night around midnight and are better if the person is out in the fresh, cool air.

Arum triphyllum
Arum triph.; jack-in-the-pulpit, Indian turnip, wild turnip, pepper turnip, dragon root, memory root

This is a common wild plant of North America and Canada, which has unusually shaped leaves that are borne on long stalks. It has a broad, flattened root that is highly irritant if eaten, causing severe symptoms of vomiting, nausea and diarrhoea and burning inflammation of the mucous membranes of the mouth and digestive tract. ('Arum' is derived from the Arabic word for 'fire', ar). The fresh root is used to make the homoeopathic remedy, which is used as a remedy for colds and hay fever with symptoms mainly on the left side. There may be cracking and bleeding of the skin around the nose and mouth and dry, sore lips. It is also given for hoarseness and laryngitis. Typically, there is a burning and profuse nasal discharge, and the person may feel hot and unwell. The symptoms may be caused by overuse of the voice, for instance if the person is a singer, or be brought on by exposure to the cold. Symptoms are made worse by cold weather, especially if exposed to biting winds, and also by lying down. They improve for drinking coffee and are also better in the morning.

Asafoetida
Ferula foetida, food of the gods, devil's dung

Ferula foetida is a large plant that is a native of eastern Iran and Afghanistan, and grows to a height of several feet. It has a thick and fleshy root, and when this is cut, a white, gumlike, milky fluid is exuded that hardens into resin. The sap of the plant smells rank and unpleasant and has an effect upon the digestive system. The hardened gum is made into a powder for use in homoeopathy, and it is used for digestive disorders and hysteria. It is a remedy for indigestion, abdominal pains and flatulence, bloatedness and hysterical symptoms.

Astacus fluviatilis
Crawfish

This homoeopathic remedy is used to treat allergic skin reactions that may have arisen as a result of eating shellfish. There is a raised, itchy skin rash (urticaria) and there may be a high temperature, malaise, chills and swollen glands. Symptoms are made worse by exposure to cold and draughts.

Avena sativa
Avena; wild oats

Oats have been cultivated for centuries as a nutritious source of food for both people and livestock. Oats are the only known food to reduce the level of cholesterol in the blood. The fresh green parts of the plant are used to make the homoeopathic remedy, and in both homoeopathy and herbal medicine the preparations are used to treat nervous complaints. The homoeopathic remedy is given as a treatment for nervous exhaustion, stress, sleeplessness and anxiety. It helps to relieve the nervous symptoms of those suffering from alcohol abuse and may be used to treat impotence. Symptoms are made worse by consumption of alcohol and relieved by a good night's sleep.

Baptisia tinctoria

Baptisia; wild indigo, indigo weed, horsefly weed, rattlebush

This is an herbaceous, perennial plant that grows throughout Canada and most of the United States in dry, upland, wooded habitats. It has a dark woody root that is pale on the inside with many small roots arising from it, and this is the part used in homoeopathy. The root was ground down and used by the Indian peoples both as a medicine and as a dye. ('Baptisia' is derived from the Greek word *bapto*, meaning 'to dye'). The plant grows to about three feet in height, producing yellow flowers in August and September. It is poisonous if eaten in large quantities but preparations of the root are valued for their antibacterial, antiseptic, astringent properties. In homoeopathy it is used to treat acute, severe infections and fevers. These include influenza, whooping cough, scarlet fever and typhoid fever. The person feels unwell and may be exhausted, confused and delirious with a discoloured tongue and bad breath. There may be diarrhoea with an offensive smell. Symptoms are made worse by hot, humid airless conditions and improve with gentle exercise in the fresh, open air, once the person is convalescent.

Baryta carbonica

Baryta carb., witherite, barium carbonate

The barium carbonate that is used to make the homoeopathic remedy is found as white crystals of witherite and barite in ancient rocks. Barium, which is derived from these minerals, is used in radiology and also in the manufacture of glassware. Witherite was once used medicinally to treat swollen glands and tuberculosis. In homoeopathy it is a useful remedy for children and elderly persons suffering from intellectual and, possibly, physical impairment. Children may have Down's syndrome or similar disorders, and often have a disproportionately large head and impairment of growth.

They tend to suffer from recurrent respiratory infections such as tonsillitis. Elderly persons who benefit from Baryta carb. may suffer from dementia or be physically and intellectually impaired because of an event such as a stroke. People suitable for this remedy are shy and unsure of themselves and they need a great deal of reassurance. They tend to be childlike, and need to be guided into making the right decisions. Symptoms are made worse by cold in any form, especially damp and chilly weather and biting cold winds. They improve with warmth in any form and with exercise in the open air. The person feels better if warm clothing is worn.

Bellis perennis

Bellis; the daisy, bruisewort, garden or common daisy

This little plant with its dark green leaves and white flowers with yellow centres, is so common as to be familiar to all. The leaves contain an acrid liquid that protects the plant from being eaten by insects or grazing animals. The daisy has a long history of medicinal use, having been used since mediaeval times to relieve bruising (hence bruisewort). The whole fresh flowering plant is used to make the homoeopathic remedy, which is mainly used to treat bruising, pain and inflammation following accidental injury, trauma or surgery. It is useful for the prevention of infection and in the treatment of boils and abscesses. Symptoms are more severe if the person becomes chilled when already too hot, and glands may be swollen. Arms and legs may feel cold or numb. Bellis may be given during pregnancy to relieve pains and cramps. Symptoms are made worse by chilling, becoming wet and for sweating and being too hot at night in bed. They improve with massage or rubbing of the painful area and for gentle exercise and movement.

Benzoicum acidum

Benz. ac.; benzoic acid

Benzoic acid is found naturally in a resinous substance, benzoin gum, that occurs in some plants. A combination of sodium and benzoic acid forms sodium benzoate, which is used in the preservation of food. The homoeopathic remedy is used for arthritic conditions and gout and also for urinary disorders, particularly kidney stones. There is a characteristic clicking of the joints in arthritic conditions and severe, searing pain. Urinary complaints are accompanied by the production of a dark urine that smells offensive and associated pain. The person is very sensitive to cold and often feels chilled. Benz. ac. may also be given as a treatment for menstrual disorders and a prolapsed uterus. Symptoms are made worse for getting cold while undressing or chilling because of winter weather or draughts. They improve with heat and hot applications to the painful part.

Berberis vulgaris

Berberis, barberry, pipperidge bush

Berberis is a common bushy shrub that grows throughout Europe, producing pale green leaves, yellow flowers and glossy red berries. The berries have always been valued for culinary purposes, and the plant also has a long history of medicinal use. The physicians of ancient Greece and Arabia used Berberis to treat feverish conditions, haemorrhage, gastroenteritis, dysentery and jaundice. In herbal medicine it is still used to treat jaundice, liver disorders, gallstones and digestive disorders. The fresh root of the plant is used to prepare the homoeopathic remedy, which is used in the treatment of kidney complaints accompanied by severe pain, such as renal colic and kidney stones. These complaints may be accompanied by the production of dark-coloured abnormal urine with an offensive odour. Also, it is used for gallstones, jaundice and biliary colic accompanied by the passing of pale faeces. People suitable for this remedy tend to have an unhealthy appearance, being pale with sunken features and dark shadows beneath the eyes. Symptoms may show rapid fluctuations and are made worse by prolonged standing. They are relieved for stretching exercise and gentle movements.

Borax

Borate of sodium

This homoeopathic remedy acts on the gastrointestinal tract and is used in the treatment of digestive disorders. It is particularly helpful as a remedy for pains, diarrhoea, nausea and vomiting. These may be accompanied by sweating, fever and giddiness. Symptoms are made worse by downward movements such as sitting or lying down.

Bothrops lanceolatus

Bothrops; *Lachesis lanceolatus*, fer-de-lance,
  yellow pit viper

This greyish-brown snake, marked with a diamond pattern, is a native animal of the Caribbean island of Martinique. It produces a deadly venom, and if a person receives a bite, the af-fected part swells and eventually becomes affected by gangrene. The venom of the snake is harvested and used to make the homoeopathic remedy, which is given for conditions of the blood such as haemorrhage and thrombosis. It is also used for strokes that affect the left side of the brain, producing symptoms of weakness and paralysis on the right side of the body and speech difficulty. People who need Bothrops are frequently exhausted, with slow, weary movements, and may be subject to tremor (involuntary trembling).

Bovista

Lycoperdon bovista; warted puffball,
  Lycoperdon giganteum

This fungus can be found in countries throughout Europe and has the shape of a round, white ball, varying in diameter from four inches to one foot. When the fungus is ripe, an irregular gash forms in its surface and dark browny/green spores are released. Young puffballs are eaten in some countries and they have a long history of use among country dwellers. The puffball was cut and applied to wounds to staunch bleeding and also burnt to produce a smoke that would stupefy bees so that honey could be collected from a hive. In homoeopathy, the remedy is used for speech disorders such as stammering and also for skin lesions, including eczema, blisters, warts, bunions, corns and nettle rash. These skin eruptions tend to weep and crust over and produce severe itching. Symptoms are made worse by heat and relieved by cold applications.

Bufo rana

Bufo, the common toad

This toad is found in many countries throughout the world and has a mottled brown and pale warty skin. When the toad is disturbed and feels threatened, it secretes a toxic irritant substance from pores in its skin, especially from the raised pouches above its eyes. This poisonous substance is noxious and prevents the toad from being eaten. It affects the mucous membranes of the mouth, throat, eyes, etc, and can produce quite severe symptoms, even in larger predators that might be tempted to attack the toad. The poison has a long history of use in Chinese medicine and is collected and prepared to make the homoeopathic remedy, which was first investigated and proved by the American homoeopath Dr James Tyler Kent. It is used to treat epilepsy, in which the person is disturbed by bright lights or music before the onset of a fit and moves the tongue rapidly (lapping). After the fit, the sufferer is left with a severe headache. Symptoms are made worse at night and for sleep and during menstruation in women. They are much better in the morning and after resting lying down. People who benefit from this remedy have a puffy appearance because of fluid retention. They are apt to lose their temper if unable to make their views understood.

Cactus grandiflorus

Cactus grand; *Selinecereus grandiflorus*, night-blooming cereus, sweet-scented cactus, vanilla cactus, large-flowered cactus

This plant grows in the parched, arid desert regions of South America, Mexico and the United States. It is a shrubby plant with thick fleshy stems and large white flowers with yellow centres. The flowers are about eight to twelve inches across and have a pleasant perfume resembling vanilla. They open in the evening and are closed during the day. The homoeopathic remedy is made from the fresh flowers and young stems, and it was investigated and proved in 1862 by Dr Rubins. He discovered that it produced effects on the heart with feelings of constriction and pain. Hence, the remedy is used to treat the unpleasant and frightening symptoms of angina. These include severe, gripping pain that is worse for physical exertion and stress, and a feeling of the chest being held and compressed by tight, constricting bands. There may be numbness, coldness and tingling in the left hand and arm and palpitations. The person feels extremely anxious and fears that death is imminent, and the pain is worse if he or she lies on the left side. Symptoms are worse from late morning until late evening and improve for lying on the right side with the head raised. A person with these symptoms needs reassurance and should not be left alone.

Calcarea hypophosphorosa

Hypophosphate of lime

This is a remedy for persons with the Calcarea constitutional type. The remedy is used for arthritic and rheumatic disorders, especially of the hands and wrists. The hands feel clammy and cold, and the symptoms are made worse by cold, damp weather. The person is very susceptible to cold and has a pale, chilly skin.

Calcarea iodata

Iodide of lime

A remedy for glandular swellings and infections in the neck, including tonsillitis, swollen adenoids and enlarged thyroid (goitre). It is also given for fibroids in the uterus and similar benign breast lumps of a fibrous nature.

Calcarea sulphurica

Calc. sulph.; calcium sulphate, plaster of Paris, gypsum

The source of calcium sulphate is the mineral deposit gypsum, which was formed as a precipitate when salt water evaporated. It is one of the SCHUSSLER TISSUE SALTS (*see* Glossary) and is used to make plaster casts for immobilizing fractured bones. It is a remedy for infected conditions of the skin in which pus is produced. Ailments include boils, carbuncles, skin ulcers and abscesses and infected eczema. The skin looks grey and unhealthy and feels cold and clammy although the soles of the feet may be hot. There may be yellow fur on the tongue, and the person may suffer from malaise and weakness. Symptoms are worse in weather that is wet and cold and improve in dry, fresh open air. They are also better for eating and for drinks of tea. A person suitable for Calc. sulph. has a tendency to be irritable and gloomy, with a jealous nature. Although symptoms are made worse by cold, Calc. sulph. people dislike heat and prefer to feel cool even to the extent of wearing inadequate clothing in winter weather.

Camphora

Camphor; *Laurus camphora*, gum camphor, laurel camphor

This remedy was investigated and proved by Hahnemann who used it to treat a cholera outbreak during the 1830s. The remedy was used again during a further epidemic in 1854 and proved to be highly successful on both occasions. Camphor is obtained from a tree that grows in central China and Japan. Chips of wood are heated with steam, and a liquid is collected from which clear deposits of camphor are precipitated out. Camphor has a characteristic pungent odour and has a range of applications in herbal medicine. In homoeopathy, it is used to treat acute conditions and fevers in which there is sweating, a cold clammy pale skin, chills and anxiety. There may be severe symptoms of very low blood pressure, collapse and convulsions. It is sometimes used in circumstances in which other homoeopathic remedies have failed to produce an improvement.

Capsicum frutescens

Capsicum; African pepper, red cayenne pepper, chilli pepper, bird pepper

The capsicum plant is a native of South America, West Indies and East Indies, but it is cultivated in many countries throughout the world. Elongated red chilli fruits, which may be used fresh or dried, are much used in Eastern cookery for their fiery properties. They cause sweating and a feeling of heat, dilate blood vessels and promote blood flow. They have been used to treat infectious disorders but are now mainly given for digestive symptoms. Cayenne is one of the most important remedies in herbal practice and is a constituent of many compound medicines. The fruits and seeds are used to prepare the homoeopathic remedy, which is used to treat ailments with hot, burning, stinging pains. It is used for indigestion, especially heartburn, piles, or haemorrhoids, diarrhoea, sore throat with painful burning sensation on swallowing, and rheumatic disorders. Symptoms are made worse by cool, draughty conditions and when the person first begins movement. They are made better for warmth and heat, and with sustained exercise and movement. People suitable for this remedy are often fair-haired and blue-eyed and tend to be obese. They are often unfit, disliking physical exercise. Overindulgence in alcohol or rich spicy foods makes them lazy and lethargic, and they tend to have a melancholy disposition. If they go away from home, they soon become depressed and homesick.

Carboneum sulphuratum
Carbon bisulphide

This remedy is used for ailments affecting the nerves, in which there may be weakness, numbness, tremor or paralysis. Also, for some disorders of the eye and vision and for indigestion, abdominal pains, wind, diarrhoea and constipation.

Caulophyllum thalictroides
Caulophyllum; papoose root, squawroot, blueberry root, blue cohosh

This is an attractive perennial plant that is a native species of Canada and North America, growing in moist conditions near creeks or in swamps. It produces greenish-yellow flowers in early summer and, later, large pea-sized seeds that were gathered, roasted and used by the Indian people to make a hot drink. The root of the plant is brown, gnarled and contorted, and this is the part that is used in homoeopathy. The preparation made from the root acts as a stimulant on the uterus, and this property was well known to the Indian people, who used the medicine to hasten a slow or painful labour. Caulophyllum was investigated and proved by an American homoeopathic doctor, Dr Hale, in the late 1800s, and one of its main uses in homoeopathy is to speed up and strengthen weak or painful ineffective contractions of the womb during labour. It is also used to treat absent menstruation and some other conditions of the uterus, such as menstrual and postpartum pain. Caulophyllum is an effective remedy for rheumatic disorders affecting the fingers, hands, wrists, toes, ankles and feet. Typically there are cramp-like stabbing pains that are intermittent in character. Symptoms are worse in women when menstruation is absent or erratic and during pregnancy. All symptoms improve in warm conditions or with the application of heat.

Causticum hahnemanni
Causticum, potassium hydrate

This remedy was prepared, investigated and proved in the early 1800s by Hahnemann, and is used only in homoeopathy. It is prepared by a chemical process in which lime that has been newly burnt is combined with potassium bisulphate in water. The mixture is heated and distilled, and the clear liquid distillate is collected and used to prepare the homoeopathic remedy. It is used for weakness of nerves and muscles that control the throat and voice box or vocal cords, bladder, eyelids and face on the right side. Typical throat complaints include hoarseness and loss of the voice and there may be a dry, unproductive cough. Bladder complaints include stress incontinence (i.e. a leakage of urine when the person coughs, sneezes, laughs loudly, etc) and wetting the bed, particularly if suffering from a chill. Other symptoms include sore, hot pains as in heartburn and rheumatic complaints. The symptoms are made worse by exposure to cold winds, physical exercise and also during the evening. They improve with warmth and are better for drinking something cold and having a wash. People suitable for Causticum are often thin, pale and with dark eyes and hair. They are able to enter into other people's suffering and feel the effects of grief very profoundly. They tend to feel the cold rather acutely and may be prone to warts on the skin. Causticum people may be rather rigid in their views and tend to have a weak constitution.

Ceanothus americanus
Ceanothus; red root, Jersey tea root, New Jersey tea, wild snowball

This shrub, which grows to a height of about five feet, is a native species of North America and Canada. It produces numerous small white flowers in June and July, and its leaves were used to make tea during the War of Independence when real tea was hard to come by. The plant has thick, reddish-coloured roots that give it one of its common names. The root is used in herbal medicine, but in homoeopathy the fresh leaves, gathered when the plant is in flower, are used to prepare the remedy. Ceanothus is given for abdominal pains and enlargement of the spleen and for symptoms on the left side of the abdomen. The pain is of a piercing nature and is made worse by lying on the left side. Exercise and movement exacerbate the symptoms, but they are relieved by rest and lying still. People who benefit from Ceanothus are extremely sensitive to the cold and like to sit as close as possible to a heat source in order to keep warm.

Chelidonium majus

Chelidonium, greater celandine, wartweed, garden celandine

This plant is a native of many countries in Europe and belongs to the same family as the poppy. The plant has a slender branching stem, large leaves that are a yellow-green colour on their upper surface and grey underneath, and yellow flowers. After flowering, long thin pods are produced containing black seeds. The plant produces a yellowish orange poisonous sap that is acrid, caustic and irritant with an unpleasant smell. The fresh flowering plant is used to prepare the homoeopathic remedy, which is mainly used to treat liver and gall bladder disorders. The types of disorder treated include gallstones, hepatitis, abdominal pain and indigestion. There may be symptoms of nausea, jaundice, vomiting and digestive upset with an aching pain located under the right shoulder blade. All symptoms are more common on the right side and are made worse by a change in the weather, for heat, in the afternoon around 4 p.m. and in the early morning around 4 a.m. They improve on eating and if firm pressure is applied to the painful area. Also for drinking hot beverages or milk and for passing stools.

People suitable for Chelidonium are often fair-haired and thin with yellowish or sallow skin. They tend to be gloomy and seldom look on the bright side of life and dislike intellectual effort. They are prone to headaches that make them feel heavy and lethargic. Chelido-

nium types enjoy hot drinks and cheese and may have one hot and one cold foot.

The Chelidonium remedy is also applied externally to remove warts, and this property has given the plant one of its common names, wartweed.

Cicuta virosa

Cicuta; water hemlock

This plant is a native species of Canada, North America, Siberia and some parts of Europe. It has highly poisonous roots that, if eaten, cause convulsions, overproduction of saliva, hyperventilation and profuse perspiration, often with a fatal outcome. The fresh root is used to prepare the homoeopathic remedy, which is used as a treatment for injuries and disorders of the central nervous system. Hence it is used to treat spasms, twitchings and muscular jerking, especially when the head and neck are thrown backwards, as may occur in epilepsy, following a head injury, meningitis and eclampsia of pregnancy. The patient may be confused, delirious, agitated and moaning unconsciously. The pupils of the eyes may be dilated. Symptoms are worse for sudden movement, cold and with touch. They improve with warmth and the elimination of abdominal wind. A person who benefits from this remedy may crave unsuitable substances as food.

Cinnamomum

Cinnamon; Cinnamomum zeylanicum

There are several varieties of cinnamon but the Cinnamomum zeylanicum tree is a native species of Sri Lanka and is also grown in several other eastern countries and the West Indies. The tree grows to about 30 feet in height, producing white flowers and, later, blue-coloured berries. The part used is the bark of the shoots, which is dried and rolled into thin brown quills. There is a characteristic pleasant, aromatic smell, and powdered cinnamon is widely used as a spice in food. In homoeopathy, the remedy is used to treat bleeding such as nosebleeds and also vomiting, nausea and diarrhoea. Some of the symptoms may be caused by stress or hysteria.

Clematis erecta

Upright virgin's bower

This poisonous perennial plant is a native of many European countries, growing to about three feet in height and having reddish-green leaves and white flowers. The leaves and flowers are acrid and irritant when crushed, producing inflammation and blistering. In homoeopathy, the remedy is used mainly in the treatment of gonorrhoea, including blockage of the urethra and a slow flow of urine because of inflammation or scarring. It may be used to treat other inflammations of the genital and urinary tract, eye disorders and neuralgia.

Cocculus
Indian cockle

This remedy, prepared from the body of the whole animal, is used to treat symptoms of nausea, sickness, giddiness and vertigo. Often there is accompanying depression, and, in women, symptoms are worse at the time of the period, which tends to be painful and may be early. A person suitable for this remedy is frequently talkative and hates wearing constricting clothing.

Coffea arabica
Coffea; coffee

The coffee tree is a native of Arabia but has been cultivated for many years in other tropical countries. In addition to having been widely used for many centuries as a drink, coffee has been valued medically for its stimulant, analgesic and diuretic properties. The plant has dark green, shiny, evergreen leaves and produces attractive white flowers. Later, berries are formed, which are bright orange-red when ripe, containing the seeds or coffee beans. The beans are roasted for use as a drink, but the unroasted beans are used to prepare the Coffea remedy. Coffea is used to treat insomnia when the brain is over-active and the person cannot relax enough to fall asleep. It is a useful remedy for any form of over-excitability and also severe pain such as toothache and painful labour. The person is very sensitive to noise, touch, disturbance or odours of any kind, and symptoms are made worse by cold winds. They improve with warmth and resting in quiet, calm, peaceful surroundings.

Colchicum autumnale
Colchicum; naked ladies, meadow saffron

This attractive flower grows from a bulbous structure called a corm, which is an underground swollen stem. The pretty light purple flowers appear in September and October (hence 'autumnale') and it grows on limestone soils throughout Europe, parts of Asia, North America and Canada. The plant has been well known since ancient times for its medicinal properties, being especially valued by Greek physicians for the treatment of painful rheumatic and gouty joints. It was known as the

'soul of joints'. It is poisonous, irritant and emetic in larger doses, having an effect on the digestive organs and kidneys. The fresh bulb is used to prepare the homoeopathic remedy, which is used to treat severe painful gout, especially of the big toe, and digestive upset including nausea, sickness, diarrhoea and abdominal pains that are relieved if the body is bent forwards. Symptoms are made worse by cold, damp weather, especially in the autumn, and by exercise or being touched. They improve with warmth, and resting in quiet surroundings.

Conium maculatum
Conium; hemlock, spotted hemlock, poison hemlock, poison parsley, beaver poison, spotted corobane, musquash root

This highly poisonous plant grows widely throughout Europe, parts of Asia, Canada, the United States of America and South America. It has been well known and used for centuries and is described in the writings of the ancient Greeks and Romans, including Pliny and Dioscorides. It was used as a means of execution of criminals, and Socrates was forced to drink the fatal poison of hemlock. Roman physicians used hemlock to treat a number of different disorders, including tumours and swellings of the joints and skin, cancer of the breast, liver diseases and as a sedative for spasms and dysfunction of nerves and muscles. Since it induces paralysis, it was used to combat pain and also to control inappropriate sexual feelings. Hemlock is a tall plant that may reach a height of four feet, producing large, indented green leaves and heads of white flowers. The stalks are streaked with purply-red, which, one old legend suggests, is a reminder of the mark on the forehead of Cain, the first murderer. Juice obtained from the leaves and stems of hemlock is used to prepare the homoeopathic remedy, which is used for enlarged and hardened glands, including the prostate gland, cancerous tumours and nodules, particularly of the breast, painful breasts before and during periods or because of pregnancy. The remedy is also used for nerve and muscle paralysis, especially that which gradually creeps up the legs and in which there may additionally be a dislike of strong light. It is used to treat premature ejaculation and dizziness that increases when the person lies down or moves the head. In general, the symptoms are made worse by suppression of sexual needs or an excess of sexual activity. Watching a moving object and drinking alcohol also make the symptoms worse. They improve with continued pressure applied to the painful part, sustained gentle exercise and if there is abdominal flatulence. People who benefit from Conium tend to have rather fixed and narrow ideas and a lack of interest in the wider world, which causes depression and a feeling of boredom and apathy. These feelings may be caused either by an over-indulgence in, or too little, sexual activity. Conium people do not cope well if forced to be celibate.

Crocus sativus

Crocus, saffron crocus, saffron

Crocus sativus is a native of the western parts of Asia but has long been cultivated throughout Europe, especially in Spain. The three long, deep orange-red stigmas within the crocus flower are the source of saffron, which has been used medicinally since ancient times. Saffron is mentioned in the Old Testament Song of Solomon (4 :14) and was described by Hippocrates as having aphrodisiac and purgative qualities. It was used to treat uterine bleeding disorders and prolonged and painful childbirth as well as diseases of the liver. Throughout history it has been used to treat a wide variety of physical and mental disorders. In homoeopathy the remedy is used to treat disorders of menstruation and nosebleeds and also emotional symptoms of weepiness, depression and mood swings. The symptoms are made worse by warm, stuffy surroundings and listening to music. They improve out in the fresh open air and after eating breakfast.

Crotalus homolus

Crotalus hor.; venom of the rattlesnake

The rattlesnake is familiar to people throughout the world, far beyond its normal habitat in the dry, semi-desert regions of the United States, Canada, Mexico and South America. Its most noteworthy characteristic is the rattling tail, which the snake uses as a warning when it is agitated or about to strike, and the animal has been widely described and depicted in books, films and nature programmes. The snake produces a potent venom that it uses to paralyse its prey, and this was investigated and proved in 1837 by Dr Constantine Hering, an outstanding American homoeopathic doctor. In modern homoeopathy the remedy is used to treat serious illnesses such as strokes affecting the right side of the body, symptoms of liver

failure including jaundice and oedema, cancer and heart disease. The remedy helps to arrest bleeding from a natural orifice of the body and is used to treat septicaemia, shock and collapse. The symptoms are worse for lying on the left side and for wearing constricting, tight clothing. Humid, warm, moist weather aggravates the symptoms but they are better out in the fresh, clean, dry air.

Croton tiglium

Croton oil seeds

This small, shrubby bush is a native species of the coastal regions of India and Asia, and produces fruits that each contain a single seed rich in oil. Croton oil is obtained by compressing the ripe seeds, and in its neat form is highly purgative if taken internally, producing colicky abdominal pains, diarrhoea and vomiting. It may prove fatal if more than one small dose is taken. Applied externally, it produces irritation and blistering of the skin. In herbal medicine it is used to treat severe constipation, often combined with castor oil, and also as a counterirritant in some rheumatic, bronchitic and other disorders. In homoeopathy, the remedy is used to treat severe digestive symptoms of colic-type abdominal pains, copious watery diarrhoea and vomiting. Also, it is used for severe skin inflammations in which there is redness, heat and blistering.

Cyclamen europaeum

Cyclamen; sowbread

There are several species of cyclamen, many of which are native to the warmer countries of southern Europe and northern Africa. The plant has a large, swollen, brown root and derives its common name from the fact that these tubers were a source of food for wild pigs. Cyclamen was used by the physicians of ancient Greece and Rome and also Arabia. It was used to treat disorders of the liver and spleen, including jaundice and hepatitis, and to regulate periods in women. The plant produces very pretty pink flowers, each borne on a single firm, fleshy stalk, and varieties of cyclamen are very popular as house plants. The fresh root is extremely acrid and acts as a purgative, and is used for this purpose in herbal medicine. In homoeopathy the sap from the fresh root is used to prepare the remedy, which is used for an irregular menstrual cycle in women. It is also helpful in the treatment of searing, hot pains in the muscles or skin and severe migraine-like headaches with disturbance of vision. People who benefit from this remedy may crave bizarre and inappropriate things to eat. They tend to have a melancholy disposition, often feeling sad and depressed or beset by guilt or remorse. Symptoms are made better by exercise and moving around and with crying. They improve in the fresh open air.

Datura stramonium

Stramonium; thorn apple, devil's apple, stinkweed, devil's trumpet, Jamestown weed, Jimson weed

There are a number of species of *Datura* distributed throughout many countries of the world, and all are poisonous with highly narcotic effects. *Datura stramonium* is found in Europe, North America and Asia, often growing as a weed on waste ground. It is a large, bushy plant, usually about three or four feet in height and producing large white flowers. Later, pebble-sized capsules protected by thorns are produced that open when ripe to reveal black or very dark brown seeds. The flowers have a pleasant scent, but the rest of the plant, especially the leaves, give off an unpleasant, rank smell that is repellent to grazing animals. The plant has been used in herbal medicine for many hundreds of years. Inhalation of the smoke from the burning plant was used as a cure for attacks of asthma, and sometimes a type of cigarette was made from the leaves for this purpose. Preparations of the plant were used externally to relieve painful rheumatism, neuralgic conditions such as sciatica, haemorrhoids, abscesses and boils, and other inflammations. It has also been used for sedation and was eaten by soldiers in medieval Europe before going into battle to calm their fears. Juice extracted from the green parts of the plant before it comes into flower are used to prepare the homoeopathic remedy. It is used to treat nervous system disorders and is a useful remedy for children. Symptoms include muscular jerking, spasms and twitches, convulsions because of epilepsy, high fever in children or meningitis and strokes. Also, for physical symptoms suffered by a person who has sustained a severe shock or fright, night terrors in children, states of great anxiety and mental agitation. A child may be terrified of the dark and the imagined creatures of the night. An adult may have a fear of water or is unreasonably afraid that he or she may suffer violence. The person often has a craving for drinks of an acidic nature and has an excessive thirst.

Symptoms are worse if the person is left alone and following sleep. Also, when the person tries to swallow liquids or food and if the weather is overcast and cloudy. The symptoms improve if the person has the reassurance and company of other people, particularly if the surroundings are light, airy and warm.

Delphinium staphysagria

Staphysagria; stavesacre, staphisagris, planted larkspur, lousewort

This plant has a long history of medicinal use going back to the civilizations of ancient Greece and Rome, being described by both Dioscorides and Pliny. It was used externally to destroy parasites such as lice and to treat insect bites and stings, and has continued to be employed for this purpose throughout history. It is highly poisonous and even in small doses causes vomiting and diarrhoea, acting as a purgative. Staphysagria is a large, annual plant with hairy stems and leaves, which grows to a height of about four feet and is a native of southern European and Asian countries. It produces spikes of light blue/purple flowers and, later, seed pods containing dark-coloured seeds. The seeds are the part used in both herbal medicine and homoeopathy. The homoeopathic remedy is used to treat neuralgic pains, toothache, pain from the incision of an operation, pressure headache, inflammation and infection of the eyes or eyelids, such as styes and blepharitis, cystitis and painful sexual intercourse in women. It may also be used for painful teething in young children and for disorders of the prostate gland in men. Usually, the person who benefits has suppressed anger or resentment and is inclined to be irritable. Symptoms are made worse for suppression of feelings, following a sleep in the afternoon and after eating breakfast. They improve with warmth and by giving voice to the emotions. People suitable for staphysagria appear equable and mild on the outside but internally seethe with suppressed emotions, especially anger. They are inclined to harbour resentment for supposed slights or insults and are somewhat driven, workaholic people. They often have a high libido and suppress their emotions because they are afraid of losing self-control, especially in front of other people. Body secretions may smell unpleasant, and they have a desire for alcoholic drinks and sweetened foods.

Digitalis purpurea

Digitalis; foxglove, fairy thimbles, fairy's gloves, witch's gloves, folk's glove

The striking and attractive foxglove, with its deep pink-purple, long, bell-shaped flowers, is a familiar plant in Britain and other European countries. One of its oldest name, folk's glove, associates it with the 'good folk', or fairies, who were believed to inhabit the woods and groves where the plant commonly grows. The name foxglove is derived from Anglo-Saxon, but the plant was given its Latin adjective of *Digitalis* in the mid-16th century, derived from *digitabulum*, meaning 'thimble'. The plant was used medicinally in ancient times as a cure for wounds and bruising. It was not until 1785, however, that its value in the treatment of dropsy (oedema, or fluid retention, which may accompany heart disease) was discovered by a Dr William Withering. Its main use, both in modern orthodox medicine and homoeopathy, is as a major remedy for heart disorders. Liquid extracted from the new fresh green leaves collected in the spring is used to prepare the homoeopathic remedy. It is used as a treatment for a slow, faint or irregular heartbeat such as may accompany heart failure and other heart and circulatory disorders. The person often experiences a sinking sensation in the pit of the stomach such as occurs with fear and may feel that the heart is about to cease to beat altogether. There may be additional problems, particularly with the liver or kidneys. The symptoms are made worse by listening to music, eating a meal and sitting in an upright position. They improve out in the fresh open air and by not eating. The person who benefits from this remedy may feel nauseated at the sight of food.

Dioscorea villosa

Dioscorea; wild yam, rheumatism root, colic root, wild yamwurzel

This perennial plant is a native species of Canada and the United States, although there are many other varieties inhabiting most tropical countries. It has a twining habit with a long, twisted, branched root that is the part used to prepare the homoeopathic remedy. Preparations of the root act upon the smooth muscle of the digestive tract, having antispasmodic properties. Hence the remedy is used to treat spasmodic colicky pains, bilious colic, morning sickness during pregnancy, abdominal wind and diarrhoea. Other types of spasmodic pain, such as neuralgia, may benefit from this remedy, and symptoms are relieved by gentle exercise and movement.

Dryopteris filix-mas

Male shield fern

A common type of fern found in the United Kingdom, Europe and many other countries with a temperate climate. The plant has a stocky, short rhizome or underground stem just beneath the surface of the soil, with a tangle of roots protruding from its under surface. This part is collected and dried and used to prepare remedies both in herbal and homoeopathic medicine. The root contains a liquid oleoresin and has been known since ancient times for its anthelmintic properties (anti-worm), being particularly useful for the expulsion of a tapeworm. One method, using the root of the fern, is described by Dioscorides, and the remedy continues to be used for this purpose today. If a tapeworm is present there may be little in the way of symptoms but abdominal cramps, slight bleeding and itching. One dose is usually sufficient to expel the parasite, and preparations have also been used in veterinary medicine.

Duboisia myoporoides

Duboisia; corkwood elm, corkwood tree

This large shrub or small tree is a native species of Australia, producing large, white flowers and green leaves that are gathered when the plant is flowering to prepare the homoeopathic remedy. The preparation made from the leaves acts on the central nervous system, having an hypnotic and sedative effect. Applied to the eye it is a mydriatic, causing dilation of the pupil. In homoeopathy, the remedy is used for eye disorders, particularly if there are one or more floating red spots (debris) causing disturbance of vision. Also, for painful, irritated and inflamed eyes such as may be caused by conjunctivitis. It may be used for symptoms of vertigo or where there are symptoms of mental confusion.

Elaps corallinus

Corallinus; coral snake

The attractive coral snake is a native animal of North and South America, especially Brazil and Canada. The snake has broad red and narrower blue bands of colour down the length of its body that are separated from one another by thin strips of white. The homoeopathic remedy is prepared from fresh snake venom and is used as a treatment for troublesome bleeding and strokes. The bleeding disorders that may benefit from Elaps include nosebleeds, heavy menstruation (menorrhagia), piles and strokes affecting the right side of the body. The person may have a feeling of being chilled inside and desire cold drinks. However, cold foods and drinks, humid weather before a thunderstorm and getting too hot in bed make the symptoms worse. Also, they are worse if the person lies on his or her front or walks around. Symptoms are generally better during the night and for staying still. People who benefit from Elaps are usually afraid of snakes and fear being left on their own and do not like the rain. They are frightened of death and the possibility of having a stroke.

Equisetum hiemale, Equisetum arvense

Equisetum; horsetail, scouring rush, pewterwort, bottlebrush, shave-grass, paddock-pipes

The horsetails are a very ancient group of plants descended from species that grew during the Carboniferous geological period. Several species are found in the British Isles. *Equisetum arvense* is the most common of these and is also distributed in many other countries of the world. *Equisetum hiemale* is found in China and other eastern countries. Horsetails produce two kinds of stems, fertile and barren, which are jointed and hollow. There are no leaves but long green spikes at the joints with jagged edges. The fruiting or fertile stem, which is produced early in the season before the barren stems appear, has a cone-like structure at the end containing numerous spores. The stems of horsetails are strengthened with silica, and the plants were formerly used for scouring and cleaning purposes (hence the names pewterwort, scouring brush, bottlebrush, etc). There is a long history of medicinal use going back to ancient times, and the plant is described by Dioscorides as being good for the healing of wounds. While the plant continued to be used for wounds and ulcers, it was also believed to be helpful in the healing of ruptures and for bowel and kidney complaints. In modern herbal medicine, it is used for kidney disorders and fluid retention (oedema) as it has diuretic as well as astringent properties. The fresh parts of the plant are used to prepare the homoeopathic remedy, which is used to treat an irritable bladder. The symptoms resemble those of cystitis but without the presence of infection. The bladder feels constantly full with an aching and dragging sensation. There is a continual feeling of the need to pass urine, which is usually released only in small amounts with pain at the end of urination. There may be kidney pain and slight incontinence. Equisetum is a useful remedy for children who wet the bed when suffering from disturbed sleep because of nightmares. The symptoms are worse if pressure is applied to the painful part and with touch, exercise or movement. They improve if the person remains still and lies on the back.

Euonymus atropurpurea

Euonymus; burning bush, wahoo, Indian arrowroot

This shrub is a native species of the United States and grows to a height of about six feet. It produces attractive deep purple flowers and dark green leaves that are edged with a purple tinge. The bark of the roots and stems is used and, in small doses, the preparation has a stimulant effect on the digestive system. However, in large doses it has an irritant and purgative effect. In herbal medicine, it is valued as a liver stimulant promoting the flow of bile juice. The homoeopathic remedy is used for digestive complaints with bloatedness and abdominal pain and swelling of the feet and ankles because of retention of fluid (oedema). There may be stomach irritation (gastritis) with diarrhoea or blood in the stools. The remedy is also used for mental symptoms of irritability or confusion.

Euonymus europea

Spindle tree, prickwood, skewerwood, fusanum, fusoria

The spindle tree grows in woods and hedges in the British Isles and other European countries. It produces clusters of white flowers tinged with green in early summer and, later, bright red fruits containing orange seeds. The leaves, fruits and bark are all harmful and are not touched by grazing animals. The fruits cause severe sickness and diarrhoea if eaten, and the seeds are used to prepare the homoeopathic remedy. It is used to treat digestive disorders with severe abdominal pains and copious diarrhoea. Also, for symptoms of angina, including constricting chest pains and breathlessness. Symptoms may occur mainly on the left side.

Eupatorium perfoliatum

Eupator; boneset, thoroughwort, agueweed, feverwort

This perennial plant is a native species of North America, being common on damp ground in low-lying situations. It is a very important plant in herbal medicine and has always been valued for its medicinal uses, firstly by the Indian native peoples and later by European and African settlers. It has a thick hairy stem and abundant white flowers throughout the summer months. Preparations made from the plant act as a tonic or stimulant of the digestive system in small doses. However, in large doses it causes sickness and diarrhoea, having a purgative effect. It is also valued for its fever-reducing qualities and, in addition, is diaphoretic, promoting perspiration. The whole green plant and flowers are used to prepare the homoeopathic remedy, which is given for feverish conditions such as colds and influenza. Accompanying symptoms include restlessness, severe aches and pains in the bones, hot, dry skin and little perspiration. The person craves ice-cold drinks and foods, such as ice cream, and may have a painful, dry cough. Symptoms are worse for exercise and movement and in the early morning between 7 a.m. and 9 a.m. Also, they are worse outside in fresh clean air. They are better inside and for talking to other people and for vomiting bile.

Ferrum metallicum

Ferrum met.; iron

Iron is a very important mineral in the body, being a part of the haemoglobin molecule. Haemoglobin is the iron-containing pigment in red blood cells that combines with oxygen in the lungs from where it is transported and supplied to all cells and tissues. If there is a deficiency of iron in the blood, which can arise for a number of different reasons, the result is anaemia. The person becomes pale, tired and breathless. especially with any form of exertion, and body systems cannot function properly. Iron is widely used in conventional medicine as well as homoeopathy. The source is iron ore, and haematite, a red-coloured bulbous deposit found in association with various rocks, particularly in North America, Canada and Venezuela, is especially rich in this mineral. The homoeopathic remedy is used for circulatory disorders and anaemia. The person is frequently tired and listless, looks pale and feels chilled and may have cold hands and feet, but at the same time is often restless. The person soon becomes exhausted and may be breathless with physical exertion. The tiredness may

cause irritability, depression and changes of mood. People suitable for Ferrum met. are frequently well built and appear robust but suffer from the symptoms described above. They dislike food rich in fat or cholesterol but enjoy pickled and sour foods. They may be allergic to eggs but like tomatoes.

Fluoricum acidum

Fluor. ac.; hydrofluoric acid

Hydrofluoric acid has several industrial uses, particularly in the manufacture of metals and glassware, being used for cleaning and etching. It is obtained by a distillation process involving sulphuric acid and calcium fluoride with the production of hydrogen fluoride gas. When this gas is passed through water it dissolves to give hydrofluoric acid, which contains fluorine. Fluorine is an important constituent of teeth and bones and is a strengthening substance. The homoeopathic remedy is used to treat disorders of connective tissue, bones and teeth. Varicose veins and ulcers, bone pain and tumours and decaying, softened teeth may benefit from Fluor ac. People suitable for this remedy are frequently rather selfish and self-centred and not inclined to commit themselves to others. They are worldly and materialistic and tend to judge success in life in financial terms. Fluor. ac. people lack spiritual and emotional understanding and may have a high sex drive. They manage with little sleep and are very active, seldom feeling cold or tired.

Formica rufa

Red ant

The homoeopathic remedy is obtained from the body of the crushed red ant. It is suitable for conditions producing symptoms of hot, burning, stabbing pains such as may affect joints, as in arthritic, rheumatic and gouty disorders. It is also used for severe headaches and numbness affecting the face. There may be an inability to concentrate, vagueness or slight forgetfulness.

Fragaria vesca

Wild strawberry, wood strawberry

This plant is a native species of most European countries, including Britain. It is a low, creeping plant with a tangle of stalks and leaves, and produces white flowers followed by small red berries that are covered with tiny seeds. The flavour of the fruit is delicious and fragrant and has long been valued as food. The fruit, and especially the leaves, have been used for hundreds of years for medicinal purposes, the plant having diuretic, astringent and laxative properties. Preparations made from the plant were used to treat kidney stones and urinary complaints, wounds, gout, tooth decay and diarrhoea. The cut strawberries rubbed on the skin help to relieve sunburn and other skin complaints and remove stains when applied to the teeth. The homoeopathic remedy is used to alleviate an allergic reaction to strawberries, especially when this causes a skin rash and itching. It is also used for stones in the kidneys or gall bladder, a build-up of tartar on the teeth and chilblains or sunburn.

Fraxinus americana
American white ash

Ash trees of the genus *Fraxinus* have been used for medicinal purposes in many different countries. Various parts of the plant have been used, especially the bark, leaves, fruit and 'keys'. The bark of the American white ash, which grows in the United States, is used to prepare a homoeopathic remedy. It has astringent and tonic properties and is used in homoeopathy to treat a prolapsed uterus with dragging lower abdominal pain and also for fibroids.

Gentiana cruciata
Cross-leaved gentian

There are many species of gentian found in most countries throughout the world. In all varieties the plant, and especially the root, is extremely bitter and is used as a tonic medicine. The cross-leaved gentian, with leaves growing in the shape of a cross, has been used in herbal medicine as a treatment for hydrophobia (rabies). In homoeopathy, the root is used to prepare the remedy, which is given for a sore throat or hoarseness, gastritis and infections of the stomach, colicky pains, nausea, sickness and diarrhoea and hernia.

Gentiana lutea
Yellow gentian

The yellow gentian is a native species of the mountainous, alpine and sub-alpine pastures of Europe although it does not occur naturally in the British Isles. It has a long root exceeding one foot in length, and the stalk grows to a height of three or four feet. The leaves are a yellow-green colour, and the plant produces attractive, large, deep orange-yellow flowers. The root is collected and dried to make medicinal preparations and has long been valued for its bitter, tonic properties. In homoeopathy, it is used as a remedy for digestive prob-

lems and gastritis with symptoms of griping abdominal pains, nausea, vomiting and diarrhoea, heartburn and bloatedness.

Glonoinum
Glonoin; nitroglycerine, glyceryl trinitrate

This substance, which occurs as a clear, poisonous, oily liquid, is derived from a chemical process and was discovered in the mid-1800s by an Italian chemist. It is prepared by mixing together certain proportions of sulphuric acid and nitric acid and then adding glycerine. The addition of diatomaceous earth or kiesel-guhr (a natural deposit of sediment composed of the silica skeletons of minute marine creatures called diatoms) to nitroglycerine, produces dynamite. This extremely dangerous explosive was first formulated by the eminent Swedish scientist, Alfred Nobel, in 1867. Nitroglycerine acts very strongly on the heart and blood circulation and is used in conventional medicine as a remedy for the symptoms of angina. In homoeopathy the remedy is also used for symptoms affecting the blood circulation and head caused by a sudden, increased rush of blood. Symptoms include a feeling of congestion in the head with a pounding, severe headache, hot flushes and sweats. The person may try to relieve the pain by holding and pressing the head between the hands. Also, it is used in the treatment of heat exhaustion and the early symptoms of heatstroke. The symptoms are made worse by any kind of movement, especially turning the head, and by heat. They are relieved by cold and being out in cool, fresh air.

Helleborus niger
Christmas rose, Christ herb, melampode, black hellebore

The Christmas rose is a highly poisonous plant that is found naturally in the mountainous regions of southern, central and eastern Europe. It is known as a garden plant in the British Isles and derives its name of black hellebore from the colour of the root. It flowers in the depths of winter, from which comes its association with Christmas and Christ. The plant has large, serrated, dark-green leaves and white flowers tinged with pink, but it is the dark-coloured rhizome and root that are used to prepare the herbal and homoeopathic remedies. The plant has been known since ancient times and is described in the writings of Pliny. It was used as a cure for various ailments in cattle and other domestic animals, and has strong purgative and narcotic effects. It also has a powerful effect on the kidneys, heart and uterus. In homoeopathy, it is used in the treatment of severe headaches with stabbing pain that may be associated with a former head injury. There may be symptoms of mental confusion, mood changes or even convulsions or epilepsy. Slight movements make the symptoms worse, as do cold draughts of air.

Hydrastis canadensis

Hydrastis; golden seal, yellow puccoon, orange root, Indian dye, Indian paint, eye balm, eye root, ground raspberry

This plant is a native species of Canada and the eastern United States, and has a long history of medicinal use, firstly by the Indian peoples, particularly the Cherokees, and later by Europeans. It is a small, perennial plant growing to a height of about six to twelve inches and producing a greenish white flower and later an inedible fruit resembling a raspberry. There is a knotty, yellow-brown tangled root system from which a dye was extracted and used by the Indians to colour their clothes and skin. The fresh root or rhizome (underground stem) is the part used medicinally. It was used by the Indian peoples to treat digestive disorders, liver complaints, eye irritations, ulcers and cancer, heart conditions and fevers. It has a particular effect on mucous membranes, making it useful in the treatment of catarrh, and has tonic, cleansing and astringent properties. The homoeopathic remedy was investigated and proved by the American homoeopath Dr Hale in 1875, although the plant had been known in Europe since the mid-18th century. In homoeopathy the remedy is used to treat catarrhal complaints such as may occur with infections of the nose and throat and chest. Typically, a thick, yellow catarrh is produced, and there may be a sore throat and other pains. It is also used for digestive disorders in which there may be persistent constipation, nausea and vomiting and loss of appetite and weight. It is particularly useful as a tonic for people who have lost weight because of a long, debilitating illness. The symptoms are worse in the evening and night and out in cold air. They are relieved by rest, quiet and warm surroundings.

Hyoscyamus niger

Hyoscyamus; henbane, henbell, hogbean

Henbane grows widely throughout Europe and western Asia, and has been introduced and become naturalized in North America, Canada and parts of South America, such as Brazil. It is believed that it may have been brought to Britain and other European countries by the Romans, and it is described by both Dioscorides and Pliny. The plant is poisonous, narcotic and sedative, and was used by ancient physicians to induce sleep and relieve pain. Henbane has a varied habit, occurring as both annual and biennial forms. Both are used medicinally, although the biennial form is generally considered to be more useful. The preparations are narcotic, hypnotic and antispasmodic in effect, and are used in conventional medicine to treat spasms of the digestive tract. Juice extracted from the fresh whole flowering plant is used to prepare the homoeopathic remedy, which is used for mental and emotional problems.

Symptoms include paranoia and suspicion of others, unreasonable behaviour and jealousy, delusions, aggressive outbursts and the use of foul and sexually suggestive language. Henbane is also used to relieve the physical symptoms of muscular spasms and cramp-like intermittent pains that may accompany epilepsy, disorders of the digestive system and bladder. Symptoms are made worse by lying down and being touched, with being covered up and for any emotional upheaval. They are relieved if the person sits in an upright position.

Iberis amara

Bitter candytuft

This small, flowering annual plant grows throughout Europe and is a familiar garden flower. It grows to a height of about six inches and produces white or pink flowers in the summer months. All parts of the plant are used in herbal medicine, but the seeds alone are gathered and prepared to make a tincture used in homoeopathy. The remedy was investigated and proved by the American homoeopath Dr Edwin Hale, and it is used to treat heart disorders. It may be given for angina, palpitations, oedema, breathlessness and chest pains. It is also a treatment for bronchitis and asthma and sickness and vertigo.

Iodum

Iodine

Iodine is a nonmetallic element that is an essential substance for the normal functioning of metabolic processes within the body. It is mainly concentrated in the thyroid gland and is a major component of thyroid hormones, which themselves regulate many body processes. A deficiency of iodine causes a gain in weight, swelling of the face and neck, a dry skin and mental apathy. The person feels excessively tired, and the hair starts to fall out. This deficiency is not usually seen in western countries because iodine is added to table salt. Iodine is found naturally in seaweed and deposits of saltpetre (an evaporate mineral found in dry, desert-like conditions, particularly in Chile). Tincture of iodine is used in homoeopathy as a remedy for hyperthyroidism (an overactive thyroid gland). The symptoms include weakness and wasting, noticed especially in the limbs, pain and bulging of the eyes, excessive hunger, restlessness, nervousness, sweating, breathlessness, intolerance of heat and rapid heart beat. It is also used for severe, hacking coughs, shortness of breath, laryngitis and throat disorders and pain in the bones. People who benefit from this remedy like to be busy and may be talkative and excitable. However, they may also be forgetful so that their activities may be inefficient and disorganized. Symptoms are made worse by heat in any form and are relieved by cool, fresh air. They also improve for movement and exercise and after meals.

Iris versicolor

The blue flag, water flag, poison flag, liver lily, flag lily, snake lily, dagger flower, dragon flower

This attractive but poisonous flowering plant is a native species of North America and Canada, growing in damp, low-lying conditions. It is a popular garden plant in the British Isles, growing to a height of about two or three feet and producing deep blue-purple flowers. Preparations made from the rhizome have a diuretic and stimulant effect and cause sickness and diarrhoea. They are mainly used for liver and digestive complaints. The fresh rhizome or underground stem is used to prepare the homoeopathic remedy, which is used for indigestion, vomiting and nausea, diarrhoea, colicky pains and also for migraine where the headache is on the right side.

Kali bromatum

Kali brom.; potassium bromide

This white, crystalline substance, which is obtained from a chemical process, is used in the photographic industry and has also been given as a remedy in conventional medicine. It was given to men to reduce an excessive libido and particularly to male prisoners. It was also given

for some other psychiatric disorders and as a treatment for epilepsy. The homoeopathic remedy is given as a treatment for severe acne and skin disorders, excessive menstrual bleeding especially during the menopause, impotence, epilepsy, nervous exhaustion and depression. People suitable for Kali brom. tend to be restless and anxious and have a need to be busy. During their teenage years they may require a lot of reassurance and tend to feel guilty about their emerging sexuality. They may have strong religious beliefs and feel that sexual needs are immoral, and this causes mental stress and conflict. They are prone to acne, especially at puberty and during times of hormonal change. In women, symptoms are worse during menstruation. All symptoms improve if the person is fully occupied.

Kali sulphuricum

Potassium sulphate

Potassium sulphate is another of the SCHUSSLER TISSUE SALTS (see Glossary), which is used in homoeopathy for catarrhal conditions in which there is a thick white or yellow discharge. This may occur in bronchitis and other infections of the nose and throat. Also, it is used to treat infected skin conditions, such as erysipelas and eczema, in which there is a pus-like discharge. It may be used as a remedy for such infectious illnesses as measles and scarlet fever, which affect the skin, and also for rheumatism. Symptoms are made worse by hot surroundings and heat in any form and are relieved by coldness and fresh air.

Kalium carbonicum

Kali carb; potassium carbonate

Potassium carbonate occurs naturally in all plants, and is obtained from the ash of burnt wood or other vegetation, or by a chemical process. Potassium carbonate was used by the ancient Egyptian civilization in the manufacture of glassware. The remedy is used for complaints affecting the mucous membranes of the upper respiratory system and digestive organs. It is used for coughs and bronchitis with stitch-like pains, menopausal and menstrual problems, pains in the back and head. The person feels cold and fluid is retained (oedema), causing swelling of the face, especially the upper eyelids. The person feels chilled and may be likely to catch colds or influenza. Symptoms are worse for physical exertion, bending the body forwards and for cool conditions. They are worse in the very early morning between 2 and 3 a.m. Symptoms improve in warm, dry conditions and weather. People who are suitable for all the Kalium remedies have a strict sense of duty and firm ideas about right and wrong. They are possessive and may be jealous and difficult to live with. They cope badly with any kind of emotional trauma and may feel as though they have been kicked in the abdomen if they receive upsetting news.

Kalium muriaticum

Kali mur.; potassium chloride

This white or colourless crystalline substance is found naturally as the mineral sylvite, which occurs in beds of evaporite deposits. It is much used as a fertilizer, and in homoeopathy is one of the SCHUSSLER TISSUE SALTS (*see* GLOSSARY). A deficiency of potassium chloride affects blood-clotting capability. The Kali mur. remedy is used to treat inflammations and infections of the mucous membranes. Typically, there is a thick, mucus discharge, and this may occur with middle ear and throat infections, glue ear in children and tonsillitis. The throat may be very sore and swallowing painful and difficult, and the person may have a fever and swollen glands. Symptoms are worse in cold, damp weather and in cold fresh air. Also, they feel worse for eating fatty foods and, in women, during a period. Symptoms are better for sipping ice-cold drinks and for gently rubbing the painful part.

Kalmia latifolia

American laurel, broad-leaved laurel, sheep laurel, calico bush, lambkill, kalmia

An attractive but poisonous evergreen shrub that is a native species of some states of the United States of America. It grows to a height of anything up to twenty feet and produces an abundance of pink flowers. The leaves are the part of the plant used medicinally, and they have narcotic and astringent properties and also sedative effects on the heart. The plant was known to the native Indian people and has been used in the treatment of skin diseases, fevers, syphilis, neuralgia, blood disorders, haemorrhages, diarrhoea and dysentery. The homoeopathic remedy is made from the fresh leaves of the plant and is used to treat symptoms occurring on the right side of the body, such as facial and other neuralgia, shingles, rheumatic pains, numbness and paralysis, and heart problems such as angina. Symptoms are made worse by cold in any form, touch or pressure, and are relieved by warmth.

Kreosotum

Creosote in spirits

This remedy is used for infected conditions in which there is pus or other discharge that often has an offensive smell. Hence it is used for skin eruptions such as boils, gum disease and tooth decay with bad breath, and infections of the womb, bladder, pelvic organs and prostate gland. The person may suffer from general weakness and debility with nausea, vomiting, diarrhoea and colicky pains. Symptoms may occur mainly on the left side.

Lac caninum

Lac. can.; milk from a female dog, bitch's milk

This is one of the oldest known remedies, being described by a physician of ancient Greece, Sextus, who used it for treating ear infections and sensitivity to light. Pliny referred to its usefulness in treating female reproductive disorders, and this is one of its uses in homoeopathy. The homoeopathic remedy is used in the treatment of erosion of the cervix, in which cells that line the neck of the womb are worn away. It is also used for sore breasts during breast-feeding or before menstruation. Another major use is in the treatment of severe sore throats, as in tonsillitis, and for diphtheria. The pains or other symptoms often switch from one side of the body to another and may be accompanied by malaise and weakness. The person may feel light-headed, experiencing a floating sensation. People suitable for Lac. can. tend to be highly sensitive, over-imaginative to the point of allowing imagined fears to take over, timid and forgetful. In contrast to this, they are capable on occasion of being unreasonable and aggressive. They have many fears and often experience nightmares, and may have a phobia about snakes. Lac. can. people enjoy spicy salty food and hot drinks. Symptoms are made worse by touch or pressure and improve out in the fresh air.

Lactrodectus mactans

Lactrodectus mac.; female black widow spider

The female black widow is one of the most poisonous of spiders, and its venom can rapidly prove fatal. The venom is injected when the spider bites and produces symptoms of severe, constricting chest pains, sweating, spasm in muscles and blood vessels, fear, collapse and death. The spider is found in a number of countries with a hot climate, particularly in some parts of the United States. The homoeopathic remedy is derived from the body of the female spider and is used to treat serious heart complaints including heart attack and angina. It is also used for states of great anxiety and fear with hyperventilation, agitation, breathlessness and collapse. Symptoms are made worse by cold, damp weather and in oppressive conditions before a storm breaks. They are worse at night but improve with reassurance and sitting still and with taking a hot bath.

Lapis albus
Calcium silico-fluoride

This remedy, which is prepared chemically, was investigated and proved by a German homoeopathic doctor, Edward von Grauvogl, in the 19th century. It is used to treat hot, stabbing pains in the womb, breasts or stomach and for burning, itchy skin.

Lilium tigrinum
Lilium; tiger lily

This striking flowering plant, which is popular in gardens, is a native species of China and Japan. It produces large, orange flowers that are funnel-shaped with the petals curved back upon themselves. The petals are covered with deep, reddish-coloured spots. The homoeopathic remedy, which is made from the whole fresh flowering plant, was investigated and proved in 1869 by the American homoeopath Dr Carroll Dunham. It is used for disorders of the female reproductive organs, including a prolapsed uterus with dragging pains, uterine fibroids (benign tumours of the womb) that may affect the bladder, increasing the desire to pass urine, swollen ovaries and ovarian pain, and itching in the genital region. Also, it is given for disorders of the bladder, rectum and veins, and for symptoms of angina. These symptoms include severe constricting chest pain, anxiety and rapid heart beat rate, and a feeling of numbness extending down the right arm. People suitable for this remedy have a very strong sense of right and wrong and set themselves very high standards of behaviour. This may result in conflict between their natural, especially sexual, needs and what they regard as the correct way to behave, leading to feelings of guilt and self-loathing. Their inner turmoil may make them irritable and liable to take offence, especially at remarks that appear to be critical. Lilium people have hot hands and are more comfortable in cool or cold weather. Symptoms are made worse by any form of heat and at night. They improve in cool surroundings and out in the cold fresh air.

Symptoms are relieved if the person lies on his or her left side.

Lycopus virginicus
Lycopus; bugleweed, Virginia water, horehound, water bugle, gipsyweed

This attractive plant is a native species of the eastern parts of the United States, growing in damp, low-lying situations in plenty of shade. The plant produces purple-coloured flowers and has smooth, green leaves. It gives off a slightly minty aromatic smell and has astringent, sedative and slightly narcotic properties. It was formerly used to treat bleeding in the lungs, as in tuberculosis, encouraging blood to be coughed up. It has also been used in place of DIGITALIS in the treatment of heart disorders. The whole fresh parts of the plant and flowers are used to prepare the homoeopathic remedy, which was first investigated and introduced by the American homoeopath, Edwin Moses Hale in the latter part of the 19th century. It is used to treat heart disorders, including abnormalities of the heartbeat and palpitations, aneurysms (balloon-like swellings of artery walls), inflammation of the membranous sac surrounding the heart (pericarditis), raised blood pressure and heart failure. It is also used to treat a disorder of the thyroid gland (goitre) that produces a protrusion of the eyes. Symptoms are made worse by physical activity and exertion, agitation or excitement and heat in any form. The symptoms are usually worse following sleep but are relieved by pressure on the affected part.

Lyssin
Hydrophobinum

This remedy is prepared from the saliva of a dog that has contracted rabies. It is used for serious disorders of the nervous system, especially convulsions that may be related to epilepsy, severe headaches and pre-eclampsia of pregnancy (a condition marked by retention of fluid and swelling of feet and ankles, high blood pressure and the presence of protein in the urine). If not treated, pre-eclampsia may lead to full eclampsia of pregnancy, which is a life-threatening condition marked by convulsions. The fits intensify if the person is in the presence of running water.

Magnesia carbonica
Mag. carb.; magnesium carbonate

Magnesium carbonate, which is a white, powdery substance, has a variety of industrial uses including the manufacture of bricks, cements, paper, paints and materials for insulation. In pharmaceutical manufacture it is used as a bulking material in some types of powder and tablets. The main source is magnesite, which is formed from altered limestones, dolomites or serpentines and is mined in China, the United States and Austria. The homoeopathic remedy was investigated and proved by Hahnemann and is used to treat loss of the sense of taste when there is a thick, whitish coating on the tongue, indigestion and heartburn and digestive complaints with diarrhoea or constipation. The person may have a longing for fruity, acidic drinks and an unpleasant taste in the mouth. This is also a remedy for weakness and failure to thrive in babies where there is a lack of muscle tone. Symptoms are made worse by touch, resting, at night and if conditions are windy. They improve for walking about and being out in fresh, clean air. People suitable for Mag. carb. are often dark-haired and pale-skinned and are prone to exhaustion with pains in the legs and feet. They are very sensitive to cold draughts and being touched and may be on edge and irritable. They are prone to having a sour, unpleasant taste in the mouth and are hypersensitive, being apt to feeling ignored and left out by others. They frequently have an intolerance such as sour smells, milk and sweat.

Magnesia phosphorica

Mag. phos.; phosphate of magnesia, magnesium phosphate

This white compound is one of the SCHUSSLER TISSUE SALTS (see GLOSSARY) and is prepared chemically from sodium phosphate and magnesium sulphate. Magnesium occurs naturally in the body and is essential for the correct functioning of nerves and muscles. A deficiency can cause cramping pains and spasms and have deleterious effects on the heart and skeletal muscles. The remedy is used to treat neuralgic pains, writer's cramp, spasms and cramps. The pains are shooting and intermittent and may be brought on by a cold draught. Often, they occur mainly on the right side of the body. Colicky pains that are relieved by doubling over or by bending and by heat and firm pressure, benefit from Mag. phos. People who benefit from this remedy are often thin, sensitive and worried and may be academic, workaholic types. Symptoms are worse for cold air, touch, at night and if the person is tired and debilitated. They improve with any form of heat, pressure and warm surroundings.

Manganum aceticum

Acetate of manganese

This remedy was investigated and proved by Hahnemann in the 19th century. It is useful for the treatment of general debility and weakness with loss of appetite and weight, anaemia and, possibly, ulcers of the skin or bed sores. The skin is a bluish colour, and the body is extremely sensitive to touch. The person has great difficulty in eating enough to maintain body weight.

Medorrhinum

A remedy prepared from gonorrhoeal discharge

Gonorrhoea, the sexually transmitted bacterial disease, has plagued humankind since ancient times, and was first given the name of gonorrhoea by Galen, a physician of the Roman civilization. The effects of gonorrhoea can be passed from a mother to her baby during birth. Hahnemann believed that gonorrhoea was responsible for inherited traits or weaknesses in subsequent generations, and he called this a 'miasm', in this case the sycotic miasm (sycosis). Two other miasms were identified, 'psora', connected with the blisters and itching of scabies (see PSORINUM), and syphilis (see SYPHILINUM). Gonorrhoea has always been a feared and devastating illness and was formerly treated with injections of silver nitrate. In conventional medicine it is treated with modern antibiotics.

The homoeopathic remedy is used to treat a variety of physical and mental symptoms. It is used to treat inflammation and infection of pelvic organs, menstrual pain and pain in the ovaries. Some other disorders of the mucous membranes, kidneys, nerves and spine, e.g. neuralgia, may benefit from this remedy. It is especially suitable for people who have a family history of gonorrhoea and some forms of heart disease. Emotional disorders may be treated with Medorrhinum, especially mood swings with the person changing from irritability and extreme impatience to passive withdrawal. In the impatient state the person is always in a hurry and is inclined to be selfish and insensitive. In the withdrawn state the person is dreamy and forgetful and very much in touch with, and moved by, the beauty of nature. In both states, the person tends to be forgetful and may feel neglected, lost or deserted. Symptoms are made worse by damp weather, heat in the early morning between 3 and 4 a.m. and after passing urine. Even slight movements make the symptoms worse, but they improve with lying on the front, in the evening and being beside the sea. Symptoms are also better if the person rests on the hands and knees ('all fours').

Mercurius corrosivus

Merc. cor.; mercuric chloride, mercury chloride HgCl$_2$

Mercuric chloride is a highly poisonous corrosive substance, causing burning and destruction of tissue if swallowed. It has antiseptic properties and is used to treat bulbs and tubers to prevent fungal attack. It is also used industrially in the manufacture of plastics. The homoeopathic remedy is used for severe symptoms of ulceration in the digestive and urinary tracts and mouth and throat. It is used for ulcerative colitis with copious diarrhoea containing blood and mucus, and abdominal pains. Also, for severe bladder infections and urethritis with painful and frequent urination, the urine containing blood and mucus. There may be thick discoloured discharges containing pus. Throat and mouth symptoms include ulcerated tonsils covered with a white, pus-containing discharge, facial pain, exhaustion and secretion of excess saliva. Symptoms are worse in the evening and if the person walks about. They are also worse if the person eats fatty meals or acidic foods. Symptoms are better after breakfast and if the person rests.

Mercurius cyanatus

Mercuric cyanide

This homoeopathic remedy is used to treat severe symptoms of diphtheria. The throat is extremely sore and the person finds swallowing and speech unbearable, and there is a covering of thick, greyish-white mucus. The person feels cold, and the skin has a blue-coloured tinge because of a lack of oxygen (cyanosis). The person may be on the verge of collapse.

Mercurius dulcis

Merc. dulc.; mercurous chloride, calomel, mercury chloride Hg$_2$Cl$_2$

This substance has laxative properties, and calomel was used as a purgative in medieval times. It is now used in the horticultural and agricultural industries as a constituent of certain insecticides and fungicides. Both *Mercurius dulcis* and *Mercurius corrosivus* are found in mineral deposits in the United States of America, Mexico, Germany and parts of central Europe. Merc. dulc. is a useful remedy for children suffering from glue ear and ca-

tarrhal problems. The child has swollen glands, and the nasal, ear and throat passages are clogged with discharges of thick, sticky mucus. Breathing may be noisy, and hearing is often affected. Symptoms are worse if the child is engaged in sport or physical exercise and also at night.

Mixed autumn moulds

MAP

This homoeopathic remedy is derived from a mixture of three moulds—mucor, aspergillus and penicillum—and it is used to treat symptoms of hay fever that arise in the autumn. These symptoms include a runny nose and catarrh, itchy, red, watery eyes, sneezing and wheezing with a tight feeling in the chest. The usual time for symptoms to appear is in the early months of autumn, especially September.

Moschus moschiferus

Moschus; musk from the musk deer

Musk is a strong-smelling, aromatic secretion produced by the male musk deer in order to attract a female. The secretion has long been used in the production of perfume and has a long-lived effect. Samuel Hahnemann was concerned about the widespread use of musk-based scents, believing that the substance made people more susceptible to disease by weakening their natural immunity. The musk deer is a small deer found in countries of central Asia, inhabiting hilly or mountainous areas. Dried musk is used to prepare the homoeopathic remedy, which is mainly given for hysterical, neurotic and emotional symptoms. Physical symptoms include giddiness and fainting, pallor and exhaustion and sweating. People suitable for this remedy have a tendency towards hypochondria and may feel that everyone is against them. They tend to talk incessantly and have hurried, clumsy movements. They tend to feel chilled, although one half of the body may seem cold and the other hot. Their exhaustion is worse for resting than for moving about, and all symptoms are aggravated by cool, fresh air and emotional upset or excitement. Symptoms improve after burping and for warm surroundings.

Murex

Purple mollusc

This homoeopathic remedy is prepared from the body of the shellfish and is useful for menopausal symptoms of irregular bleeding. It is also used to treat emotional and hysterical symptoms and stress. A person suitable for this remedy dislikes being touched and especially having a medical examination.

Mygale lasiodora

Mygale las.; *Mygale avicularia, Aranea avicularia*, Cuban spider

This spider, which is a large variety native to Cuba, has a highly poisonous bite used to immobilize its prey. If a person is bitten, the area becomes inflamed and discoloured, turning purple and green, and the effects spread outwards as the poison drains along the lymph vessels. The person experiences a high fever, tremor, chills, dry skin and mouth, severe anxiety and breathing difficulties and is very thirsty. The person fears that he or she will die. The homoeopathic remedy is used to treat involuntary twitching and jerking of the muscles, which may be caused by nerve disorders such as various forms of chorea. The remedy is sometimes used to treat sexually transmitted venereal diseases. Symptoms are worse during the morning but improve when the person is sleeping.

Naja naja

Naja; *Naja tripudians*, venom of the cobra

The cobra, which has the habit of drawing itself erect and extending the skin below its neck to form a hood before it strikes, has long been both revered and feared. The snake is capable of shooting its venom into the eyes of its prey from a distance of six feet away, which causes blindness. The bite of the cobra may prove fatal, affecting the heart and lungs, causing collapse and death. The dried venom, which is bright yellow, is used to prepare the homoeopathic remedy. It is used to treat left-sided symptoms, particularly of the heart, but also of the left ovary. Symptoms include crushing, choking pain as in angina, with the pain extending to the left shoulder and down the arm and hand. The pulse may be slow and the person feels breathless and oppressed. Ovarian pain may extend to the upper left-hand side of the body. Asthma that comes on after an attack of hay fever may be treated with Naja. The symptoms are made worse by lying on the left side, by cold draughts and following sleep. They are also aggravated by wearing tight, constricting clothing and drinking alcohol. For women, symptoms are worse following the monthly period.

Natrum carbonicum

Nat. carb.; sodium carbonate, soda ash

Sodium carbonate was once derived from the ashes of burnt seaweed but is now obtained from a chemical process. It is used industrially in the manufacture of detergents, soaps and glass-making. Sodium carbonate has various uses in conventional medicine, being used in creams and ointments to treat burns, eczema and other skin conditions. Also, it is used in preparations to clear up catarrh and vaginal discharge. The homoeopathic remedy was investigated and proved by Hahnemann. It is used to treat a variety of skin disorders such as eczema, chapped, dry, sore skin, cold sores, moles, warts, corns and blisters. Also, for sore throats and catarrh, headache and indigestion. Symptoms are made worse by warm, humid weather, heat in any form, including being out in the hot sun. They are relieved by eating. People suitable for Nat. carb. have a sensitive, kind and intuitive nature, always ready to provide a sympathetic audience to others. They are devoted to their family and friends and give generously of themselves, endeavouring to be cheerful even when feeling unwell or depressed. They tend to be delicate and prone to digestive upsets, especially being intolerant of milk and dairy products. Ankles are another weak point, tending to be easily strained or sprained. Nat. carb. people are highly sensitive to music and are upset by noise and thunderstorms. They are soon exhausted by physical activity.

Natrum phosphoricum

Nat. phos.; sodium phosphate

Sodium phosphate occurs naturally in body cells and is one of the SCHUSSLER TISSUE SALTS (*see* GLOSSARY). It is involved in the regulation of acidity in body tissues and fluids, and in complex metabolic chemical processes utilizing fatty acids. It is derived from a chemical reaction between sodium carbonate and phosphoric acid. It is a useful remedy for symptoms caused by an excess of lactic acid or uric acid. Excess lactic acid may be caused by a diet too rich in milk, dairy products or fatty foods. Also, there may be an excess of gastric or stomach acid, and this may be connected with eating too much sour food. The symptoms are those of acid indigestion with a sour taste in the mouth, wind and abdominal pains. An excess of uric acid is present in people suffering from gout with painful, inflamed stiff joints. Symptoms are made worse by thunderstorms and by eating fatty, sour or sweet foods and with physical exertion. They improve for being out in the fresh, clean air and for cool, airy surroundings. People suitable for this remedy tend to be refined and somewhat timid and prone to blush easily. They are easily exhausted but are inclined to be restless or slightly agitated. They do not accept advice readily and are prone to dissatisfaction and depression.

Natrum sulphuricum

Nat. sulph.; sodium sulphate, Glauber's salt, sal mirabile

Sodium sulphate is a naturally occurring substance within the body and is involved in the regulation of the salt/water balance in tissues and fluids. It is found in natural brines associated with salt lakes or can be manufactured by a chemical process. Sodium sulphate is used in industry in the manufacture of wood pulp and paper, glass, chemicals and detergents. It was investigated and proved by Schussler and is one of the tissue salts (see GLOSSARY). It is used in the treatment of liver disorders including jaundice, digestive complaints with indigestion and colicky pains, severe chesty conditions such as bronchitis and asthma, and bladder problems with urinary frequency. It is also used to relieve mental symptoms that arise after a head injury, such as depression or personality changes. Symptoms are made worse by damp, cold weather or surroundings and by lying on the back. The symptoms are worse at night and during the morning. Symptoms are relieved by cool, fresh, dry conditions and being out in the fresh air. Symptoms improve if the person changes position. People suitable for Nat. sulph. may either be very serious, keeping their emotions tightly controlled and putting up a front that may hide severe depression and suicidal thoughts. Or the depression may be more apparent, and they can become emotional on hearing music or contemplating art. These types are less repressed but still tend to suffer from depression. Nat. sulph. people are often somewhat materialistic and are very sensitive to damp weather with a tendency for asthma and chesty complaints with catarrh.

Nicotiana tabacum

Tabacum; tobacco

The tobacco plant derives its Latin name from Jean Nicot, a Portuguese diplomat who was an ambassador for France in South America during the 1500s. He brought tobacco to France in about 1560, but it had long been used by the Indian peoples. The plant has a hairy stem and leaves, giving off a narcotic odour. It contains nicotine, which is a powerful poison causing sickness and nausea, palpitations, sweating, headache and giddiness. It is now well established that smoking tobacco is a major cause of premature death. The homoeopathic remedy is prepared from the fresh leaves of the plant and is given as a remedy for nausea and vomiting, such as in travel sickness, vertigo and disorders affecting the organs of balance in the ears. Symptoms are made worse by even slight movements such as turning the head, and for heat and tobacco smoke. They improve in cold surroundings and after vomiting.

Nitric acidum

Nitric ac; nitric acid, aqua fortis

This is a burning, extremely corrosive, clear liquid that gives off choking fumes that cause death by inhalation. Its industrial uses are mainly in the manufacture of agricultural fertilizers and high explosives. It has been used medicinally in extremely dilute form to treat severe infections and fevers, and to dissolve stones in the kidneys or bladder. It has been applied externally to the skin to burn away warts. Nitric acid is derived from a chemical reaction between sulphuric acid and sodium nitrate.

The homoeopathic remedy is used to treat sharp, stabbing pains that may be intermittent in nature and are associated with piles, or haemorrhoids, anal fissure, ulcers in the mouth or on the skin, severe sore throat with ulceration, thrush infections and ulcers in the stomach or duodenum. Usually, the affected person suffers from broken, cracked skin with a tendency for ulcers and warts, and usually feels cold. The urine and other bodily secretions have a strong, pungent odour. Symptoms are worse for acidic fruits and drinks, milk, touch or pressure and movement. They are more severe at night and improve with heat and warm, dry surroundings. People suitable for Nitric ac. tend to be selfish, self-centred and apt to hold long grudges against others. They feel that everyone is against them but are themselves apt to fly into a rage and take offence very easily. They like to re-examine events and slights of the past and may be suspicious of other people. When ill, they are very fearful and worry that they may die.

Nux moschata

Nux mosch.; Myristica fragrans, nutmeg

The nutmeg tree grows mainly on an Indonesian island called Banda, which is one of the

Molucca group, and also in the Far East and India. It was introduced to Constantinople (Istanbul) from India in about 540 AD and soon became widely used both for culinary, cosmetic and medicinal purposes. It was used to treat digestive upsets and headache and rheumatic pain. In herbal medicine, the remedy is given for sharper, clearer eyesight. In large doses, nutmeg produces hallucinogenic symptoms of drowsiness, giddiness and unsteadiness, with unco-ordinated movements and fainting. The homoeopathic tincture is made from the inner seeds without their outer tough husks. The remedy is mainly given for mental and emotional disorders and digestive upsets. Symptoms include hysteria, agitation, excitement and exhaustion and drowsiness and confusion that may follow an epileptic attack or stroke. Also, for abdominal pains and indigestion, constipation and inflammation of the gastro-intestinal tract. People who benefit from this remedy have a need for fluids being somewhat dehydrated, but do not feel any great desire to drink. Symptoms are made worse by sudden changes in the weather and damp and cool conditions. They improve for being warm, wearing plenty of clothes and for high humidity.

Ocymum canum
Alfavaca, bush basil

This is a low-growing bushy plant that is a native of India and has a sweet scent. The homoeopathic tincture is made from fresh leaves, and it is used as a remedy for renal colic and stones affecting the right kidney. The symptoms are pain and vomiting, a cloudy urine because of a deposit of reddish 'sand', and urinary frequency. There may be infection present and a sharp pain on passing urine, as in cystitis. The urine has a strong, pungent smell.

Oleander
Rose laurel

The fresh leaves are used to make the homoeopathic remedy, which was first investigated and proved by Hahnemann. It is given for heart symptoms including palpitations, weakness, great anxiety and fainting. The person may feel giddy or be on the point of collapse. Also, for symptoms of gastroenteritis including diarrhoea, nausea and sickness and abdominal pains. The person often has sore, dry, chapped skin and is liable to suffer from depression, lack of concentration and clumsiness with a tendency for falls and even accidents. Physical symptoms that may benefit from this rem-

edy include vertigo, headache, blurred vision, muscular weakness, and lack of co-ordination.

Oleum petrae
Petroleum

Petroleum, or liquid crude oil, is found trapped in oil-bearing rocks in the earth's crust and is derived from decayed organic material from the Carboniferous geological period. Petroleum is a vital fuel resource upon which people throughout the world are heavily reliant. In conventional medicine, petroleum jelly is used as an external treatment for minor skin abrasions. Purified petroleum is used to prepare the homoeopathic remedy, which was first investigated and proved by Hahnemann and which is given for skin complaints. These include dry, cracked, chafed skin, particularly on the fingers, and eczema. These complaints are worse in cold weather, when the skin is subjected to chilling and heating. The remedy is also used for sickness, nausea and vomiting, especially as a result of travel sickness. There is a tendency for headaches to occur, especially in the back of the head. People who benefit from this remedy may be irritable because of having constantly inflamed, itchy, sore skin. They may fly into a rage and tend to have an excitable temperament. They dislike and are upset by fatty foods and their sweat has a strong odour. Symptoms are made worse by cold, windy weather, particularly during the winter months, and by thunderstorms. They improve with warmth and warm, dry weather and following a meal.

Onosmodium
False gromwell

The whole fresh parts of the green plant are needed to make the homoeopathic remedy, which is used for mental symptoms including anxiety, tension and irritability. Also, for depression, lack of concentration and clumsiness, with a tendency for accidental and even accidents. Physical symptoms that may benefit from this remedy include vertigo, headache, blurred vision, muscular weakness and lack of co-ordination.

Ornithogalum umbrellatum
Star of Bethlehem

This remedy is used for severe, persistent, digestive upsets and is made from the whole green parts of the plant. There may be burning pains and regurgitation of stomach acid. The abdomen tends to be bloated with air, and there is flatulence. The person may suffer from depression and severe anxiety and is irritable and short-tempered with others. There is a tendency for peptic or duodenal ulcers to occur.

Oxalic acid

Sorrel acid, common wood sorrel, *Oxalis acetosella*

This remedy is derived from the leaves of sorrel, which have long had a culinary use. The leaves have a sour, sharp quality and can be used in place of vinegar. The plant itself is small and delicate and grows in Britain and other European countries. It produces delicate, white flowers shaped like little bells, which are veined with purple. Preparations made from the plant have cooling and diuretic properties. The homoeopathic remedy is used for painful, rheumatic disorders, mainly affecting the left side of the body. The pains are severe and sharp, and the person becomes weak and cold. There is a tendency for small haemorrhages called petechiae to occur, which have the appearance of dark red spots beneath the skin. The person may have a tendency to bleed easily and to vomit blood.

Paeonia officinalis

Peony

This plant is well known in the British Isles as a pretty, deep pink garden flower, but it has been used medicinally since ancient times. It is believed to derive its name from a Greek physician called Paos, who, according to mythology, used it to cure the gods, including Pluto, of wounds sustained during the Trojan War. Many ancient superstitions and charms were connected with the plant, which was believed to have come from the moon and to have divine origins. The root of the peony has been used to prevent nightmare and epilepsy, as a cure for madness and to combat infection after childbirth. The fresh root, which is used to prepare both the herbal and homoeopathic remedies, has antispasmodic, sedative and antiseptic qualities. In homoeopathy, it is used as a remedy for itchy piles, or haemorrhoids, with discomfort and swelling. Also, it is used for sleep disturbance because of nightmares and indigestion and the need to sleep during the afternoons.

Papaver somniferum

Opium poppy, mawseed

The opium poppy is a native of Asia but is widely cultivated in other countries. In the wild, the poppy flowers are a pale mauve colour with a deeper purple spot at the base of the petals. Cultivated flowers have a variety of colours, from white to red/purple. The unripened green seed capsules that develop at the base of the flowers are the part used in herbal medicine and homoeopathy. An incision is made into the capsule, and a milky white juice is exuded that darkens as it dries. This is collected by scraping the capsules. The principal constituents of the opium juice are the alkaloids morphine and codeine, which are widely used in conventional medicine for their potent analgesic properties. Opium was used by the physicians of ancient Greece and Rome as a painkiller. It was probably introduced into India and hence to Europe by Arabian physicians. Dark grey poppy seeds, from the red/purple coloured flowers (called mawseed) are used in cooking and do not contain opium or morphine. They are also a constituent of bird seed. Opium has narcotic, sedative, hypnotic and antispasmodic properties. In homoeopathy the remedy is used to treat symptoms of mental shock following a severe emotional shock or frightening experience. The symptoms may either be those of withdrawal and apathy, or of great agitation, excitement and sleeplessness with a greatly enhanced acute sense of hearing. It is also given for respiratory and breathing problems, constipation, alcohol withdrawal symptoms (delirium tremens) and following a stroke. Symptoms are worse for sleep and heat and improve with movement and exercise and in cool surroundings.

Pareira brava

Ice vine, velvet leaf

This climbing vine is a native species of Peru, Brazil and the West Indies and has very large leaves and flowers. It has a twisted, knotty root, and it is this part that is used to prepare the homoeopathic remedy. Preparations made from the root have a stimulant effect on the kidneys and bowels and have diuretic and tonic properties. The homoeopathic remedy is used for the treatment of urinary tract infections and disorders including cystitis, urethritis, urine retention and urinary frequency. There may be hot, burning pains on passing urine with abdominal pain or discomfort.

Paris quadrifolia

One berry, true love, herba Paris

This herbaceous, perennial plant flourishes in moist, shady conditions in woodlands throughout Europe and in Russia. A single stem is produced, which grows to a height of about ten inches or one foot, near the top of which are four pointed leaves. A single flower is produced in early summer, which is a whitish-green in colour and has an unpleasant rank smell. Later, a purple-black fruit is produced, which splits to release its seeds when ripe. The whole plant is used to prepare the homoeopathic remedy, and it was first investigated and proved by Hahnemann. The plant is poisonous and has narcotic properties. If eaten in large quantities, it produces vomiting and diarrhoea, giddiness, dry throat, sweating and possibly convulsions and death. In homoeopathy, it is used as an eye remedy for conjunctivitis and inflamed, irritated, itchy, watery eyes. Symptoms are mainly on the left side and the person is often excitable and talkative.

Parotidinum
The mumps nosode

This homoeopathic remedy is derived from mumps-infected parotid salivary gland secretion. It is usually given as a preventative medicine to adults at risk of contracting mumps.

Passiflora incarnata
Passionflower, maypops

There are a number of species of passionflower, which gain their name from the resemblance of the blooms to the crown of thorns worn by Jesus. The plant produces large, sweet-scented flowers that are white or whitish-peach coloured with tinges of purple. Later, large berries with many seeds are produced, which are edible. The green parts of the plant are used to prepare herbal and homoeopathic remedies. Preparations derived from the passionflower have sedative, narcotic and antispasmodic properties. In homoeopathy, the remedy is used for convulsions, as in epilepsy, and also for illnesses in which there are severe spasms, such as whooping cough, asthmatic attacks and tetanus. Also, for serious mental disturbance, including delirium tremens resulting from alcoholism, and excited manic states.

Pertussin
Coqueluchin

This remedy is a nosode of whooping cough and is derived from material contaminated with the virus. It is given to treat the symptoms of whooping cough but also as a preventative measure for those at risk of contracting the disease.

Phellandrium aquaticum
Water fennel, fine-leaved water dropwort

This plant grows in ditches or on the banks of rivers near to the water; the lower parts may be submerged. The plant produces fruits that yield a yellow liquid from which the herbal and homoeopathic remedies are derived. The preparations have expectorant and diuretic properties and are useful for treating chesty, bronchitic complaints. In homoeopathy, the remedy is used for chest and respiratory disorders, with symptoms mainly on the right side. Conditions treated include bronchitis and emphysema with breathlessness, a severe cough and the production of thick mucus. Headache is another common symptom.

Phleum pratense
Timothy grass

This is a remedy for hay fever that is triggered by exposure to the pollen of flowering grasses. The person has the typical symptoms of watering, itchy eyes and running nose and sneezing. Breathlessness and asthma may also occur. The remedy is sometimes given to prevent the occurrence of an attack of hay fever.

Phosphoricum acidum
Phos. ac.; phosphoric acid

Phosphoric acid is a clear, crystalline substance that is obtained by a chemical process from a naturally occurring mineral, apatite. Apatite is rich in phosphate and occurs in various igneous (volcanic) and metamorphic rocks (ones altered by high temperatures and pressures) and mineral veins. Phosphoric acid has various industrial uses in the manufacture of fertilizers and detergents. It is used in the food industry as a flavouring for soft drinks and in the refining of white sugar. Also, it is used in the production of various pharmaceutical drugs. In conventional medicine it is used in the treatment of parathyroid gland tumours, acting to reduce blood calcium levels.

The homoeopathic remedy was first investigated and proved by Hahnemann and is used to treat emotional and physical symptoms of apathy, exhaustion, listlessness and depression. These symptoms may arise from overwork or study or follow on after a debilitating illness that has caused dehydration. Other symptoms are a loss of appetite, feeling continually cold and shivery, dizziness, especially in the evening, and a feeling of pressure pushing downwards on the head. Phos. ac. is also given for growing pains in children or who suffer from sleep disturbance because of an awareness of sexual feelings. Symptoms are worse for cold, damp, draughty conditions and for loud noises. They improve following restful sleep and with warm surroundings.

Physostigma veneriosum
Calabar bean, chop nut, ordeal bean

This perennial climbing plant grows to a height of about 50 feet and is a native species of West Africa. It was introduced into Britain (and grown in the Botanical Gardens in Edinburgh) in 1846. It produces purple-coloured elongated flowers and later, dark brown seeds in pods about 6 inches in length. The seeds are extremely poisonous and were given as a test for witchcraft by West African peoples. If the accused person vomited after being forced to swallow the seeds, he or she was deemed innocent, but if death was the outcome then the accusation of being a witch was upheld. The poison causes depression of the central nervous system, slowing of the pulse and a rise in blood pressure, and death may follow because of respiratory collapse. Preparations made from the seeds are also miotic, causing a rapid contraction of the pupil of the eye, and its main use in herbal medicine is in the treatment of eye diseases. The ripe beans or seeds are used to prepare the homoeopathic remedy, which is given for serious disorders in which there are muscular spasms. These include tetanus, meningitis and poliomyelitis. Also, for other disorders characterized by muscular and nervous degeneration or paralysis including Friedrich's ataxia, motor neurone disease and multiple sclerosis. The remedy may also be given for diarrhoea, vomiting, fever, sweating, prostration, and palpitations in which the pupils of the eye are very much contracted.

Phytolacca deccandra
Phytolacca; Virginian poke root, garget, reading plant, pocon, branching grape, pigeon berry

This plant is a native species of the United States and Canada, but is also found in Mediterranean countries, China and North Africa. It has a striking appearance and produces white flowers followed by clusters of shiny black berries. The orange-coloured fleshy root is the part used to prepare the homoeopathic remedy, but both the root and berries are used in herbal medicine. Preparations derived from the plant have purgative, emetic and restorative properties. Native American Indians used poke root to cause vomiting and to encourage movement of the bowels and as a heart stimulant. It was

also used as a remedy for skin disorders. Europeans used the plant to treat breast lumps and tumours and for mastitis (inflammation). In herbal medicine it is used to treat skin disorders, ringworm and scabies, chronic rheumatism, granular conjunctivitis (eye inflammation), ulcers and severe menstrual pain.

In homoeopathy the remedy is given for small hard lumps or tumours in the breasts, which may be either benign or cancerous, and for mastitis. The breasts may be hot, swollen and painful to touch with stabbing pains. Also, it is used to treat severe sore throats and swallowing difficulty in which there is great pain, redness and inflammation. These symptoms may occur with tonsillitis, pharyngitis and diphtheria. The symptoms are made worse by swallowing, movement, hot drinks and in cold, damp draughty conditions. They improve with warmth and sunny, dry weather, cold drinks and having plenty of rest.

Picricum acidum
Picric acid

This poisonous substance is obtained by chemical reactions between nitric, sulphuric and carbolic acids. Since it was first investigated and proved for homoeopathic use in 1868, it has been used to treat extreme exhaustion with mental and intellectual indifference and apathy. It usually occurs after an extended period of intense intellectual activity such as may occur among students cramming for exams. The person feels generally heavy and lethargic and is too tired to engage in conversation or to think clearly. Often, a numbing headache and aching eyes occur, or there may be a boil in the outer part of the ear. These symptoms may also arise as a result of grief. Symptoms are made worse with any physical or intellectual activity and in hot surroundings. They improve with rest and in cool conditions and if the weather is sunny but not hot.

Pilocarpus jaborandi, Pilocarpus microphyllus
Jaborandi

The drug known as Jaborandi is extracted from the leaves of Pilocarpus, which are shrubs native to Brazil. The leaves contain a volatile oil, and the most important active constituent of this is an alkaloid substance called pilocarpine. Preparations made from the leaves have diaphoretic properties, causing sweating, and are also stimulant and expectorant. Pilocarpine is mydriatic, causing contraction of the pupil of the eye. In herbal medicine, Jaborandi is used to treat diabetes, asthma, skin disorders such as psoriasis, catarrh and oedema (fluid retention). Also it is used as a tonic in preparations to stimulate new hair growth in the treatment of baldness. The homoeopathic remedy is given for various eye and vision disorders, sweating because of the menopause or in hyperthyroidism (an overactive thyroid gland) and mumps.

Plantago major

Common plantain, broad-leaved plantain, waybread, ripple grass

This is a very familiar weed that grows throughout Britain and Europe and was introduced by colonists into the New World continents. The use of plantain in medicine goes back to ancient times, and it is described by Erasmus and Pliny. In Britain, plantain was an ingredient of many old remedies. It has been used in the past to treat wounds and external bleeding, for venomous bites and for disorders of the bowels and kidneys. It was used as a remedy for piles, or haemorrhoids, and to treat diarrhoea. Plantain is still used to treat these ailments in modern herbal medicine and homoeopathy. The whole fresh plant is used to prepare the homoeopathic remedy, which is sometimes used as the mother tincture. It is given for piles, toothache and tooth abscess and facial neuralgia. It is also used in the treatment of conditions such as diabetes, characterized by large quantities of urine being passed. Most symptoms occur on the left side and are worse for movement, cold and heat and draughts.

Platinum metallicum

Platinum

Platinum was discovered in South America during the 1700s. It is regarded as a very precious metal and is used to make jewellery. It is used in the electrical industry, in dentistry for fillings, and to make surgical pins to repair fractured bones. The homoeopathic remedy is used almost entirely for female reproductive disorders that may have associated emotional problems. These include pain in the ovaries, spasm in vaginal muscles, making it difficult for the woman to have sexual intercourse (vaginisimus), heavy menstrual bleeding, absence of periods and genital itching. The woman may experience feelings of numbness, chilling and constriction of muscles and has a great fear of gynaecological examinations and procedures. Symptoms are made worse by touch and physical contact and by tiredness. They are worse in the evening but are relieved by being out in fresh clean air.

Women suitable for platinum set themselves and others extremely high standards of achievement that are not possible to attain. Hence they feel let down by apparent failures and tend to become depressed and irritable, feeling that the past was better than the present. They may become cynical and contemptuous of the efforts of others.

Plumbum metallicum

Plumbum met.; lead

Lead has been useful to humans for centuries and was used extensively by the Romans, especially to make pipes for plumbing systems. Lead continued to be mined and used throughout the ages, and has had many uses, e.g. in roofing, to make weights and lead shot, pencils, pottery glazes, paint and as an additive in fuel for vehicle engines. It has been known for some time, however, that lead is an insidious poison if present above a certain level in the human body. Early symptoms of poisoning are constipation that persists, weakness of muscles, pale skin and a blue line (because of lead sulphide) along the margin of gums and teeth. There is intellectual dullness and impairment and behavioural changes, and these are especially noticeable in children. Later, there are severe abdominal pains of a colicky nature, drooping wrists and feet, tremors, increasing muscular weakness and paralysis. Convulsions and lead encephalopathy affecting the brain may occur, leading to death if not diagnosed and treated.

The homoeopathic remedy is used to treat long-term diseases of a sclerotic nature, i.e. leading to hardening of the affected tissues. These conditions include arteriosclerosis and atherosclerosis, Parkinson's disease and multiple sclerosis. Also for colic, constipation, muscular weakness and tremor and retention of urine. Symptoms are made worse by movement and are more severe at night. They improve with warmth and firm pressure or massage on the affected area. People suitable for Plumbum met. may have poor concentration and intellectual capabilities dulled by illness. They may have a poor memory and find it difficult to express themselves clearly. This intellectual impairment may make the person lethargic or short-tempered with others.

Podophyllum peltatum

Podophyllum; May apple, hog apple, American mandrake, duck's foot, wild lemon, racoonberry.

This herbaceous perennial plant is a native of the United States and Canada. The stalks grow to a height of about one or two feet and produce large, divided leaves and white flowers that have an unpleasant scent. Later, yellow fruits are produced that are edible although the leaves and roots are poisonous. The plant has a yellowish-brown rhizome and roots, and these are the parts used both in herbal medicine and homoeopathy. Preparations made from the plant have purgative and emetic properties and act strongly on the liver and digestive organs. The plant was used by the native American peoples to eliminate parasitic worms and as a cure for deafness. The homoeopathic remedy is given for digestive disorders such as vomiting and diarrhoea in gastroenteritis, gallstones, colicky pain and flatulence. There may be alternate bouts of diarrhoea and constipation. Symptoms are worse first thing in the morning and during hot weather. They are better for massaging the abdomen and for lying on the front.

Primula veris
Cowslip, herb Peter, key flower, mayflower, key of heaven, pargle, peggle

This familiar and pretty wild flower is common in shady woodlands in Europe and Great Britain. It produces delicate yellow flowers, and it is these that are used to prepare the herbal and homoeopathic remedies. Preparations made from the plant have a sedative and antispasmodic effect. The flowers have been used to make cowslip wine, and the leaves were once valued as a salad vegetable. The homoeopathic remedy is used for serious symptoms of high blood pressure and threatened stroke. These include confusion and giddiness, headache and a feeling of throbbing heat.

Prunus laurocerasus
Cherry laurel, cherry bay, common laurel

This fairly small evergreen shrub is a native species of Russia but also grows in Europe and some parts of Asia. It produces dark green shiny leaves and white flowers followed by clusters of black, cherry-like fruits. The fresh leaves are used to prepare the herbal and homoeopathic remedies and give off a characteristic bitter almonds smell because of the presence of prussic acid. The shrubs are popular in gardens in Europe, having been first introduced in the late 16th century. The leaves are mainly used to produce cherry laurel water in herbal medicine, and preparations have a sedative

effect. They are used for coughs and spasms, particularly whooping cough and asthma. The homoeopathic remedy is used to treat severe symptoms of breathlessness and cyanosis (a blue tinge to the skin because of lack of oxygen in the blood) with a spasmodic cough. The symptoms are caused by serious disorders of the heart or lungs.

Psorinum
This remedy is derived from the fluid of scabies blisters and was first investigated and proved by Hahnemann. Hahnemann wrote extensively about the development of chronic diseases. He believed that in certain people the blisters produced in scabies were a manifestation of a deeper disorder. While the scabies blisters themselves might heal and disappear, this suppressed disease, or MIASM, still continued to cause disruption within the body and might even be passed on to subsequent generations. The symptoms or disorder associated with the scabies miasm are called psora and mainly affect the skin. The skin is dry, cracked and sore and there may be infections with pus-filled blisters. Also, digestive upsets, particularly diarrhoea and indigestion, exhaustion, depression and a pessimistic outlook on life are believed to be common manifestations of psora. The psorinum remedy is given to treat the symptoms described above and also for some respiratory ailments, especially hay fever, and general debility. Digestive ailments treated include irritable bowel syndrome and diverticulitis. Skin conditions such as eczema, acne, dermatitis, boils and ulceration may all respond to psorinum.

People suitable for this remedy are generally worried, pessimistic and gloomy, with a fear of all that may go wrong in life. They are very sensitive to cold and often feel chilled, even during the height of summer. They often experience a gnawing hunger and have a headache that is relieved by eating. They may feel that friends and family have deserted them. Symptoms are worse for cold winter weather and also for becoming too hot, either in bed or through physical exercise or wearing too many clothes. They improve in summer, with resting with the limbs spread out and with warm surroundings.

Ptelea trifoliata
Wafer ash, swamp dogwood, hop tree, wingseed, shrubby trefoil, ptelea

This small, shrubby tree, which grows to a

height of six to eight feet, is a native species of the United States and Canada. The bark of the root is the part used to prepare remedies used in herbal medicine and homoeopathy. The bark has a fairly pungent smell and a bitter taste and has a tonic effect, acting mainly on the liver and digestive organs. The homoeopathic remedy is used mainly for liver disorders such as hepatitis and enlargement and tenderness. There is discomfort and heaviness in the region of the liver. Also, for digestive disorders, particularly indigestion, and rheumatism. All symptoms are mainly on the right side of the body and are made worse if the person lies on his or her right side.

Pyrogenium

Pyrogenium is a remedy introduced to homoeopathy by Dr John Drysdale in 1880. It was a mixture of raw beef and water left to stand for three weeks. After straining, a straw-coloured liquid, called sepsin, was left, which, when mixed with glycerine, was called pyrogen. Dr Drysdale believed that pyrogen had profound effects upon the blood if taken in large amounts, causing septicaemia or blood poisoning. In modern homoeopathy, the pyrogenium remedy is given for blood poisoning and septic conditions in which the healing process is rather slow. Characteristically, the person is feverish and has aching bones, a rapid pulse with feelings of heat and burning. The person is uncomfortable and restless and may have considerable pain if suffering from a septic condition such as an abscess. Symptoms are made worse by cold and draughts but improve with moving about.

Radium bromatum

Radium brom.; radium bromide

Radium bromide is derived from radium, which was discovered by Pierre and Marie Curie at the end of the 19th century. Radium is used in conventional medicine in radiotherapy for the treatment of cancer. It is obtained from the radioactive mineral uranite, which is also the main ore of uranium. Radium bromide is obtained by a chemical process from radium, and the homoeopathic remedy is used to treat skin complaints in which there is itching and burning. Ailments include eczema, moles, skin ulcers, acne, skin cancer, rosacea (a red, flushed face and enlargement of the skin's sebaceous glands) and dry, chafed, sore skin. Also, for aching painful bones as in lumbago, rheumatic and arthritic disorders and bone cancer. Pains

may move from one side of the body to the other, and symptoms are worse at night and on first moving after resting. They improve if the person lies down or moves about for a prolonged period. They are also better for lying down and for having a hot bath.

Rananculus bulbosus

Buttercup, bulbous buttercup, crowfoot, St Anthony's turnip, gold cup, frogsfoot

The familiar bright yellow buttercup is a familiar summer flower in Great Britain and other European countries. Small, bulbous swellings that resemble little turnips occur at the base of the stems. The plant can cause blistering and inflammation of the skin and has been used in a similar way to Cantharis (Spanish fly). The homoeopathic remedy is used for skin irritation and blistering, as in shingles and eczema, and for rheumatism with hot, tearing pains. Also, for pleurisy with severe pains during breathing. All symptoms are made worse by cold and damp and if the person feels afraid. The person tends to be generally rundown and unwell.

Raphanus sativus

Black radish, black Spanish radish

There are many varieties of radish that are cultivated as salad vegetables. In herbal medicine, the juice obtained from the radish is used as a cure for gallstones and other stones or gravel. In homoeopathy the remedy is used for abdominal flatulence and may be given post-operatively if there is sluggishness or some degree of paralysis of the digestive tract.

Rhatanhy

Krameria triandra, krameria root, Peruvian rhatany, rhantania

This low-growing shrub, which produces attractive large, red flowers, is a native species of Peru, growing in dry sandy soils in mountainous regions up to about 8,000 feet. The plant has strong roots, and it is these that are used to prepare the herbal and homoeopathic remedies. Preparations made from the plant have astringent and tonic properties and have been used to treat anal fissure and haemorrhage, diarrhoea, urinary incontinence, and excessive menstrual bleeding. The homoeopathic remedy is used to treat constipation with the development of painful haemorrhoids, or piles. The pains feel like glass splinters in the rectum and are very sharp. The person may have an odd sensation as though cold water is flowing over the molar teeth.

Rhododendron chrysanthemum

Rhododendron; yellow rhododendron, snow
rose, rosebay

This low shrub or bush has a highly branched,
reddish stem and grows to a height of about
eighteen inches or two feet. The leaves are oval
and resemble those of laurel. Large, attractive,
golden yellow flowers are produced, and the
plant is a native of the mountainous regions of
Siberia, Asia and Europe. In herbal medicine
the plant has long been used to treat rheumatic
disorders and gout. The fresh leaves are used
to prepare the herbal and homoeopathic remedies. In homoeopathy, the remedy is also used
to treat gout, rheumatism and arthritis. Main
symptoms are hot, painful swollen joints with
severe pains. The remedy is additionally used
for stabbing neuralgic pains around the eyes
and in the face, pain in the testicles, high fever
with confusion and delirium, and severe headaches. People who benefit from this remedy
tend to have an anxious temperament. Symptoms are worse during the approach of a thunderstorm and at night. They are also made
worse by standing still for a long period of time,
by resting and at the start of movement. They
improve with warmth and following a meal.

Rosa canina

The familiar dog-rose is an attractive bush producing pretty, delicately perfumed white or
pink flowers in summer. Later, scarlet-coloured
hips are produced containing the seeds that are
used to make rose hip syrup. The hips have
astringent and cooling properties and are a
good source of vitamin C. They have been used
in herbal medicine to treat diarrhoea, coughs
and the coughing up of blood, as in consumption (tuberculosis), colic and kidney stones. In
homoeopathy, the remedy made from the ripe
hips is used to treat disorders of the bladder
and prostate gland, characterized by difficult
and slow release of urine.

Rosmarinus officinalis

Rosemary, compass weed, polar plant,
compass plant

This small, evergreen herb is a native of the
arid, rocky hills along the Mediterranean coast
but may also grow inland. It has been grown
in Britain for centuries and has been important for both culinary and medicinal purposes.
It was believed to affect the brain, strengthening the memory, and became associated with
the virtues of remembrance, fidelity and friendship. It was included in bridal and funeral

wreaths and flowers, burned as incense in religious festivals and believed to have magical
properties. It was burnt or hung up as an antiseptic in sick rooms and hospitals, and strewn
among clothes and linen to prevent attack by
moths. Oil of rosemary was used externally to
treat baldness, dandruff and gout in the hands
and feet, and in wine for headaches, palpitations and dropsy (fluid retention or oedema).
Oil of rosemary is obtained from the flowering sprigs or tops of the plant. The homoeopathic remedy is used for memory loss and lack
of concentration and for baldness.

Rumex crispus

Yellow dock, curled dock

This dock is commonly found on wasteland
and along roadsides in the British Isles and has
leaves that are curled and crisp at the edges. It
grows to a height of about three feet and has
large green leaves. The root is used in herbal
medicine and has laxative and tonic properties. The homoeopathic remedy is prepared
from the whole flowering plant. It is used to
treat itching skin conditions, nasal congestion
with an abundance of thick, sticky catarrh, and
diarrhoea and digestive disorders. Symptoms
are made worse by cold and draughts and are
better for warmth and heat.

Sabadilla officinarum

Sabadilla; *Asagraea officinalis*, cevadilla,
cebadilla, *Veratum sabadilla*

These rushlike plants grow in the southern
states of the United States, Mexico and Central America (Venezuela and Guatemala). The
seeds are used to prepare herbal and homoeopathic remedies, and these have been known
in Europe since the 16th century. The preparations can be poisonous if taken internally, causing severe vomiting and diarrhoea. They were
formerly used in Europe to kill intestinal parasitic worms and to eliminate lice. They were
also used to treat rheumatism, gout and neuralgia. Sabadilla produces respiratory symptoms, resembling those of a cold, i.e. sneezing, running nose, watering, itchy eyes, coughing, headache and a painful sore throat. The
homoeopathic remedy is used to treat these
symptoms and also to eliminate an infestation
of threadworms. The symptoms are worse for
cold and draughts and better for warmth and
wearing warm clothes.

Sabal semilata

Sabal; the sabal palm, saw palmetto, palmetto
scrub

This palm-like tree grows to a height of six to ten feet and has a crown of large, serrated leaves. It grows in the coastal regions of South Carolina and Florida and in southern California. Irregularly shaped, oval, dark brown berries are produced containing seeds, and these are a source of fatty oil. They are a valuable food source for wild animals, promoting weight gain. The fresh berries and seeds are used to prepare the remedies used in herbal medicine and homoeopathy, and they have sedative, tonic and diuretic properties. The homoeopathic remedy is mainly used to treat enlargement of the prostate gland, causing difficult, slow urination with sharp pains. Sexual intercourse may be painful, and there is general tiredness and loss of libido. Also, for inflammation of the testicles and breasts (mastitis) with heat, swelling and tenderness.

People who are suitable for sabal are afraid of going to sleep, and their symptoms are made worse by cold, damp conditions and the sympathy of others. Symptoms improve with warm, dry weather and surroundings.

Sabina cacumina
Savine; savine tops

The shrub or small evergreen tree *Juniperus sabina* is a native species of the northern states of North America and some European countries. This plant is grown in gardens in Britain, and the fresh spring growth is used to prepare herbal and homoeopathic remedies. Preparations derived from the plant are irritant and poisonous in large doses and have powerful effects upon the uterus, causing bleeding. In herbal medicine the remedy is used externally for skin conditions, especially to encourage the drawing out of infection. In homoeopathy the remedy is given for rectal and uterine bleeding with pains that may be stabbing or burning. Also, for cystitis, heavy menstrual periods and varicose veins.

Salvia officinalis
Sage, garden sage

Sage is a familiar garden herb that has been cultivated in Europe for many centuries. There are several varieties, but the wild form of sage is found in the warmer parts of Europe and along the Mediterranean coast. Sage has long been valued as a herb for flavouring food and to make a form of 'tea'. It has been used medicinally since ancient times and was used to treat liver diseases, wounds, ulcers and bleeding, especially the coughing up of blood,

headache and rheumatic pains, throat infections, as a remedy for snake bites and to strengthen the brain and memory. The homoeopathic remedy is made from the fresh leaves and flowers, and preparations derived from sage have astringent and tonic properties and calming effects on the digestive organs. The remedy is used to treat hoarseness and sore throats, mouth ulcers or ulcerated throat and bleeding or infected gums.

Sanguinaria canadensis
Sanguinaria; red puccoon, blood root, coon root, sweet slumber, snakebite, Indian paint

This attractive, perennial plant is a native species of North America and Canada, growing in rich soils in woodlands. It produces beautiful, white flowers and has thick, bulbous fleshy roots containing orange-red sap. This juice was used by the native Indian peoples as dye for clothes and body paint. The root, green parts of the plant, fruit and seeds are used to prepare herbal and homoeopathic remedies. The plant contains a potent alkaloid substance called sanguinarine, which forms colourless crystals. This is toxic in large doses, causing burning in the stomach with vomiting, thirst, giddiness, disturbed vision and possible collapse and death. In smaller doses the preparations have emetic and expectorant properties and also act on the uterus, promoting menstruation. In both herbal and homoeopathy, the remedies are used for chest and respiratory ailments, including bronchitis, pharyngitis (inflammation of the pharynx), asthma and polyps (small, fleshy projections) in the nose or throat. Symptoms include dryness and soreness, thirst, chest pain that may extend to the right shoulder, and croup-like cough. Also, for whooping cough, colds and influenza, hay fever, severe migraine-like headaches with visual disturbance and rheumatic pains in the right shoulder. Symptoms often occur mainly on the right side and are worse if the person lies on that side of the body. They are made worse by cold, damp weather, touch and movement and by eating sweet foods. Symptoms improve in the evening and following sleep and if the person lies on the left side.

Sanicula aqua
Sanicula

Sanicula is a spring of water in Ottawa in Canada and Illinois in the United States of America. The water contains various salts and minerals that are themselves used to make homoeopathic remedies. The sanicula remedy is mainly given to children with delicate stomachs and a tendency to suffer from constipation or diarrhoea after eating, vomiting and sickness, travel sickness and wetting the bed. Children who need this remedy are usually thin in spite of eating heartily and may have rapidly changing moods. Often there is a tendency for the head and feet to be hot and sweaty. Symptoms are made worse by downward, falling movements but improve if the child rests with little clothing or covering.

Secale comutum
Secale; ergot, spurred rye

The condition known as ergot is a form of fungus that grows on rye, wheat and various other grasslike cereals. The spores of the fungus germinate and grow on the stigmas and ovaries of the head of the grass. They form small, curved, black seed-like bodies (sclerotia, singular sclerotium) that eventually fall off when the ears of the cereal crop are ripe. The sclerotia are collected when immature before the grain is ripe to prepare the homoeopathic remedy. Ergot has been known as a poison for many centuries. Cases of poisoning occurred because of eating foods made from contaminated cereals. Ergot contains several potent alkaloid substances, and symptoms of poisoning include burning pains, a crawling feeling on the skin, delirium, convulsions, gangrene, collapse and death. The substances have a powerful effect on the uterus and other smooth muscle, causing it to contract, and also on the central nervous system.

In modern homoeopathy the remedy is used to treat spasms in the arteries, as in Raynaud's phenomena (numbness and blanching, redness and burning in fingers and toes), cramp-like pain in leg muscles, uterine pains and contractions leading to bleeding irregularities, and ineffective contractions during labour. The person has cold, numb skin but feels hot and burning inside. (In orthodox medicine, ergot is used to control postpartum haemorrhage following childbirth or abortion). Symptoms are worse for any form of heat or covering and better in cool, fresh air and surroundings.

Senecio aureus
Golden groundsel, life root, golden senecio, squaw weed

This perennial plant, which grows to a height of one or two feet, is a native of North America and Canada and also grows in Europe. It produces golden yellow flowers, and the whole plant is used to prepare the remedies used in herbal medicine and homoeopathy. Preparations made from the plant have astringent and diuretic properties and also act on the uterus, chest and lungs. The homoeopathic remedy is used for absent or suppressed periods that may be accompanied by pain, chesty catarrhal complaints, urinary problems such as kidney stones and cystitis, and bleeding problems, e.g. nosebleeds.

Smilax officinalis, Smilax medica
Sarsaparilla; red-bearded sarsaparilla, Jamaica sarsaparilla

The unusual name of this plant was derived from two Spanish words, *sarza* for 'bramble' and *parilla* for 'vine'. The plant has prickly, thorny stems and is a native of Central and South America. It is thought to have been exported via Jamaica to Europe, but it does not grow in the West Indies. It was once used as a treatment for syphilis, and smoke from the burning plant was considered beneficial in the treatment of asthma. Preparations made from the plant have diuretic and tonic properties and promote perspiration. The fresh root is used to prepare the herbal and homoeopathic remedies. In homoeopathy sarsaparilla is used to treat bladder, kidney and urinary disorders, especially kidney stones causing renal colic and cystitis. There is a frequent need to urinate, although only small amounts may be passed, and sharp burning pains. The urine frequently appears cloudy, containing small deposits or stones. There may be a slight degree of incontinence of urine, especially if sitting down. The remedy is also used for rheumatism with pains that are worse at night and in cold, damp, draughty conditions. Also, for eczema and dry skin with painful deep cracks and fissures. People who benefit from this remedy feel cold and have a tendency to have dry scaly skin and spots. Skin conditions are worse in the months of spring. Symptoms are worse at night and in cold, damp, draughty conditions. They improve if the person is standing and uncovers the chest and neck.

Solanum dulcamara
Dulcamara; woody nightshade, scarlet berry, bittersweet, felonwort, felonberry, violet bloom

This rambling, trailing plant grows over bushes and hedges, extending for a considerable distance and supported by other plants. It is a native species of many European countries, including Britain. The young stems of the plant are green and furry, but they become more woody and smooth with age. The plant produces purple-blue flowers and, later, berries that are bright red when ripe. The stems taste bitter at first if chewed and then sweet (hence, bittersweet). Felon is an old name for a whitlow (an abscess on a finger or toe) and the name felonwort refers to the fact that the plant was used to cure these. Woody nightshade has a long history of medicinal use going back to ancient times. It has been used to treat a wide variety of disorders, especially skin complaints, asthma and chesty, catarrhal conditions, rheumatism and absent menstruation. The young shoots and twigs, leaves and flowers are used to prepare the homoeopathic remedy. This is given for ailments that are made worse, or are brought on, by exposure to cold and damp or sudden cooling, including colds and coughs, catarrhal complaints and conjunctivitis. Also, for skin conditions such as eczema, itchy rashes, ringworm, nettle rash (urticaria) and warts. Symptoms are worse for cold, damp weather and changes of temperature. They improve with exercise, movement, warmth and heat.

Solidago virgaurea
Golden rod, woundwort, Aaron's rod, solidago
This familiar garden plant grows in Europe, Asia and North America. It produces green leaves and golden yellow flowers and has long been valued as a remedy for kidney and urinary disorders, especially kidney stones. The green parts are used to prepare the homoeopathic remedy, which is used to treat problems of urine retention and lack of urination and renal colic.

Spigelia anthelmia
Spigelia; pink root, annual worm grass
This perennial plant is a native of the northern countries of South America and the West Indies, and a related type, *Spigelia marylandica*, grows in some states of North America. It was used by the native Indian peoples to expel intestinal parasitic worms, and is narcotic and a potent poison if taken in large amounts. The fresh plant has an unpleasant smell and is gathered and dried to prepare the homoeopathic remedy, which is given especially for left-sided symptoms and particularly heart disorders. These include angina and coronary artery disease with severe pain. Also given for neuralgia, left-sided headache and

migraine, iritis (inflammation of the iris of the eye), all of which are accompanied by sharp pains. People who benefit from this remedy have a phobia about long, pointed, sharp objects, e.g. needles. Symptoms are worse for lying on the left side, cold air, touch and movement, and during the approach of a thunderstorm. They improve with warm, dry conditions, lying on the right side, in the evening and for having the head raised when resting.

Spongia tosta
Spongia; natural sponge
Natural sponge has been used since the early Middle Ages to treat the enlargement of the thyroid gland, known as goitre, that results from a deficiency in iodine. The condition may result from a dietary lack of iodine or by some disorder of metabolism or of the thyroid gland itself. In more recent times, scientists discovered that sponges are naturally rich in iodine. Roasted sponge is used to prepare the homoeopathic remedy, which is used to treat thyroid gland disorders and goitre. There may be symptoms of palpitations, flushing, sweating, breathlessness, heat intolerance, anxiety and nervousness. Also, for heart disorders, including an enlarged heart or disease of the valves. Symptoms include palpitations, pain, breathlessness, exhaustion and a feeling of being crushed by a heavy weight. The person may be flushed and anxious with a fear of death. The Spongia remedy is useful in the treatment of a hoarse, dry sore throat, as in laryngitis, and particularly where respiratory illnesses such as tuberculosis are associated with the family. Symptoms are worse for movement, touch, trying to talk and for cold drinks and cold surroundings. They improve with warmth and warm meals and drinks, and for sitting propped up. People suitable for Spongia are often thin with a fair complexion and light-coloured hair.

Stannum metallicum
Stannum met.; tin
Tin is obtained from the mineral cassiterite, which occurs as dark-coloured crystals in such rocks as pegmatites and granites and in the alluvial deposits of streams and rivers. Tin is a soft, silver-coloured metal that has long been useful to humankind and has had many industrial uses. Medicinally, it was once given to expel intestinal tapeworms. In modern homoeopathy, the remedy is used for severe catarrhal chest complaints, including bronchitis,

laryngitis, asthma and inflammation of the windpipe (tracheitis). There is a thick, yellowish catarrh and a hoarse, dry cough. The person is sometimes weak and debilitated, suffering from loss of weight and exhaustion with associated depression and weepiness. The remedy is also given for neuralgic pain and headache, particularly on the left side. The pains may have a gradual onset and also be slow to disappear. Symptoms are made worse if the person lies on his or her right side and drinks warm fluids. They improve for coughing up catarrh and for firm pressure on the painful part.

Sticta pulmonaria
Sticta; lungwort, oak lungs, lung moss, Jerusalem cowslip

This plant, which is familiar in gardens in Great Britain and other European countries, has rough, oval green leaves speckled with white, reminiscent of lungs. The stalks grow to a height of about one foot, and the flowers are a pinky-red at first but purply-blue when fully open. Preparations of the plant have astringent properties and act on the mucous membranes of the respiratory tract. The homoeopathic remedy is prepared from the whole fresh plant and is used to treat colds, asthma, lung inflammation and rheumatic disorders. The catarrh is difficult to cough up and persistent. Symptoms are worse at night and for cold, damp conditions. They are worse for lying down and better for warmth.

Strophanthus kombe, Strophanthus hispidus
Kombé seeds

These climbing plants are native to tropical parts of East Africa. The name is derived from two Greek words, *strophos*, 'rope' or 'twisted cord', and *anthos*, 'flower'. They produce seeds that are extremely poisonous, and the poison was used on arrows for hunting by African tribal peoples. The most active constituents are a glucoside substance called strophanthin and an alkaloid, inoeine. Preparations made from the seeds have a similar effect to digitalis, and are used to treat heart and circulatory disorders. The homoeopathic remedy is used to treat palpitations, irregular heartbeat and breathlessness. It is a useful remedy for those whose health has been compromised by smoking or drinking alcohol.

Sulphuric acid
This remedy is used for mental exhaustion and depression, the person being restless and agitated. There is a tendency for skin problems to occur, including ulcers and boils. Other symptoms include mouth ulcers, bleeding gums and depression.

Symphoricarpus racemosa
Snowberry, wolf berry, coal berry, wax berry

Preparations made from this North American plant have emetic and purgative properties. The homoeopathic remedy is used for cases of severe vomiting and nausea, including morning sickness in pregnancy. There is a loss of appetite and there may also be a loss of weight.

Syphilinum
This remedy is derived from material obtained from a syphilitic lesion. Syphilis is a serious sexually transmitted bacterial disease that has plagued humankind for centuries. Hahnemann believed that syphilis was one of three main MIASMS, having an inherited element from earlier generations affected with the illness. The homoeopathic remedy is used to treat chronic ulcers and abscesses, especially in the genital area. Also for menstrual pains, neuralgia, varicose ulcers, constipation and inflammation of the iris of the eyes (iritis). The person may experience pain in the long bones and have weak teeth. Symptoms are worse for great heat or cold, at night, near the sea and during a thunderstorm. They improve with gentle walking and through the day and for being in a mountainous region.

People suitable for this remedy tend to be anxious and on edge, with nervous mannerisms such as exaggerated blinking or a muscular twitch or tic. They may show obsessive behaviour, such as a need to recheck constantly on something or to keep on washing their hands. They may find it difficult to concentrate and have a poor memory. They may have a problem with alcohol, drugs or smoking.

Tammus communis
Black bryony, blackeye root

This poisonous climbing plant is common in hedges, copses and open woodlands in the British Isles. It has heart-shaped leaves and white flowers, with bright red berries produced in the autumn. The plant has a dark-coloured root that is the part most often used in herbal medicine and homoeopathy. Preparations made from the plant have diuretic and blistering properties and are helpful for clearing the discoloration of a bruise (hence blackeye root). The homoeopathic remedy is used to treat chilblains with soreness, redness, inflammation and itching.

Terebinthinae oleum
Terebinth; turpentine

Turpentine is obtained from pine and other coniferous trees in the form of an oily, aromatic resin. It has many industrial uses, especially as a cleaning agent, in paint strippers and thinners and in products containing pine oil. It causes burning if swallowed and produces vomiting and diarrhoea. It also causes external burning and blistering if applied to the skin, and choking, sneezing and coughing if the fumes are inhaled. It was once used in the treatment of genital infections, including gonorrhoea. The homoeopathic remedy is used to treat similar types of infection involving inflammation and infection of the bladder and kidneys. These include cystitis with frequent urination, blood in the urine and burning pains, and kidney inflammation with stabbing back pains. The urine is usually cloudy or contains blood and may have a strong smell. Also, for other forms of kidney disease with symptoms of puffiness because of retention of fluid (oedema). Symptoms are worse at night and in cold, damp, draughty conditions. They are better for walking about in fresh clean air and for warmth.

Teucrium marum venum
Teucrium mar. ver.; cat thyme, marum

This strongly aromatic plant is a native of Spain but grows in many countries throughout the world. It has branching stalks and forms a bush or shrub about two to four feet in height. The small, oval leaves are sage green in colour and slightly furred, and the flowers are an attractive deep pink. Both flowers and leaves have a pungent aromatic smell, especially when rubbed. The plant has stimulant and astringent properties and has long been used in herbal medicine for a variety of disorders. All the fresh parts of the plant are used to prepare the homoeopathic remedy, which is used to treat polyps, which are small growths or tumours on mucous membranes. These may occur in the rectum, bladder or nasal passages. Also, the remedy is used for conditions producing thick catarrh that is persistent and difficult to eliminate. The remedy may be given to treat threadworm infestation in children. Symptoms are worse for cold, damp conditions and sudden weather changes. Also, if the person becomes hot and sweaty in bed. Symptoms improve for being out in the cool, fresh clean air.

Theridion curassavicum
Orange spider of Curaçao and other parts of the West Indies

This is a small spider about the size of a pea that has a body covered with orange spots. There is a larger yellow spot on its under surface, and it is particularly found in Curaçao. It has a poisonous bite and causes unpleasant symptoms of tremor, chilling, sweating, fainting and great anxiety. The whole spider is used to prepare the homoeopathic remedy, which was first investigated and proved in the early 1830s by Dr Constantine Hering. The remedy is used to treat ailments of the spine and nerves and bone disorders. All these ailments are very sensitive to movement, vibration and noise, which set off sensations of great pain. Disorders treated include Ménière's disease, a disease of the inner ear with deafness and tinnitus (ringing in the ear) with symptoms of vertigo, nausea and vomiting. Also, toothache, degeneration of bones and spine with inflammation and pain, morning sickness, travel sickness, vertigo, severe headache, chills and fainting. Symptoms are made worse by closing the eyes, by any kind of movement or vibration, bending, touch and during the night. They improve for rest with the eyes open and with warmth and quiet surroundings.

Trillium erectum, Trillium pendulum
Bethroot, Indian balm, birthroot, Indian shamrock, lamb's quarters, wake-robin

Plants belonging to this group are all native species of North America. Trillium erectum, which flourishes in rich, moist soils in woodlands and grows to a height of between one foot and sixteen inches, produces white flowers. Preparations made from the plant have astringent, antiseptic and tonic properties and were used by the native Indian peoples for childbirth and haemorrhage, especially from the womb. The homoeopathic remedy is used to treat heavy bleeding from the womb, which may be associated with fibroids or the menopause. It may be given to prevent an early threatened miscarriage.

Tuberculinum koch, Tuberculinum bovum
Dead, sterile tuberculous tissue derived from cattle or human beings

This remedy was extensively investigated and researched by Dr Compton Burnett in the late 1800s, following an earlier discovery by Dr Robert Koch, that dead tuberculous material was effective in the prevention and treatment of tuberculosis. The homoeopathic remedy is given for chronic conditions characterized by wasting, pallor, a persistent racking cough, drenching sweats at night and pains in the left lung. The glands in the neck are enlarged, and the whites of the eyes (sclera) may appear slightly blue. Symptoms are erratic and may move about. Often there is a family history of tuberculosis or other severe respiratory disorder such as asthma. People who benefit from this remedy are usually thin, fair-haired and blue-eyed, prone to colds and chest ailments and lacking physical strength and stamina. They tend to be restless, seeking constant change in their personal life and surroundings, yearning for excitement, travel and new romantic attachments. They may be afraid of dogs or cats and enjoy milk and the taste of smoked foods.

Valerian officinalis

Great wild valerian; all-heal, setwall, capon's tail

Valerian species grow throughout Europe and northern Asia, and *Valerian officinalis* flourishes in marshy, wet ground in ditches and near rivers and streams. The stems reach a height of three to four feet, producing dark green leaves and light pink flowers. The rhizome or root is the part used in herbal medicine and homoeopathy, and the plant has a long history of medicinal use. It was valued so highly in the Middle Ages as to be given the name all-heal, while its Latin name may be derived from *valere*, meaning 'to be in health'. Preparations made from the plant have powerful effects on the central nervous system, acting as sedatives and antispasmodics. The homoeopathic remedy is given for excitable, mental symptoms including agitation and restlessness. Also, for muscular spasms, hysteria, headache and pains that may move from one part to another. The person may suffer from sleeplessness, headaches, diarrhoea and restlessness with gnawing hunger and nausea.

Veratum album

Verat. alb.; white hellebore

This plant grows throughout Europe, although not in the British Isles, and produces a creamy-white flower. The rhizome or root is the part used in herbal medicine and homoeopathy, and it is extremely poisonous. If swallowed it causes diarrhoea and vomiting and may result in collapse, convulsions and death. Preparations made from the plant have irritant and cardiac depressant properties. There is a long history of medicinal use going back to the time of Hippocrates, and the remedy was investigated and proved for homoeopathy by Hahnemann during the late 1820s.

The homoeopathic remedy is used for severe conditions of collapse and shock in which there is pallor, dehydration, chilling and possibly cyanosis (a blue tinge to the skin because of a lack of oxygen in the blood and tissues). The person may be cold with clammy skin because of sweating. Also, for diarrhoea, severe throbbing headache and mental symptoms of extreme agitation or severe depression, suicidal feelings, mania and aggression. It may be given for severe cramping menstrual pain or cramp during pregnancy leading to fainting, and collapse because of mental shock or trauma. Symptoms are made worse by movements and cold drinks, and also during the night. They improve with warmth, heat and hot meals and drinks. They are also better for rest and lying down.

Viburnum opulus

Guelder rose, high cranberry, dog rowan tree, cramp bark, snowball tree, rose elder

The guelder rose is a bush or small tree found in copses and hedges in England, Europe and North America. It produces abundant heads of white flowers and, later, bright red berries that have a bitter taste. The bark, which contains a bitter glucoside substance called viburnine, is used to prepare remedies in herbal medicine and homoeopathy. Preparations of the bark are very effective in the relief of cramp-like pains and spasms. The homoeopathic remedy is used to treat menstrual cramps, pain in the ovaries at ovulation and prevention of early threatened miscarriage.

Vinca minor

Lesser periwinkle

This trailing plant grows in Great Britain and other European countries, producing dark-green leaves and purply-blue flowers. Periwinkles have a long history of use in herbal medicine and were used to treat bleeding, cramps, piles and skin inflammations. There are also many ancient superstitions attached to the plant, and it was believed to ward off evil spirits. Preparations made from the plant have astringent and tonic properties. In homoeopathy it is used for heavy menstrual bleeding and haemorrhage and for inflammations of the scalp.

Viola tricolor

Wild pansy, love-lies-bleeding, love-in-idleness, heartsease, and many other country names

This pretty flower is abundant throughout the British Isles, with rounded green leaves and purple, yellow and white flowers. The whole plant is used to prepare herbal and homoeopathic remedies that have a long history of medicinal use. The plant has been used to treat a wide variety of ailments, including asthma, epilepsy, skin disorders, convulsions, heart and blood disorders. Preparations made from the plant have diuretic properties. In homoeopathy, the remedy is used for skin conditions such as infected eczema or impetigo. There is a thick pus-containing discharge and crusts and scabs on the skin. Also, the remedy is used to treat bed-wetting and urinary incontinence.

Vipera communis

Venom of the adder or viper

This attractively patterned snake is a greyish colour with a dark zig-zag pattern down the length of its back. Its bite is painful but rarely serious, causing swelling, inflammation and bleeding in the veins, which then become enlarged. The homoeopathic remedy made from the venom of the snake, is used to treat phlebitis and varicose veins and ulcers with swelling, inflammation and pain. The leg feels heavy, as though it might burst. Symptoms are worse for touch, pressure or tight clothing and are relieved by raising the affected part.

Viscum album

Mistletoe

This parasitic plant grows in the British Isles and throughout Europe, trailing over fruit and other trees. It produces white berries that ripen in December, but the leaves and twigs are used to prepare the remedies for herbal medicine and homoeopathy. Preparations derived from the plant act on the central nervous system and have tonic, antispasmodic and narcotic properties. It has been used to treat epilepsy, spasms and haemorrhage. Many ancient superstitions are attached to mistletoe, which was a sacred plant for the Druids. In homoeopathy, the remedy is used as a last resort to treat extreme conditions of collapse, weak pulse and respiration and low blood pressure.

Vitex agnus castus

Agnus castus; chaste tree; monk's pepper, wild lavender

This aromatic shrub is a native plant of the shores of the Mediterranean and also grows in other part of Europe and North America. It has flexible fine twigs that are used to weave baskets, dark green leaves and fragrant flowers. Dark, purply-red berries are produced containing seeds, and these are used to prepare herbal and homoeopathic remedies. The plant was associated with chastity by the ancient Greeks. The plant was used to treat muscular weakness and paralysis and is used in herbal medicine to stimulate hormone production during the menopause. The homoeopathic remedy is given for menopausal symptoms and for physical disorders arising from alcohol or drug abuse or sexual excess. Symptoms may include fatigue, depression, loss of sexual desire, apathy and inability to concentrate. Also for postnatal depression with loss of libido and drying up of the breast milk. Symptoms are worse in the morning and for exercise and movement and are relieved by firm pressure on an affected part.

Zincum metallicum

Zinc. met.

Zinc is an essential trace element in the human body, being a constituent of digestive enzymes and essential for normal growth. Zinc is used in conventional medicine as a constituent of creams and ointments for a variety of skin complaints. It is also taken internally for some nervous complaints, spasms and neuralgia. The homoeopathic Zinc. met. remedy is prepared from zinc sulphide and is used for conditions of restlessness, agitation and nervous twitching. The person is usually suffering from great mental and physical exhaustion and is irritable and highly sensitive to the least noise, interruption or touch. Symptoms are worse for suppression of natural discharges (e.g. by using a suppressant remedy in the case of a cold). Also, they are made worse by noise, touch, vibration and alcoholic drinks, particularly wine. Symptoms improve when natural body functions take place and are not suppressed.

Glossary of Terms used in Homoeopathy

aggravations a term first used by Dr Samuel Hahnemann to describe an initial worsening of symptoms experienced by some patients, on first taking a homoeopathic remedy, before the condition improved. In modern homoeopathy this is known as a *healing crisis*. To prevent the occurrence of aggravations, Hahnemann experimented with further dilutions of remedies and, in particular, vigorous shaking (SUCCUSSING) of preparations at each stage of the process.

allopathy a term first used by Dr Samuel Hahnemann meaning 'against disease'. It describes the approach of conventional medicine, which is to treat symptoms with a substance or drug with an opposite effect in order to suppress or eliminate them. This is called the 'law of contraries' and is in direct contrast to the 'like can cure like', the 'law of similars' or *similia similibus curentur* principle, which is central to the practice of homoeopathy.

centesimal scale of dilution the scale of dilution used in homoeopathy based on one part (or drop) of the remedy in 99 parts of the diluent liquid (a mixture of alcohol and water).

classical the practice of homoeopathy based on the work of Dr Samuel Hahnemann and further developed and expanded by other practitioners, particularly Dr Constantine Hering and Dr James Tyler Kent.

constitutional prescribing and constitutional types the homoeopathic concept, based on the work of Dr James Tyler Kent, that prescribing should be based on the complete make-up of a person, including physical and emotional characteristics, as well as on the symptoms of a disorder.

decimal scale of dilution the scale of dilution used in homoeopathy based on one part (or drop) of the remedy in nine parts of the diluent liquid (a mixture of alcohol and water).

healing crisis the situation in which a group of symptoms first become worse after a person has taken a homoeopathic remedy, before they improve and disappear. The healing crisis is taken to indicate a change and that improvement is likely to follow. It is usually short-lived (*see also* AGGRAVATIONS).

homoeopathy the system of healing based on the principle of 'like can cure like' and given its name by Samuel Hahnemann. The word is derived from the Greek *homeo* for 'similar' and *pathos* for 'suffering' or 'like disease'.

laws of cure, law of direction of cure three concepts or 'laws' formulated by Dr Constantine Hering to explain the means by which symptoms of disease are eliminated from the body.

(1) Symptoms move in a downwards direction.

(2) Symptoms move from the inside of the body outwards.

(3) Symptoms move from more important vital organs and tissues to those of less importance.

Hering was also responsible for the view in homoeopathy that more recent symptoms disappear first before ones that have been present for a longer time. Hence symptoms are eliminated in the reverse order of their appearance.

materia medica detailed information about homoeopathic remedies, listed alphabetically. The information includes details of the symptoms that may respond to each remedy, based on previous research and experience. Details about the source of each remedy are also included. This information is used by a homoeopathic doctor when deciding upon the best remedy for each particular patient and group of symptoms.

miasm a chronic constitutional weakness that is the aftereffect of an underlying suppressed disease that has been present in a previous generation or earlier in the life of an individual. The concept of miasm was formulated by Samuel Hahnemann who noted that some people were never truly healthy but always acquired new symptoms of illness. He believed that this was because of a constitutional weakness that he called a miasm, which may have been inherited and was caused by an illness in a previous generation. These theories were put forward in his research writings entitled *Chronic Diseases*. Three main miasms were identified, PSORA, SYCOSIS and SYPHILIS.

modalities a term applied to the responses of the patient, when he or she feels better or worse, depending upon factors in the internal and external environment. These are unique from one person to another, depending upon the individual characteristics that apply at the time, although there are common features within each constitutional type. Modalities include responses, fears and preferences to temperature, weather, foods, emotional responses and relationships, etc, which all contribute to a person's total sense of wellbeing. Modalities are particularly important when a person has symptoms of an illness in prescribing the most beneficial remedy.

mother tincture (symbol O) the first solution obtained from dissolving a substance in a mixture of alcohol and water (usually in the ratio of 9/10 pure alcohol to 1/10 distilled water). It is subjected to further dilutions and SUCCUSSIONS (shakings) to produce the homoeopathic remedies.

nosode a term used to describe a remedy prepared from samples of infected diseased tissue, often to treat or prevent a particular illness. They were first investigated by Wilhelm Lux, not without considerable controversy. Examples are *Medorrhinum* and *Tuberculinum*.

organon *The Organon of Rationale Medicine*. is one of the most important works of Samuel Hahnemann, published in Leipzig in 1810, in which he set out the principles and philosophy of modern homoeopathy. The *Organon* is considered to be a classic work and basic to the study of homoeopathy.

polycrest a remedy suitable for a number of illnesses, disorders or symptoms.

potency the dilution or strength of a homoeopathic remedy. Dr Samuel Hahnemann discovered that by further diluting and SUCCUSSING (shaking) a remedy, it became more effective or potent in bringing about a cure. It is held that the process of diluting and shaking a remedy releases its innate energy or dynamism, even though none of the original molecules of the substance may remain. Hence the greater the dilution of a remedy, the stronger or more potent it becomes. Hahnemann called his new dilute solutions

'potentizations'.

potentiate the release or transfer of energy into a homoeopathic solution by succussing or vigorous shaking of the mixture.

principle of vital force 'vital force' was the term given by Samuel Hahnemann to the inbuilt power or ability of the human body to maintain health and fitness and fight off illness. Illness is believed to be the result of stresses, causing an imbalance in the vital force, which assail all people throughout life and include inherited, environmental and emotional factors. The symptoms of this 'disorder' are illness and are held to be the physical indications of the struggle of the body's vital force to regain its balance. A person with a strong vital force will tend to remain in good health and fight off illness. A person with a weak vital force is more likely to suffer from long-term, recurrent symptoms and illnesses. Homoeopathic remedies are believed to act upon the vital force, stimulating it to heal the body and restore the natural balance.

provings the term given by Samuel Hahnemann to experimental trials he carried out to test the reactions of healthy people to homoeopathic substances. These trials were carried out under strictly controlled conditions (in advance of the modern scientific approach), and the symptoms produced, the results, were meticulously recorded. Quinine was the first substance that Hahnemann investigated in this way, testing it initially on himself and then on close friends and family members. Over the next few years he investigated and proved many other substances, building up a wealth of information on each one about the reactions and symptoms produced. After conducting this research, Hahnemann went on to prescribe carefully the remedies to those who were sick. Provings are still carried out in modern homoeopathy to test new substances that may be of value as remedies. Usually, neither the prescribing physician nor those taking the substance — the 'provers' — know the identity of the material or whether they are taking a placebo.

psora one of three MIASMS identified by Samuel Hahnemann, believed to be because of suppression of scabies (an itchy skin infection caused by a minute burrowing mite). Psora was believed to have an inherited element or to be because of suppression of an earlier infection in a particular individual.

Schussler tissue salts Wilhelm Heinrich

Schussler was a German homoeopathic doctor who introduced the biochemic tissue salt system in the late 1800s. Schussler believed that many symptoms and ailments resulted from the lack of a minute, but essential, quantity of a mineral or tissue salt. He identified twelve such tissue salts that he regarded as essential and believed that a cure could be obtained from replacing the deficient substance. Schussler's work was largely concentrated at the cell and tissue level rather than embracing the holistic view of homoeopathy.

similia similibus curentur the founding principle of homoeopathy that 'like can cure like' or 'let like be treated by like', which was first put forward by Hippocrates, a physician of ancient Greece. This principle excited the interest of Paracelsus in the Middle Ages, and was later restated and put into practice by Hahnemann with the development of homoeopathy.

simillimum a homoeopathic remedy that in its natural, raw state is able to produce the same symptoms as those being exhibited by the patient.

succussion vigorous shaking of a homoeopathic remedy at each stage of dilution, along with banging the container holding it against a hard surface causing further release of energy.

sycosis one of the three major MIASMS identified by Samuel Hahnemann and believed to result from a suppressed gonorrhoeal infection. Sycosis was believed to have an inherited element or to be because of suppression of an earlier infection in a particular individual.

syphilis the third of the three major MIASMS identified by Samuel Hahnemann believed to result from a suppressed syphilis infection. Syphilis was believed to have an inherited element or to be because of suppression of an earlier infection in a particular individual.

trituration the process, devised by Samuel Hahnemann, of rendering naturally insoluble substances soluble so that they can be made available as homoeopathic remedies. The process involves repeated grinding down of the substance with lactose powder until it becomes soluble. The substance usually becomes soluble at the third process of trituration. Each trituration is taken to be the equivalent of one dilution in the centesimal scale. Once the substance has been rendered soluble, dilution can proceed in the normal way.

Useful Addresses

Stress Centres
Centre for Stress Management
156 Westcombe Hill
London
SE3 7GB
Tel: 0208 293 4114

International Stress Management
  Association
PO Box 348
Waltham Cross
Cheshunt
EN8 8ZL
Tel: 07000 780 430
www.isma.org

Counselling Services
The British Association of Counselling
1 Regent Place
Rugby
Warwickshire
CV21 2PJ
Tel: 01788 550 899
www.bac.co.uk

MIND (National Association for Mental
  Health)
Granta House
15–19 Broadway
London
E15 4BQ
Tel: 0208 519 2122
www.mind.org.uk

Samaritans
10 The Grove
Slough
Berks SL1 1QP
Tel: 01753 216 500
www.samaritans.org.uk
(or look up in your local phone book)

Complementary Medicine
The Institute for Complementary
  Medicine (ICM)
PO Box 194
London
SE16 7QZ
Tel: 0207 237 5165
www.icmedicine.co.uk
icm@icmedicine.co.uk

The British Complementary Medicine
  Association (BCMA)
Kensington House
33 Imperial Square
Cheltenham
GL50 1QZ
(Address soon to change to PO Box
  number; please phone for details or
  consult the website)
Tel: 0845 345 5977
www.bcma.co.uk

The British Holistic Medical Association
59 Lansdowne Place
Hove
East Sussex
BN3 1FL
Tel: 01273 725951
www.bhma.org

UK College for Complementary Health
  Care Studies
St Charles Hospital
Exmoor Street
London
W10 6DZ
Tel: 0208 964 1205/6
www. ukcollege.com
info@ukcollege.com

Acupuncture
British Acupuncture Council
63 Jeddo Road
London
W12 9HQ
Tel: 0208 735 0400
www.acupuncture.org.uk

International College of Oriental
  Medicine
Green Hedges House
Green Hedges Avenue
East Grinstead
West Sussex
RH19 1OZ
Tel: 01342 313 106/7
www.orientalmed.ac.uk
info@orientalmed.ac.uk

The Alexander Technique
The Professional Association of
  Alexander Teachers (PAAT):

Mrs P Hebblethwaite
Hon Sec PAAT
40 The Southend
Ledbury
Herefordshire
HR8 2HD
Tel: 01531 632 502
priska@tesco.net

The Recreational Course Director
PAAT
Room 706
'The Big Peg'
120 Vyse Street
Birmingham
B18 6NF
Tel: 0121 248 1133
fred.o@virgin.net

Allergy Therapy
The Institute of Allergy Therapists
Ffynnonwen
Llangwryfon
Aberystwyth
Dfyed
SY23 4EY
Tel: 01974 241 376

Aromatherapy
Aromatherapy Trade Council
PO Box 387
Ipswich
IP2 9AN
Tel: 01473 603 630
www.a-t-c.cwc.net

International Society of Professional
  Aromatherapists
ISPA House
82 Ashby Road
Hinckley
Leics
LE10 1SN
Tel: 01455 637 987
www.ispa.demon.co.uk

Register of Qualified Aromatherapists
PO Box 3431
Danbury
Chelmsford
Essex
CM3 4UA
Te: 01245 227 957
www.rqa-uk.org
admin@rqa-uk.org
(List of recognized schools available)

International Federation of
  Aromatherapists
182 Chiswick High Road
London W4 1PP
Tel: 0208 742 2605
www.int-fed-aromatherapy.co.uk

Bach Flower Remedies
The Dr Edward Bach Foundation
The Bach Centre
Mount Vernon
Bakers Lane
Sotwell
Wallingford
Oxon   OX10 0PZ
Tel: 01491 834 678
www.bachcentre.com

Chiropractic
The British Chiropractic Association
Blagrave House
17 Blagrave Street
Reading
Berkshire RG1 1QB
Tel: 0118 950 5950
www.chiropractic-uk.co.uk

British Association for Applied
Chiropractic (BAAC)
BAAC Register of Members
The Old Post Office
Cherry Street
Stratton Audley
Bicester
Oxford
OX6 9BA
(Send an SAE for a list of the
McTimoney-Corley practitioners)
Tel: 01869 277 111
BAAC.Admin@btinternet.com

McTimoney Chiropractic Association
21 High Street
Eynsham
Oxford
OX18 1HE
Tel: 01865 880 974
(Please send SAE for information)
www.mctimoney-chiropratic.org
admin@mctimoney-chiropractic.org

Colonic Hydrotherapy
Colonic International Association
Admin Department
16 Drummond Ride
Tring
Herts
HP23 5DE
(For a list of local practitioners please
send an SAE to the address above or
consult the website)
Tel: 01442 827 687
www.colonic-association.com

Holistic Massage
The London College of Massage
5–6 Newman Passage
London
W1T 1EH
Tel: 0207 323 3574
www.massagelondon.com
admin@massagelondon.com
See also:
www.londonhealth.co.uk/massage.asp

Holistic Medicine
British Holistic Medical Association
59 Lansdowne Place
Hove
East Sussesx
BN3 1FL
Tel/Fax: 01273 725 951
www.bhma.org

Homoeopathy
The Society of Homoeopaths
4a Artizan Road
Northampton NN1 4HU
Tel: 01604 621 400
Fax 01604 622 622
(Register of qualified professional
homoeopaths)

The United Kingdom Homoeopathic
Medical Association
Administration Office
6 Livingstone Road
Gravesend
Kent DA12 5DZ
Tel/Fax: 01474 560 336

Hypnotherapy
British Society of Clinical Hypnothera-
pists
229a Sussex Gardens
Lancaster Gate
London
W2 2RL
Tel: 0207 402 9037
(For a nationwide list of practitioners)
www.XLR.com/hypnosis

National Register of Hypnotherapists
and Psychotherapists
Suite B
12 Cross Street
Nelson
BB9 7EN
Tel: 01282 716 839
www.nrhp.co.uk

British Society of Experimental and
Clinical Hypnosis
Mr G Callow
Westview
Westport
Near Langport
Somerset
TA10 0BH
(For details of private therapists in your
area)

British Society of Clinical Hypnosis
The Organising Secretary
125 Queensgate
Bridlington
East Yorkshire
YO16 7JQ
Tel: 01262 403 103
www.bsch.org.uk
sec@bsch.org.uk

British Council of Hypnotist Examiners
Tel: 01723 585 960
(For details of qualified hypnotherapists
in your area)

Iridology
Guild of Naturopathic Iridologists
94 Grosvenor Road
London
SW1V 3LF
Tel: 0207 834 3579

Kinesiology
The Kinesiology Federation:
PO Box 17153
Edinburgh
EH11 3WQ
Tel: 08700 113 545
www.kinesiologyfederation.org
kfadmin@kinesiologyfederation.org

Also:
Ms Carol Smith
PO Box 17
Woolmer Green
Herts
Tel/Fax: 01438 817 998
kinesiology@btinternet.com

Association of Systematic Kinesiology
39 Browns Road
Surbiton
Surrey
KT5 8ST
(SAE and four loose first class stamps
for information)
www.kinesiology.co.uk
info@kinesiology.co.uk

Nutritional Therapy
Society for the Promotion of Nutritional
Therapy (SPNT)
PO Box 47
Heathfield
East Sussex
TN21 8ZX
Tel: 01435 867 007
(Send SAE and £1.00 for information
and a list of your nearest nutritional
therapists)

British Association of Nutritional
Therapists
BCM BANT
London
WC1N 3XX
(Send £2.00 and a SAE to obtain a
register of therapists)

The Institute of Optimum Nutrition
13 Blades Court
Deodar Road
London
SW15 2LR
Tel: 0208 877 9993
www.ion.ac.uk

Osteopathy
British Osteopathic Association
Langham House East
Luton
Bedfordshire
LU1 2NA
www.osteopathy.org
enquiries@osteopathy.org

Reflexology
The Philip Salmon Reflexology Course
PO Box 145
59 The Enterprise Centre
Potters Bar
EN6 3EW
(For a prospectus and information on
the course)

The British Reflexology Association
Monks Orchard
Whitbourne
Worcester
WR6 5RB
Tel:/Fax 01886 821 207
(Register of members £2.00; for details
of training courses, books, charts
send SAE)
www.britreflex.co.uk
bra@britreflex.co.uk

Shiatsu

The European Shiatsu School
Central Administration
Highbanks
Lockeridge
Marlborough
Wiltshire
SN8 4EQ
Tel: 01672 513 444
www.shiatsu.co.uk

Yoga

The British School of Yoga
Stanhope Square
Holsworthy
Devon
EX22 6DF
Tel: 0800 731 9271
www.bsygroup.co.uk

The British Wheel of Yoga
25 Jermyn Street
Sleaford
Lincs.
NG34 7RU
Tel: 01529 306 851
www.bwy.org.uk

Relationship Stress, Counselling and support

Childline
Freepost 1111
London N1 0BR
Freephone 0800 1111
www.childline.org.uk

CRUSE
Cruse House
126 Sheen Road
Richmond
Surrey
TW9 1UR
Tel: 0870 167 1677
www.crusebereavementcare.org.uk
info@crusebereavementcare.org.uk

Support for families who have gone through divorce

Gingerbread
7 Sovereign Court
Sovereign Close
London
E1W 3HW
Tel: 0800 018 4318
To find out the contact number of your local Gingerbread group:
Tel: 0207 488 9300
www.gingerbread.org.uk
office@gingerbread.org.uk

Help for single parents

National Association of Widows
Tel: 0247 6634 848

National Council for One-Parent Families
255 Kentish Town Road
London
NW5 2LX
Tel: 0207 428 5400

RELATE
Herbert Gray College
Little Church Street
Rugby
Warwicks
CV21 3AP
Tel: 01788 573 241
www.relate.org.uk

Health

Sports Council
16 Upper Woburn Place
London
WC1H 0QP
Tel: 0207 273 1500

Alcoholism

Alcoholics Anonymous
PO Box 1
Stonebow House
Stonebow
York
YO1 7NJ
Tel: 01904 644026

Drug Addiction

Westminster Drugs Project
470 Harrow Road
London
W9 3RU
Tel: 0207 286 3339

Council for Involuntary Tranquilizer Addiction (CITA)
Cavendish House
Brighton Road
Waterloo
Liverpool
L22 5NG
Tel: 0151 949 0102

Families Anonymous
Doddington and Rollo Community Association (DRCA)
Charlotte Despard Avenue
London
SW11 5HD
Tel: 0207 498 4680

Tranquillizer and Anxiety Self-help Association (TASHA)
Tel: 0208 569 9933

Smoking

Action on Smoking and Health (ASH)
102 Clifton Street
London
EC2A 4HW
Tel: 0207 759 5902
www.ash.org.uk

ASH Scotland
8 Frederick Street
Edinburgh
EH2 2HB
Tel: 0131 225 4725
www.ashscotland.org.uk

Stress-related Illnesses

Arthritis

The Arthritic Association
First Floor Suite
2 Hyde Gardens
Eastbourne
BN21 4PN
Tel: 01323 416 550 and 0207 491 0233
(Provides dietary guidance with homoeopathic and herbal treatment to help relieve those suffering from arthritis and rheumatitis)
www.arthriticassociation.org.uk

Asthma

National Asthma Campaign
Providence House
Providence Place
London
N1 0NT
0207 226 2260
www.asthma.org.uk

Diabetes

Diabetes UK Central Office
10 Queen Anne Street
London
W1G 9LH
Tel: 0207 323 1531
www.diabetes.org.uk

Heart Disease

British Heart Foundation
14 Fitzhardinge Street
London
W1H 6DH
Tel: 0207 935 0185
www.bhf.org.uk

The Coronary Prevention Group
102 Gloucester Place
London
W1H 3DA
Tel: 0207 927 2125

Migraine

Migraine Action Association
178a High Road
Byfleet
West Byfleet
Surrey
KT14 7ED
Tel: 01932 352 468
www.migraine.org.uk

Migraine Trust
45 Great Ormond Street
London
WC1N 3HZ
Tel: 0207 831 4818
www.migrainetrust.org

British Association for the Study of Headache
The Princesss Margaret Migraine Clinic
Charing Cross Hospital
Fulham Place Road
London
W6 8RF
Tel: 0208 846 1191

PMS
National Association for Premenstrual
   Syndrome
7 Swift's Court
High Street
Seal
Kent
TN15 0EG
Tel: 01732 760 011
Helpline: 01732 760 012
www.pms.org.uk

Skin Disorders
National Eczema Society
Hill House
Highgate Hill
London
N19 5NA
Tel: 0207 281 3553
Helpline: 0870 241 3604
www.eczema.org

The Psoriasis Association
7 Milton Street
Northampton
NN2 7JG
Tel: 01604 711 129

Alternative and Spiritual Healing
Acorn Christian Healing Trust
Whitehill Chase
High Street
Bordon
Hampshire
GU35 0AP
Tel: 01420 478 121/472 779
www.acornchristian.org

Ayurvedic Medicine and Transcendental
   Meditation
Freepost
London
SW1P 4YY
Tel: 0800 269 303

College of Healing
Runnings Park
Croft Bank
West Malvern
Worcestershire
WR14 4BP
Tel: 01684 566 450

College of Psychic Studies
16 Queensberry Place
London
SW7 2EB
Tel: 0207 589 3292/3
www.psychic-studies.org.uk

Centre for Alternative Education and
   Research
Rosemerryn
Lamorna
Penzance
Cornwall
TR19 6BN
Tel: 01736 810 530

Confederation of Healing Organizations
Suite J
The Red and White House
113 High Street
Berkhamsted
Hertfordshire BP4 2DJ
01442 244 296

Eagle's Wing Centre for Contemporary
   Shamanism
58 Westbere Road
London
NW2 3RU
Tel: 0207 435 8174
www.shamanism.co.uk

Council for Alternative and Comple-
   mentary Medicine
For information on:
Acupuncture: 0208 735 0400
Homoeopathy: 01604 621 400
Medical Herbalism: 01392 526 022
Naturopathy: 01458 840 072

The National Federation of Spiritual
   Healers (NFSH)
Old Manor Farm Studio
Church Street
Sunbury-on-Thames
Middlesex
TW16 6RJ
Tel: 01932 783 164/5
www.nfsh.org.uk

The Radionic Association
Baerlein House
Goose Green
Deddington
Banbury
Oxfordshire
OX15 0SZ
Tel: 01869 338 852
www.radionic.co.uk

The Shiatsu Society UK
Eastlands Court
St Peter's Road
Rugby
Warwickshire
CV21 3QP

Soul Directed Astrology
5a Cedar Road
Sutton
Surrey
SM2 5DA
Tel: 0208 643 4898

Spiritualist Association of Great Britain
33 Belgrave Square
London
SW1X 8QL
Tel: 0207 235 3351

Westbank Natural Health
Strathmiglo
Cupar
Fife
Scotland
KY14 7QP
Tel: 01337 860 233

The Association of Natural Medicine
19a Collingwood Road
Witham
Essex
CM8 2DY
Tel: 01376 502 762

Matthew Manning Centre
PO Box 100
Bury St Edmund's
Suffolk
IP29 4DE
Tel: 01284 830 222

Index